Stedman's
CARDIOLOGY &
PULMONARY
WORDS

SECOND EDITION

Edited by
Helen Littrell

Stedman's

CARDIOLOGY & PULMONARY WORDS

SECOND EDITION

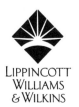

LIPPINCOTT
WILLIAMS
& WILKINS

BALTIMORE • PHILADELPHIA • LONDON • PARIS • BANGKOK
BUENOS AIRES • HONG KONG • MUNICH • SYDNEY • TOKYO • WROCLAW

Series Editor: Elizabeth B. Randolph
Associate Managing Editor: Maureen Barlow Pugh
Editor: Helen Littrell
Production Coordinator: Marette Magargle-Smith
Cover Design: Reuter & Associates

Copyright © 1997
Williams & Wilkins
351 West Camden Street
Baltimore, Maryland 21201-2436 USA

Printed in the United States of America

First Edition, 1993

Library of Congress Cataloging-in-Publication Data

Stedman's cardiology & pulmonary words / edited by Helen Littrell.—
2nd ed.
   p.   cm—(Stedman's word book series)
   Rev. ed. of: Stedman's cardiology words. c1993.
   Developed from the database of Stedman's medical dictionary and
supplemented by terminology found in the current medical literature.
   Includes bibliographical references.
   ISBN 0-683-40081-9
   1. Cardiopulmonary system—Diseases—Terminology.
2. Cardiopulmonary system—Terminology. Ι Littrell, Helen E. II. Stedman, Thomas Lathrop, 1853–1938. Medical dictionary. Iιı. Stedman's cardiology words. IV. Series: Stedman's word books.
   [DNLM: 1. Cardiology—terminology. 2. Pulmonary disease
(Specialty)—terminology.   WG 15 S8124 1997]
RC702.S74   1997
616.1′2′0014—dc21
DNLM/DLC
for Library of Congress   96–45978
                                     CIP

Developed from the database of Stedman's medical dictionary and supplemented by
terminology found in the current medical literature.
      Includes bibliographical references.

98 99 00
3 4 5 6 7 8 9 10

Contents

Acknowledgments

An important part of our editorial process is the involvement of medical transcriptionists—as advisors, reviewers and/or editors.

Special thanks are due Helen Littrell for editing and proofing the manuscript (and doing the necessary research involved with that large task) as well as proofreading the first edition of the book and helping to compile the appendices. We also would like to extend our thanks to Donna Taylor, CMT, who reviewed all the new terms that were added to *Stedman's Cardiology & Pulmonary Words, Second Edition,* and to Martha Richards, who reviewed the combined manuscript.

Thanks also to our *Stedman's Cardiology & Pulmonary Words* MT Editorial Advisory Board, consisting of Ann Donnelly, CMT; Gail Schoolcraft, CMT; Pamela Maykulsky; and Judith Patterson, CMT. These medical transcriptionists served as editors and advisors, and spent hours perusing texts, journals, and manufacturers' information to compile the latest terms in the specialties of cardiology, pulmonary, and respiratory therapy.

Other important contributors to this revised edition include: Ellen Atwood, Patricia Collins, CMT; Betsy Dearborn; Robin Koza; LeVerne Randol, CMT; and Christa Scott, all of whom gathered new words and/or provided invaluable suggestions. Barb Ferretti played an integral role in the process by updating the database and providing a final quality check.

As with all our *Stedman's* word references, we have benefitted from the suggestions and expertise of our many contacts in the medical transcriptionist community. Thanks to all our advisory board participants, reviewers and editors, AAMT meeting attendees, and others who have written in with requests and comments—keep talking, and we'll keep listening.

Preface to the Second Edition

The terminology of cardiology and pulmonology frequently overlaps that of the closely-related areas of respiratory therapy and asthma. Reliable, up-to-date references for these interlinked fields have been few and far between. For years, we medical transcriptionists have had to rely on either our "little black books" or our memories, neither of which was entirely satisfactory.

When Williams & Wilkins contacted me about their plans to revise *Stedman's Cardiology Words,* we discussed how adding related pulmonary and respiratory terms would make a truly comprehensive second edition. Plans were set in motion to implement some major changes in *Stedman's Cardiology & Pulmonary Words, Second Edition.* With the help of myself and other medical transcriptionists, many entries in the first edition were consolidated, obsolete terms were deleted, and many, many new entries were added. It has taken a great deal of collaboration, painstaking research, and fine-tuning to accomplish our objective. We feel satisfied that we have accomplished what we set out to do—provide a comprehensive user-friendly word book that completely covers its subject matter with the latest terminology available. I feel that this second edition of *Stedman's Cardiology & Pulmonary Words* will meet the needs of not only medical transcriptionists but a diverse group of other medical professionals as well.

In the preface of *Stedman's Ob-Gyn Words, Second Edition,* I stated that it was a rare privilege to be associated with a company that listens carefully to the input from its readers and responds by producing a superb word book series targeted directly to our needs. In the intervening time, I have continued to work closely with the editorial staff at Williams & Wilkins, and can honestly say that this is indeed a publisher that considers the needs and concerns of medical transcriptionist as their highest priority in constantly updating and improving their entire word book series. I am once again honored to be associated with this current project, *Stedman's Cardiology & Pulmonary Words, Second Edition.*

Helen Littrell

Publisher's Preface

Stedman's Cardiology & Pulmonary Words, Second Edition offers an authoritative assurance of quality and exactness to the wordsmiths of the health care professions — medical transcriptionists, medical editors and copy editors, health information management personnel, court reporters, and the many other users and producers of medical documentation.

Users of the first edition of *Stedman's Cardiology Words* will notice the addition of terms in the areas of pulmonary, respiratory, and asthma in this second edition. In this "combined" word book, we have edited, updated, and expanded the cardiology content from the first edition and have added both basic and cutting edge pulmonary and respiratory terms.

Stedman's Cardiology & Pulmonary Words, Second Edition, can be used to validate both the spelling and the accuracy of terminology specific to cardiac catheterization, angiography, atherectomy, electrophysiology studies, stress tests, echocardiography, rehabilitation, and exercise. Pulmonary and respiratory-related terms include: flexible fiberoptic bronchoscopy, pulmonary function tests, incentive spirometry, respiratory therapy, and pediatric and adult respiratory equipment. In addition, the user will find terminology related to these specialties, such as asthma and allergy.

The user will find listed thousands of drugs, diagnostic and therapeutic procedures, new techniques and maneuvers, lab tests, and equipment, instrument and prosthesis names. Abbreviations and acronyms are also included. For quick reference, anatomy illustrations, a list of drug names by indication, a list of terms by commonly performed procedures, and sample reports of common procedures appear in the appendices at the back of the book.

Because our goal has been to provide a comprehensive yet streamlined reference tool, we have omitted terminology that is not specific to these specialties. Thus, some terms (such as anatomy and physiology terms) that are often dictated in these specialties are not included in this text, as they can be found in general medical dictionaries.

This compilation of over 48,600 entries, fully cross-indexed for quick access, was built from a base vocabulary of over 28,200 medical words, phrases, abbreviations and acronyms. The extensive A-Z list was developed from the database of *Stedman's Medical Dictionary* and supplemented by terminology found in current medical literature (please see list of References on page xvi).

We at Williams & Wilkins strive to provide you with the most up-to-date and accurate word references available. Your use of this word book will prompt new editions, which will be published as often as justified by updates and revisions. We welcome your suggestions for improvements, changes, corrections, and additions — whatever will make this *Stedman's* product more useful to you. Please use the postpaid card at the back of this book and send your recommendations care of "Stedmans" at Williams & Wilkins.

Explanatory Notes

Medical transcription is an art as well as a science. Both are needed to correctly interpret a physician's dictation, whose language is a product of education, training, and experience. This variety in medical language means that there are several acceptable ways to express certain terms, including jargon. This second edition of *Stedman's Cardiology & Pulmonary Words* provides variant spellings and phrasings for many terms. This, in addition to complete cross-indexing, makes *Stedman's Cardiology & Pulmonary Words, Second Edition* a valuable resource for determining the validity of terms as they are encountered.

Alphabetical Organization
Alphabetization of entries is letter by letter as spelled, ignoring punctuation, spaces, prefixed numbers, Greek letters, or other characters. For example:

acid-fast staining methods

acid formaldehyde hematin

α-acid glycoprotein

acid hematin

In subentries, the abbreviated singular form or the spelled-out plural form of the noun main entry word is ignored in alphabetization.

Format and Style
All main entries are in **boldface** to speed up location of a sought-after entry, to enhance distinction between main entries and subentries, and to relieve the textual density of the pages.

Irregular plurals and variant spellings are shown on the same line as the singular or preferred form of the word. For example:

scolex, pl. **scoleces**

curette, curet

Hyphenation

As a rule of style, multiple eponyms (e.g., Green-Kenyon corneal marker) are hyphenated. Also, hyphens have been added between a manufacturer and one or more eponyms (e.g., Vital-Metzenbaum dissecting scissors). Please note that hyphenation is a question of style, not of accuracy, and thus is a matter of choice.

Possessives

Possessive forms have been dropped in this reference for the sake of consistency and to conform to the guidelines outlined by the American Association for Medical Transcription (AAMT) and other groups. Please note, however, that retaining the possessive is a question of style, not of accuracy, and thus is a matter of choice. To form the possessive of a word, simply add the apostrophe or apostrophe "s" to the end of the word.

Cross-indexing

The word list is in an index-like main entry-subentry format that contains two combined alphabetical listings:

(1) A *noun* main entry-subentry organization typical of the A-Z section of medical dictionaries like **Stedman's:**

dyspnea
    exertional d.
    functional d.
    inspiratory d.
    nocturnal d.

endoscope
    AccuSharp e.
    Endocam e.
    Messerklinger e.
    lung imaging fluorescence e.

(2) An *adjective* main entry-subentry organization, which lists words and phrases as you hear them. The main entries are the adjectives or modifiers in a multi-word term. The subentries are the nouns around which the terms are constructed and to which the adjectives or modifiers pertain:

metabolic
    m. acidosis
    m. alkalosis
    m. encephalopathy
    m. rate meter

embolic
    e. abscess
    e. aneurysm
    e. pneumonia
    e. stroke

This format provides the user with more than one way to locate and identify a multi-word term. For example:

disease	**Paget**
Paget d.	P. disease
aneurysm	**cardiac**
cardiac a.	c. aneurysm
fusiform a.	c. tamponade
saccular a.	c. valve prosthesis

It also allows the user to see together all terms that contain a particular descriptor as well as all types, kinds, or variations of a noun entity. For example:

balloon	**angioplasty**
b. laser angioplasty	balloon laser a.
b. occlusion	complex a.
Blue Max b.	a. guiding catheter
Brandt cytology b.	high-risk a.
Express b.	transluminal coronary a.

Wherever possible, abbreviations are separately defined and cross-referenced. For example:

AICD
automatic implantable cardioverter-defibrillator

automatic
a. implantable cardioverter-defibrillator (AICD)

cardioverter-defibrillator
automatic implantable c.-d. (AICD)

References

In addition to the manufacturers' literature we gather at various medical meetings, scientific reports from hospitals, and our MT Editorial Advisory Board members' lists (from their daily transcription work), we used the following sources for new words for *Stedman's Cardiology & Pulmonary Words, Second Edition:*

Books

Cardiology words and phrases, 2ed. Modesto: Health Professions Institute, 1995.

Khan MG, Marino PL, Pingleton SK, Saksena S. Cardiac and pulmonary management. Philadelphia: Lea & Febiger, 1993.

Lance LL. Quick look drug book. Baltimore: Williams & Wilkins, 1996.

Mandell GL, Bennett JE, Dolin R. Principles and practice of infectious diseases, 4th ed. New York: Churchill Livingstone, 1995.

Middleton Jr. E, et al. Allergy: Principles and practice, 4th ed. St. Louis: Mosby-Yearbook, Inc., 1993.

Pyle V. Current medical terminology, 5th ed. Modesto: Health Professions Institute, 1994.

Stedman's medical dictionary. 26th ed. Baltimore: Williams & Wilkins, 1995.

Sloane SB. The medical word book, 3rd ed. Philadelphia: WB Saunders Company, 1991.

Stedman's medical & surgical equipment words. Baltimore: Williams & Wilkins, 1996.

Stedman's cardiology words. Baltimore: Williams & Wilkins, 1993.

Journals

The American Journal of Cardiology, Belle Mead, NJ: Excerpta Medica, Inc., 1992–1996.

Cardiology in Review, Baltimore: Williams & Wilkins, 1994–1996.

Clinical Pulmonary Medicine, Baltimore: Williams & Wilkins, 1994–1996.

Internal Medicine. Montvale, NJ: Medical Economics, 1995–1996.

Journal of the American Association for Medical Transcription. Modesto: American Association for Medical Transcription, 1995–1996.

Journal of the American College of Cardiology. New York, Elsevier Science Inc., 1992–1996.

The Latest Word. Philadelphia: WB Saunders Company, 1994–1996.

Perspectives on the Medical Transcription Profession. Modesto: Health Professions Institute, 1993–1996.

A
    A wave
A2
    A2 multipurpose catheter
    A2 to opening snap interval
A23187
    calcium ionophore A23187
A₂
    aortic second sound
AA
    ascending aorta
A-a
    alveolar-arterial
AAA
    abdominal aortic aneurysm
AACD
    abdominal aortic counterpulsation
      device
AAI
    atrial demand-inhibited
      AAI pacemaker
      AAI pacing
A-A interval
A₁-A₂ interval
AAI-RR pacing
AAL
    anterior axillary line
AARC
    American Association for
      Respiratory Care
AAT
    alpha-1 antitrypsin
    atrial demand-triggered
    automatic atrial tachycardia
      human pooled AAT
      AAT pacemaker
      AAT pacing
AAVNRT
    atypical atrioventricular nodal
      reentrant tachycardia
abacterial thrombotic endocarditis
Abbe
    A. flap
    A. operation
Abbokinase
    A. injection
    A. Open-Cath
Abbott infusion pump
ABC
    airway, breathing, and circulation

    aspiration biopsy cytology
    ABC leads
    ABC protocol
abciximab
ABD
    automated border detection
    automatic boundary detection
abdominal
    a. angina
    a. aorta
    a. aortic aneurysm (AAA)
    a. aortic counterpulsation
      device (AACD)
    a. aortography
    a. asthma
    a. bruit
    a. heart
    a. jugular test
    a. left ventricular assist device
      (ALVAD)
    a. pocket
    a. respiration
abdominalis
    aorta a.
abdominocardiac reflex
abdominojugular reflux
abdominothoracic
    a. arch
    a. pump
ABE
    acute bacterial endocarditis
ABECB
    acute bacterial exacerbation of
      chronic bronchitis
Abee support
Abelcet
Abell-Kendall equivalent
Abelson cannula
aberrancy
    acceleration-dependent a.
    bradycardia-dependent a.
    postextrasystolic a.
    tachycardia-dependent a.
aberrant
    a. artery
    a. QRS complex
    a. thyroid
    a. ventricular conduction
aberrantly conducted beat

aberration
> intraventricular a.
> ventricular a.

abetalipoproteinemia
> Bassen-Kornzweig a.
> familial a.

ABG
> arterial blood gas

ABI
> ankle-brachial index

ability
> torquing a.

Abiomed
> A. biventricular support system
> A. BVAD 5000
> A. Cardiac device

ABL
> ABL 520 blood gas
> measurement system
> ABL 625 system

ablater
> radiofrequency a.

ablation
> Ablatr temperature control
> device a.
> accessory conduction a. (ACA)
> atrioventricular junctional a.
> catheter a.
> continuous-wave laser a.
> coronary rotational a.
> direct-current shock a.
> electrical catheter a.
> fast-pathway radiofrequency a.
> His bundle a.
> Kent bundle a.
> laser a.
> percutaneous radiofrequency
> catheter a.
> pulsed laser a.
> radiofrequency a. (RFA)
> radiofrequency catheter a.
> RF a.
> rotational a.
> slow-pathway a.
> tissue a.
> transcatheter a.

ablative
> a. cardiac surgery
> a. device
> a. laser angioplasty
> a. technique

Ablatr
> A. temperature control device

A. temperature control device
> ablation

ABLC
> amphotericin B lipid complex

abnormal
> a. cleavage of cardiac valve
> a. left axis deviation (ALAD)
> a. right axis deviation (ARAD)

abnormality
> atrioventricular conduction a.
> clotting a.
> electrical activation a.
> figure-of-8 a.
> hemodynamic a.
> immunochemical a.'s
> left ventricular wall motion a.
> lusitropic a.
> neurogenic a.'s
> sinus node/AV conduction a.
> snowman a.
> ventricular depolarization a.
> wall motion a.

aborted systole
abortive pneumonia
abouchement
ABP
> arterial blood pressure
> automated boundary protection

ABPA
> allergic bronchopulmonary
> aspergillosis

Abraham laryngeal cannula
Abrahams sign
Abrams
> A. heart reflex
> A. needle
> A. pleural biopsy punch

Abrams-Lucas flap heart valve
abrasion
> pleural a.

abreuography
ABS
> acrylonitrile-butadiene-styrene

abscess
> Brodie a.
> embolic a.
> lung a.
> myocardial a.
> papillary muscle a.
> periaortic a.
> retropharyngeal a.
> ring a.

abscessus
    Mycobacterium a.
absent
    a. breath sounds
    a. pericardium
    a. respiration
Absidia
absolute
    a. cardiac dullness (ACD)
    a. refractory period (ARP)
absorbable
    a. gelatin
absorption
    fluorescent treponemal
        antibody a. (FTA-ABS)
absorption atelectasis
abuse
    alcohol a.
    cocaine a.
    drug a.
AC
    alternating current
AC137
ACA
    accessory conduction ablation
acacia
    gum a.
ACAD
    atherosclerotic carotid artery disease
acadesine
Acanthamoeba
    A. astronyxis
    A. castellani
    A. culbertsoni
    A. glebae
    A. hatchetti
    A. palestinensis
    A. polyphaga
    A. rhysodes
acanthocytosis
acapnia
ACAPS
    Asymptomatic Carotid
    Atherosclerosis Plaque Study
acarbia
acarbose
acardiotrophia

ACAS
    Asymptomatic Carotid
    Atherosclerosis Study
ACBG
    aortocoronary bypass graft
ACC
    American College of Cardiology
accelerated
    a. conduction
    a. hypertension
    a. idioventricular rhythm
       (AIVR)
    a. idioventricular tachycardia
    a. junctional rhythm
    a. respiration
acceleration-dependent aberrancy
acceleration time
accelerator
    proconvertin prothrombin
       conversion a.
    serum prothrombin
       conversion a. (SPCA)
accelerometer
    Caltrac a.
Accent-DG balloon
accentuated antagonism
access
    A-Port vascular a.
    Low Profile Port vascular a.
    side-entry a. (SEA)
    venous a.
accessory
    a. arteriovenous connection
    a. artery
    a. atrium
    a. conduction ablation (ACA)
    a. cusp
    a. muscles of respiration
    a. pathway
    a. pathway effective refractory
       period (APERP)
    a. thyroid
accident
    cardiac a.
    cardiovascular a.
    cerebrovascular a. (CVA)
accidental murmur

NOTES

Accolate
accretio
    a. cordis
    a. pericardii
accrochage
Accucap CO_2/O_2 monitor
Accu-Chek
    A.-C. II Freedom
Accucom cardiac output monitor
Accudynamic adjustable damping
Accufix
    A. pacemaker
    A. pacemaker lead
Acculith pacemaker
AccuMark calibrated infant feeding
tube
accumulation
    lipid a.
    phytanic acid a.
Accupressure infusion pump
Accupril
Accurbron
AccurOx mask
Accustaple
Accutorr
    A. A1, 3 blood pressure
        monitor
Accutracker
    A. blood pressure device
    A. II ambulatory blood
        pressure monitor
ACD
    absolute cardiac dullness
    Active Compression-Decompression
    arrhythmia control device
    Res-Q ACD
    ACD resuscitator
ACE
    angiotensin-converting enzyme
    ACE balloon
    ACE fixed-wire balloon
    catheter
    ACE inhibitor
Ace
    A. Cloud Enhancer
acebutolol
    a. hydrochloride
acecainide hydrochloride
acedapsone
ACEI
    angiotensin-converting enzyme
    inhibitor
Acel-Imune

acenocoumarol
Aceon
ace of spades sign
acetaldehyde
acetaminophen
    a. and dextromethorphan
    hydrocodone and a.
acetate
    anaritide a.
    carbon-11 a.
    cortisone a.
    desmopressin a. (DDAVP)
    Florinef A.
    fludrocortisone a.
    guanabenz a.
    guanfacine a.
    Hydrocortone A.
    paramethasone a.
    pirbuterol a.
acetazolamide
acetohexamide
acetylcarnitine
acetylcholine
    a. test
acetylcholinesterase
    a. deficiency
acetyl-CoA
acetylcysteine
    N-a.
acetyldigitoxin
N-acetylprocainamide
acetylsalicylic acid (A.S.A.)
acetylstrophanthidin (AcS)
ACG
    angiocardiography
    apexcardiogram
    apexcardiography
achalasia
    esophageal a.
Aches-N-Pain
Achiever balloon dilatation catheter
Acholeplasma laidlawii
Achromobacter xylosoxidans
Achromycin V Oral
ACI
    asymptomatic cardiac ischemia
acid
    N-acetylneuraminic a.
    acetylsalicylic a. (A.S.A.)
    amino a.
    aminocaproic a.
    aminosalicylic a.
    amoxicillin and clavulanic a.

arachidonic a.
ascorbic a.
aspartic a.
carbon-11-labeled fatty a.'s
cystidine monophospho-*N*-
acetylneuraminic a. (CMP-
NANA)
deoxyribonucleic a. (DNA)
diethylenetriamine pentaacetic a.
(DPTA)
docosahexaenoic a.
eicosapentaenoic a. (EPA)
enalaprilic a.
ethacrynic a.
ethylenediaminetetraacetic a.
(EDTA)
fatty a.
ferrous salt and ascorbic a.
ferrous sulfate, ascorbic a.,
vitamin B-complex, and
folic a.
fibric a.
folic a.
fosinoprilic a.
free fatty a.'s (FFA)
fusidic a.
gadolinium-diethylenetriamine
pentaacetic a. (Gd-DTPA)
gamma-aminobutyric a.
glycyrrhizinic a.
hydrochloric a.
hydrocyanic a.
a. infusion test
lactic a.
linoleic a.
a. maltase deficiency
mefenamic a.
messenger ribonucleic a.
(mRNA)
mevalonate a.
a. mucopolysaccharide (AMP)
nalidixic a.
n-3 fatty a.
n-6 fatty a.
nicotinic a.
nonesterified fatty a. (NEFA)
omega-3 unsaturated fatty a.'s

palmitic a.
paraaminobenzoic a.
paraaminosalicylic a. (PAS,
PASA)
perchloric a.
a. phosphatase
phosphinic a.
pyruvic a.
ribonucleic a. (RNA)
sialic a.
ticarcillin and clavulanic a.
tranexamic a.
trans fatty a.'s
uric a.
urocanic a.
zofenoprilic a.
acid-base
a.-b. disorder
a.-b. imbalance
acidemia
acid-fast bacilli (AFB)
**acidic fibroblast growth factor
(aFGF)**
acidity
total a.
acidosis
hypercapnic a.
hyperchloremic a.
lactic a.
metabolic a.
respiratory a.
acid-reactive
thiobarbituric a.-r.
acinar
a. adenocarcinoma
a. nodule
Acinetobacter
A. anitratus
A. calcoaceticus
A. calcoaceticus-baumannii
complex
A. lwoffi
A-C interval
acinus
lung a.
acipimox

NOTES

ACIPS
Asymptomatic Cardiac Ischemia
Pilot Study
acitretin
aCLa
anticardiolipin antibodies
Acland-Banis arteriotomy set
Acland-Buncke counterpressor
Acland microvascular clamp
acleistocardia
ACLS
advanced cardiac life support
ACME
Angioplasty Compared to Medicine
Evaluation
acnes
Propionibacterium a.
aconitine
Acorn II nebulizer
Acosta disease
Acoustascope esophageal stethoscope
acoustic
a. imaging
a. microscope
a. quantification (AQ)
a. shadow
a. shadowing
a. window
ACPE
acute cardiogenic pulmonary edema
acquired
a. atelectasis
a. immunodeficiency syndrome
(AIDS)
acquisition
a. gate
gated equilibrium
ventriculography, frame-
mode a.
gated equilibrium
ventriculography, list-mode a.
multiple gated a. (MUGA)
a. time
Acra-Cut Spiral craniotome blade
acradinium-ester-labeled nucleic acid
probe
Acremonium
acroasphyxia
acrocephalopolysyndactyly
acrocyanosis
acromegalic heart disease
acromegaly
Acrotheca aquaspera

acrotic
acrotism
acrylonitrile
acrylonitrile-butadiene-styrene (ABS)
ACS
Advanced Cardiovascular Systems
Advanced Catheter Systems
ACS Alpha balloon
ACS Amplatz guidewire
ACS Angioject
ACS angioplasty catheter
ACS angioplasty Y connector
ACS balloon catheter
ACS Concorde over-the-wire
catheter system
ACS Endura coronary dilation
catheter
ACS Enhanced Torque 8/7.5 F
Taper Tip catheter
ACS extra-support guidewire
ACS Gyroscan
ACS Indeflator
ACS JL4 French catheter
ACS LIMA guidewire
ACS microglide wire
ACS Mini catheter
ACS Monorail catheter
ACS Multi-Link coronary stent
ACS OTW Lifestream
coronary dilatation catheter
ACS percutaneous introducer
set
ACS RX LifeStream coronary
dilatation catheter
ACS RX perfusion balloon
catheter
AcS
acetylstrophanthidin
ACT
activated clotting time
axial computed tomography
ACTH
adrenocorticotropic hormone
Acthar
ActHIB vaccine
Actifed Allergy Tablet
Actigraph
Mini-Motionlogger A.
Actilyse
Actimmune
α-actinin
actin monomer
actin-myosin crossbridge

Actinobacillus
    A. *actinomycetemcomitans*
    A. *equuli*
    A. *hominis*
    A. *suis*
    A. *ureae*
Actinomyces
    A. *bovis*
    A. *israelii*
actinomycetemcomitans
    Actinobacillus a.
actinomycetoma
actinomycosis
action
    catecholamine a.
    mechanism of a.
    a. potential
    a. potential duration (APD)
Activase
    A. injection
activated
    a. balloon expandable
      intravascular stent
    a. clotting time (ACT)
    a. partial thromboplastin time
      (aPTT)
activation
    eccentric atrial a.
    length-dependent a.
    a. map-guided surgical
      resection
    myofilament contractile a.
activation-sequence mapping
activator
    2-chain urokinase
      plasminogen a. (tcu-PA)
    plasminogen a.
    recombinant tissue
      plasminogen a. (rt-PA)
    recombinant tissue-type
      plasminogen a.
    tissue plasminogen a. (t-PA)
    tissue-type plasminogen a.
    urokinase-type plasminogen a.
      (uPA)
    vampire bat plasminogen a.

Active
    A. Compression-Decompression
      (ACD)
active
    a. congestion
    a. dynamic stiffness
    a. hyperemia
    a. tuberculosis
active-site inhibited factor VIIa
Activitrax II pacemaker
activity
    intrinsic sympathomimetic a.
    membrane-stabilizing a.
    muscle sympathetic nerve a.
      (MSNA)
    myocyte metabolic a.
    plasma renin a. (PRA)
    pulseless electrical a. (PEA)
    a. scale
    sinoaortic baroreflex a.
    snooze-induced excitation of
      sympathetic triggered a.
      (SIESTA)
    spike a.
    sympathetic a.
    triggered a.
activity-sensing pacemaker
actocardiotocograph
Actron
actuarial survival curve
actuation
    direct mechanical ventricular a.
      (DMVA)
Acuson
    A. cardiovascular system
    A. computed sonography
    A. echocardiographic equipment
    A. V5M multiplane TEE
      transducer
    A. V5M transesophageal
      echocardiographic monitor
    A. XP-5 ultrasonoscope
ACUTE
    Assessment of Cardioversion Using
      Transesophageal Echocardiography
acute
    a. allograft rejection

NOTES

acute *(continued)*
  a. bacterial endocarditis (ABE)
  a. bacterial exacerbation of chronic bronchitis (ABECB)
  a. cardiogenic pulmonary edema (ACPE)
  a. chest syndrome
  a. compression triad
  a. fibrinous pericarditis
  a. glomerulonephritis (AGN)
  a. hemorrhagic bronchopneumonia
  A. Infarction Ramipril Efficacy (AIRE)
  a. infective endocarditis (AIE)
  a. intermittent porphyria (AIP)
  a. interstitial pneumonia
  a. interstitial pneumonitis
  a. isolated myocarditis
  a. laryngotracheal bronchitis
  a. lung rejection
  a. miliary tuberculosis
  a. myocardial infarction (AMI)
  a. obliterating bronchiolitis
  a. pharyngitis
  a. physiologic assessment and chronic health evaluation (APACHE)
  a. pleurisy
  a. pulmonary embolism
  a. radiation pneumonitis
  a. renal failure
  a. respiratory distress syndrome
  a. respiratory failure (ARF)
  a. response
  a. retroviral syndrome
  a. rheumatic arthritis
  a. rheumatic fever
  a. severe hypotension
  a. tamponade
  a. ventricular assist device (AVAD)
Acutrim Precision Release
ACX
  A. balloon
  A. II balloon catheter
acyanotic
  a. heart disease
acyclovir
acylcarnitine
acyl-CoA
acyl-CoA:cholesterol acyltransferase inhibitor

acyl-coenzyme A
acyltransferase
  lecithin-cholesterol a. (LCAT)
ADA
  adenosine deaminase
  ADA deficiency
Adagen
Adalat
Adamkiewicz artery
Adams-DeWeese
  A.-D. device
  A.-D. vena caval serrated clip
Adams disease
Adams-Stokes
  A.-S. attack
  A.-S. disease
  A.-S. syncope
  A.-S. syndrome
adapter
  Bodai a.
  catheter a.
  Harris a.
  Peep-Keep II a.
  Protex swivel a.
  Rosenblum rotating a.
  Tuohy-Borst a.
  Venturi jet a.
Addison
  A. disease
  A. maneuver
  A. plane
adenine nucleotide translocator
adenocarcinoma
  acinar a.
  bronchiolar a.
  bronchioloalveolar a.
  bronchogenic a.
  papillary a.
Adenocard
  A. injection
adenoid
  hypertrophic a.'s
adenoma
  bronchial a.
adenopathy
  hilar a.
Adenoscan
  A. contrast medium
adenosine
  a. deaminase (ADA)
  a. deaminase deficiency
  a. diphosphate (ADP)
  a. echocardiography

a. monophosphate (AMP)
a. nucleotide translocator (ANT)
a. radionuclide perfusion imaging
a. ^{99m}Tc sestamibi SPECT
a. thallium test
a. triphosphatase (ATPase)
a. triphosphate (ATP)
a. triphosphate disodium
adenosquamous carcinoma
adenoviral
a. pneumonia
a. type 40/41 infection
Adenoviridae
adenovirus
adenovirus-mediated gene transfer
adenylate
a. cyclase
a. cyclase stimulator forskolin
a. cyclase toxin
ADH
antidiuretic hormone
adherence assay
adherent pericardium
adhesin-receptor interaction
adhesins
adhesiolysis
adhesion
fibrinous a.
pleural a.
adhesive
Biobrane a.
Histocryl Blue tissue a.
a. pericarditis
a. phlebitis
a. pleurisy
adiabatic fast passage
adiastole
adiemorrhysis
"a" dip
adipose tissue
adiposis
a. cardiaca
a. universalis
adipositas cordis

adiposum
cor a.
adjunctive balloon angioplasty
Adlone injection
admixture
venous a.
ADP
adenosine diphosphate
ADR-529
adrenal
a. hyperplasia
a. hypertension
a. medulla
Adrenalin
adrenaline
adrenergic
α-a., alpha-a.
a. antagonist
β-a., beta-a.
a. nervous system
a. receptor
a. stimulant
β-adrenergic
β-a. stimulation
adrenoceptor
beta a.
a. blocker
adrenocorticotropic hormone (ACTH)
adrenogenital syndrome
adrenomedullary triad
adrenomedullin peptide
adrenoreceptor
Adriamycin cardiotoxicity
Adrucil injection
ADR Ultramark 4 ultrasound
Adson
A. forceps
A. test
Adson-Coffey scalenotomy
adult
Coronary Artery Risk Development in Young A.'s (CARDIA)
a. respiratory distress syndrome (ARDS)

NOTES

adult *(continued)*
    A. Star 1010 ventilator
    a. tuberculosis
adultorum
    scleredema a.
advanced
    a. cardiac life support (ACLS)
    A. Cardiovascular Systems (ACS)
    A. Care cholesterol test
    A. Catheter Systems (ACS)
    a. life support (ALS)
    a. trauma life support (ATLS)
adventitia
    aortic tunica a.
    esophageal a.
adventitial
    a. bed
    a. layer
adventitious
    a. breath sounds
Advil Cold & Sinus Caplets
AE-60-I-2 implantable pronged unipolar electrode
AE-60-K-10 implantable unipolar endocardial electrode
AE-60-KB implantable unipolar endocardial electrode
AE-60-KS-10 implantable unipolar endocardial electrode
AE-85-I-2 implantable pronged unipolar electrode
AE-85-K-10 implantable unipolar endocardial electrode
AE-85-KB implantable unipolar endocardial electrode
AE-85-KS-10 implantable unipolar endocardial electrode
AECG
    ambulatory ECG
AEC pacemaker
AED
    automatic external defibrillator
Ae-H interval
AEM
    ambulatory electrocardiographic monitoring
Aequitron pacemaker
aequorin
aeremia
aerendocardia
aeroallergen
Aerobacter

aerobic
    a. capacity
    a. exercise stress test
    a. metabolism
    a. respiration
    a. threshold
AerobiCycle
AeroBid Oral Aerosol Inhaler
Aerochamber
    A. mask
    A. spacing device
Aerodyne bicycle
aeroembolism
aeroemphysema
aerogenes
    Pasteurella a.
aerogenic tuberculosis
aerogenosum
    sputum a.
aerogenous
Aerolate
Aeromonas
    A. caviae
    A. sobria
    A. veronii
Aeropent
aerophagia
aerosol
    Brethaire Inhalation A.
    A. Cloud Enhancer
    Duo-Medihaler A.
    Nasalide Nasal A.
    a. nebulizer
    steroid a.
    Tilade Inhalation A.
    Virazole A.
aerosolization
aerosolized
    a. bronchodilator
    a. pentamidine
Aerosomes
AeroSonic personal ultrasonic nebulizer
AeroTech II nebulizer
aerotherapy
aerothorax
aeruginosa
    Pseudomonas a.
AET
    atrial ectopic tachycardia
AF
    atrial fibrillation

AFB
  acid-fast bacilli
AFBG
  aortofemoral bypass graft
AFF
  atrial fibrillation-flutter
afferent
  a. arteriole
  a. artery
  a. impulse
  a. nerve fibers
afferentia
affinity
  a. chromatography
  a. maturation
afflux, affluxion
aFGF
  acidic fibroblast growth factor
AFORMED
  alternating, failure of response,
  mechanical, to electrical
  depolarization
  AFORMED phenomenon
AFP
  alpha-fetoprotein
  AFP II pacemaker
African
  A. Burkitt lymphoma
  A. cardiomyopathy
  A. endomyocardial fibrosis
  A. histoplasmosis
  A. sleeping sickness
  A. tick typhus
Afrin Tablet
afterdepolarization
  delayed a.
  early a. (EAD)
afterload
  a. matching
  a. mismatching
  a. reduction
  a. resistance
  ventricular a.
afterpotential
  diastolic a.
  oscillatory a.
  a. oversensing

  pacemaker a.
  positive a.
Ag
  silver
agalactiae
  Streptococcus a.
agammaglobulinemia
agar diffusion assay
agarose
  a. gel electrophoresis
  MetaPhor a.
agenesis
  pulmonary a.
agent
  Albunex contrast a.
  alpha blocking a.
  AlphaNine clotting a.
  antianginal a.
  antiarrhythmic a.
  antidiabetic a.
  antihypertensive a.
  antiplatelet a.
  beta-adrenergic blocking a.
  beta blocking a.
  calcium channel blocking a.
  chemotherapeutic a.
  cholinergic a.
  contrast a.
  diuretic a.
  dopaminergic a.
  Eaton a.
  histocompatibility a. B27
  hypoglycemic a.
  imaging a.
  inhalation a.
  inotropic a.
  macrolide antimicrobial a.
  nonglycoside inotropic a.
  nonsteroidal anti-
    inflammatory a.
  Norwalk a.
  psychotropic a.
  saluretic a.
  sclerosing a.
  SHU 508A contrast a.
  sonicated contrast a.
  steroid-sparing a.

NOTES

11

agent *(continued)*
 thrombolytic a.
 toxic a.
 TWAR a.
 vasodilator a.
age-undetermined myocardial
 infarction
agglutinating antibody
agglutination
agglutinative thrombus
agglutinins
 cold a.
aggregation
 platelet a.
aggregometer
 Alivi a.
aggregometry
 Born a.
 impedance a.
aglycon
AGN
 acute glomerulonephritis
agonal
 a. clot
 a. respiration
 a. rhythm
 a. thrombosis
 a. thrombus
agonist
 alpha a.
 alpha-adrenoreceptor a.
 beta a.
 beta-adrenergic a.
 beta-adrenoreceptor a.
 calcium channel a.
 muscarinic a.
agony clot
agranulocytosis
A greater than E
agricultural anthrax
Agrobacterium
AH
 artificial heart
A-H
 A-H conduction time
 A-H curve
 A-H interval
AHA
 American Heart Association
AH:HA ratio
AHI
 apnea-hypopnea index
Ahlquist-Durham embolism clamp

AHM
 ambulatory Holter monitoring
A-hydroCort
AI
 apical impulse
AICA
 anterior inferior communicating
 artery
 AICA riboside
AICD
 automatic implantable cardioverter-
 defibrillator
 automatic internal cardioverter-
 defibrillator
 Cadence AICD
 Guardian AICD
 AICD plus Tachylog device
 Res-Q AICD
 Ventak P3 AICD
AICD-B pacemaker
AICD-BR pacemaker
AID
 automatic implantable defibrillator
AID-Check monitor
AIDS
 acquired immunodeficiency
 syndrome
AIE
 acute infective endocarditis
A-II receptor
AIOD
 aortoiliac obstructive disease
AIP
 acute intermittent porphyria
air
 a. bronchogram
 a. bronchogram sign
 a. clamp inflatable vessel
 occluder
 a. embolization
 a. embolus
 a. entry
 a. exchange
 expiratory trapping of a.
 extrapleural a.
 high-efficiency particulate a.
 (HEPA)
 a. hunger
 a. movement
 a. pulmonary embolism
 a. space
 A. Supply
 tidal a.

a. trapping
a. trousers
A. Viva
air-borne transmission
air-driven artificial heart
AIRE
Acute Infarction Ramipril Efficacy
Aire-Cuf tracheostomy tube
Airet
airflow obstruction
air-fluid level
Airlie House criteria
Air-Lon
A.-L. inhalation cannula
A.-L. tracheal tube brush
air-powered nebulizer
air-puff tonometer
airspace
a. consolidation
a. disease
peripheral a.'s
airtrapping
airway
a. bacterial colonization
Beck mouth tube a.
Berman a.
a. branching
a. clearance
Combitube a.
Connell a.
esophageal obturator a.
flabby a.
Foerger a.
Guedel a.
nasal a.
a. obstruction
a. occlusion technique
a. pressure release ventilation (APRV)
a. reactivity index (ARI)
a. resistance
Safar-S a.
a. stenosis
upstream a.'s
airway, breathing, and circulation (ABC)

AIVR
accelerated idioventricular rhythm
Ajellomyces dermatitidis
ajmaline test
Akaike information criteria
AK-Chlor Ophthalmic
A-K diamond knife
akinesia
akinesic
akinesis
akinetic
Akutsu III total artificial heart
AL
AL II guiding catheter
Al
aluminum
AL-1 catheter
ALAD
abnormal left axis deviation
Aladdin infant flow system
alanine aminotransferase (ALT)
alar
a. chest
a. flaring
alaryngeal speech
AlaSTAT latex allergy test
Alatest Latex-specific IgE allergen test kit
Alazide
Alazine Oral
alba
pneumonia a.
albendazole
a. sulfoxide
Albertini treatment
Albert slotted bronchoscope
albicans
Candida a.
Monilia a.
albida
macula a.
Albini nodules
Albright syndrome
albumin
perfluorocarbon-exposed sonicated dextrose a. (PESDA)

NOTES

albumin *(continued)*
    radioactive iodinated serum a.
    (RISA)
    sonicated dextrose a.
albumin-coated vascular graft
albuminized woven Dacron tube
    graft
albuminoid sputum
albuminuria
Albunex
    A. contrast agent
albuterol
    a. inhaler
    a. sulfate syrup
Alcalgenes odorans
Alcaligenes
    A. bookeri
    A. dentrificans
    A. faecalis
    A. piechaudii
    A. xylosoxidans
ALCAPA
    anomalous origin of the left
    coronary artery from the
    pulmonary artery
Alcatel pacemaker
Alcock catheter plug
alcohol
    a. abuse
    ethyl a.
    a. intoxication
alcoholic
    a. cardiomyopathy
    a. malnutrition
    a. myocardiopathy
    a. pneumonia
alcoholism, leukopenia,
    pneumococcal sepsis (ALPS)
Alcon Closure System
Aldactazide
Aldactone
aldehyde-tanned bovine carotid
    artery graft
aldesleukin
Aldoclor
Aldomet
Aldoril
aldosterone
    a. antagonist
    a. depression
aldosteronism
aldosteronoma

Aldrete needle
Aldrich score
Alexander-Farabeuf periosteotome
Alexander rib stripper
alexandrite laser
alexithymia
    A. Provoked Response
    Interview
alfa
    dornase a.
alfa-2a
    interferon a.
alfa-2b
    interferon a.
alfentanil hydrochloride
Alfred M. Large vena cava clamp
alglucerase
algorithm
    Levenberg-Marquardt a.
algovascular
aliasing
    a. artifact
    image a.
alignment mark
alinidine
aliquot
Alivi aggregometer
Alkaban-AQ
alkaline
    a. phosphatase
alkaloid
    ergot a.
    Rauwolfia a.
alkalosis
    altitude a.
    metabolic a.
    respiratory a.
alkaptonuria
Alkeran
Alladin InfantFlow nasal continuous
    positive air pressure
Allain method
allantoic
    a. circulation
    a. vein
allele
    mutant a.
Allen-Brown
    A.-B. criteria
    A.-B. shunt
Allen test
Aller-Chlor Oral

allergen
environmental a.
a. exposure
allergen-induced
a.-i. asthma
a.-i. mediator release
allergic
a. alveolitis
a. asthma
a. bronchopulmonary
aspergillosis (ABPA)
a. bronchospasm
a. diathesis
a. granulomatosis
a. granulomatous angiitis
a. reaction
a. rhinitis
a. salute
a. shiners
a. vasculitis
allergy
bronchial a.
seasonal a.'s
AllerMax Oral
ALLHAT
Antihypertensive Lipid Lowering
Heart Attack Trial
alligator pacing cable
Allis clamp
Allison
A. hiatal hernia repair
A. lung retractor
Alliston procedure
allogeneic transplant
allograft
bovine a.
cardiac a.
cryopreserved heart valve a.
cryopreserved human aortic a.
CryoVein saphenous vein a.
a. vasculopathy
allometric
allorhythmia
all-or-none law
allosteric modification of enzyme
Allport-Babcock searcher

ALMCA
anomalous left main coronary artery
almitrine bismesylate
almokalant
Aloka
A. color Doppler
A. color Doppler system for
blood flow imaging
A. echocardiograph machine
A. ultrasound
alpha
a. agonist
a. blocking agent
a. lipoprotein
a. receptor
alpha-1
a.-1 antitrypsin (AAT)
a.-1 antitrypsin deficiency
a.-1 proteinase inhibitor
alpha-2 macroglobulin
alpha-adrenergic
a.-a. blocker
a.-a. stimulation
alpha-adrenoreceptor
a.-a. agonist
a.-a. blocker
alpha-alpha homodimer
alpha-fetoprotein (AFP)
alpha-hydroxybutyrate
dehydrogenase
alpha-methyldopa
AlphaNine
A. clotting agent
alpha-tocopherol
Alphavirus
Alport syndrome
alprazolam
alprenolol
alprostadil
ALPS
alcoholism, leukopenia,
pneumococcal sepsis
ALPS syndrome
ALS
advanced life support
ALT
alanine aminotransferase

NOTES

15

alternans *(continued)*
 discordant a.
 electrical a.
 parvus a.
 pulsus a.
 QRS a.
 ST segment a.
 systole a.
 total a.
 T wave a.
 U wave a.
alternating
 a. bidirectional tachycardia
 a. current (AC)
 a. pulse
alternating, failure of response,
  mechanical, to electrical
  depolarization (AFORMED)
alternation
 cardiac a.
 concordant a.
 cycle length a.
 discordant a.
 electrical a. of heart
 mechanical a.
altitude
 a. alkalosis
 a. hypoxia
 a. simulation study
aluminum (Al)
 a. hydroxide gel
Alupent
ALVAD
 abdominal left ventricular assist
  device
 ALVAD artificial heart
Alvarez prosthesis
Alvarez-Rodriguez cardiac catheter
alvei
 Bacillus a.
alveobronchiolitis
alveolar
 a. asthma
 a. bronchiole
 a. capillary
 a. carbon dioxide pressure
 a. carbon dioxide tension
 a. cell carcinoma
 a. dead space
 a. duct emphysema
 a. ectasia
 a. edema
 a. flooding

a. hypertension
a. hyperventilation
a. hypoventilation
a. hypoxia
a. leak
a. opacification
a. oxygen partial pressure
  (PAO$_2$)
a. oxygen tension
a. proteinosis
a. ventilation
a. ventilation per minute (V$_A$)
alveolar-arterial (A-a)
 a.-a. oxygen tension gradient
alveolar-capillary
 a.-c. block
 a.-c. membrane
alveolar-septal amyloidosis
alveoli (*pl. of* alveolus)
 a. pulmonis
alveolitis
 allergic a.
 cryptogenic fibrosing a. (CFA)
 desquamative a.
 diffuse sclerosing a.
 extrinsic allergic a.
 fibrosing a.
 lymphoid a.
alveoloarterial oxygen tension
 gradient
alveolocapillary
 a. membrane
 a. partial pressure gradient
alveolus, pl. alveoli
 ventilated alveoli
Alzate catheter
Amadeus
AMA-Fab
 antimyosin monoclonal antibody
  with Fab fragment
 AMA-Fab scintigraphy
amalonaticus
 Citrobacter a.
amantadine hydrochloride
Amapari virus
amaurosis partialis fugax
amaurotic
amazon thorax
Amba
ambasilide
Ambenyl
Amberlite particles
Ambien

Amapari virus
amaurosis partialis fugax
amaurotic
amazon thorax
Amba
ambasilide
Ambenyl
Amberlite particles
Ambien
ambiguus
  situs a.
AmBisome
Amblyomma americanum
Ambrose plaque type
Ambu
  A. bag
  A. CardioPump
  A. respirator
ambulatory
  a. ECG (AECG)
  a. electrocardiographic
    monitoring (AEM)
  a. electrocardiography
  a. Holter monitoring (AHM)
  a. nuclear detector
Amcath catheter
Amcort
amdinocillin
amebiasis
  pulmonary a.
amebic
  a. pericarditis
  a. pneumonia
ameboid cell
ameboma
American
  A. Association for Respiratory
    Care (AARC)
  A. Cancer Society
  A. College of Cardiology
    (ACC)
  A. Heart Association (AHA)
  A. Heart Association
    classification
  A. Heart Association diet
  A. Optical Cardiocare
    pacemaker

  A. Optical oximeter
  A. Optical R-inhibited
    pacemaker
  A. Thoracic Society (ATS)
  A. tracheotomy tube
  A. trypanosomiasis
americanum
  Amblyomma a.
americanus
  Necator a.
Amesec
A-methaPred injection
AMI
  acute myocardial infarction
  anterior myocardial infarction
Amicar
Amidate
amifloxacin
amikacin
  a. sulfate
Amikin
  A. injection
amiloride
  a. hydrochloride
  a. and hydrochlorothiazide
amine
  sympathomimetic a.
amino acid
aminocaproic acid
aminoethyl ethanolamine
aminoglutethimide
aminoglycoside
aminoguanidine
aminopenicillin
aminophylline
aminophylline, amobarbital, and
  ephedrine
aminosalicylate sodium
aminosalicylic
  a. acid
  a. acid hypersensitivity
aminoterminal propeptide
aminotransferase
  alanine a. (ALT)
  aspartate a. (AST)
amiodarone
  desethyl a.

NOTES

amiodarone *(continued)*
  a. hydrochloride
  a. pulmonary fibrosis
amiodarone-induced hyperthyroidism
Amipaque
Amis 2000 respiratory mass spectrometer
Ami-Tex LA
amitriptyline
amlodipine
  a. and benazepril
  a. besylate
ammonia
  N-13 a.
  nitrogen-13 a.
ammonium chloride
amnesia
  global a.
amniocentesis
amniotic
  a. fluid embolism
  a. fluid syndrome
A-mode
  A.-m. echocardiography
  A.-m. echo-tracking device
Amorolfine
amorphous parenchymal opacification
amoxapine
amoxicillin
  a. and clavulanic acid
  a. and potassium clavulanate
Amoxil
AMP
  acid mucopolysaccharide
  adenosine monophosphate
  average mean pressure
ampere
amphetamine
  a. sulfate
  a. toxicity
amphipathic helix
Amphojel
amphoric
  a. echo
  a. murmur
  a. rales
  a. respiration
  a. voice
amphoriloquy
amphotericin
  a. B
  a. B lipid complex (ABLC)

ampicillin
  a. and sulbactam
Amplatz
  A. coronary catheter
  A. dilator
  A. Hi-Flo torque-control catheter
  A. left I, II catheter
  A. right coronary catheter
  A. right I, II catheter
  A. Super Stiff guidewire
  A. technique
  A. torque wire
  A. tube guide
Amplex guidewire
Amplicor *Mycobacterium tuberculosis* **test**
Amplified *Mycobacterium tuberculosis* **Direct test**
amplitude
  apical interventricular septal a.
  atrial pulse a.
  C to E a.
  contractile a.
  D to E a.
  a. image
  a. linearity
  pulse a.
  P wave a.
  R wave a.
  ventricular pulse a.
  wall a.
  wave a.
amprolium hydrochloride
ampulla, pl. **ampullae**
  Bryant a.
  Thoma a.
ampullary aneurysm
amrinone
  a. lactate
AMS
  automatic mode switching
amsacrine
Amtech-Killeen pacemaker
amyl
  a. nitrite
  a. nitrite study
amylase
  serum a.
amyloid
  a. A protein
  a. heart disease

A

amyloidosis
 alveolar-septal a.
 cardiac a.
 familial a.
 mediastinal a.
 nodular pulmonary a.
 parenchymal a.
 pleural a.
 primary systemic a.
 pseudotumoral mediastinal a.
 pulmonary a.
 senile a.
 tracheobronchial a.
amyocardia
amyotrophic chorea
ANA
 antinuclear antibody
anabolic steroid
anacrotic
 a. limb
 a. notch
 a. pulse
anacrotism
anadicrotic
 a. pulse
anadicrotism
anadicrotus
 pulsus a.
anaerobe
anaerobic
 a. empyema
 a. metabolism
 a. Pulsator syringe
 a. respiration
 a. threshold
anaerobiosis
Anaerobiospirillum
anaerobius
 Peptostreptococcus a.
analgesic
 a. nephropathy
 patient-controlled a. (PCA)
analog-to-digital conversion
analysis, pl. **analyses**
 backscatter a.
 beat-to-beat a.

 centerline method of wall
  motion a.
 Doppler spectral a.
 Doppler waveform a.
 fast Fourier spectral a.
 forced vital capacity a.
  (FVCA)
 Fourier series a.
 Fourier transform a.
 frequency-domain a.
 hydroxyproline a.
 immunoprecipitin a.
 multilinear regression a.
 phase image a.
 pressure-volume a.
 probability a.
 quantitative coronary
  angiographic a.
 regression a.
 Scatchard plot a.
 sensitivity a.
 spectral a.
 sputum a.
 time-domain a.
 Van Slyke a.
 a. of variance (ANOVA)
 wall motion a.
analyzer
 Beckman O_2 a.
 Cat-a-Kit a.
 Cobas Fara centrifugal a.
 Criticare $ETCO_2$ multigas a.
 Datex $ETCO_2$ multigas a.
 DMI a.
 Enzymun-Test System ES22 a.
 $ETCO_2$ multigas a.
 Marquette Series 8000
  Holter a.
 Medigraphics 2000 a.
 MiniOX 1A oxygen a.
 MiniOX 1000 oxygen a.
 Nellcor N2500 $ETCO_2$
  multigas a.
 Novametrix $ETCO_2$ multigas a.
 Ohmeda $ETCO_2$ multigas a.
 pacing system a.
 pulse-height a.

NOTES

analyzer *(continued)*
    Puritan Bennett ETCO$_2$
      multigas a.
    Sole Primeur 33D a.
anapamil
anaphylactic
    a. antibody
    a. crisis
anaphylactoid
    a. purpura
    a. reaction
anaphylatoxin
anaphylaxis
    eosinophil chemotactic factors
      of a. (ECF-A)
    slow-reacting substance of a.
      (SRS-A)
anaplastic carcinoma
anaplerosis
anaplerotic sequence
anapnea
anapneic
anapnotherapy
Anaprox
anaritide acetate
anastomose
anastomosis, pl. **anastomoses**
    aortic a.
    arterial a.
    arteriovenous a.
    Baffe a.
    bidirectional cavopulmonary a.
      (BCA)
    bidirectional superior
      cavopulmonary a. (BSCA)
    cavopulmonary a.
    cobra-head a.
    Cooley intrapericardial a.
    Cooley modification of
      Waterston a.
    distal a.
    Fontan atriopulmonary a.
    Glenn a.
    Kugel a.
    Nakayama a.
    portacaval a.
    portoportal a.
    portosystemic a.
    Potts a.
    Potts-Smith a.
    a. of Riolan
    Sucquet-Hoyer a.

    systemic to pulmonary
      artery a.
    Waterston extrapericardial a.
anatomic
    a. assessment
    a. block
    a. localization
anatomical dead space
anatomy
    coronary a.
    designed after natural a.
    native coronary a.
anatricrotic
anatricrotism
ANCA
    antineutrophil cytoplasmic
      antibodies
Ancef
anchor
    Harpoon suture a.
Ancobon
ANCOR imaging system
Ancrod
Ancylostoma
    A. braziliense
    A. caninum
Andersen
    A. syndrome
    A. triad
Anderson
    A. procedure
    A. test
Anderson-Keys method
Andral decubitus
Andrews
    A. retractor
    A. suction tip
Andrews-Pynchon tube
Androsov vascular stapler
anechoic
Anectine
    A. Chloride
Anel operation
anemia
    aplastic a.
    chronic hemolytic a.
    Cooley a.
    hemolytic a.
    Mediterranean a.
    megaloblastic a.
    microangiopathic a.
    sickle cell a.
    splenic a.

anemic
- a. hypoxia
- a. murmur

anergy

Anestacon

anesthesia
- Bier block a.
- MacIntosh blade a.

anesthetic

aneurysm
- abdominal aortic a. (AAA)
- ampullary a.
- aortic a.
- aortoiliac a.
- arterial a.
- arteriovenous pulmonary a.
- atherosclerotic a.
- atrial septal a.
- Berard a.
- berry a.
- brain a.
- cardiac a.
- cerebral a.
- Charcot-Bouchard a.
- cirsoid a.
- congenital aortic a.
- coronary a.
- Crisp a.
- cylindroid a.
- descending thoracic a.
- dissecting aortic a.
- dolichoectatic a.'s
- ectatic a.
- embolic a.
- embolomycotic a.
- false aortic a.
- fusiform aortic a.
- infected a.
- infrarenal abdominal aortic a.
- innominate a.
- interventricular septum a.
- intracranial a.
- left ventricular a.
- luetic a.
- mitral valve a.
- mixed a.
- mural a.
- mycotic aortic a.
- Park a.
- phantom a.
- popliteal a.
- Pott a.
- racemose a.
- Rasmussen a.
- Richet a.
- Rodriguez a.
- ruptured aortic a.
- saccular a.
- serpentine a.
- Shekelton a.
- sinus of Valsalva a.
- spurious a.
- suprasellar a.
- syphilitic aortic a.
- thoracic aortic a.
- thoracoabdominal aortic a.
- traction a.
- traumatic aortic a.
- true aortic a.
- ventricular a.
- verminous a.
- windsock a.
- a. wrapping

aneurysmal, aneurysmatic
- a. bone cyst
- a. bruit
- a. cough
- a. dilation
- a. hematoma
- a. murmur
- a. phthisis
- a. thrill

aneurysmectomy
- Matas a.

aneurysmography

aneurysmoplasty

Anexsia

ANF
- atrial natriuretic factor

AngeLase combined mapping-laser probe

Angelchik antireflux prosthesis

NOTES

Angell-Shiley
  A.-S. bioprosthetic valve
  A.-S. xenograft prosthetic valve
angel's trumpet
Ange-Med Sentinel ICD device
Anger scintillation camera
Angestat hemostasis introducer
Angetear tearaway introducer
angialgia
angiasthenia
angiectasis
angiitis
  allergic granulomatous a.
  Churg-Strauss a.
  leukocytoclastic a.
  necrotizing a.
  nonnecrotizing a.
angina
  abdominal a.
  anxiety a.
  bandlike a.
  benign croupous a.
  Bretonneau a.
  chronic stable a.
  classic a.
  cold-induced a.
  a. cordis
  coronary spastic a.
  crescendo a.
  a. crouposa
  a. cruris
  decubitus a.
  a. decubitus
  a. dyspeptica
  effort a.
  ergonovine maleate
    provocation a.
  esophageal a.
  exercise-induced a.
  exertional a.
  false a.
  first-effort a.
  food a.
  a. gangrenosa
  Heberden a.
  hippocratic a.
  hypercyanotic a.
  hysteric a.
  a. inversa
  ischemic rest a.
  lacunar a.
  a. laryngea
  Ludwig a.

  a. membranacea
  microvascular a.
  mixed a.
  neutropenic a.
  nocturnal a.
  nonexertional a.
  a. nosocomii
  a. notha
  office a.
  pacing-induced a.
  a. pectoris
  a. pectoris decubitus
  a. pectoris sine dolore
  a. pectoris vasomotoria
  a. phlegmonosa
  postinfarction a.
  postprandial a.
  preinfarction a.
  Prinzmetal variant a.
  A. Prognosis Study in
    Stockholm (APSIS)
  pseudomembranous a.
  Randomized Intervention in the
    Treatment of A. (RITA)
  rate-dependent a.
  rebound a.
  reflex a.
  rest a.
  a. rheumatica
  a. scarlatinosa
  Schultz a.
  sexual a.
  silent a.
  a. simplex
  smoking-induced a.
  a. spuria
  stable a.
  Thrombolysis and Angioplasty
    in Unstable A. (TAUSA)
  toilet-seat a.
  a. tonsillaris
  a. trachealis
  treadmill-induced a.
  a. ulcerosa
  unstable a.
  variable threshold a.
  variant a. (VA)
  variant a. pectoris
  vasomotor a.
  vasospastic a.
  vasotonic a.
  Vincent a.

A

walk-through a.
white-coat a.
anginae
    Saccharomyces a.
angina-guided therapy
angina inversa
anginal
    a. equivalent
    a. perceptual threshold
anginiform
anginoid
anginophobia
anginosa
    syncope a.
anginose, anginous
anginosus
    status a.
    Streptococcus a.
angiocardiogram
angiocardiography (ACG)
    first-pass radionuclide a.
    radionuclide a.
    transseptal a.
angiocardiokinetic
angiocardiopathy
angiocarditis
Angiocath
    A. PRN catheter
angiocatheter
    Brockenbrough a.
    Corlon a.
    Deseret a.
    Eppendorf a.
Angio-Conray
Angiocor
    A. prosthetic valve
    A. rotational thrombolizer
angiodermatitis
angiodynagraphy
angiodynia
angiodysplasia
    a. of colon
angioedema
Angioflow high-flow catheter
angiogenesis
Angiografin

angiogram
    ECG-synchronized digital
      subtraction a.
    gated nuclear a.
    venous digital a.
    wedge a.
angiograph
    3DFT magnetic resonance a.
angiographic
    a. assessment
    a. catheter
    a. contrast
    a. instrumentation
angiographically occult intracranial
  vascular malformation (AOIVM)
angiography
    aortography a.
    balloon-occlusion pulmonary a.
    biplane orthogonal a.
    carotid a.
    cerebral a.
    color power a.
    coronary a.
    digital subtraction a. (DSA)
    digitized subtraction a.
    equilibrium radionuclide a.
      (ERNA)
    fluorescein a.
    gated blood-pool a.
    gated radionuclide a.
    indocyanine green a.
    internal mammary artery
      graft a.
    intraoperative digital
      subtraction a. (IDSA)
    intraoperative vascular a. (IVA)
    intravenous digital
      subtraction a. (IVDSA)
    left aortic a.
    left atrial a.
    left ventricular a.
    mesenteric a.
    multigated a.
    noncardiac a.
    nonselective coronary a.
    pulmonary wedge a.
    quantitative coronary a. (QCA)

NOTES

angiography *(continued)*
  radionuclide a.
  renal a.
  renovascular a.
  rest and exercise gated
    nuclear a.
  rest radionuclide a.
  saphenous vein bypass graft a.
  selective a.
  subtraction a.
  surveillance a.
  synchrotron-based
    transvenous a.
  thermal a.
  ultrasound a.
  ventricular a.
  wedge pulmonary a.
Angioject
  ACS A.
Angio-Jet rapid thrombectomy system
angiokeratoma
  a. corporis diffusum
angiokinesis
Angio-Kit catheter
angioleiomyoma
angioma
  cherry a.
  spider a.
angiomatosis
  bacillary a.
Angiomedics catheter
angionecrosis
angioneurotic edema
Angiopac
angiopigtail catheter
angioplasia
angioplasty
  ablative laser a.
  adjunctive balloon a.
  balloon catheter a. (BCA)
  balloon coarctation a.
  balloon coronary a.
  balloon laser a.
  bootstrap two-vessel a.
  brachiocephalic vessel a.
  A. Compared to Medicine
    Evaluation (ACME)
  complementary balloon a.
  coronary a.
  culprit lesion a.
  excimer laser coronary a.
  (ELCA)

  facilitated a.
  high-risk a.
  Ho:YAG laser a.
  Kinsey rotation atherectomy
    extrusion a.
  kissing balloon a.
  laser-assisted balloon a.
  (LABA)
  Osypka rotational a.
  patch-graft a.
  percutaneous balloon a.
  percutaneous transluminal
    coronary a. (PTCA)
  peripheral laser a. (PLA)
  rescue a.
  salvage balloon a.
  Tactilaze a.
  thermal/perfusion balloon a.
  (TPBA)
  Thrombolysis and A. in
    Myocardial Infarction (TAMI)
  thulium:YAG laser a.
  tibioperoneal vessel a.
  transluminal coronary a.
  vibrational a.
angioplasty-related vessel occlusion
angiopneumography
angiosarcoma
angioscintigraphy
angiosclerotic gangrene
angioscope
  Imagecath rapid exchange a.
  Masy a.
angioscopy
  percutaneous transluminal a.
  (PTAS)
Angio-Seal hemostatic puncture closure device
Angioskop-D
Angiosol
angiostomy
angiotensin
  renin a.
angiotensinase
angiotensin-converting
  a.-c. enzyme (ACE)
  a.-c. enzyme inhibitor (ACEI)
angiotensin-I converting enzyme
angiotensin-II
  a.-II receptor blockade
  a.-II receptor blocker
angiotensinogen
  a. gene

angiotomy
Angiovist
angle
    blunted costophrenic a.
    cardiodiaphragmatic a.
    cardiophrenic a.
    costophrenic a.
    costovertebral a. (CVA)
    Ebstein a.
    flip a.
    intercept a.
    Louis a.
    Ludwig a.
    nail-to-nail bed a.
    phase a.
    Pirogoff a.
    a. port pump
    QRS-T a.
    sternoclavicular a.
    xiphoid a.
angled
    a. balloon II catheter
    a. pigtail catheter
    a. pleural tube
angor
    a. animi
    a. pectoris
Ang-O-Span
angulated multipurpose catheter
angulation
    RAO a.
angusta
    aorta a.
Anhydron
Anichkov, Anitschkow
    A. myocyte
animal dander
animi
    angor a.
A-N interval
anion
    a. exchange resin
    a. gap
    superoxide a.
anisa
    Legionella a.
anisopiesis

anisorrhythmia
anisosphygmia
anisotropic conduction
anisotropy
anisoylated plasminogen streptokinase activator complex (APSAC)
anistreplase
anitratus
    Acinetobacter a.
Anitschkow (*var. of* Anichkov)
ankle
    a. edema
    a. exercise
ankle-arm index
ankle-brachial
    a.-b. blood pressure ratio
    a.-b. index (ABI)
ankylosing spondylitis (AS)
anlagen
annihilation photon
annular
    a. array transducer
    a. dehiscence
    a. phased array system (APAS)
    a. thrombus
annuli (*pl. of* annulus)
    a. fibrosi cordis
annuloaortic ectasia
annulocuspid hinge
annuloplasty
    Carpentier a.
    DeVega tricuspid valve a.
    Gerbode a.
    prosthetic ring a.
    tricuspid valve a.
    Wooler-type a.
annulus, anulus, pl. **annuli**
    aortic a.
    a. fibrosus
    mitral valve a.
    a. ovalis
    tricuspid valve a.
anodal
    a. closure contraction
    a. opening contraction

NOTES

anode
anomalous
  a. atrioventricular excitation
  a. bronchus
  a. complex
  a. conduction
  a. first rib thoracic syndrome
  a. left main coronary artery (ALMCA)
  a. mitral arcade
  a. origin
  a. origin of the left coronary artery from the pulmonary artery (ALCAPA)
  a. pulmonary vein
  a. pulmonary venous connection
  a. pulmonary venous drainage (APVD)
  a. pulmonary venous return
  a. rectification
anomaly
  atrioventricular connection a.
  coloboma, heart anomaly, choanal atresia, retardation, and genital and ear a.'s (CHARGE)
  congenital conotruncal a.
  conotruncal a.
  coronary artery a.
  Ebstein cardiac a.
  Freund a.
  pulmonary valve a.
  pulmonary venous connection a.
  pulmonary venous return a.
  Shone a.
  Taussig-Bing a.
  Uhl a.
  ventricular inflow a.
  vertebral, vascular, anal, cardiac, tracheoesophageal, renal, and limb a.'s (VACTERL)
  viscerobronchial cardiovascular a.
Anopheles
anorexia nervosa
ANOVA
  analysis of variance
anoxemia test
anoxia
  cerebral a.

  myocardial a.
  stagnant a.
ANP
  atrial natriuretic polypeptide
AN region
Anrep
  A. effect
  A. phenomenon
ansa cervicalis
ansamycin
ANT
  adenosine nucleotide translocator
antacid
antagonism
  accentuated a.
  Coronary Artery Restenosis Prevention on Repeated Thromboxane A. (CARPORT)
antagonist
  adrenergic a.
  aldosterone a.
  beta a.
  beta$_1$ a.
  beta$_2$ a.
  calcium a.'s
  calcium channel a.
  dihydropyridine calcium a.
  thromboxane receptor a.
  vitamin K a.
antasthmatic
antecedent
  plasma thromboplastin a.
antecubital
  a. fossa
  a. space
antegrade
  a. aortography
  a. approach
  a. block cycle length
  a. conduction
  a. double balloon/double wire technique
  a. internodal pathway
  a. refractory period
antegrade/retrograde cardioplegia technique
antemortem
  a. clot
  a. thrombus
anterior
  a. anodal patch electrode
  a. approach
  a. axillary line (AAL)

a. chamber
a. descending coronary artery
a. inferior communicating
   artery (AICA)
a. internodal pathway
a. leaflet
a. myocardial infarction (AMI)
a. oblique projection
a. papillary muscle (APM)
a. sandwich patch technique
a. table
a. wall (AW)
a. wall dyskinesis
a. wall myocardial infarction
anteriorly-directed jet
anteroapical
   a. dyskinesis
anterograde
   a. APERP
   a. block
   a. conduction
   a. flow
   a. transseptal technique
anteroinferior myocardial infarction
anterolateral myocardial infarction
anteromesial hypokinesis
anteroposterior
   a. paddles
   a. projection
   a. thoracic diameter
anteroseptal myocardial infarction
   (ASMI)
antesystole
anthopleurin-A
anthracis
   Bacillus a.
anthraconecrosis
anthracosilicosis
anthracosis
anthracotic tuberculosis
anthracycline-induced
   cardiomyopathy
anthracycline toxicity
anthraquinone
anthrax
   agricultural a.
   industrial a.

a. pneumonia
pulmonary a.
Anthron
   A. heparinized antithrombogenic
      catheter
   A. II catheter
anthropi
   Ochrobacterium a.
anthropometric evaluation
antiadhesin antibody
antiadrenergic
antialdosterone therapy
anti-aliasing technique
antianginal
   a. agent
   a. treatment
antiarrhythmic
   a. agent
   a. drug classification (Ia, Ib,
      Ic, II, III, IV)
   a. therapy
Antiarrhythmics versus Implantable
   Defibrillators (AVID)
antiatherogenic
antiatherosclerotic
antibacterial
antibasement membrane
antibiotic
   antipseudomonas a.
   azalide class of a.'s
   macrolide a.'s
   prophylactic a.
antibody, pl. antibodies
   agglutinating a.
   anaphylactic a.
   antiadhesin a.
   anticardiolipin antibodies
      (aCLa)
   anti-DNA a.
   antidystrophin a.
   antiglomerular basement
      membrane antibodies
   anti-La antibodies
   antineutrophil cytoplasmic
      antibodies (ANCA)
   antinuclear a. (ANA)
   antiphospholipid a.

NOTES

antibody *(continued)*
  antireceptor a.
  anti-Ro SS-A antibodies
  anti-Sm a.
  anti-SSA/Ro antibodies
  anti-SSB/La antibodies
  B cell a.
  CD18 antibodies
  cross-reactive a.
  digitalis-specific a.
  direct fluorescent a. (DFA)
  7E3 glycoprotein IIb/IIIa
    platelet a.
  7E3 monoclonal Fab a.
  fibrin-specific a.
  fluorescent antimembrane a.
    (FAMA)
  monoclonal antimyosin a.
  monoclonal a. 3G4
  myosin-specific a.
  OKT3 a.
  platelet a.
  Rh a.
  sheep antidigoxin Fab a.
  streptococcal a.
  streptokinase a.
  teichoic acid a.
  thyroid a.
  tissue-specific antibodies
  treponemal a.
  TR-R9 antithrombin receptor
    polyclonal a.
  Y2B8 a.
antibradycardia
anticardiolipin antibodies (aCLa)
anticholinergic
  a. bronchodilator
anticipated systole
anticoagulant
  lupus a.
  a. therapy
Anticoagulants in the Secondary
  Prevention of Events in
  Coronary Thrombosis (ASPECT)
anticoagulation
anti-deoxyribonuclease B
antidepressant
  tricyclic a.
antidiabetic agent
antidiuretic hormone (ADH)
anti-DNA antibody
anti-DNase B

antidromic circus-movement
  tachycardia
antidysrhythmic
antidystrophin antibody
antielastase
antiembolism stockings
antiendotoxin therapy
antifibrillatory
antifibrin antibody imaging
antifilarial
antifoaming inhalant
antifungal
antigen
  Australia a.
  avian a.
  carcinoembryonic a. (CEA)
  Epstein-Barr nuclear a.
    (EBNA)
  human leukocyte a. (HLA)
  human lymphocyte a. (HLA)
  inhalant a.
  KI a.
  O a.
  p24 a.
  PLA-I platelet a.
  proliferating cell nuclear a.
    (PCNA)
antigen-binding
  a.-b. diversity
  fragment a.-b.
antigenicity
antiglomerular basement membrane
  antibodies
anti-G suit
antiheart antibody titer
antihemophilic
  a. factor
  a. factor (human)
  a. factor (recombinant)
Antihist-1
antihistamine
antihypertensive
  a. agent
  A. Lipid Lowering Heart
    Attack Trial (ALLHAT)
antihypotensive
anti-inflammatory
anti-inhibitor coagulant complex
anti-La
  a.-L. antibodies
antilymphocyte serum
antimalarial
  primaquine phosphate a.

antimicrobial
a. catheter cuff
macrolide a.
a. therapy
Antiminth
antimony
a. compound
a. toxicity
antimycobacterial
a. chemotherapy
antimycotic
antimyosin
a. antibody imaging
a. infarct-avid scintigraphy
a. monoclonal antibody with
Fab fragment (AMA-Fab)
**antineutrophil cytoplasmic antibodies
(ANCA)**
antinuclear antibody (ANA)
antioxidative
antiparasitic
antiphospholipid
a. antibody
a. syndrome
antiplasmin
antiplatelet
a. agent
a. therapy
antipneumococcal
antipseudomonas antibiotic
antireceptor antibody
antireflux prosthesis
anti-Rho-D titer
anti-Ro SS-A antibodies
Anti-Sept bactericidal scrub solution
antishock garment
antisialagogue
anti-Sm antibody
anti-SSA/Ro antibodies
anti-SSB/La antibodies
antistasin
antistreptokinase
antistreptolysin O (ASO)
antistreptozyme (ASTZ)
antitachycardia
a. pacemaker (ATP)
a. pacing

antithrombin
antithrombin III (AT-III)
antithromboplastin
antithrombotic
**Antithrombotics in the Prevention
of Reocclusion in Coronary
Thrombolysis (APRICOT)**
antithymocyte
a. globulin
antitoxin
diphtheria a.
antitrypsin
alpha-1 a. (AAT)
M-type alpha 1-a.
plasma alpha 1-a. (pAAT)
recombinant alpha$_1$ a. (rAAT)
α1-antitrypsin
antituberculin
antituberculous
a. chemotherapy
a. drug
antitussive
antler sign
antrectomy
antrum, pl. **antra**
cardiac a.
Anturane
Antyllus method
anulus (*var. of* annulus)
anxiety
a. angina
a. attack
a. neurosis
anxiolytic
any-plane echocardiography
AoBP
aortic blood pressure
AOD
arterial occlusive disease
AOIVM
angiographically occult intracranial
vascular malformation
A-OK ShortCut knife
AOO
A. pacemaker
A. pacing
aorta, pl. **aortae**

NOTES

aorta *(continued)*
abdominal a.
a. abdominalis
a. angusta
arch of a.
arcus aortae
a. ascendens
ascending a. (AA)
bifurcation of a.
buckled a.
buckling of a.
button of a.
a. chlorotica
coarctation of a.
a. descendens
descending a.
dextropositioned a.
dissecting a.
dissection of a.
double-barreled a.
dynamic a.
kinked a.
medionecrosis of a.
overriding a.
porcelain a.
primitive a.
pseudocoarctation of a.
recoarctation of a.
retroesophageal a.
sacrococcygeal a.
straddling a.
terminal a.
a. thoracalis
thoracic a.
a. thoracica
aorta-left atrium ratio
aortalgia
aortarctia
aortartia
aortectasis, aortectasia
aortectomy
aortic
a. anastomosis
a. aneurysm
a. aneurysmal disease
a. aneurysm clamp
a. annulus
a. arch
a. arch interruption
a. arch syndrome
a. arteritis syndrome
a. assist balloon introducer
a. atresia

a. balloon pump
a. bifurcation
a. blood pressure (AoBP)
a. bulb
a. closure sound
a. coarctation
a. commissure
a. compliance
a. cross-clamp
a. cuff
a. cusp
a. cusp separation
a. dicrotic notch pressure
a. dissection (type A, type B)
a. dwarfism
a. embolism
a. envelope
a. facies
a. hiatus
a. homograft
a. impedance
a. incompetence
a. intramural hematoma
a. isthmus
a. jet velocity
a. knob
a. knuckle
left atrial to a. (La:A)
a. nipple
a. notch
a. obstruction
a. orifice
a. override
a. perfusion cannula
a. pressure gradient
a. prosthesis
a. pullback
a. pullback pressure
a. pulmonary window
a. reflex
a. regurgitation (AR)
a. regurgitation murmur
a. ring
a. root
a. root dimension
a. root ratio
a. rupture
a. sac (AS)
a. sclerosis
a. second sound (A_2)
a. septal defect
a. sinus
a. spindle

a. stenosis (AS)
a. stenosis jet
a. stenosis murmur
a. thrill
a. thromboembolic disease
a. thrombosis
a. triangle
a. tube graft
a. tunica adventitia
a. tunica intima
a. tunica media
a. valve
a. valve area
a. valve disease
a. valve gradient (AVG)
a. valve leaflet
a. valve regurgitation
a. valve replacement (AVR)
a. valve resistance
a. valve restenosis
a. valve vegetation
a. valve velocity profile
a. valvotomy
a. valvular insufficiency
a. valvulitis
a. valvuloplasty
a. vasa vasorum
a. window
aortic-left ventricular tunnel murmur
aortic-mitral combined disease murmur
aorticopulmonary
a. septal defect
a. window
aorticus
torus a.
aortismus abdominalis
aortitis
arthritis-associated a.
Döhle-Heller a.
giant cell a.
luetic a.
nummular a.
rheumatic a.
syphilitic a.
Takayasu a.

aortoannular ectasia
aortobifemoral
aortobi-iliac bypass
aortocarotid bypass
aortocaval fistula
aortocoronary
a. bypass graft (ACBG)
a. snake graft
aortocoronary-saphenous vein bypass
aortofemoral
a. arterial runoff
a. arteriography
a. artery shunt
a. bypass graft (AFBG)
aortogram
digital subtraction supravalvular a.
flush a.
a. with distal runoff
aortography
abdominal a.
a. angiography
antegrade a.
arch a.
ascending a.
atherosclerotic a.
biplane a.
caudally-angled balloon occlusion a.
digital subtraction supravalvular a.
flush a.
laid-back balloon occlusion a.
mycotic a.
retrograde a.
selective a.
single-plane a.
sinus of Valsalva a.
thoracic arch a.
transbrachial a.
translumbar a.
traumatic a.
true vs. false aneurysm a.
aortoiliac
a. aneurysm
a. bypass graft
a. obstructive disease (AIOD)

NOTES

aortoiliac *(continued)*
    a. occlusive disease
    a. thrombosis
aortoiliofemoral
    a. bypass
    a. circuit
aorto-ostial lesion
aortopathy
aortoplasty
aortoptosia, aortoptosis
aortopulmonary
    a. collateral
    a. fenestration
    a. shunt
    a. window
aortorenal bypass
aortorrhaphy
aortosclerosis
aortostenosis
aorto-subclavian-carotid-axilloaxillary
  bypass
aortotomy
aortovelography
    transvenous a. (TAV)
APACHE
    acute physiologic assessment and
    chronic health evaluation
      APACHE II, III score
apallic syndrome
APAS
    annular phased array system
apathetic hyperthyroidism
APB
    atrial premature beat
APC
    atrial premature contraction
APD
    action potential duration
APERP
    accessory pathway effective
    refractory period
      anterograde APERP
Apert syndrome
aperture
    transducer a.
apex, pl. **apices**
    a. beat
    cardiac a.
    a. cordis
    a. impulse
    left ventricular a.
    a. murmur

    a. pneumonia
    right ventricular a. (RVA)
apexcardiogram (ACG)
    upstroke pattern on a. (dP/dt)
apexcardiography (ACG)
aphasia
    ataxic a.
    expressive a.
    global a.
    receptive a.
    Wernicke a.
aphasic
apheresis
aphonic pectoriloquy
aphrophilus
    Haemophilus a.
apical
    a. bronchus
    a. five-chamber view
      echocardiogram
    a. four-chamber view
    a. four-chamber view
      echocardiogram
    a. impulse (AI)
    a. interventricular septal
      amplitude
    a. left ventricular puncture
    a. lordotic roentgenogram
    a. mid-diastolic heart murmur
    a. pneumonia
    a. scarring
    a. systolic heart murmur
    a. two-chamber view
    a. two-chamber view
      echocardiogram
apices (*pl. of* apex)
apicolysis
    extrapleural a.
    Semb a.
apicoposterior segment
aplasia
    pulmonary a.
aplastic anemia
Aplisol
APM
    anterior papillary muscle
apnea
    a. alarm mattress
    deglutition a.
    initial a.
    late a.
    a. monitor
    a. neonatorum

obstructive sleep a. (OSA)
posthyperventilation a.
sleep a.
traumatic a.
apnea-hypopnea index (AHI)
apneic
apneumatosis
apneumia
apneusis
apneustic
a. breathing
a. respiration
Apo A-1 deficiency
Apo E3 isoform
Apo E test
Apogee CX 100 Interspec
ultrasound machine
apolipoprotein
a. A-I Milano, B, D, E
aponeurosis
aponeurotic
apoplectic
a. coma
a. cyst
apoplexy
asthenic a.
capillary a.
cerebral a.
ingravescent a.
apoprotein A, B, C, D, E
apoptosis
apoptotic cell death
A-Port vascular access
aposthematosa
pneumonia a.
apo-zidovudine
apparatus
Davidson pneumothorax a.
Fell-O'Dwyer a.
Jacquet a.
Langendorff a.
V-Vac suction a.
appearance
cluster-of-grapes a.
cottage-loaf a.
dirty-lung a.
finger-in-glove a.

ground-glass a.
hazy a.
salt-and-pepper a.
tree-in-winter a.
appendage
atrial a.
auricular a.
left atrial a. (LAA)
right atrial a. (RAA)
appendectomy
auricular a.
applanation tonometry
apple picker's disease
applesauce sign
appliance
TheraSnore oral a.
apposition
mitral-septal a.
stent a.
approach
antegrade a.
anterior a.
brachial artery a.
central a.
femoral a.
Lortat-Jacob a.
percutaneous a.
posterior a.
retrograde femoral a.
transradial a.
transxiphoid a.
trap-door a.
approximation
Friedewald a.
approximator
rib a.
Wolvek sternal a.
Apresazide
Apresoline
A. injection
A. Oral
APRICOT
Antithrombotics in the Prevention of
Reocclusion in Coronary
Thrombolysis
aprindine
Aprinox

NOTES

aprotinin
APRV
    airway pressure release ventilation
APSAC
    anisoylated plasminogen
    streptokinase activator complex
APSIS
    Angina Prognosis Study in
    Stockholm
aPTT
    activated partial thromboplastin time
Apt test
APVD
    anomalous pulmonary venous
    drainage
AQ
    acoustic quantification
aquagenic urticaria
AquaMEPHYTON
    A. injection
Aquaphyllin
AquaShield
aquaspera
    Acrotheca a.
Aquatag
Aquatensen
Aquatherm II
Aquazide
aqueous
    penicillin g, parenteral, a.
AR
    aortic regurgitation
AR-1 catheter
arabinoside
    cytosine a. (CA)
arachidic bronchitis
arachidonate metabolism
arachidonic
    a. acid
    a. acid metabolites
arachnodactyly
ARAD
    abnormal right axis deviation
Araki-Sako technique
araldehyde-tanned bovine carotid
artery graft
Aralen Phosphate
Aramine
araneus
    nevus a.
Arani double-loop guiding catheter
Arantii
    ductus A.

Arantius
    bodies of A.
    A. body
    canal of A.
    A. nodule
arborization block
arbovirus
Arbrook Hemovac
arbutamine
arcade
    anomalous mitral a.
    a. collateral
    septal a.
arcanobacterial pharyngitis
arch
    abdominothoracic a.
    a. of aorta
    aortic a.
    a. aortography
    a. arteriography
    axillary a.
    azygos a.
    carotid a.
    cervical aortic a.
    circumflex aortic a.
    congenital interrupted aortic a.
    double aortic a.
    FemoStop femoral artery
    compression a.
    interrupted aortic a.
    jugular venous a.
    Langer axillary a.
    palmar a.
    pharyngeal a.
    pulmonary a.
    right aortic a.
    Zimmermann a.
architecture
    lung a.
Arco
    A. atomic pacemaker
    A. lithium pacemaker
Arcomax
    A. FMA cardiac angiography
    system
arcus
    a. aortae
    a. corneae
    corneal a.
    a. cornealis
    a. costarum
    a. lipoides corneae
    a. senilis

arc-welder lung
ARDS
    adult respiratory distress syndrome
Arduan
area, pl. **areae, areas**
    aortic valve a.
    Bamberger a.
    body surface a. (BSA)
    a. of cardiac dullness
    echo-spared a.
    effective balloon-dilated a.
    (EBDA)
    end-diastolic a. (EDA)
    Erb a.
    Krönig a.
    mitral valve a. (MVA)
    proximal isovelocity surface a.
    (PISA)
    pulmonary valve a.
    pulmonic a.
    regurgitant jet a. (RJA)
    secondary aortic a.
    subxiphoid a.
    tricuspid valve a.
    truncoconal a.
    valve orifice a.
area-length method
Arelix
Arenaviridae virus
AREx inhaler
ARF
    acute respiratory failure
ArF excimer laser
Arfonad injection
argatroban
Argesic-SA
arginine vasopressin (AVP)
argipressin
argon
    a. beam coagulator
    a. ion laser
    a. needle
    a. vessel dilator
Argyle
    A. catheter
    A. CPAP nasal cannula
    A. Sentinel Seal chest tube

    A.-Turkel safety thoracentesis
    system
    A.-Turkel thoracentesis
Argyll Robertson pupils
ARI
    airway reactivity index
Aria CPAP system
ARIC
    Atherosclerotic Risk in Communities
A-ring
    esophageal A.-r.
Aristocort
    A. Forte
    A. Intralesional Suspension
    A. Tablet
Aristospan
Arkin-Z
Arloing-Courmont test
arm
    chest and left a. (CL)
    chest and right a. (CR)
    dissected tissue a.
    a. ergometry treadmill
    a. exercise stress test
Arm-a-Med
    A.-a.-M. endotracheal tube
    A.-a.-M. Isoetharine
    A.-a.-M. isoproterenol
    A.-a.-M. Metaproterenol
arm-ankle indices
arm-leg gradient
armored heart
arm-tongue
    a.-t. time
    a.-t. time test
Aromatic Ammonia Aspirols
ARP
    absolute refractory period
array
    convex linear a.
    multi-element linear a.
    PRx Endotak-Sub-Q a.
    sock a.
    symmetrical phased a.
arrest
    asystolic a.
    bradyarrhythmic a.

NOTES

arrest *(continued)*
 cardiac a. (CA)
 cardioplegic a.
 cardiopulmonary a.
 cardiorespiratory a.
 circulatory a.
 cold ischemic a.
 deep hypothermia circulatory a.
  (DHCA)
 heart a.
 hypothermic fibrillating a.
 intermittent sinus a.
 respiratory a.
 sinoatrial a.
 sinus a.
 total circulatory a.
Arrhigi
 point of A.
arrhythmia
 atrial a.
 atrioventricular junctional a.
 A-V nodal Wenckebach a.
 baseline a.
 cardiac a.
 a. circuit
 continuous a.
 a. control device (ACD)
 exercise-induced a.
 a. focus
 hypokalemia-induced a.
 inducible a.
 inotropic a.
 juvenile a.
 lethal a.
 Lown a.
 malignant ventricular a. (MVA)
 Mönckeberg a.
 A. Net
 A. Net arrhythmia monitor
 nodal a.
 nonphasic sinus a.
 paroxysmal supraventricular a.
 pause-dependent a.
 perpetual a.
 phasic sinus a.
 postperfusion a.
 reentrant a.
 reperfusion a.
 respiratory a.
 senile a.
 Singh-Vaughan Williams
  classification of a.'s
 sinus a.

 stress-related a.
 supraventricular a.
 tachybrady a.
 vagus a.
 ventricular a.
arrhythmic
arrhythmogenesis
arrhythmogenic
 a. right ventricular disease
 a. right ventricular dysplasia
  (ARVD)
 a. substrate
arrhythmogenicity
arrhythmokinesis
Arrow
 A. balloon wedge catheter
 A. Berman angiographic
  balloon
 A. Flex intra-aortic balloon
  catheter
 A. Hi-flow infusion set
 A. pneumothorax kit
 A. QuadPolar electrode
  catheter
 A. sheath
 A. TwinCath multilumen
  peripheral catheter
Arrow-Clarke thoracentesis device
Arrow-Fischell EVAN needle
ArrowFlex sheath
ARROWgard
 A. Blue antiseptic-coated
  catheter
 A. Blue Line catheter
 A. central venous catheter
Arrow-Howes multilumen catheter
arsenic (As)
 a. poisoning
arsine gas poisoning
artegraft
artemisin
arteria, pl. **arteriae** *(See* artery)
 a. anastomotica auricularis
  magna
arterial
 a. anastomosis
 a. aneurysm
 a. bleeding
 a. blood flow
 a. blood gas (ABG)
 a. blood pressure (ABP)
 a. calcification
 a. carbon dioxide pressure

a. carbon dioxide tension
a. cone
a. coupling
a. cutdown
a. decortication
a. dicrotic notch pressure
a. dissection
a. embolectomy catheter
a. embolism
a. entry site
a. filter
a. groove
a. hyperemia
a. hypertension
a. hypotension
a. hypoxemia
a. impedance
a. insufficiency
a. mean
a. mean line
a. media
a. murmur
a. needle
a. occlusive disease (AOD)
a. oscillator endarterectomy instrument
a. oxygen partial pressure (PaO$_2$)
a. oxygen saturation (SaO$_2$)
a. partial pressure of CO$_2$ (PaCO$_2$)
a. pulse
a. remodeling
a. runoff
a. saturation
a. sclerosis
a. sheath
a. spasm
a. spider
a. stick
a. switch operation
a. switch procedure
a. thrill
a. thrombosis
a. vein of Soemmerring
a. wave
a. wedge

arterialization
arteriarctia
arteriectasis, arteriectasia
arteries (*pl.* of artery)
arterioatony
arteriocapillary sclerosis
arteriogram
  brachial a.
  runoff a.
arteriographic
  a. regression
arteriography
  aortofemoral a.
  arch a.
  biplane pelvic a.
  biplane quantitative coronary a.
  carotid a.
  catheter a.
  coronary a.
  digital subtraction a.
  femoral a.
  quantitative a.
  renal a.
  selective a.
  Sones selective coronary a.
arteriohepatic dysplasia syndrome
arteriolar
  a. hyalinosis
  a. sclerosis
arteriole
  afferent a.
  efferent a.
  precapillary a.'s
arteriolith
arteriolitis
  necrotizing a.
arteriolonecrosis
arteriolosclerosis
arteriolovenular bridge
arteriomalacia
arteriometer
arterionecrosis
  hyaline a.
arteriopalmus
arteriopathy
  hypertensive a.
  plexogenic pulmonary a.

NOTES

arterioplania
arteriopressor
arteriorrhexis
arteriosclerosis
 cerebral a.
 coronary a.
 decrudescent a.
 hyaline a.
 hypertensive a.
 Mönckeberg a.
 nodose a.
 nodular a.
 a. obliterans
 peripheral a.
 senile a.
arteriosclerotic
 a. cardiovascular disease
  (ASCVD)
 a. heart disease (ASHD)
 a. peripheral vascular disease
  (ASPVD)
 a. vascular disease (ASVD)
arteriospasm
arteriosum
 cor a.
 ligamentum a.
arteriosus
 conus a.
 ductus a.
 patent ductus a. (PDA)
 persistent ductus a.
 persistent truncus a.
 pseudotruncus a.
 reversed ductus a.
 truncus a.
arteriotomy
 brachial a.
arteriotony
arteriovenous (A-V, AV)
 a. anastomosis
 a. communication
 a. crossing changes
 a. fistula (AVF)
 a. malformation (AVM)
 a. nicking
 a. oxygen difference (AVD O$_2$)
 a. pulmonary aneurysm
 a. shunt
arteritis, pl. arteritides
 brachiocephalic a.
 coronary a.
 cranial a.
 a. deformans

fibrinoid a.
giant cell a.
granulomatous a.
Horton a.
a. hyperplastica
infantile a.
mesenteric a.
a. nodosa
a. obliterans
rheumatic a.
rheumatoid a.
syphilitic a.
Takayasu a.
temporal a.
tuberculous a.
a. umbilicalis
a. verrucosa
artery, pl. arteries
 aberrant a.
 accessory a.
 Adamkiewicz a.
 afferent a.
 anomalous left main
  coronary a. (ALMCA)
 anomalous origin of the left
  coronary artery from the
  pulmonary a. (ALCAPA)
 anterior descending coronary a.
 anterior inferior
  communicating a. (AICA)
 atrioventricular node a.
 A-V nodal a.
 axillary a.
 banding of pulmonary a.
 beading of arteries
 blocked heart a.
 brachial a.
 brachiocephalic a.
 bronchial a.
 carotid a.
 celiac a.
 cephalic a.
 circumflex a.
 coarctation of pulmonary a.
 common carotid a.
 common femoral a.
 common hepatic a.
 common iliac a.
 complete transposition of great
  arteries
 copper-wire arteries
 corkscrew arteries
 coronary a.

cricothyroid a.
diagonal a.
diaphragmatic a.
D-loop transposition of the
  great arteries
Drummond marginal a.
D-transposition of great arteries
  (D-TGA)
a. ectasia
efferent a.
end a.
esophageal a.
external carotid a.
external mammary a.
femoral a.
first obtuse marginal a. (OM-
  1)
gastroepiploic a. (GEA)
Global Utilization of
  Streptokinase and t-PA for
  Occluded Coronary Arteries
  (GUSTO)
great a.
hepatic a.
iliac a.
inferior epigastric a. (IEA)
inferior mesenteric a.
innominate a.
intermediate circumflex a.
  (ICXA)
internal carotid a. (ICA)
internal mammary a. (IMA)
internal thoracic a. (ITA)
intersegmental arteries
intramural coronary arteries
jejunal a.
Kugel anastomotic a.
left anterior descending a.
  (LAD)
left circumflex a. (LCX)
left common carotid a.
left coronary a. (LCA)
left internal mammary a.
  (LIMA)
left main coronary a. (LMCA)
left subclavian a. (LSCA)
main pulmonary a. (MPA)

mainstem coronary a.
malposition of great arteries
  (MGA)
mammary a.
marginal circumflex a.
mesenteric a.
Neubauer a.
nodal a.
obtuse marginal a. (OMA)
parieto-occipital a.
perforating arteries
pericardiophrenic a.
perineal a.
peroneal a.
pharyngeal a.
phrenic a.
popliteal a.
posterior circumflex a. (PC)
posterior descending a. (PDA)
posterior inferior
  communicating a. (PICA)
Pravastatin Limitation of
  Atherosclerosis in Coronary
  Arteries (PLAC)
profunda femoris a.
pulmonary a. (PA)
radial a.
ramus intermedius a.
renal a.
retinal a.
right common carotid a.
right coronary a. (RCA)
right internal mammary a.
  (RIMA)
right pulmonary a. (RPA)
second obtuse marginal a.
  (OM-2)
septal perforating arteries
silver-wiring of retinal arteries
sinoatrial nodal a.
sinus node a.
sternocleidomastoid a.
subclavian a.
superficial femoral a.
superior carotid a.
superior thyroid a.
thoracodorsal a.

NOTES

artery *(continued)*
    tibial a.
    transposition of great arteries (TGA)
    umbilical a.
Artha-G
Arthritis
    A. Foundation Ibuprofen
    A. Foundation Pain Reliever
arthritis, pl. arthritides
    acute rheumatic a.
    juvenile rheumatoid a.
    rheumatoid a. (RA)
arthritis-associated aortitis
arthropod venom
Arthus-type reaction
articulation
Articulose-50 injection
artifact
    aliasing a.
    baseline a.
    beam width a.
    catheter impact a.
    catheter whip a.
    coin a.
    cupping a.
    end-pressure a.
    flow a.
    pacemaker a.
    reverberation a.
    side lobe a.
    T a.
    view-aliasing a.
    wrap-around ghosting a.
    zebra a.
artifactual bradycardia
artificial
    a. blood
    a. cardiac valve
    a. heart (AH)
    a. larynx
    a. lung
    a. pacemaker
    a. pneumothorax
    a. respiration
    a. ventilation
ARVD
    arrhythmogenic right ventricular dysplasia
Arvidsson dimension-length method
Arvin
arylsulfatase
arytenoid

Arzco
    A. model 7 cardiac stimulator
    A. pacemaker
    A. TAPSUL pill electrode
AS
    ankylosing spondylitis
    aortic sac
    aortic stenosis
AS-800
As
    arsenic
A.S.A.
    acetylsalicylic acid
asaccharolyticus
    Peptostreptococcus a.
asbestiform
asbestos
    a. bodies
    a. pneumoconiosis
asbestosis bodies
Asbron G
ASCAD
    atherosclerotic coronary artery disease
A-scan echography
ascariasis
ascendens
    aorta a.
ascending
    a. aorta (AA)
    a. aorta-to-pulmonary artery shunt
    a. aortic pressure
    a. aortography
    a. loop of Henle
    a. polyneuropathy
Ascension Bird
Aschner
    A. phenomenon
    A. reflex
    A. sign
Aschner-Dagnini reflex
Aschoff
    A. bodies
    A. cell
    A. nodules
Aschoff-Tawara node
ascites
    a. praecox
ascorbate dilution curve
ascorbic acid
Ascriptin

ASCVD
arteriosclerotic cardiovascular
disease
atherosclerotic cardiovascular
disease
ASD
atrial septal defect
asequence
ASH
asymmetric septal hypertrophy
ASHD
arteriosclerotic heart disease
Asherman chest seal
Asherson syndrome
Ashley phenomenon
Ashman
A. beat
A. phenomenon
Asian influenza
ASIS-1
First American Study of Infarct
Survival
ASIST
Atenolol Silent Ischemia Trial
Ask-Upmark
A.-U. kidney
A.-U. syndrome
Asmalix
ASMI
anteroseptal myocardial infarction
ASO
antistreptolysin O
asparaginase
aspartate aminotransferase (AST)
aspartic acid
ASPECT
Anticoagulants in the Secondary
Prevention of Events in Coronary
Thrombosis
aspergilloma formation
aspergillosis
allergic bronchopulmonary a.
(ABPA)
bronchopulmonary a.
invasive pulmonary a.
pulmonary a.

Aspergillus
A. avenaceus
A. caesiellus
A. candidus
A. carneus
A. flavus
A. fumigatus
A. nidulans
A. oryzae
A. restrictus
A. sydowi
A. terreus
A. ustus
A. versicolor
aspergillustoxicosis
asphygmia
asphyxia
blue a.
a. carbonica
cyanotic a.
a. cyanotica
a. livida
local a.
a. neonatorum
a. pallida
secondary a.
symmetric a.
traumatic a.
white a.
asphyxiate
asphyxiating thoracic dystrophy
(ATD)
asphyxiation
aspirate
bronchotracheal a.
endotracheal a.
needle a.
tracheal a.
aspirated and flushed
aspirating needle
aspiration
a. biopsy
a. biopsy cytology (ABC)
fine-needle a. (FNA)
fluid a.
a. of foreign body
a. pneumonia

NOTES

A

aspiration *(continued)*
a. pneumonitis
transbronchial needle a.
transthoracic needle a. (TTNA)
transtracheal a.
aspirator
Bovie ultrasound a.
bronchoscopic a.
Cavitron ultrasonic surgical a.
(CUSA)
Cook County a.
Vac-Pak-II ultra-lite portable a.
aspirin
Bayer Buffered A.
buffered a.
enteric-coated a.
Extra Strength Bayer Enteric
500 A.
St. Joseph Adult Chewable A.
Aspirols
Aromatic Ammonia A.
asplenia
Asprimox
ASPVD
arteriosclerotic peripheral vascular
disease
assay
adherence a.
agar diffusion a.
Asserachrom D-DI ELISA a.
Asserachrom t-PA
immunologic a.
Bioclot protein S a.
Cardiac T Rapid a.
cardiac troponin I a.
Cardiac T a. for troponin T
Clauss a.
CoA-set fibrin monomer a.
cTn-I a.
Enzygnost TAT ELISA a.
enzyme-linked
immunosorbent a. (ELISA)
Hemochron high-dose thrombin
time a.
Hybritech immunoradiometric a.
immune adherence
immunosorbent a. (IAIA)
immunoradiometric a. (IRMA)
immunoturbidimetric a.
MonoClone
immunoenzymetric a.
multimer a.

myoglobin a.
Opus cardiac troponin I a.
PCR a.
radioligand binding a.
sandwich enzyme-linked
immunosorbent a.
serum Mgb a.
Stachrom PAI chromogenic a.
thyrotoxin radioisotope a.
assembly
Collins SurveyTach with
MicroTach a.
infant nasal cannula a. (INCA)
Asserachrom
A. D-DI ELISA assay
A. t-PA immunologic assay
assessment
anatomic a.
angiographic a.
cardiovascular function a.
causality a.
echocardiographic a.
functional a.
hemodynamic a.
invasive a.
jugular bulb catheter
placement a.
noninvasive a.
transposition a.
**Assessment of Cardioversion Using
Transesophageal Echocardiography
(ACUTE)**
Assess peak flow meter
assist/control mode ventilation
assisted
a. circulation
a. ventilation
Assmann
A. focus
A. tuberculous infiltrate
association
American Heart A. (AHA)
CHARGE a.
AST
aspartate aminotransferase
Astech peak flow meter
Astelin nasal spray
astemizole
asterixis
asteroid body
asteroides
Nocardia a.

asthenia
neurocirculatory a.
vasoregulatory a.
asthenic apoplexy
asthenicus
thorax a.
asthma
abdominal a.
allergen-induced a.
allergic a.
alveolar a.
atopic a.
bacterial a.
baker's a.
bronchial a.
cardiac a.
cat a.
catarrhal a.
Cheyne-Stokes a.
chronic a.
cotton-dust a.
a. crystals
cutaneous a.
diisocyanate a.
dust a.
Elsner a.
emphysematous a.
essential a.
exercise-induced a. (EIA)
extrinsic a.
a. flare
food a.
grinders' a.
Heberden a.
horse a.
humid a.
infective a.
intrinsic a.
isocyanate-induced a.
Kopp a.
meat-wrapper's a.
Millar a.
miller's a.
miner's a.
mixed a.
nasal a.
nervous a.

nocturnal a.
occupational a.
a. paper
pollen a.
poorly reversible a.
potter's a.
reflex a.
Rostan a.
sexual a.
spasmodic a.
steam-fitter's a.
steroid-dependent a.
stone a.
stone-stripper's a.
subclinical a.
symptomatic a.
thymic a.
triad a.
true a.
Wichmann a.
AsthmaHaler
AsthmaNefrin
Asthmastik
Bird A.
asthmatic
a. bronchitis
steroid-dependent a.
tight a.
asthmaticus
status a.
asthmatiform
asthmogenic
asthmoid
a. respiration
a. wheeze
Astler-Coller classification
Astra
A. profile
A. T4, T6 pacemaker
Astrand bicycle exercise stress test
Astrand-Rhyming protocol
astrocyte
astronyxis
Acanthamoeba a.
Astropulse cuff
Astro-Trace Universal adapter clip
Astroviridae virus

NOTES

Astrup blood gas value
ASTZ
   antistreptozyme
   ASTZ test
ASVD
   arteriosclerotic vascular disease
asymmetric
   a. septal hypertrophy (ASH)
asymptomatic
   a. cardiac ischemia (ACI)
   A. Cardiac Ischemia Pilot
   Study (ACIPS)
   A. Carotid Atherosclerosis
   Plaque Study (ACAPS)
   A. Carotid Atherosclerosis
   Study (ACAS)
   a. complex ectopy
asynchronous
   a. pacing
   a. pulse generator
asynchrony
   a. index
asynergy
asystole
   atrial a.
   Beau a.
asystolia
asystolic
   a. arrest
AT
   atrial tachycardia
   MemoryTrace AT
α_1-**AT**
   α_1-proteinase inhibitor
Atakr system
A-T antiembolism stockings
ataxia
   a. cordis
   Friedreich a.
   hereditary a.
   spinocerebellar a.
ataxic
   a. aphasia
   a. gait
ATD
   asphyxiating thoracic dystrophy
atelectasis
   absorption a.
   acquired a.
   bibasilar a.
   compression a.
   congenital a.
   lobar a.

   obstructive a.
   patchy a.
   platelike a.
   postobstructive a.
   primary a.
   relaxation a.
   resorption a.
   rounded a.
   secondary a.
   segmental a.
   tricuspid a.
atelectatic
   a. band
   a. rales
atelocardia
atenolol
   a. and chlorthalidone
Atenolol Silent Ischemia Trial
(ASIST)
Atgam
   lymphocyte immune globulin
atherectomy
   Auth a.
   a. catheter
   coronary a.
   coronary angioplasty versus
   excisional a.
   coronary rotational a. (CRA)
   directional coronary a. (DCA)
   high-speed rotational a.
   (HSRA)
   a. index
   Kinsey a.
   percutaneous coronary
   rotational a. (PCRA)
   rotational coronary a. (RCA)
   transluminal extraction a.
   (TEA)
atheroblation laser
AtheroCath
   Simpson peripheral A.
   A. spinning blade catheter
atheroembolism, pl. atheroemboli
atherogenesis
   monoclonal theory of a.
   response-to-injury hypothesis
   of a.
atherogenic
   a. dyslipidemia
atherogenicity index
atherolytic reperfusion guidewire
atheroma
   coronary a.

atheromatous
    a. embolism
    a. plaque
atherosclerosis
    cardiac allograft a. (CAA)
    coronary artery a.
    de novo a.
    encrustation theory of a.
    lipogenic theory of a.
    a. obliterans
    premature a.
atherosclerotic
    a. aneurysm
    a. aortic disease
    a. aortography
    a. cardiovascular disease (ASCVD)
    a. carotid artery disease (ACAD)
    a. coronary artery disease (ASCAD)
    a. narrowing
    a. plaque
    A. Risk in Communities (ARIC)
atherosis
atherothrombosis
atherothrombotic
atherotome
athlete's heart
athletic heart
AT-III
    antithrombin III
Ativan
Atkins-Cannard tracheal tube
Atkinson tube stent
Atlas
    A. LP PTCA balloon dilatation catheter
    A. ULP balloon dilatation catheter
Atlee clamp
ATLS
    advanced trauma life support
ATL Ultramark 7 echocardiographic device

atm
    atmosphere
atmosphere (atm)
atmospheres of pressure
atmotherapy
ATnativ
atomizer
atopic asthma
atopy
atorvastin
atovaquone
ATP
    adenosine triphosphate
    antitachycardia pacemaker
        ATP hydrolysis
ATPase
    adenosine triphosphatase
    myofibrillar ATPase
    SR calcium ATPase
ATRAC-II double-balloon catheter
ATRAC multipurpose balloon catheter
atracurium
Atra-grip clamp
Atraloc needle
Atrauclip hemostatic clip
atraumatic needle
atresia
    aortic a.
    bronchial a.
    esophageal a.
    glottic a.
    Gross tracheoesophageal a.
    laryngeal a.
    membranous pulmonary a.
    mitral a.
    pulmonary a.
    tricuspid a.
atria (*pl. of* atrium)
atrial
    a. activation mapping
    a. anomalous bands
    a. appendage
    a. arrhythmia
    a. asynchronous pacemaker
    a. asystole
    a. baffle operation

NOTES

45

atrial *(continued)*
a. balloon septostomy
a. bigeminy
a. bolus dynamic computer tomography
a. capture
a. capture beat
a. capture threshold
a. chaotic tachycardia
a. cuff
a. defibrillation threshold
a. demand-inhibited (AAI)
a. demand-inhibited pacemaker
a. demand-triggered (AAT)
a. demand-triggered pacemaker
a. diastole
a. diastolic gallop
a. dissociation
a. echo
a. ectopic beat
a. ectopic tachycardia (AET)
a. ectopy
a. effective refractory period
a. ejection force
a. escape interval
a. extrastimulus method
a. extrasystole
a. fibrillation (AF)
a. fibrillation-flutter (AFF)
a. filling pressure
a. flutter
a. fusion beat
a. infarction
a. kick
a. lead impedance
a. liver pulse
a. myocardial infarction
a. myxoma
a. natriuretic factor (ANF)
a. natriuretic peptide
a. natriuretic polypeptide (ANP)
a. non-sensing
a. notch
a. ostium primum defect
a. overdrive pacing
a. pacing stress test
a. pacing study
a. pacing wire
a. paroxysmal tachycardia
a. premature beat (APB)
a. premature complexes
a. premature contraction (APC)
a. premature depolarization
a. pulse amplitude
a. pulse width
a. reentry tachycardia
a. repolarization wave
a. rhythm
a. ring
a. sensing configuration
a. sensitivity
a. septal aneurysm
a. septal defect (ASD)
a. septal defect single disk closure device
a. septal defect umbrella
a. septectomy
a. septostomy
a. septum
a. shear
a. sound
a. standstill
a. stasis index
a. synchronous pulse generator
a. synchronous ventricular inhibited pacemaker
a. synchrony
a. systole
a. tachycardia (AT)
a. thrombus
a. tracking pacemaker
a. train pacing
a. transport function
a. triggered pulse generator
a. triggered ventricular-inhibited pacemaker
a. valve
a. vector loop
a. venous pulse
a. ventricular nodal reentry tachycardia
a. ventricular reciprocating tachycardia (AVRT)
a. ventricular shunt
a. VOO pacemaker
atrial-axis discontinuity
atrialized chamber
atrial-paced cycle length
atrial-well technique
Atricor Cordis pacemaker
atriocarotid interval
atriocommissuropexy
atriocyte
atriodextrofascicular tract
atriodigital dysplasia

atriofascicular tract
atriography
atrio-Hisian
   a.-H. bypass tract
   a.-H. fiber
   a.-H. interval
atrio-His pathway
atrionodal bypass tract
atriopressor reflex
atriopulmonary shunt
atrioseptal
   a. defect
   a. sign
atriosystolic murmur
atriotomy
atrioventricular (A-V, AV)
   a. block
   a. bundle
   a. canal
   a. canal cushion
   a. canal defect
   a. conduction (AVC)
   a. conduction abnormality
   a. conduction defect
   a. conduction system
   a. conduction tissue
   a. connection anomaly
   a. discordance
   a. dissociation (AVD)
   a. extrasystole (AVE)
   a. flow rumbling murmur
   a. furrow
   a. gradient
   a. groove
   a. interval
   a. junction
   a. junctional ablation
   a. junctional arrhythmia
   a. junctional bigeminy
   a. junctional escape beat
   a. junctional heart block
   a. junctional reciprocating
     tachycardia
   a. junctional rhythm
   a. junction motion
   a. malformation (AVM)
   a. nodal bigeminy

   a. nodal extrasystole
   a. nodal reentrant tachycardia
     (AVNRT)
   a. nodal reentry
   a. nodal rhythm
   a. nodal tachycardia (AVNT)
   a. node (AVN)
   a. node artery
   a. node pathways
   a. orifice
   a. reciprocating tachycardia
   a. refractory period
   a. ring
   a. septal defect
   a. sequential pacemaker
   a. situs concordance
   a. sulcus
   a. synchrony
   a. time
   a. valve
   a. valve insufficiency
atrioventricularis
   crus dextrum fasciculi a.
   crus sinistrum fasciculi a.
   crux dextrum fasciculi a.
   crux sinistrum fasciculi a.
   nodus a.
Atri-pace I bipolar flared pacing
  catheter
Atrium
   A. Blood Recovery System
atrium, pl. atria
   accessory a.
   common a.
   congenital single a.
   a. cordis
   a. dextrum
   a. of heart
   high right a.
   left a. (LA)
   low septal a.
   a. of lungs
   a. pulmonale
   right a. (RA)
   single a.
   a. sinistrum
   stunned a.

NOTES

Atromid-S
atrophic
    a. cardiomyopathy
    a. catarrh
    a. emphysema
    a. laryngitis
    a. papulosis
    a. pharyngitis
    a. thrombosis
atrophy
    brown a.
    cardiac a.
    cyanotic a. of liver
    Erb a.
    multiple system a.
    olivopontocerebellar a.
    optic a.
    peroneal muscular a.
    red a.
    spinal muscular a.
atropine
    a. sulfate
    a. test
Atrostim phrenic nerve stimulator
Atrovent
    A. Aerosol Inhalation
    A. Inhalation Solution
ATS
    American Thoracic Society
attack
    Adams-Stokes a.
    anxiety a.
    heart a.
    transient ischemic a. (TIA)
    vagal a.
    vasovagal a.
attenuation
    heterogeneous a.
attenuator
attrition murmur
atypical
    a. atrioventricular nodal
      reentrant tachycardia
      (AAVNRT)
    a. chest pain
    a. mycobacterial colonization
    a. pneumonia
    a. tamponade
    a. tuberculosis
    a. verrucous endocarditis
Au
    gold

auditory
    a. alternans
    a. fremitus
Auenbrugger sign
Aufrecht sign
Aufricht elevator
auger wire
augmentation therapy
Augmentin
auranofin
aureomycin
    a. sensitivity
aureus
    Staphylococcus a.
auricle
auricular
    a. appendage
    a. appendectomy
    a. complex
    a. extrasystole
    a. fibrillation
    a. flutter
    a. premature beat
    a. standstill
    a. systole
    a. tachycardia
Auriculin
auriculopressor reflex
auriculoventricular
    a. extrasystole
    a. groove
    a. interval
Aurora
    A. dual-chamber pacemaker
    A. pulse generator
aurothiomalate
Ausculscope
auscultation
    cardiac a.
    Korányi a.
    percussion and a. (P&A)
auscultatory
    a. alternans
    a. gap
    a. sign
    a. sound
Austin
    A. Flint murmur
    A. Flint phenomenon
    A. Flint respiration
    A. Flint rumble
Australia antigen

Australian
  A. Q fever
  A. Therapeutic Trial
australis
  Rickettsia a.
Austrian syndrome
autacoid
Auth
  A. atherectomy
  A. atherectomy catheter
Autima II dual-chamber pacemaker
autoanalyzer
Autoclix
autoclot
autocrine
autodecremental pacing
autodigestion of connective tissue
autogenic graft
autogenous
  a. vein
autograft
autohypnosis
autoimmune disorder
Auto-Injector
  Lido-Pen A.-I.
Autolet
autologous
  a. blood
  a. clot
  a. fat graft
  a. pericardial patch
  a. transfusion
automated
  a. border detection (ABD)
  a. boundary protection (ABP)
  a. cervical cell screening
    system
  a. edge detection
automatic
  a. atrial tachycardia (AAT)
  a. beat
  a. boundary detection (ABD)
  a. ectopic tachycardia
  a. exposure system
  a. external defibrillator (AED)
  a. implantable cardioverter-
    defibrillator (AICD)

  a. implantable defibrillator
    (AID)
  a. internal cardioverter-
    defibrillator (AICD)
  a. internal defibrillator
  a. intracardiac defibrillator
  a. mode switching (AMS)
  a. oscillometric blood pressure
    monitor
  a. pacemaker
  a. ventricular contraction
automaticity
  enhanced a.
  pacemaker a.
  sinus nodal a.
autonomic
  a. dysreflexia
  a. hyperreflexia
  a. modulation
  a. nervous system
  a. sensory innervation
autoperfusion balloon catheter
Autoplex Factor VIII inhibitor
  bypass product
Autoplex T
autoregulation
  heterometric a.
  homeometric a.
autosome
Autostat ligating and hemostatic
  clip
Auto Suture Surgiclip
autotoxic cyanosis
Autotransfuser
  Biosurge Synchronous A.
autotransfusion system
autotransplantation
Autotrans system
autumnal catarrh
auxocardia
A-V, AV
  arteriovenous
  atrioventricular
  A-V block
  A-V bundle
  A-V conduction
  A-V conduction defect

NOTES

A-V *(continued)*
    A-V delay interval
    A-V dissociation
    A-V extrasystole
    A-V Gore-Tex fistula
    A-V groove
    A-V junction
    A-V junctional escape beat
    A-V junctional escape complex
    A-V junctional extrasystole
    A-V junctional rhythm
    A-V junctional tachycardia
    A-V Miniclinic
    A-V nodal artery
    A-V nodal bigeminy
    A-V nodal conduction
    A-V nodal extrasystole
    A-V nodal modification
    A-V nodal reentry
    A-V nodal reentry tachycardia
    A-V nodal rhythm
    A-V nodal tachycardia
    A-V nodal Wenckebach
      arrhythmia
    A-V node
    A-V node reentrant tachycardia
    A-V node Wenckebach
      periodicity
    A-V reciprocating tachycardia
    A-V sequential pacemaker
    A-V synchronous pacemaker
    A-V synchrony
    A-V Wenckebach block
AVAD
    acute ventricular assist device
Avanti introducer
avascular necrosis
AVC
    atrioventricular conduction
AVCO
    A. aortic balloon
    A. balloon pump
AVD
    atrioventricular dissociation
    AVD O$_2$
AVE
    atrioventricular extrasystole
    AVE Micro stent
avenaceus
    Aspergillus a.
Avenue insertion tool

average
    a. mean pressure (AMP)
    a. pulse magnitude
averaging
    digital a.
    signal a.
AVF
    arteriovenous fistula
aVF, aVL, aVR leads
AVG
    aortic valve gradient
Avian
avian
    a. antigen
    a. tuberculosis
aviators' disease
AVID
    Antiarrhythmics versus Implantable
      Defibrillators
avidin-biotin peroxidase
Avitene
avium
    Mycobacterium a.
avium-intracellulare
    Mycobacterium a.-i. (MAI)
Avius sequential pacemaker
AVL OPTI 1
Avlosulfon
AVM
    arteriovenous malformation
    atrioventricular malformation
AVN
    atrioventricular node
AVNRT
    atrioventricular nodal reentrant
      tachycardia
AVNT
    atrioventricular nodal tachycardia
AVP
    arginine vasopressin
AV-Paceport thermodilution catheter
AVR
    aortic valve replacement
AVRT
    atrial ventricular reciprocating
      tachycardia
avulsion
AW
    anterior wall
axes (*pl. of* axis)
axial
    a. computed tomography
      (ACT)

a. control
a. plane
axillary
  a. arch
  a. artery
  a. block
  a. lymph nodes
  a. triangle
  a. vein
axilloaxillary bypass
axillofemoral bypass
Axiom
  A. DG balloon angioplasty
    catheter
  A. double sump pump
  A. thoracic trocar
Axios 04 pacemaker
axis, pl. **axes**
  clockwise rotation of
    electrical a.
  a. deviation
  electrical a.
  hypophyseal-pituitary adrenal a.
  instantaneous electrical a.
  J point electrical a.
  junctional a.
  long a. (LAX)
  mean electrical a.
  mean QRS a.
  normal electrical a.
  P wave a.
  QRS a.
  rightward a.
  a. shift
  short a. (SAX)
  Strong unbridling of celiac
    artery a.

  superior QRS a.
  thoracic a.
  X a.
  Y a.
Ayers
  A. cardiovascular needle holder
  A. sphygmomanometer
  A. T-piece
Ayerza
  A. disease
  A. syndrome
Aygestin
Azactam
azalide
  a. class of antibiotics
azapetine phosphate
azatadine maleate
azathioprine
azidothymidine (AZT)
azithromycin
Azlin
azlocillin
Azmacort
azotemia
  extrarenal a.
  postrenal a.
  prerenal a.
  renal a.
AZT
  azidothymidine
aztreonam
azurophil granule
azygography
azygoportal interruption
azygos
  a. arch
  a. vein

NOTES

B

B bump
B cell
B cell antibody
B cell lymphoma
B1 cell
B4
leukotriene B4 (LTB4)
B6 bronchus sign
Babcock
B. operation
B. thoracic tissue-holding
forceps
Babesia
B. bigemina
B. bovis
B. canis
B. divergens
B. major
B. microti
B. rodhaini
Babinski
downgoing B.
B. reflex
B. syndrome
upgoing B.
baby
blue b.
BABYbird respirator
babygram x-ray
BAC
bronchioloalveolar carcinoma
bacampicillin hydrochloride
Baccelli sign
Bachmann
B. bundle
internodal tract of B.
B. pathway
Baci-IM injection
bacillary
b. angiomatosis
b. embolism
b. phthisis
b. pneumonia
**Bacille bilié de Calmette-Guérin
(BCG)**
bacilli (*pl. of* bacillus)
bacilliformis
Bartonella b.

Bacillus
B. alvei
B. anthracis
B. Calmette-Guérin Live
B. cereus
B. circulans
B. laterosporus
B. licheniformis
B. megaterium
B. pneumoniae
B. polymyxa
B. pseudodiphtheriticum
B. pumilus
B. sphaericus
B. stearothermophilus
B. subtilis
B. subtilis enzymes
bacillus, pl. bacilli
acid-fast bacilli (AFB)
enteric gram-negative bacilli
gram-negative bacilli (GNB)
gram-positive bacilli
Klebs-Löffler b.
Löffler b.
Warthin-Starry-staining bacilli
bacitracin
back-bleeding
backflush
background subtraction technique
backscatter
b. analysis
two-dimensional integrated b.
backward heart failure
BACTEC
B. radiometry
B. system
bacteremia
bacteremic
bacteria (*pl. of* bacterium)
facultative b.
**bacteria-free stage of bacterial
endocarditis**
bacterial
b. asthma
b. endocarditis (BE)
b. infection
b. myocarditis
b. pericarditis
b. pneumococcal pneumonia
b. vegetation

B

bactericidal titer
bacterioid
bacteriophage
bacterium, pl. bacteria
Bacteroides
    B. corrodens
    B. oralis
Bactocill
    B. injection
    B. Oral
Bactrim
Bactroban Topical
BAE
    bronchial artery embolization
Baffe anastomosis
baffle
    fabric b.
    b. fenestration
    Gore-Tex b.
    intra-atrial b.
    b. leak
    Mustard atrial b.
    pericardial b.
    Senning intra-atrial b.
bag
    Ambu b.
    Douglas b.
    eXtract specimen b.
    Hope b.
    Lifesaver disposable
      resuscitator b.
    rebreathing b.
    Sones hemostatic b.
    SureGrip breathing b.
    Voorhees b.
bagassosis
BagEasy disposable manual
  resuscitator
bagged
baggy heart
bagpipe sign
bag-valve-mask (BVM)
Bahnson
    B. aortic clamp
    B. sternal retractor
Bailey
    B. aortic clamp
    B. catheter
    B. rib spreader
Bailey-Gibbon rib contractor
Bailey-Glover-O'Neill
  commissurotomy knife

bailout
    b. autoperfusion balloon
    catheter
    b. stent
    b. stenting
    b. valvuloplasty
Baim pacing catheter
Baim-Turi
    B.-T. cardiac device
    B.-T. monitoring/pacing catheter
Bainbridge
    B. effect
    B. reflex
Bair Hugger
baker's asthma
Bakes dilator
Bakst valvulotome
BAL
    bronchoalveolar lavage
balance
    sympathovagal b.
Balectrode pacing catheter
BALF
    bronchoalveolar lavage fluid
Balke
    B. exercise stress test
    B. treadmill protocol
Balke-Ware
    B.-W. test
    B.-W. treadmill protocol
ball
    fungus b.
    pleural fibrin b.'s
    b. poppet
    b. thrombus
    b. valve
    b. valve prosthesis
    b. valve thrombus
    b. variance
    b. wedge
ball-and-cage prosthesis
ball-cage
    b.-c. prosthesis
    b.-c. valve
ballerina-foot pattern
ballet
    cardiac b.
ball-in-cage prosthetic valve
ballistocardiogram
ballistocardiograph (BCG)
ballistocardiography
ball-occluder valve

balloon

Accent-DG b.
ACE b.
ACS Alpha b.
ACX b.
b. angioplasty catheter
b. aortic valvotomy (BAV)
b. aortic valvuloplasty (BAV)
Arrow Berman angiographic b.
b. atrial septostomy
AVCO aortic b.
Baxter Intrepid b.
bifoil b.
Blue Max high-pressure b.
Brandt cytology b.
b. catheter angioplasty (BCA)
b. coarctation angioplasty
b. coronary angioplasty
counterpulsation b.
b. counterpulsation
Cribier-Letac aortic
  valvuloplasty b.
Datascope b.
b. dilation
Distaflex b.
b. embolectomy catheter
Epistat double b.
Express b.
Extractor three-lumen
  retrieval b.
Hadow b.
Helix b.
Hunter-Sessions b.
b. inflation
Inoue self-guiding b.
Integra II b.
intra-aortic b. (IAB)
14K b.
Kay b.
Kontron b.
b. laser angioplasty
latex b.
Mansfield b.
Micross SL b.
b. mitral commissurotomy
  (BMC)
b. mitral valvotomy (BMV)

b. mitral valvuloplasty (BMV)
Monorail Speedy b.
NoProfile b.
b. occlusion
b. occlusive intravascular lysis
  enhanced recanalization
  (BOILER)
Olbert b.
Omega-NV b.
Omniflex b.
Omni SST b.
Orion b.
Owens b.
PET b.
Piccolino b.
pillow-shaped b.
POC b.
polyethylene terephthalate b.
polyolefin copolymer b.
polyvinyl chloride b.
Prime b.
b. pulmonary valvotomy
b. pulmonary valvuloplasty
  (BPV)
b. pump
QuickFurl SL b.
radiofrequency hot b.
b. rupture
Schneider-Shiley b.
Shadow b.
Short Speedy b.
b. shunt
sizing b.
Slalom b.
Slider b.
Slinky b.
Solo b.
Spears laser b.
Stack autoperfusion b.
Stretch b.
b. tamponade
Ten b.
thigh b.
Thruflex b.
trefoil b.
trefoil Schneider b.
b. tricuspid valvotomy

B

NOTES

balloon *(continued)*
  Tyshak b.
  b. valvuloplasty (BV)
  b. valvuloplasty catheter
  B. Valvuloplasty Registry
  B. versus Optimal Atherectomy
    Trial (BOAT)
  waisting of b.
  windowed b.
balloon-centered argon laser
balloon-expandable
  b.-e. flexible coil stent
  b.-e. intravascular stent
balloon-flotation pacing catheter
balloon-imaging catheter
ballooning mitral cusp syndrome
balloon-occlusion pulmonary
  angiography
Balloon-on-a-Wire
balloon-shaped heart
balloon-tipped
  b.-t. angiographic catheter
  b.-t. flow-directed catheter
  b.-t. thermodilution catheter
ball-wedge catheter
Balme cough
Baltaxe view
Baltherm catheter
Bamberger
  B. area
  B. bulbar pulse
  B. sign
Bamberger-Marie disease
bamiphylline
Bamyl
Bancap HC
bancrofti
  Wuchereria b.
band
  atelectatic b.
  atrial anomalous b.'s
  contraction b.
  CPK-BB b.'s
  CPK-MB b.
  CPK-MM b.
  I b.
  moderator b.
  myocardial b. (MB)
  Parham b.'s
  pulmonary artery b.
  b. saw effect
  Vesseloops rubber b.
  Z b.

bandage
  Tricodur Epi compression
    support b.
  Tricodur Omos compression
    support b.
  Tricodur Talus compression
    support b.
bandbox
  b. resonance
  b. sound
banding
  Muller b.
  PA b.
  pulmonary artery banding
  b. of pulmonary artery
  pulmonary artery b. (PA
    banding)
  Trusler rule for pulmonary
    artery b.
bandlike angina
bandpass filter
bandwidth
bangungot syndrome
bank
  tissue b.
Bannister disease
Bannwarth syndrome
Banophen Oral
BAR
  beta-adrenergic receptor
Baratol
barbed
  b. epicardial pacing lead
  b. hook
barbiturate
barb-tip lead
Bard
  B. balloon-directed pacing
    catheter
  B. cardiopulmonary support
    pump
  B. cardiopulmonary support
    system
  B. Clamshell septal occluder
  B. Clamshell septal umbrella
  B. electrophysiology catheter
  B. guiding catheter
  B. nonsteerable bipolar
    electrode
  B. PDA umbrella
  B. percutaneous
    cardiopulmonary support
    system

B. probe
B. sign
B. TransAct intra-aortic
balloon pump
Bardco catheter
Bardenheurer ligation
Bardic cutdown catheter
Bard-Parker
B.-P. blade
B.-P. U-Mid/Lo humidifier
BARI
Bypass Angioplasty
Revascularization Investigation
barium
b. enema
b. swallow
barium-impregnated poppet
barking cough
Barlow syndrome
Barnard
B. mitral valve prosthesis
B. operation
barometer-maker's disease
barometric pressure
baroreceptor
cardiac b.
carotid b.
perturbed carotid b.
b. reflex
b. sensitization
baroreflex
barosinusitis
barospirator
barotrauma
pulmonary b.
Barraya forceps
barrel-hooping compression
barrel-shaped
b.-s. chest
b.-s. thorax
Barrett esophagus
barrier
blood-air b.
blood-brain b.
blood-retina b.
placental b.
Barron pump

Barsony-Polgar syndrome
Barth syndrome
Bartonella bacilliformis
Bartter syndrome
basal
b. cell carcinoma
b. diastolic murmurs
b. segmental bronchus
b. tuberculosis
basal-septal hypertrophy
base
whole blood buffer b.
baseline
b. arrhythmia
b. artifact
b. echocardiography
b. EKG
b. rhythm
b. variability
b. variability of fetal heart
rate
wandering b.
basement membrane
baseplate
winged b.
basic
b. cardiac life support (BCLS)
b. cycle length (BCL)
b. drive cycle length
b. fibroblast growth factor
(bFGF)
b. life support (BLS)
Basidiomycetes
basilar
b. rales
basilic vein
basis pulmonis
Basix pacemaker
basket
Medi-Tech multipurpose b.
pericardial b.
basophil
Bassen-Kornzweig
abetalipoproteinemia
Batch least-squares method
bath
film fixer b.

B

NOTES

bath *(continued)*
  film wash b.
  fixer b.
  Haake water b.
  Nauheim b.
  wash b.
bathycardia
bathypnea
batrachotoxin
Batson plexus
battery
  Celsa b.
  lithium b.
  nickel-cadmium b.
battery-assisted heart assist device
Battey-avium complex
bat wing shadow
Bauer syndrome
Baumès symptom
bauxite
  b. pneumoconiosis
  b. pneumonoconiosis
BAV
  balloon aortic valvotomy
  balloon aortic valvuloplasty
  bicommissural aortic valve
Baxter
  B. angioplasty catheter
  B. Flo-Gard 8200 volumetric
    infusion pump
  B. Intrepid balloon
  B. mechanical valve
  B. mechanical valve prosthesis
Bayer
  B. Buffered Aspirin
  B. Low Adult Strength
  B. Select Chest Cold Caplets
  B. Select Pain Relief Formula
Bayes theorem
BAY k 8644
Bayle granulations
Bayliss theory
Baylor
  B. autologous transfusion
    system
  B. cardiovascular sump tube
  B. rapid autologous transfusion
    (BRAT)
  B. total artificial heart
Baypress
Bazett
  B. corrected QT interval
  B. formula

Bazin disease
BBB
  bundle-branch block
BBBB
  bilateral bundle-branch block
BCA
  balloon catheter angioplasty
  bidirectional cavopulmonary
    anastomosis
BCD Plus cardioplegic unit
BCG
  Bacille bilié de Calmette-Guérin
  ballistocardiograph
  bronchocentric granulomatosis
    TICE BCG
BCKD
  branched chain alpha ketoacid
    dehydrogenase
BCL
  basic cycle length
BCLS
  basic cardiac life support
BCO$_2$
  Cardiac Stimulator BCO$_2$
B-complex
  ferrous sulfate, ascorbic acid,
    and vitamin B.-c.
B-D
  Becton-Dickinson
    B-D Potain thoracic trocar
BE
  bacterial endocarditis
Bead
  Digoxin RIA B.
beading of arteries
Beall
  B. disk valve prosthesis
  B. mitral valve
  B. mitral valve prosthesis
  B. scissors
Beall-Surgitool
  B.-S. ball-cage prosthetic valve
  B.-S. disk prosthetic valve
beam
  b. splitter
  b. width artifact
bean
  castor b.
  green coffee b.
Bear
  B. 1, 2 adult volume
    ventilator

B

B. Cub infant ventilator
B. 5 respirator
Beardsley aortic dilator
beat
aberrantly conducted b.
apex b.
Ashman b.
atrial capture b.
atrial ectopic b.
atrial fusion b.
atrial premature b. (APB)
atrioventricular junctional
  escape b.
auricular premature b.
automatic b.
A-V junctional escape b.
capture b.'s
combination b.
coupled b.'s
dependent b.
Dressler b.
dropped b.
echo b.
ectopic b.
entrained b.
escape b.
extrasystolic b.
fascicular b.
forced b.
fusion b.
heart b.
interference b.
interpolated b.
junctional escape b.
Lown class 4a or b
  ventricular ectopic b.'s
malignant b.
missed b.
mixed b.
nodal b.
paired b.'s
parasystolic b.
b.'s per minute (bpm)
postextrasystolic b.
premature atrial b.
premature junctional b.
premature ventricular b. (PVB)

pseudofusion b.
reciprocal b.
retrograde b.
salvo of b.'s
skipped b.
summation b.
unifocal ventricular ectopic b.
  (UVEB)
ventricular ectopic b. (VEB)
ventricular escape b.
ventricular fusion b.
ventricular premature b. (VPB)
beats per minute (bpm)
beat-to-beat
b.-t.-b. analysis
b.-t.-b. variability
b.-t.-b. variability of fetal heart
  rate
Beatty-Bright friction sound
Beau
B. asystole
B. disease
B. lines
Beaver blade
BEB
blind esophageal brushing
Beck
B. cardiopericardiopexy
B. Depression Inventory
B. epicardial poudrage
B. I, II operation
B. miniature aortic clamp
B. mouth tube airway
B. triad
Becker
B. accelerator cannula
B. disease
Becker-type tardive muscular
dystrophy
Beckman O₂ analyzer
Beck-Potts aortic and pulmonic
clamp
Beclard hernia
Becloforte
beclomethasone
b. dipropionate

NOTES

Beclovent · bent

Beclovent
    B. Oral Inhaler
Beconase AQ Nasal Inhaler
becquerel (Bq)
Becton-Dickinson (B-D)
    B.-D. guidewire
    B.-D. Teflon-sheathed needle
bed
    adventitial b.
    b. blocks
    capillary b.
    cyanosis of nail b.'s
    myocardial b.
    nail b.
    perfusion b.
    pulmonary b.
    Sanders b.
    Stress Echo b.
    vascular b.
    venous capacitance b.
Bedfont carbon monoxide monitor
Bedge antireflux mattress
beef insulin
beef-lung heparin
Beepen-VK Oral
beep-o-gram
beer
    b. and cobalt syndrome
    b. heart
beer-drinker's cardiomyopathy
Beer-Lambert principle
bee venom
behavior
    contractile b.
    type A, B b.
behavioral
    b. factor
    b. therapy
Behçet
    B. disease
    B. syndrome
Béhier-Hardy sign
bejel syphilis
Belix Oral
bell
    b. sound
    b. tympany
Bellavar medical support stockings
belli
    Isospora b.
bell-metal resonance
bellows
    chest b.

b. murmur
b. sound
Belsey
    B. esophagoplasty
    B. Mark II, IV fundoplication
    B. two-thirds wrap
        fundoplication
Belzer solution
Bena-D injection
Benadryl
    B. injection
    B. Oral
    B. Topical
Benahist injection
benazepril
    amlodipine and b.
    b. hydrochloride
bendrofluazide
bendroflumethiazide
bends
Benedict retractor
Benedict-Roth spirometer
BENESTENT trial
Bengash needle
Bengolea forceps
benign
    b. croupous angina
    b. early repolarization (BER)
    b. intracranial hypertension
benigna
    endocarditis b.
benignum
    empyema b.
Benjamin
    B. binocular slimline
        laryngoscope
    B. pediatric laryngoscope
Benjamin-Havas fiberoptic light clip
Bennett
    B. Cascade II Servo
        Controlled Heated Humidifier
    B. MA-1, PR-2 ventilator
    B. monitoring spirometer
    B. pressure-cycled ventilator
    B. Slip/Stream
    B. Twin
Benoject injection
Bentall
    B. cardiovascular prosthesis
        inclusion technique of B.
    B. inclusion technique
    B. procedure
bent bronchus sign

60

Bentley
    B. Duraflo II
    B. oxygenator
    B. transducer
Bentson
    B. exchange straight guidewire
    B. floppy-tip guidewire
Bentson-Hanafee-Wilson catheter
Benylin
    B. DM
    B. Expectorant
benzathine
    b. benzyl penicillin
    penicillin g b.
benzoate
    caffeine and sodium b.
benzocaine
benzodiazepine
benzonatate
benzothiadiazide
benzthiazide
benzylpenicillin
benzyl-thiourea
bepridil hydrochloride
BER
    benign early repolarization
beractant
Berard aneurysm
**Berenstein occlusion balloon
catheter**
Berger operation
Bergmeister papilla
beriberi
    cerebral b.
    dry b.
    b. heart
    infantile b.
    wet b.
**Berkovits-Castellanos hexapolar
electrode**
Berlin
    B. nosology
    B. TAH
Berman
    B. airway
    B. angiographic catheter
    B. balloon flotation catheter

Bernheim syndrome
**Berning and Steensgaard-Hansen
score**
Bernoulli
    B. equation
    B. theorem
Bernstein test
Berotec
berry
    b. aneurysm
    B. sternal needle holder
berylliosis
beryllium disease
besylate
    amlodipine b.
    cisatracurium b.
Beta-2
beta
    b. adrenoceptor
    b. adrenoceptor stimulation
    b. agonist
    b. antagonist
    b. blockade
    b. blocker
    b. blocking agent
    b. lactamase
    b. lipoprotein
    b. ray
    b. receptor
    b. thromboglobulin
beta-adrenergic
    b.-a. agonist
    b.-a. blocker
    b.-a. blocking agent
    b.-a. receptor (BAR)
    b.-a. stimulation
beta-adrenoreceptor
    b.-a. agonist
    b.-a. blocker
beta$_2$ antagonist
beta$_1$ antagonist
beta-beta homodimer
beta-blockade
beta-blocker therapy
Beta-Cath system
Betacel-Biotronik pacemaker
Betachron E-R

NOTES

Betadine Helafoam solution
beta-endorphin
betaine diet
beta-lactam
beta-lactamase
    CAZ b.-l.
    b.-l. inhibitor
Betaloc
betamethasone
beta-myosin heavy-chain gene
Betapace
    B. Oral
Betapen-VK Oral
beta-thromboglobulin
    plasma b.-t.
betaxolol
    b. hydrochloride
bethanechol chloride
bethanidine
Bethea sign
Bethesda Conference
Bethune
    B. lobectomy tourniquet
    B. rib shears
Betimol Ophthalmic
Betoptic
    B. Ophthalmic
Bettman-Fovash thoracotome
Beuren syndrome
bevantolol
beveled thin-walled needle
bezafibrate
    B. Infarction Prevention (BIP)
Bezalip
Bezold-Jarisch reflex
bFGF
    basic fibroblast growth factor
BF large core bronchoscope
B-H interval
Bianchi
    B. nodules
    B. valve
biatrial
    b. enlargement
biatriatum
    cor pseudotriloculare b.
Biaxin
    B. Filmtabs
bibasally
bibasilar
    b. atelectasis
    b. coarse crackles
    b. rales

bible printer's lung
BICAP
    Bipolar Circumactive Probe B unit
    BICAP unit
bicarbonate (HCO₃)
    sodium b.
bicarbonaturia
Bicarbon Sorin valve
bicardiogram
bicaval
Bicer-val prosthetic valve
Bichat tunic
Bicillin
    B. L-A injection
Bickel ring
BiCNU
bicommissural aortic valve (BAV)
Bicor catheter
bicuspid aortic valve
bicuspidization
bicycle
    Aerodyne b.
    b. dynamometer
    b. echocardiography
    b. ergometer exercise stress test
    b. ergometry
    Tredex b.
bidimensional
bidirectional
    b. cavopulmonary anastomosis (BCA)
    b. four-pole Butterworth high-pass digital filter
    b. shunt
    b. shunt calculation
    b. superior cavopulmonary anastomosis (BSCA)
    b. ventricular tachycardia
Bier block anesthesia
Biermer sign
bifascicular
    b. heart block
biferious (var. of bisferious)
biferious pulse
Bifidobacterium
bifid P waves
bifocal demand DVI pacemaker
bifoil
    b. balloon
    b. balloon catheter

bifurcated
> b. J-shaped tined atrial pacing and defibrillation lead
> b. vein graft for vascular reconstruction

bifurcation
> b. of aorta
> aortic b.
> carotid b.
> coronary b.
> b. lesion
> b. of pulmonary trunk
> b. of trachea

bifurcatio tracheae
bigemina (*var. of* bigeminy)
> *Babesia b.*

bigeminal
> b. bisferious pulse
> b. pulse
> b. rhythm

bigeminus
> pulsus b.

bigeminy, *bigemina*
> atrial b.
> atrioventricular junctional b.
> atrioventricular nodal b., A-V nodal b.
> escape-capture b.
> junctional b.
> nodal b.
> reciprocal b.
> rule of b.
> ventricular b.

bilateral
> b. adrenal hyperplasia
> b. bundle-branch block (BBBB)
> b. lung transplant (BLT)
> b. sequential lung transplant

bile
> b. acid binding resin
> b. acid sequestrant

bileaflet tilting-disk prosthetic valve
bi-level positive airway pressure (BiPAP)
Bilharzia
bilharziasis

biliary
> b. cirrhosis
> b. colic
> b. disease

BiliBlanket phototherapy system
Bili mask
bilious pneumonia
bilirubin
bilirubinemia
Billingham criteria
billowing
> cusp b.
> b. mitral valve syndrome

bilobate
bilobectomy
biloculare
> cor b.

Biltricide
bimanual precordial palpation
binding
> guanine nucleotide modulatable b.

Bing stylet
Bing-Taussig heart procedure
Binswanger disease
bioabsorbable
> b. closure device

bioassay
bioavailability
Biobrane adhesive
Biobrane/HF graft material
Biocef
Biocell RTV implant
Bioclate
Bioclot protein S assay
biocompatibility
Biocor prosthetic valve
biodegradable stent
Biodex System
bioelectric
> b. current
> b. potential

bioelectricity
biofeedback
Biofilter cardiovascular hemoconcentrator

NOTES

biograft
   B. bovine heterograft material
   Dakin b.
   Dardik B.
   B. graft
bioimpedance
   b. electrocardiograph
      thoracic electrical b.
biological
   b. fitness
   b. half-life
Biomatrix ocular implant
Bio-Medicus
   B.-M. arterial catheter
   B.-M. pump
**Bio-Med MVP-10 pediatric
   ventilator**
biomembrane
Biomox
Bionit
   B. vascular graft
   B. vascular prosthesis
Bioplus dispersive electrode
BioPolyMeric
   B. vascular graft
bioprosthesis
   Carpentier-Edwards Perimount
      RSR pericardial b.
   Freestyle aortic root b.
   Hancock M.O. II porcine b.
   Mosaic cardiac b.
   pericarbon b.
   Perimount RSR pericardial b.
   PhotoFix alpha pericardial b.
   porcine b.
   SJM X-Cell cardiac b.
   Toronto SPV b.
bioprosthetic
   b. heart valve
   b. prosthetic valve
biopsy
   aspiration b.
   bite b.
   bronchial brush b.
   bronchoscopic needle b.
   brush b.
   catheter-guided b.
   cytological b.
   endomyocardial b. (EMB)
   endoscopic b.
   excisional b.
   fine-needle aspiration b.
   b. forceps

   lung b.
   mediastinal lymph node b.
   open lung b.
   percutaneous needle b.
   pericardial b.
   pleural b.
   punch b.
   scalene fat pad b.
   scalene lymph node b.
   supraclavicular lymph node b.
   transbronchial lung b.
   transthoracic needle
      aspiration b.
   ventricular b.
   wedge b.
bioptic sampling
bioptome
   Bycep PC Jr b.
   Caves b.
   Caves-Schultz b.
   Cordis b.
   Kawai b.
   King b.
   Konno b.
   Mansfield b.
   Olympus b.
   Scholten endomyocardial b.
   Stanford b.
   Stanford-Caves b.
Bio-Pump
Biorate pacemaker
bioresorbable implant
Biosound
   B. 2000 II ultrasound unit
   B. Phase 2 ultrasound system
   B. Surgiscan echocardiograph
   B. wide-angle monoplane
      ultrasound scanner
Biostent
**Biosurge Synchronous
   Autotransfuser**
Biot
   B. breathing
   B. respiration
   B. sign
Bio-Tab Oral
Biotrack coagulation monitor
Biotronik
   B. lead connector
   B. pacemaker
Bio-Vascular prosthetic valve
BI-OX III ear oximeter

BIP
  Bezafibrate Infarction Prevention
BiPAP
  bi-level positive airway pressure
  BiPAP nasal continuous
    positive airway pressure
  BiPAP unit
biperiden
biphasic
  b. shock
  b. stridor
biplanar tomography
biplane
  b. aortography
  b. fluoroscopy
  b. formula
  b. imaging
  b. orthogonal angiography
  b. pelvic arteriography
  b. quantitative coronary
    arteriography
  b. ventriculography
bipolar
  b. esophageal recording
  b. limb leads
  b. myocardial electrode
  b. pacemaker
Bipolar Circumactive Probe B unit (BICAP)
BiPort hemostasis introducer sheath kit
Bird
  Ascension B.
  B. Asthmastik
  B. low-flow blender
  B. machine
  B. micronebulizer
  B. neonatal CPAP generator
  B. sign
  B. 8400STi ventilator
  B. VDR ventilator
bird-breeder's lung
bird's-eye catheter
bird's nest
  b.n. lesion
  b.n. vena cava filter
birefringence

birminghamensis
  Legionella b.
Birtcher defibrillator
bis(chloromethyl) ether
bisferiens
  pulsus b.
bisferient
bisferious, biferious
  b. pulse
bishop's
  b. hat
  b. nod
Bishop sphygmoscope
bishydroxycoumarin
bismesylate
  almitrine b.
bismuth
  b. subsalicylate
Bisolvon
bisoprolol
  b. fumarate
  b. and hydrochlorothiazide
Bisping electrode
bistoury
  Jackson b.
bitartrate
  hydrocodone b.
  metaraminol b.
  norepinephrine b.
bite biopsy
bitolterol mesylate
Bitpad digitizer
BIVAD centrifugal left and right ventricular assist device
bivalve
biventricular
  b. assist device (BVAD)
  b. endomyocardial fibrosis
  b. support (BVS)
Bivona
  B. Fome-Cuff tube
  B. TTS tracheostomy tube
Bivona-Colorado voice prosthesis
Bizzari-Guiffrida laryngoscope
Björk method of Fontan procedure
Björk-Shiley
  B.-S. aortic valve prosthesis

B

NOTES

65

Björk-Shiley *(continued)*
- B.-S. convexoconcave 60-degree valve prosthesis
- B.-S. floating disk prosthesis
- B.-S. graft
- B.-S. heart valve holder
- B.-S. heart valve sizer
- B.-S. mitral valve
- B.-S. monostrut valve
- B.-S. prosthetic valve

b knuckle
black
- b. lung
- b. lung disease
- b. phthisis
- b. pleura
- b. pleura sign
- b. widow spider venom

Blackfan-Diamond syndrome
blackout
- shallow water b.
- b. spell

blade
- Acra-Cut Spiral craniotome b.
- b. atrial septostomy
- Bard-Parker b.
- Beaver b.
- CLM articulating laryngoscope b.
- b. control wire holder
- Cooley-Pontius sternal b.
- Lite B.
- SCA-EX ShortCutter catheter with rotating b.'s
- b. septostomy catheter

Blake exercise stress test
Blalock-Hanlon
- B.-H. atrial septectomy
- B.-H. operation

Blalock-Niedner pulmonic stenosis clamp
Blalock pulmonary stenosis clamp
Blalock-Taussig
- B.-T. operation
- B.-T. procedure
- B.-T. shunt

blanche
- tache b.

blanch test
bland
- b. edema
- b. embolism

Bland-Altman method

Bland-Garland-White syndrome
blanket
- bronchial mucus b.
- circulating water b.
- cooling b.
- hypothermia b.

blast
- b. chest
- b. lung

blastoma
- pulmonary b.

Blastomyces dermatitidis
blastomycosis
- North American b.

BLB
- Boothby-Lovelace-Bulbulian
- BLB oxygen mask

bleb
- emphysematous b.
- pleural b.
- b. stapling

bleeding
- arterial b.
- back-b.
- b. diathesis

blender
- Bird low-flow b.
- Virtis b.

blennothorax
Blenoxane
bleomycin
- b. sulfate

BLES
- bovine lavage extract surfactant

blind
- b. coronary dimple
- b. esophageal brushing (BEB)
- b. thoracentesis

bloater
- blue b.

bloc
- en b.
- heart-lung b.

Blocadren
- B. Oral

Bloch equation
Block
- B. cardiac device
- B. right coronary guiding catheter

block
- alveolar-capillary b.
- anatomic b.

anterograde b.
arborization b.
atrioventricular b., A-V b.
atrioventricular junctional
  heart b.
A-V Wenckebach b.
axillary b.
bed b.'s
bifascicular heart b.
bilateral bundle-branch b.
  (BBBB)
bundle-branch b. (BBB)
complete A-V b.
complete heart b. (CHB)
conduction b.
congenital heart b.
b. cycle length
divisional heart b.
entrance b.
exit b.
fascicular heart b.
first-degree A-V b.
first-degree heart b.
focal b.
functional b.
heart b.
3:1 heart b.
3:2 heart b.
heparin b.
His bundle heart b.
incomplete atrioventricular b.
infra-Hisian b.
intra-atrial b.
intra-Hisian b.
intraventricular b. (IVB)
left bundle-branch b. (LBBB)
Luciani-Wenckebach
  atrioventricular b.
Mobitz type I, II
  atrioventricular b.
paraffin b.
partial heart b.
peri-infarction b.
protective b.
pseudo-A-V b.
retrograde b.
right bundle-branch b. (RBBB)

second-degree A-V b.
second-degree heart b.
shock b.'s
sinoatrial b., sinoauricular b.
sinoatrial exit b.
sinus exit b.
subjunctional heart b.
supra-Hisian b.
third-degree heart b.
transient heart b.
trifascicular b.
unidirectional b.
vagal b.
voltage-dependent b.
Wenckebach atrioventricular b.
Wenckebach A-V b.
Wenckebach periodicity b.
Wilson b.
blockade
  angiotensin-II receptor b.
  beta b., β-b.
  stellate ganglion b.
blocked
  b. heart artery
  b. pleurisy
blocker
  adrenoceptor b.
  alpha-adrenergic b.
  alpha-adrenoreceptor b.
  angiotensin-II receptor b.
  beta b.
  beta-adrenergic b.
  beta-adrenoreceptor b.
  calcium channel b.
  calcium entry b.
  ganglionic b.
  renin-angiotensin b.
  slow channel b.
blocking
  b. vagal afferent fibers
  b. vagal efferent fibers
Blom-Singer
  B.-S. indwelling low-pressure
    voice prosthesis
  B.-S. valve
blood
  artificial b.

NOTES

blood *(continued)*
  autologous b.
  b. cardioplegia
  clot of b.
  b. clot
  b. coagulation factor (I-XIII)
  b. count
  b. dyscrasia
  b. expander
  b. flow
  b. flow measurement
  Fluosol artificial b.
  b. gas
  mixed venous b.
  b. murmur
  b. oxygen
  b. oxygen level
  oxygen saturation of the
    hemoglobin of arterial b.
  b. patch injection
  b. perfusion
  b. perfusion monitor (BPM)
  b. platelet thrombus
  b. plate thrombus
  b. pool
  b.-pool imaging
  b. pressure (BP)
  b. pressure cuff
  b. pump
  b. sampling
  shear rate of b.
  shunted b.
  sludged b.
  tonometered whole b.
  b. urea nitrogen (BUN)
  b. viscosity
  b. volume
  b. volume distribution
  b. warmer
blood-air barrier
blood-brain barrier
blood-flow probe
bloodless phlebotomy
bloodletting
blood-retina barrier
bloodstream
blood-tinged sputum
Bloodwell forceps
bloody
  b. sputum
  b. tap

Bloom
  B. programmable stimulator
  B. syndrome
blooming effect
blot
  b. test
  Western b.
blow
  diastolic b.
blow-by
  b.-b. oxygen
  b.-b. ventilator
blowing
  b. murmur
  b. wound
BLS
  basic life support
BLT
  bilateral lung transplant
blubbery diastolic murmur
blue
  b. asphyxia
  b. baby
  b. bloater
  b. disease
  b. finger syndrome
  B. FlexTip catheter
  B. Line cuffed endotracheal
    tube
  B. Max high-pressure
    balloon
  B. Max triple-lumen catheter
  methylene b.
  b. phlebitis
  b. sclera
  Sulphan B.
  b. toe syndrome
  b. velvet syndrome
Blum arterial scissors
Blumenau test
Blumenthal lesion
blunt
  b. eversion
  b. eversion carotid
    endarterectomy
  b. injury
  b. trauma
blunted costophrenic angle
blush
  capillary b.
  myocardial b.
  b. phenomenon
  tumor b.

BMC
  balloon mitral commissurotomy
BMI
  body mass index
B-mode
  B.-m. echocardiography
  B.-m. ultrasonography
  B.-m. ultrasound
BMP-2
  bone morphogenetic protein type 2
BMV
  balloon mitral valvotomy
  balloon mitral valvuloplasty
BNP
  brain natriuretic peptide
BOAT
  Balloon versus Optimal
    Atherectomy Trial
boat-shaped heart
Bochdalek hernia
Bock ganglion
Bodai adapter
body
  B. of Arantius
  Arantius b.
  asbestos b.'s
  asbestosis b.'s
  Aschoff b.'s
  aspiration of foreign b.
  asteroid b.
  Bracht-Wachter b.'s
  carotid b.
  central fibrous b.
  creola b.'s
  Döhle inclusion b.'s
  b. fat
  ferruginous b.'s
  fibrous b.
  foreign b.
  Gamna-Gandy b.'s
  gelatin compression b.
  Gordon elementary b.
  Heinz b.
  LCL b.'s
  b. mass index (BMI)
  Masson b.'s
  Medlar b.'s

multilamellar b.
Negri b.'s
para-aortic b.'s
b. plethysmograph
b. position
psammoma b.'s
b. surface area (BSA)
b. surface Laplacian mapping
  (BSLM)
thoracic vertebral b.
vagal b.
Weibel-Palade b.'s
Zuckerkandl b.'s
Boeck
  B. disease
  B. sarcoid
Boehringer Mannheim standard
Boerema hernia repair
Boerhaave
  B. syndrome
  B. tear
Boettcher forceps
Bogalusa criteria
boggy edema
Bohr
  B. formula
  B. isopleth method
BOILER
  balloon occlusive intravascular lysis
    enhanced recanalization
bois
  bruit de b.
bolometer
bolt
  Camino microventricular b.
Boltzmann distribution
bolus injection
Bonchek-Shiley
  B.-S. cardiac jacket
  B.-S. vein distention system
bond
  soldered b.
bone
  fibrous dysplasia of b.
  b. marrow embolism
  b. marrow transplant

NOTES

bone *(continued)*
    b. morphogenetic protein type
      2 (BMP-2)
    Paget disease of b.
Bonferroni
    B. correction
    B. test
bony heart
Bonzel Monorail balloon catheter
bookeri
    Alcaligenes b.
Bookwalter retractor
booming rumble
BOOP
    bronchiolitis obliterans organizing
      pneumonia
booster heart
boot
    Bunny b.
    compression b.
    Cryo/Cuff pressure b.
    gelatin compression b.
    IPC b.'s
    PNS Unna b.
    sheepskin b.
    Unna paste b.
Boothby-Lovelace-Bulbulian (BLB)
    Boothby-Lovelace-Bulbulian
      oxygen mask
boot-shaped heart
bootstrap
    b. dilation
    b. two-vessel angioplasty
    b. two-vessel technique
border
    b. of cardiac dullness
    b. rales
    sternal b.
borderline
    b. cardiomegaly
    b. EKG
    b. hypertension
Bordetella
    B. pertussis
Bordet-Gengou test
Borg
    B. numerical scale
    B. treadmill exertion scale
Born aggregometry
Bornholm disease
Boros esophagoscope
Borrelia burgdorferi

borreliosis
    Lyme b.
Borst side-arm introducer set
Bosch ERG 500 ergometer
Bosher commissurotomy knife
BosPac cardiopulmonary bypass
    system
Bostock
    B. catarrh
    B. disease
Botallo duct
botryomycosis
    pulmonary b.
bottle
    Castaneda b.
    b. sound
bottle-neck stenosis
Bouchut respiration
bougie
    bronchoscopic b.
    Celestin b.
    EndoLumina illuminated b.
bougienage
    esophageal b.
Bouillaud
    B. disease
    B. sign
    B. tinkle
bounding pulse
bouquet of vessels
Bourassa catheter
Bourns
    B. infant respirator
    B. infant ventilator
Bourns-Bear I ventilator
Boutin thoracoscope
Bouveret disease
Bovie
    B. electrocautery
    B. ultrasound aspirator
bovied
bovine
    b. allograft
    b. biodegradable collagen
    b. collagen plug device
    b. heart
    b. heart valve
    b. heterograft
    b. lavage extract surfactant
      (BLES)
    pegademase b. (PEG-ADA)
    b. pericardial heart valve
    xenograft

B

b. pericardial valve
b. pericardium strips
bovinum
cor b.
bovis
Actinomyces b.
Babesia b.
Mycobacterium b.
Bowditch
B. law
B. phenomenon
B. staircase effect
bowing of mitral valve leaflet
box
bronchoscopic battery b.
digital constant-current
pacing b.
Elecath switch b.
Boyce sign
Boyd
B. perforating vein
B. point
boydii
Pseudallescheria b.
bozemanii
Legionella b.
Bozzolo sign
BP
blood pressure
British Pharmacopoeia
bronchopulmonary
BPD
bronchopulmonary dysplasia
BPM
blood perfusion monitor
bpm
beats per minute
BPV
balloon pulmonary valvuloplasty
BQ-123
Bq
becquerel
BR
breathing reserve
brachial
b. arteriogram
b. arteriotomy

b. artery
b. artery approach
b. artery cutdown
b. artery thrombosis
b. bypass
b. catheter
b. dance
b. plexus
b. pulse
b. syndrome
b. vein
brachial-ankle index
brachioaxillary bridge graft fistula
brachiocephalic
b. arteritis
b. artery
b. ischemia
b. system
b. vein
b. vessel angioplasty
brachiogram
Bracht-Wachter
B.-W. bodies
B.-W. lesion
brachycardia
brachytherapy
endobronchial b.
Bradbury-Eggleston syndrome
bradied down
Bradilan
Bradshaw-O'Neill aorta clamp
bradyarrhythmia
bradyarrhythmic arrest
bradycardia
artifactual b.
Branham b.
cardiomuscular b.
central b.
clinostatic b.
essential b.
fetal b.
idiopathic b.
idioventricular b.
junctional b.
nodal b.
postinfectious b.
postinfective b.

NOTES

bradycardia *(continued)*
pulseless b.
sinoatrial b.
sinus b.
vagal b.
ventricular b.
bradycardiac
bradycardia-dependent aberrancy
bradycardia-tachycardia syndrome
bradycrotic
bradydiastole
bradydysrhythmia
bradykinin
bradypnea
bradyrhythmia
bradysphygmia
bradytachycardia
   b. syndrome
bradytachydysrhythmia
brady-tachy syndrome
Bragg-Paul respirator
braid-like lesion
brain
   b. aneurysm
   b. death
   b. infarct
   b. murmur
   b. natriuretic peptide (BNP)
   b. wave
brain-heart infusion
branch
   b. lesion
   obtuse marginal b. (OMB)
   b. pulmonary artery stenosis
   b. retinal vein occlusion
      (BRVO)
   b. vessel occlusion
   b. vessel pruning
branched chain alpha ketoacid
   dehydrogenase (BCKD)
branching
   airway b.
   mirror-image brachiocephalic b.
Brandt cytology balloon
Branham
   B. bradycardia
   B. sign
Branhamella catarrhalis
Brasdor method
Brasfield chest radiograph score
brash
   water b.

brasiliensis
   Nocardia b.
   Paracoccidioides b.
brassy cough
BRAT
   Baylor rapid autologous transfusion
   BRAT system
Brauer cardiolysis
Braunwald
   B. classification (I-IIIB)
   B. sign
Braunwald-Cutter
   B.-C. ball prosthetic valve
   B.-C. ball valve prosthesis
brawny edema
braziliense
   Ancylostoma b.
bread-and-butter
   b.-a.-b. pericardium
   b.-a.-b. textbook sign
bread knife valvulotome
breakaway splice
breast
   b. pang
   thrush b.
breath
   b. excretion test
   b. pentane test
   shortness of b. (SOB)
Breathe Right nasal strip
breath-holding test
breathing
   apneustic b.
   Biot b.
   bronchial b.
   Cheyne-Stokes b.
   controlled b.
   frog b.
   glossopharyngeal b.
   intermittent positive pressure b.
      (IPPB)
   Kussmaul b.
   Ondine curse b.
   b. pacemaker
   periodic b.
   pursed-lip b.
   b. reserve (BR)
   sign mechanism for
      ventilator b.
   sleep-disordered b.
   work of b. (WOB)
Brechenmacher fiber
Brecher and Cronkite technique

bregmocardiac reflex
Brehmer treatment
Bremer AirFlo Vest
Brenner carotid bypass shunt
brequinar sodium
Brescia-Cimino A-V fistula
Brethaire
    B. Inhalation Aerosol
Brethine
    B. injection
    B. Oral
Bretonneau angina
Bretschneider-HTK cardioplegic
    solution
Brett syndrome
bretylium
    b. tosylate
Bretylol
Breuer-Hering inflation reflex
Brevibloc
    B. injection
Brevital
Bricanyl
    B. injection
    B. Oral
bridge
    arteriolovenular b.
    muscle b.
    myocardial b.
    Wheatstone b.
bridging
    myocardial b. (MB)
bright
    B. disease
    b. echo
    B. murmur
brightness modulation
Brill-Zinsser disease
B-ring
    esophageal B.-r.
Brisbane method
British Pharmacopoeia (BP)
Broadbent inverted sign
Brock
    B. infundibulectomy
    B. operation

    B. procedure
    B. syndrome
Brockenbrough
    B. angiocatheter
    B. cardiac device
    B. curved needle
    B. curved-tip occluder
    B. effect
    B. mapping catheter
    B. sign
    B. transseptal catheter
    B. transseptal commissurotomy
Brockenbrough-Braunwald sign
Broders index
Brodie abscess
Brodie-Trendelenburg tourniquet
    test
bromazepam
Bromfed
bromhexine
bromide
    ethidium b.
    ipratropium b.
    pancuronium b.
    pipecuronium b.
bromocriptine
Brompton
    B. cocktail
    B. solution
Brom repair
Bronalide
bronchadenitis, bronchoadenitis
bronchi (*pl. of* bronchus)
    4th/5th/6th order b.
Bronchial
bronchial
    b. adenoma
    b. allergy
    b. artery
    b. artery embolization (BAE)
    b. asthma
    b. atresia
    b. breathing
    b. breath sounds
    b. brush biopsy
    b. brushings
    b. bud

NOTES

bronchial *(continued)*
b. carcinoma
b. challenge test
b. collateral
b. collateral artery murmur
b. crisis
b. cyst
b. dehiscence
b. epithelial cell
b. fremitus
b. hyperreactivity
b. lavage
b. lumen
b. markings
b. meniscus sign
b. mucous membrane
b. mucus blanket
b. mucus inhibitor
b. pneumonia
b. provocation
b. rales
b. respiration
b. sleeve resection
b. smooth muscle
b. smooth muscle tone
b. spasm
b. stenosis
b. stump
b. toilet
b. tree
b. tube
b. washings
b. wheezing
bronchiectasis
chemical b.
cylindrical b.
cystic b.
dry b.
follicular b.
fusiform b.
pseudocylindrical b.
saccular b.
traction b.
bronchiectatic
b. rales
bronchiloquy
bronchiocele
bronchiolar
b. adenocarcinoma
b. carcinoma
bronchiole
alveolar b.

bronchiolitis
acute obliterating b.
b. exudativa
follicular b.
b. obliterans
b. obliterans organizing
pneumonia (BOOP)
obliterative b.
vesicular b.
viral b.
bronchioloalveolar
b. adenocarcinoma
b. carcinoma (BAC)
bronchiolocentric
bronchitic
bronchitis
acute bacterial exacerbation of
chronic b. (ABECB)
acute laryngotracheal b.
arachidic b.
asthmatic b.
capillary b.
Castellani b.
catarrhal b.
cheesy b.
chronic asthmatic b.
croupous b.
dry b.
epidemic capillary b.
ether b.
exudative b.
fibrinous b.
hemorrhagic b.
infectious asthmatic b.
mechanic b.
membranous b.
b. obliterans
phthinoid b.
plastic b.
polypoid b.
productive b.
pseudomembranous b.
putrid b.
secondary b.
b. sicca
smoker's b.
staphylococcal b.
streptococcal b.
suffocative b.
vegetal b.
verminous b.
vesicular b.
winter b.

B

Bronchitrac L flexible suction catheter
bronchoadenitis (*var. of* bronchadenitis)
bronchoalveolar
    b. carcinoma
    b. lavage (BAL)
    b. lavage fluid (BALF)
    b. washings
bronchoalveolitis
bronchoaspergillosis
bronchoblastomycosis
bronchoblennorrhea
bronchocandidiasis
Broncho-Cath
    B.-C. double-lumen endotracheal tube
bronchocavernous respiration
bronchocentric granulomatosis (BCG)
bronchoconstriction
bronchoconstrictor
bronchodilatation
bronchodilation
bronchodilator
    aerosolized b.
    anticholinergic b.
    inhaled b.
    Marax b.
    nebulized b.
bronchoegophony
bronchoesophageal
bronchoesophagoscopy
bronchofiberscope
bronchogenic
    b. adenocarcinoma
    b. carcinoma
    b. cyst
bronchogram
    air b.
    tantalum b.
bronchography
    Cope method b.
    inhalation b.
    percutaneous transtracheal b.
bronchophony
    pectoriloquous b.

    sniffling b.
    whispered b.
bronchopleural fistula
bronchopleuropneumonia
bronchopneumonia
    acute hemorrhagic b.
    confluent b.
    diffuse b.
    focal b.
    hemorrhagic b.
    hypostatic b.
    necrotizing b.
    sequestration b.
    subacute b.
    virus b.
bronchopneumonic infiltrate
bronchopneumonitis
bronchoprovocation test
bronchopulmonary (BP)
    b. aspergillosis
    b. cyst
    b. dysplasia (BPD)
    b. fistula
    b. segment
    b. spasm
    b. washings
bronchorrhea
Broncho Saline
bronchoscope
    Albert slotted b.
    BF large core b.
    Broyles b.
    Bruening b.
    Chevalier Jackson b.
    Davis b.
    Dumon b.
    Dumon-Harrell b.
    Emerson b.
    fiberoptic b.
    flexible fiberoptic b.
    Fujinon flexible b.
    Kernan-Jackson b.
    Michelson b.
    Moersch b.
    Negus b.
    Negus-Broyles b.
    Overholt-Jackson b.

NOTES

bronchoscope *(continued)*
Pentax b.
Pilling b.
respiration b.
Riecker respiration b.
Safar b.
Storz b.
Tucker b.
ventilation b.
Waterman b.
Yankauer b.
bronchoscopic
b. aspirator
b. battery box
b. bougie
b. brush
b. face shield
b. magnet
b. needle biopsy
bronchoscopy
fiberoptic b. (FB, FOB)
flexible fiberoptic b. (FFB)
rigid b.
ultrasound-guided b.
bronchospasm
allergic b.
exercise-induced b.
reversible b.
bronchospastic component
bronchospirometry
differential b.
bronchotracheal aspirate
bronchovesicular
b. breath sounds
b. markings
b. respiration
bronchus, pl. bronchi
anomalous b.
apical b.
basal segmental b.
cardiac b.
b. intermedius
lingular b.
lobar b.
lower lobe b.
main stem b.
middle lobe b.
pig b.
b. principalis dexter
b. principalis sinister
secondary b.
segmental b.
stem b.

subsegmental b.
tracheal b.
upper lobe b.
bronchus-grasping forceps
Bronitin
Bronkaid
B. mist
Bronkephrine
B. injection
Bronkodyl
Bronkolid
Bronkometer
Bronkosol
Brontex
B. Liquid
B. Tablet
Brookfield viscometer
broth
b. test
Todd-Hewitt b.
Broviac atrial catheter
brown
b. atrophy
b. edema
b. induration of lung
b. sputum
Brown-Adson forceps
Brown-Dodge method
Brown-McHardy pneumatic dilator
Broyles
B. anterior commissure
laryngoscope
B. bronchoscope
Brozek formula
Bruce
B. bundle
B. exercise stress test
B. treadmill protocol
brucei
Trypanosoma b.
Brucella
B. melitensis
brucellosis
Bruening bronchoscope
Brughleman needle
Brugia
B. malayi
B. timori
bruit
abdominal b.
aneurysmal b.
carotid b.
b. d'airain

b. de bois
b. de canon
b. de choc
b. de clapotement
b. de claquement
b. de craquement
b. de cuir neuf
b. de diable
b. de drapeau
b. de froissement
b. de frottement
b. de galop
b. de grelot
b. de la roue de moulin
b. de lime
b. de moulin
b. de parchemin
b. de piaulement
b. de pot felé
b. de rappel
b. de Roger
b. de scie
b. de scie ou de rape
b. de soufflet
b. de tabourka
b. de tambour
b. de triolet
epigastric b.
false b.
musical b.
Roger b.
seagull b.
systolic b.
thyroid b.
Traube b.
Verstraeten b.

brunescent
Brunner rib shears
brush
Air-Lon tracheal tube b.
b. biopsy
bronchoscopic b.
Edwards-Carpentier aortic
valve b.
Mill-Rose Protected Specimen
microbiology b.
protected b.

Brush electrocardiographic score
Brushfield spot
brushing
blind esophageal b. (BEB)
bronchial b.'s
double-sheath bronchial b.'s
washings and b.'s
brusque dilatation of esophagus
BRVO
branch retinal vein occlusion
Bryant
B. ampulla
B. mitral hook
BSA
body surface area
BSCA
bidirectional superior
cavopulmonary anastomosis
B-scan frame
BSLM
body surface Laplacian mapping
BTF-37 arterial blood filter
bubble
b. humidifier
b. oxygenation
b. oxygenator
Bubble-Jet
Puritan B.-J.
bubbling rales
bubbly lung syndrome
bubonic plague
bucardia
Buccal
Nitrogard B.
buccalis
Leptotrichia b.
Buchbinder
B. Omniflex catheter
B. Thruflex over-the-wire
B. Thruflex over-the-wire
catheter
bucindolol
buckled aorta
buckling
b. of aorta
chordal b.
midsystolic b.

NOTES

bud
    bronchial b.
Budd-Chiari syndrome
budesonide
Bueleau empyema trocar
Buerger-Allen exercise
Buerger disease
buffer
    Krebs-Henseleit b.
buffered aspirin
Bufferin
buffy coat smear
Buhl desquamative pneumonia
bulb
    aortic b.
    carotid b.
bulbar pulse
bulboventricular
    b. fold
    b. foramen
    b. groove
    b. loop
    b. sulcus
    b. tube
bulbus cordis
bulge
    precordial b.
bulging
    infarct b.
bulla, pl. **bullae**
    emphysematous b.
Bullard intubating laryngoscope
bulldog clamp
bullectomy
    transaxillary apical b.
bullet-tip catheter
bullet wound
bullous emphysema
bull's-eye
    b.-e. plot
    b.-e. polar coordinate mapping
bumetanide
Bumex
bump
    B b.
    ductus b.
BUN
    blood urea nitrogen
bundle
    atrioventricular b.
    A-V b.
    Bachmann b.

    b.-branch block (BBB)
    b.-branch fibrosis
    b.-branch reentrant tachycardia
    b.-branch reentry
    Bruce b.
    commissural b.
    His b., bundle of b.
    image b.
    James b.
    Keith b.
    Kent b.
    Kent-His b.
    Mahaim b.
    main b.
    neurovascular b.
    b. of Stanley Kent
    Thorel b.
    vascular b.
Bunnell-Howard arthrodesis clamp
Bunny boot
Bunyaviridae
bupivacaine
bur
    diamond-coated b.
bur-bearing catheter
burden
    ischemic b.
Burdick
    B. EKG machine
    B. electrocardiogram
Burette multiple patient delivery system
Burford-Finochietto rib spreader
Burford rib retractor
burgdorferi
    Borrelia b.
Burger
    B. scalene triangle
    B. technique for
        scapulothoracic disarticulation
Bürger-Grütz
    B.-G. disease
    B.-G. syndrome
Burghart symptom
Burhenne steerable catheter
Burinex
Burkholderia cepacia
Burkitt lymphoma
burnetii
    Coxiella b.
Burns
    space of B.

Burow
- B. quantitative method
- B. solution

bursa
- Calori b.

burst
- b. atrial pacing
- paroxysmal b.
- respiratory b.
- b. shock
- spider b.

Buschke
- B. disease
- scleredema of B.

buspirone

Busse-Buschke disease

busulfan
- b. lung syndrome

butanedione monoxime

butorphanol

butterfly
- b. needle
- b. shadow

Butterworth bidirectional filter

buttock claudication

button
- b. of aorta
- cell b.
- DiaTAP vascular access b.
- b. electrode
- Kistner tracheal b.
- Moore tracheostomy b.
- Panje voice b.
- Perspex b.
- skin b.
- b. technique
- tracheal b.
- tracheostomy b.

buttoned device

buttonhole
- b. deformity
- mitral b.
- b. mitral stenosis

buttress
- Teflon pledget suture b.

BV
- balloon valvuloplasty

BVAD
- biventricular assist device

BV-ARA-U

BvgAS regulon

BvgS protein

BVM
- bag-valve-mask
- BVM device

BVS
- biventricular support
- BVS pump

BW755C
- cyclooxygenase-lipoxygenase blocking agent B.

Bycep
- B. biopsy forceps
- B. PC Jr bioptome

bypass
- B. Angioplasty Revascularization Investigation (BARI)
- aortobi-iliac b.
- aortocarotid b.
- aortocoronary-saphenous vein b.
- aortoiliofemoral b.
- aortorenal b.
- aorto-subclavian-carotid-axilloaxillary b.
- axilloaxillary b.
- axillofemoral b.
- brachial b.
- cardiopulmonary b. (CPB)
- carotid-axillary b.
- carotid-carotid b.
- carotid-subclavian b.
- b. circuit
- coronary artery b. graft (CABG)
- cross femoral-femoral b.
- crossover b.
- descending thoracic aortofemoral-femoral b.
- fem-fem b.
- femoral-femoral b.
- femoral-popliteal b.
- femoral-tibial b.
- femoral-tibial-peroneal b.

NOTES

bypass *(continued)*
   femoroaxillary b.
   femorofemoral crossover b.
   femoropopliteal b.
   femorotibial b.
   fem-pop b.
   b. graft
   b. graft catheter
   b. graft catheterization
   heart-lung b.
   iliopopliteal b.
   infracubital b.
   internal mammary artery b.
   left heart b.
   Litwak left atrial-aortic b.
   b. machine
   percutaneous
     cardiopulmonary b. (PCPB)

   percutaneous left heart b.
     (PLHB)
   renal artery-reverse saphenous
     vein b.
   reversed b.
   right heart b.
   subclavian-carotid b.
   subclavian-subclavian b.
   superior mesenteric artery b.
   b. surgery
   b. time
   b. tract
bypassable
by-products
   eosinophil b.-p.
Byrel SX pacemaker
Byrel-SX/Versatrax pacemaker
byssinosis

C
C to E amplitude
C wave
C-11
C-11 hydroxephedrine
C-11 palmitate
c
c wave
c7E3 Fab
CA
cancer
carcinoma
cardiac-apnea
cardiac arrest
croup-associated
cytosine arabinoside
CA monitor
CA virus
C3a
CAA
cardiac allograft atherosclerosis
CAAS
Cardiovascular Angiography Analysis System
CABG
coronary artery bypass graft
cabinet respirator
cable
alligator pacing c.
OxyLead interconnect c.
Cabot-Locke murmur
Cabral coronary reconstruction
CABRI
Coronary Angioplasty versus Bypass Revascularization Investigation
cachectic
c. endocarditis
cachexia
cancer c.
cardiac c.
thyroid c.
CAD
coronary artery disease
CADD-Plus intravenous infusion pump
Cadence
C. AICD
C. biphasic ICD
C. implantable cardioverter-defibrillator

C. tiered therapy defibrillator system
C. TVL nonthoracotomy lead
Cadet V-115 implantable cardioverter-defibrillator
cadmiosis
cadmium (Cd)
c. fumes
CADs
computer-assisted diagnostics
caesiellus
Aspergillus c.
CAF
continuous atrial fibrillation
Cafatine
café-au-lait spot
café coronary
Cafergot
Cafetrate
caffeine
citrated c.
c. and sodium benzoate
cage
c. catheter device
chest c.
rib c.
thoracic c.
titanium c.
caged
caged ball valve
caged ball valve prosthesis
CAGEIN
catheter-guided endoscopic intubation
c-a interval
caisson disease
Calan
calcicardiogram
calcicosilicosis
calcicosis
calcific
c. debris
c. mitral stenosis
c. nodular aortic stenosis
c. pericarditis
calcification
arterial c.
dystrophic c.
mitral annular c.
napkin-ring c.

81

calcification *(continued)*
   pericardial c.
   valvular c.
calcified
   c. aortic valve
   c. lesion
   c. mitral leaflet
   c. nodule
   c. pericardium
   c. plaque
   c. thrombus
calcineurin
calcinosis
calciphylaxis
calcitonin gene-related peptide
calcium
   c. antagonists
   c. channel
   c. channel agonist
   c. channel antagonist
   c. channel blocker
   c. channel blocking agent
   c. chloride
   c. entry blocker
   fenoprofen c.
   c. gluceptate
   c. gluconate
   c. ion
   c. ionophore A23187
   mitral annular c.
   myoplasmic c.
   nadroparin c.
   c. oxalate
   c. oxalate deposition
   c. paradox
   c. product
   c. rigor
   c. score
   c. sign
   c. transient
Calciviridae virus
calcoaceticus
   Acinetobacter c.
calcofluor stain
Calcort
Calculair spirometer
calculation
   bidirectional shunt c.
calculosa
   pericarditis c.
calculus, pl. calculi
   cardiac c.

calf
   c. claudication
   c. lung surfactant extract
   (CLSE)
calibration
calibrator
   Fogarty c.
Califf score
California disease
calipers
   digital c.
   Lange c.
   Mipron digital computer-
   assisted c.
   Tenzel c.
callosa
   pericarditis c.
Calman
   C. carotid clamp
   C. ring clamp
Calmers
   Robitussin Cough C.
   Sucrets Cough C.
Calmette-Guérin
   Bacille bilié de C.-G. (BCG)
calmodulin
Calm-X Oral
Calori bursa
Calot triangle
calphostin C
Caltrac accelerometer
Caluso PEG tube
CAM
   child-adult-mist
   CAM tent
Cam-ap-es
Cambridge
   C. defibrillator
   C. electrocardiograph
   C. jelly electrode
camera
   Anger scintillation c.
   cine c.
   gamma scintillation c.
   multicrystal gamma c.
   multiwire gamma c.
   scintillation c.
   Siemens Orbiter gamma c.
   single-crystal gamma c.
   Sopha Medical gamma c.
   video c.
cameral fistula
Cameron-Haight elevator

CAMIAT
Canadian Amiodarone Myocardial Infarction Arrhythmia Trial
Camino
C. intracranial catheter
C. microventricular bolt
C. microventricular bolt catheter
cAMP
cyclic adenosine monophosphate
Campbell de Morgan spots
Camp-Sigvaris stockings
CAMP test
Campylobacter
camsylate
trimethaphan c.
CAN
continuous albuterol nebulization
Canadian
C. Amiodarone Myocardial Infarction Arrhythmia Trial (CAMIAT)
C. Amlodipine/Atenolol in Silent Ischemia (CASIS)
C. Cardiovascular Society (CCS)
C. Cardiovascular Society classification
C. Cardiovascular Society grading
C. Coronary Atherectomy Trial (CCAT)
C. Coronary Atherosclerosis Intervention Trial (CCAIT)
C. Heart Classification (CHC)
canal
c. of Arantius
atrioventricular c.
carotid c.
c. of Cuvier
femoral c.
His c.
Hunter c.
c.'s of Lambert
partial atrioventricular c.
perivascular c.

persistent common atrioventricular c.
pulmoaortic c.
Van Hoorne c.
ventricular c.
Verneuil c.
canalization
cancer (CA)
c. cachexia
metachronous lung c.
non-small cell lung c. (NSCLC)
Candida
C. albicans
C. glabrata
C. guilliermondii
C. lusitaniae
C. parapsilosis
candidiasis
oral c.
candidus
Aspergillus c.
candoxatril
candoxatrilat
caninum
Ancylostoma c.
canis
Babesia c.
Toxocara c.
Cann-Ease moisturizing nasal gel
Cannon
C. endarterectomy loop
C. formula
C. theory
cannon
c. sound
c. a wave
cannonball
c. metastases
c. pulse
cannula
Abelson c.
Abraham laryngeal c.
Air-Lon inhalation c.
aortic perfusion c.
Argyle CPAP nasal c.
Becker accelerator c.

C

NOTES

cannula · Caplan

cannula *(continued)*
cardiovascular c.
Churchill cardiac suction c.
Cimochowski cardiac c.
Cobe small vessel c.
femoral perfusion c.
Flexicath silicone subclavian c.
Floyd loop c.
Fluoro Tip c.
Gregg c.
Grüntzig femoral stiffening c.
nasal c.
O_2 via nasal c.
Research Medical straight
multiple-holed aortic c.
Rockey mediastinal c.
saphenous vein c.
Sarns soft-flow aortic c.
2-stage c.
Tibbs arterial c.
vein graft c.
vena cava c.
venous c.
Wallace Flexihub central
venous pressure c.
cannulate
cannulation
canola oil
canon
bruit de c.
canrenoate potassium
canrenone
cantering rhythm
Cantlie line
Cantrell pentalogy
CAP
community-acquired pneumonia
cap
pleural c.
capacitance
c. vessel
capacitor forming time
capacity
aerobic c.
diffusing c.
diffusion c.
exercise c.
forced expiratory c. (FEC)
forced expiratory volume in 1
second to forced vital c.
ratio (FEV₁/FVC)
forced inspiratory c. (FIC)

forced inspiratory vital c.
(FIVC)
forced vital c. (FVC)
functional residual c. (FRC)
inspiratory c. (IC)
inspiratory reserve c. (IRC)
inspiratory vital c. (IVC)
lung c.
maximal breathing c.
maximal sustainable
ventilatory c. (MSVC)
maximal vital c. (MVC)
maximum breathing c. (MBC)
metabolic vasodilatory c.
normal vital c. (NVC)
oxygen-binding c.
oxygen-carrying c.
oxygen-diffusing c.
residual lung c.
residual volume/total lung c.
(RV/TLC)
respiratory c.
slow vital c. (SVC)
timed vital c.
total lung c. (TLC)
ventilatory c.
vital c. (VC)
work c.
Capastat Sulfate
Capetown
C. aortic prosthetic valve
C. aortic valve prosthesis
capillaropathy
capillary, pl. **capillaries**
alveolar c.
c. apoplexy
c. bed
c. blood gas (CBG)
c. blood sugar (CBS)
c. blush
c. bronchitis
c. embolism
c. filtration coefficient
c. leak syndrome
c. pulse
c. wedge pressure
Capintec
C. nuclear VEST monitor
C. VEST system
Capiox-E bypass system oxygenator
Capiscint
Caplan syndrome

84

Caplets
Advil Cold & Sinus C.
Bayer Select Chest Cold C.
Dimetapp Sinus C.
Dristan Sinus C.
Capnocheck
Capnocytophaga
capnograph
capnography
**Capnostat Mainstream carbon
dioxide module**
Capoten
Capozide
capped lead
capreomycin
c. sulfate
CAPRI
Cardiopulmonary Research Institute
CAPRI program
caprisans
pulsus c.
caprizant
caproate
hydroxyprogesterone c.
CAPS
Cardiac Arrhythmia Pilot Study
Caps
Drixoral Cough & Congestion
Liquid C.
Drixoral Cough Liquid C.
Drixoral Cough & Sore Throat
Liquid C.
capsulatum
Histoplasma c.
capsule
Glisson c.
Neoral cyclosporine c.'s
Tiazac extended-release c.'s
CapSure cardiac pacing lead
captopril
c. and hydrochlorothiazide
**Captopril and Thrombolysis Study
(CATS)**
capture
atrial c.
c. beats

c. complex
pacemaker c.
ventricular c.
Carabelli tube
Carabello sign
carbachol
carbamazepine
carbapenem
carbenicillin
indanyl c.
carbide
cobalt in tungsten c.
carbinoxamine and pseudoephedrine
Carbiset-TR Tablet
Carbocaine
carbocholine
Carbodec
C. Syrup
C. TR Tablet
carbohydrate intolerance
CarboMedics
C. bileaflet prosthetic heart
valve
C. cardiac valve prosthesis
C. top-hat supra-annular valve
C. valve device
carbomethoxyisopropyl isonitrile
carbon
c. dioxide (CO_2)
c. dioxide dissociation curve
c. dioxide pressure
c. dioxide production
c. dioxide tension
c. disulfide
c. monoxide (CO)
pyrolytic c.
carbon-11
c. acetate
c. hydroxyephedrine
c. palmitic acid radioactive
tracer
carbon-11-labeled fatty acids
carbonica
asphyxia c.
carbonic anhydrase inhibitor
carboplatin

NOTES

Carbo-Seal
C.-S. cardiovascular composite graft
C.-S. graft material
carboxyhemoglobin (HbCO)
carcinoembryonic antigen (CEA)
carcinogen
carcinogenicity
carcinoid
c. heart disease
c. murmur
c. plaque
c. syndrome
c. tumor
c. valve disease
carcinoma, pl. carcinomata (CA)
adenosquamous c.
alveolar cell c.
anaplastic c.
basal cell c.
bronchial c.
bronchiolar c.
bronchioloalveolar c. (BAC)
bronchoalveolar c.
bronchogenic c.
clear cell c.
ductal cell c.
epidermoid c.
giant cell c.
hair-matrix c.
infiltrating lobular c.
large cell c.
large cell undifferentiated c.
lung c.
lymphangitic c.
melanotic c.
metastatic c.
mucinous c.
mucoepidermoid c.
nasopharyngeal c.
non-small cell c.
oat cell c.
papillary c.
poorly-differentiated c.
prickle cell c.
reserve cell c.
scirrhous c.
signet-ring cell c.
c. simplex
c. in situ
small cell c.
spindle cell c.
squamous cell c.

transitional cell c.
undifferentiated c.
undifferentiated small cell c.
verrucous c.
well-differentiated c.
carcinomatosa
lymphangitis c.
carcinomatous pericarditis
CARD
cardiac automatic resuscitative device
Cardabid
Cardak percutaneous catheter introducer
Cardarelli sign
Cardec-S Syrup
Carden bronchoscopy tube
Cardene
CARDIA
Coronary Artery Risk Development in Young Adults
cardiac
c. accident
c. action potential
c. adjustment scale
c. allograft
c. allograft atherosclerosis (CAA)
c. allograft vasculopathy (CAV)
c. alternation
c. amyloidosis
c. aneurysm
c. antrum
c. apex
c. arrest (CA)
c. arrhythmia
C. Arrhythmia Pilot Study (CAPS)
C. Arrhythmia Suppression Trial (CAST)
c. asthma
c. atrophy
c. auscultation
c. automatic resuscitative device (CARD)
c. ballet
c. balloon pump
c. baroreceptor
c. blood-pool imaging
c. border of dullness
c. bronchus
c. cachexia

c. calculus
c. catheter
c. catheterization
c. chamber
c. cirrhosis
c. cocktail
c. compensation
c. competence
c. compression
c. conduction
c. conduction system
c. contraction
c. contusion
c. cooling jacket
c. crisis
c. cushion
c. cycle
c. death
c. decompensation
c. decompression
c. defibrillation
c. depressant
c. depressor reflex
c. diastole
c. dilation
c. diuretic
c. dropsy
c. dyspnea
c. dysrhythmia
c. edema
c. enlargement
c. enzyme
c. event
c. examination
c. failure
c. fibrillation
c. function
c. gap junction protein
c. gating
c. glycogenosis
c. glycoside
c. hemoptysis
c. herniation
c. heterotaxia
c. hypertrophy
c. impulse
c. incisura

c. index (CI)
c. infarction
c. insufficiency
c. insult
c. interstitium
c. ischemia
c. jelly
c. liver
c. lung
c. mapping
c. mass
c. massage
c. memory
c. metastasis
c. monitor
c. murmur
c. muscle
c. muscle wrap
c. myosin
c. myxoma
c. neural crest
c. neurosis
c. notch
c. orifice
c. output (CO)
c. output index
c. output measurement
c. pacemaker
c. patch
c. perforation
c. performance
c. perfusion
c. polyp
c. probe
c. rehabilitation
c. reserve
c. resuscitation
c. retraction clip
c. rhythm
c. risk factor
c. risk index
c. rupture
c. sarcoidosis myocarditis
c. sarcoma
c. sensory nerve
c. shadow
c. shock

NOTES

cardiac *(continued)*
   c. shunt
   c. silhouette
   c. sling
   c. souffle
   c. sound
   c. standstill
   c. status
   C. Stimulator BCO$_2$
   c. stump
   c. surgery
   c. symphysis
   c. syncope
   c. systole
   c. tamponade
   C. T assay for troponin T
   c. telemetry
   c. thrombosis
   c. thrust
   c. transplant
   C. T Rapid assay
   c. troponin I assay
   c. tumor
   c. tumor plop
   c. ultrasound
   c. valve
   c. valve prosthesis
   c. valvular incompetence
   c. variability
   c. vein
   c. volume   *Cardiofar*
   c. waist
   c. wall hypokinesis
   c. wall thickening
   c. work index (CWI)
cardiaca
   adiposis c.
   steatosis c.
cardiac-apnea (CA)
Cardiac Pacemakers, Incorporated (CPI)
cardiacwise
cardialgia
cardiataxia
cardiatelia
CardiData Prodigy system
cardiectasia
cardiectopia
Cardilate
cardinal vein
cardioacceleration
cardioaccelerator
   c. center

cardioactive
cardioangiography
cardioarterial interval
cardioauditory syndrome
Cardiobacterium hominis
cardioballistic
cardiocairograph
Cardio-Care
cardiocele
cardiocentesis
cardiochalasia
CardioCoil coronary stent
Cardio-Cool myocardial protection pouch
Cardio-Cuff
   Childs C.-C.
cardiocyte
CardioData
   C. Mark IV computer
   C. MK-3 Holter scanner
cardiodiaphragmatic angle
CardioDiary
   C. heart monitor
cardiodynamics
cardiodynia
cardioembolic
   c. stroke
cardioesophageal
   c. junction
   c. reflux
   c. sphincter
cardiofacial syndrome
Cardioflon suture
Cardiofreezer cryosurgical system
cardiogenesis
cardiogenic
   c. pulmonary edema
   c. shock
   c. syncope
Cardiografin
cardiogram
   esophageal c.
cardiograph
cardiography
   Doppler c.
   echo-Doppler c.
   ultrasonic c.
   ultrasound c.
   vector c.
Cardio-Green
   C.-G. dye
Cardioguard 4000
   electrocardiographic monitor

cardiohemothrombus
cardiohepatic triangle
cardiohepatomegaly
cardioinhibitory
    c. center
    c. syncope
    c. type
cardiokinetic
cardiokymogram
cardiokymograph
cardiokymography
Cardiolite
    C. cardiac perfusion study
    C. stress test
cardiolith
cardiologist
cardiology
    American College of C.
    (ACC)
cardiolysis
    Brauer c.
cardiomalacia
Cardiomarker catheter
cardiomediastinal silhouette
cardiomegaly
    borderline c.
    false c.
    glycogen c.
    idiopathic c.
Cardiomemo device
Cardiometrics cardiotomy reservoir
cardiometry
cardiomotility
cardiomuscular bradycardia
cardiomyocyte
cardiomyoliposis
cardiomyopathy
    African c.
    alcoholic c.
    anthracycline-induced c.
    atrophic c.
    beer-drinker's c.
    cobalt c.
    concentric hypertrophic c.
    congestive c.
    diabetic c.
    dilated c. (DCM)

    doxorubicin c.
    drug-induced c.
    false c.
    familial hypertrophic
      obstructive c.
    fibroplastic c.
    genetic hypertrophic c.
    HIV c.
    hypertensive hypertrophic c.
    hypertrophic c. (HCM)
    hypertrophic obstructive c.
    (HOCM)
    idiopathic dilated c. (IDC)
    idiopathic restrictive c.
    infiltrative c.
    ischemic c.
    metoprolol dilated c. (MDC)
    mitochondrial c.
    nephropathic c.
    nonischemic dilated c.
    obliterative c.
    obstructive hypertrophic c.
    parasitic c.
    pediatric c.
    peripartum c.
    postpartum c.
    primary c.
    rejection c.
    restrictive c.
    right ventricular c.
    secondary c.
    tachycardia-induced c.
    viral c.
    X-linked dilated c.
cardiomyoplasty
    dynamic c.
cardiomyostimulator
Cardiomyostimulator SP1005
cardioneural
cardioneuropathy
cardioneurosis
cardio-omentopexy
Cardio-Pace Medical Durapulse
    pacemaker
cardiopaludism
cardiopath
cardiopathia nigra

C

NOTES

cardiopathy
cardiopericardiopexy
  Beck c.
cardiopexy
  ligamentum teres c.
cardiophobia
cardiophone
cardiophony
cardiophrenia
cardiophrenic angle
cardioplegia
  blood c.
  cold blood c.
  cold crystalloid c.
  cold potassium c.
  c. cooling
  crystalloid potassium c.
  hyperkalemic c.
  normothermic c.
  nutrient c.
  St. Thomas Hospital c.
  whole blood c.
cardioplegic
  c. arrest
  c. solution
Cardiopoint cardiac surgery needle
cardiopressor
cardioprotection
cardioptosia
CardioPulmonary
  C. eXercise (CPX)
cardiopulmonary
  c. arrest
  c. bypass (CPB)
  c. exercise test (CPET, CPX test)
  c. murmur
  C. Research Institute (CAPRI)
  c. reserve
  c. resuscitation (CPR)
  c. support (CPS)
CardioPump
  Ambu C.
Cardioquin
  C. Oral
cardiorespiratory
  c. arrest
  c. murmur
cardiorrhaphy
cardiorrhexis
cardioschisis
cardioscope
  Carlens c.

Siemens BICOR c.
Siemens HICOR c.
c. U system
cardioselectivity
Cardioserv defibrillator
cardiosphygmograph
CardioSync cardiac synchronizer
cardiotachometer
Cardio Tactilaze peripheral angioplasty laser catheter
CardioTec
  C. scan
Cardio-Tel
Cardiotest portable electrograph
Cardiothane 51
cardiothoracic
  c. ratio (CT, CTR)
  c. surgery (CTS)
cardiothrombus
cardiothyrotoxicosis
cardiotocography
cardiotomy
  c. reservoir
cardiotonic
  c. drug
cardiotoxic
  c. myolysis
cardiotoxicity
  Adriamycin c.
  doxorubicin c.
cardiotoxin
Cardiotrast
cardiovalvotomy
cardiovalvulitis
cardiovalvulotomy
Cardiovascular
  C. Angiography Analysis System (CAAS)
cardiovascular
  c. accident
  c. cannula
  c. clamp
  c. collapse
  c. complication
  c. disability
  c. disease (CVD)
  c. excitatory centers
  c. fitness
  c. function
  c. function assessment
  c. inhibitory centers
  c. pressure
  c. silk suture

c. steady state
c. stylet
c. syphilis
c. system

cardioversion
chemical c.
direct-current c.
elective c.
electrical c.
low-energy synchronized c.
c. paddles
pharmacological c.

cardioverter
cardioverter-defibrillator (*See* defibrillator)
cardiovirus
Cardiovit
C. AT-10 ECG/spirometry combination system
C. AT-10 monitor

Cardiovue
Diasonics C. 3400 and 6400
CardioWest TAH
carditis
coxsackievirus c.
rheumatic c.
Sterges c.
streptococcal c.
verrucous c.

Cardizem
C. Injectable
C. Lyo-Ject
C. Tablet

Cardura
CARE
Cholesterol and Recurrent Events
Care
American Association for Respiratory C. (AARC)
Carey Coombs short mid-diastolic murmur
Carfin
carina, pl. **carinae**
c. not splayed
c. sharp and mobile
c. of trachea

carinatum
pectus c.
carindacillin
Carinia domestica
carinii
Pneumocystis c.
Carlens
C. cardioscope
C. double-lumen endotracheal tube
Carmalt forceps
Carmeda BioActive Surface
C-arm fluoroscopy
Carmody valvulotome
carmustine
carneae
trabeculae c.
carneus
Aspergillus c.
carnitine
Carolina color spectrum CW Doppler
Carolon life support antiembolism stockings
caroticovertebral stenosis
Carotid
C. Artery Stenosis with Asymptomatic Narrowing: Operation Versus Aspirin Study (CASANOVA)
carotid
c. angiography
c. arch
c. arteriography
c. artery
c. artery disease
c. artery murmur
c. artery shunt
c. baroreceptor
c. bifurcation
c. body
c. bruit
c. bulb
c. canal
c. Doppler
c. duplex scan
c. ejection time

C

NOTES

carotid *(continued)*
    c. endarterectomy
    c. occlusive disease
    c. phonoangiography
    c. plaque
    Pravastatin, Lipids, and
      Atherosclerosis in the C.'s
      (PLAC)
    c. pulse
    c. pulse tracing
    c. sheath
    c. shudder
    c. sinus
    c. sinus hypersensitivity
    c. sinus massage
    c. sinus nerve
    c. sinus reflex
    c. sinus syncope
    c. sinus syndrome
    c. sinus test
    c. siphon
    c. steal syndrome
    c. stenosis
    c. stent
    c. triangle
    c. upstroke
carotid-axillary bypass
carotid-carotid bypass
carotid-cavernous fistula
carotid-subclavian bypass
carotidynia
carotodynia
Carpenter syndrome
Carpentier
    C. annuloplasty
    C. annuloplasty ring prosthesis
    C. pericardial valve
    C. ring
    C. stent
    C. tricuspid valvuloplasty
Carpentier-Edwards
    C.-E. aortic valve prosthesis
    C.-E. bioprosthesis
    C.-E. glutaraldehyde-preserved
      porcine xenograft prosthesis
    C.-E. mitral annuloplasty valve
    C.-E. pericardial valve
    C.-E. Perimount RSR
      pericardial bioprosthesis
    C.-E. porcine prosthetic valve
    C.-E. porcine supra-annular
      valve

Carpentier-Rhone-Poulenc mitral ring prosthesis
carpopedal spasm
CARPORT
    Coronary Artery Restenosis
    Prevention on Repeated
    Thromboxane Antagonism
Carrel patch
Carrington pneumonia
Carr lobectomy tourniquet
Carswell grapes
cart
    MedGraphics CPX/D
      metabolic c.
    metabolic c.
    resuscitation c.
Carten mitral valve retractor
carteolol
    c. hydrochloride
Carter
    C. equation
    C. retractor
Cartilade
cartilage
    xiphoid c.
Cartrol
    C. Oral
Cartwright
    C. heart prosthesis
    C. valve prosthesis
carumonam
Carvallo sign
carvedilol
Carwin
CAS-8000V general angiography positioner
Casale-Devereux criteria
CASANOVA
    Carotid Artery Stenosis with
    Asymptomatic Narrowing:
    Operation Versus Aspirin Study
cascade
    c. phenomenon
    renin-angiotensin-aldosterone c.
caseated tissue
caseating
caseation
    tuberculous c.
CASE computerized exercise EKG system
case-control study

caseous
    c. pneumonia
    c. tonsillitis
CASIS
    Canadian Amlodipine/Atenolol in
    Silent Ischemia
Casoni test
CASS
    Coronary Artery Surgery Study
CAST
    Cardiac Arrhythmia Suppression
    Trial
Castaneda
    C. anastomosis clamp
    C. bottle
    C. principle
Castellani
    C. bronchitis
    C. disease
    C. point
castellani
    Acanthamoeba c.
Castellino sign
Castillo catheter
Castleman disease
castor bean
Castroviejo needle holder
CAT
    computerized axial tomography
catabolism
    c. of rt-PA
catacrotic
    c. pulse
    c. wave
catacrotism
catacrotus
    pulsus c.
catadicrotic
    c. pulse
    c. wave
catadicrotism
catadicrotus
    pulsus c.
Cat-a-Kit
    C.-a.-K. analyzer
catalase
catamenial hemothorax

cataplectic
cataplexy
Catapres
    C. Oral
Catapres-TTS Transdermal
catarrh
    atrophic c.
    autumnal c.
    Bostock c.
    hypertrophic c.
    Laennec c.
    postnasal c.
    sinus c.
    suffocative c.
catarrhal
    c. asthma
    c. bronchitis
    c. croup
    c. laryngitis
    c. pharyngitis
    c. pneumonia
catarrhalis
    Branhamella c.
    Moraxella c.
    Neisseria c.
cat asthma
catatricrotic
    c. pulse
catatricrotism
Catatrol
CATCH 22 syndrome
catecholamine
    c. action
    plasma c.
0 to 10 category ratio (CR-10)
catenoid
catheter
    c. ablation
    ACE fixed-wire balloon c.
    Achiever balloon dilatation c.
    ACS angioplasty c.
    ACS balloon c.
    ACS Endura coronary
    dilation c.
    ACS Enhanced Torque 8/7.5 F
    Taper Tip c.
    ACS JL4 French c.

C

NOTES

catheter *(continued)*
ACS Mini c.
ACS Monorail c.
ACS OTW Lifestream
coronary dilatation c.
ACS RX LifeStream coronary
dilatation c.
ACS RX perfusion balloon c.
c. adapter
AL-1 c.
AL II guiding c.
Alvarez-Rodriguez cardiac c.
Alzate c.
Amcath c.
Amplatz coronary c.
Amplatz Hi-Flo torque-
control c.
Amplatz left I, II c.
Amplatz right coronary c.
Amplatz right I, II c.
A2 multipurpose c.
Angiocath PRN c.
Angioflow high-flow c.
angiographic c.
Angio-Kit c.
Angiomedics c.
angiopigtail c.
angioplasty guiding c.
angled balloon II c.
angled pigtail c.
angulated multipurpose c.
Anthron heparinized
antithrombogenic c.
Anthron II c.
AR-1 c.
Arani double-loop guiding c.
Argyle c.
Arrow balloon wedge c.
Arrow Flex intra-aortic
balloon c.
ARROWgard Blue antiseptic-
coated c.
ARROWgard Blue Line c.
ARROWgard central venous c.
Arrow-Howes multilumen c.
Arrow QuadPolar electrode c.
Arrow TwinCath multilumen
peripheral c.
arterial embolectomy c.
c. arteriography
atherectomy c.
AtheroCath spinning blade c.

Atlas LP PTCA balloon
dilatation c.
Atlas ULP balloon
dilatation c.
ATRAC-II double-balloon c.
ATRAC multipurpose
balloon c.
Atri-pace I bipolar flared
pacing c.
Auth atherectomy c.
autoperfusion balloon c.
AV-Paceport thermodilution c.
Axiom DG balloon
angioplasty c.
Bailey c.
bailout autoperfusion balloon c.
Baim pacing c.
Baim-Turi monitoring/pacing c.
Balectrode pacing c.
balloon angioplasty c.
balloon embolectomy c.
balloon-flotation pacing c.
balloon-imaging c.
balloon-tipped angiographic c.
balloon-tipped flow-directed c.
balloon-tipped thermodilution c.
balloon valvuloplasty c.
ball-wedge c.
Baltherm c.
Bard balloon-directed pacing c.
Bardco c.
Bard electrophysiology c.
Bard guiding c.
Bardic cutdown c.
Baxter angioplasty c.
Bentson-Hanafee-Wilson c.
Berenstein occlusion balloon c.
Berman angiographic c.
Berman balloon flotation c.
Bicor c.
bifoil balloon c.
Bio-Medicus arterial c.
bird's-eye c.
blade septostomy c.
Block right coronary
guiding c.
Blue FlexTip c.
Blue Max triple-lumen c.
Bonzel Monorail balloon c.
Bourassa c.
brachial c.
Brockenbrough mapping c.
Brockenbrough transseptal c.

Bronchitrac L flexible
suction c.
Broviac atrial c.
Buchbinder Omniflex c.
Buchbinder Thruflex over-the-
wire c.
bullet-tip c.
bur-bearing c.
Burhenne steerable c.
bypass graft c.
Camino intracranial c.
Camino microventricular
bolt c.
cardiac c.
Cardiomarker c.
Cardio Tactilaze peripheral
angioplasty laser c.
Castillo c.
Cath-Finder c.
Cathlon IV c.
Cathmark suction c.
central venous c. (CVC)
Cereblate c.
Chemo-Port c.
Clark expanding mesh c.
Clark helix c.
Clark rotating cutter c.
Cloverleaf c.
Cobra over-the-wire balloon c.
coil-tipped c.
conductance c.
Cook arterial c.
Cook TPN c.
Cook yellow pigtail c.
Cordis BriteTip guiding c.
Cordis Ducor I, II, III c.
Cordis Ducor pigtail c.
Cordis guiding c.
Cordis Lumelec c.
Cordis Predator balloon c.
Cordis Son-II c.
Cordis Titan balloon
dilatation c.
Cordis Trakstar PTCA
balloon c.
Cordis TransTaper tip c.
coronary angiographic c.

coronary seeking c.
corset balloon c.
Cournand quadpolar c.
C. R. Bard c.
Cribier-Letac c.
CritiCath thermodilution c.
Critikon balloon temporary
pacing c.
Critikon balloon
thermodilution c.
Critikon balloon-tipped end-
hole c.
Critikon balloon wedge
pressure c.
cutdown c.
Cynosar c.
Dacron c.
c. damping
Datascope DL-II percutaneous
translucent balloon c.
decapolar electrode c.
decapolar pacing c.
deflectable quadripolar c.
DeKock two-way bronchial c.
Deseret flow-directed
thermodilution c.
diagnostic ultrasound
imaging c.
Diasonics c.
Digiflex high flow c.
c. dilation
dog-leg c.
Doppler c.
Dorros brachial internal
mammary guiding c.
Dorros infusion/probing c.
Dotter caged-balloon c.
double-balloon c.
double-chip micromanometer c.
double-J c.
double-lumen c.
double-thermistor coronary
sinus c.
drill-tip c.
dual balloon perfusion c.
(DBPC)

C

NOTES

catheter *(continued)*
dual-sensor micromanometric
high-fidelity c.
Dualtherm dual thermistor
thermodilution c.
Ducor balloon c.
Ducor-Cordis pigtail c.
Ducor HF c.
EAC c.
echo c.
EchoMark angiographic c.
EDM infusion c.
Edwards c.
EID c.
eight-lumen manometry c.
Elecath thermodilution c.
electrode c.
El Gamal coronary bypass c.
El Gamal guiding c.
Elite guide c.
embolectomy c.
c. embolectomy
c. embolism
c. embolus
Encapsulon epidural c.
end-hole balloon-tipped c.
end-hole #7 French c.
EndoSonics IVUS/balloon
dilatation c.
Endosound endoscopic
ultrasound c.
Endotak C lead transvenous c.
Enhanced Torque 8F
guiding c.
Eppendorf c.
Erythroflex hydromer-coated
central venous c.
c. exchange
expandable access c. (EAC)
Explorer 360-degree rotational
diagnostic EP c.
Explorer pre-curved diagnostic
EP c.
Express over-the-wire
balloon c.
FACT coronary balloon
angioplasty c.
Falcon single-operator exchange
balloon c.
FAST balloon flotation c.
FAST right heart
cardiovascular c.
fiberoptic c. delivery system

fiberoptic oximeter c.
fiberoptic pressure c.
Finesse guiding c.
Flexguard Tip c.
Flexxicon Blue dialysis c.
flow-directed balloon
cardiovascular c.
fluid-filled balloon-tipped flow-
directed c.
fluid-filled pigtail c.
Fogarty adherent clot c.
Fogarty-Chin extrusion
balloon c.
Fogarty embolectomy c.
Fogarty graft thrombectomy c.
Foltz-Overton cardiac c.
Forerunner coronary sinus
guiding c.
c. fragment
Franz monophasic action
potential c.
French double-lumen c.
French JR4 Schneider c.
French SAL c.
French shaft c.
Ganz-Edwards coronary
infusion c.
Gensini coronary
arteriography c.
Gensini Teflon c.
Gentle-Flo suction c.
Glidecath hydrophilic coated c.
Goeltec c.
Goodale-Lubin c.
Gorlin c.
Gould PentaCath 5-lumen
thermodilution c.
graft-seeking c.
Grollman pulmonary artery-
seeking c.
Groshong double-lumen c.
Grüntzig c.
c. guide holder
c. guidewire
guiding c.
Hakko Dwellcath c.
Halo c.
Hancock embolectomy c.
Hancock fiberoptic c.
Hancock hydrogen detection c.
Hancock luminal
electrophysiologic recording c.
Hancock wedge-pressure c.

Hartzler ACX II c.
Hartzler balloon c.
Hartzler dilatation c.
Hartzler Excel c.
Hartzler LPS dilatation c.
Hartzler Micro-600 c.
Hartzler Micro II c.
Hartzler Micro XT c.
Hartzler RX-014 balloon c.
headhunter angiography c.
helical-tip Halo c.
helium-filled balloon c.
Helix PTCA dilatation c.
hexapolar c.
high-flow c.
high-speed rotation dynamic
    angioplasty c.
Hilal modified headhunter c.
His c.
hockey-stick c.
c. hub
HydroCath c.
Hydrogel-coated PTCA
    balloon c.
IAB c.
Illumen-8 guiding c.
ILUS c.
Imager Torque selective c.
imaging-angioplasty balloon c.
c. impact artifact
impedance c.
Infiniti c.
Inoue balloon c.
c. instability
Integra c.
Intellicath pulmonary artery c.
internal mammary artery c.
Interpret ultrasound c.
Intimax vascular c.
intra-aortic balloon c.
intracardiac c.
intravascular ultrasound c.
Intrepid balloon c.
c. introduction method
ITC balloon c.
Jackman coronary sinus
    electrode c.

Jackman orthogonal c.
Josephson quadripolar c.
Jostra c.
JR4, JR5 c.
Judkins coronary c.
Judkins curve LAD c.
Judkins curve LCX c.
Judkins curve STD c.
Judkins guiding c.
Judkins torque control c.
Katzen long balloon
    dilatation c.
Kensey atherectomy c.
King guiding c.
King multipurpose c.
Kinsey atherectomy c.
Konigsberg c.
Kontron balloon c.
large-bore c.
laserprobe c.
left coronary c.
left heart c.
left Judkins c.
left ventricular sump c.
Lehman ventriculography c.
lensed fiber-tip laser
    delivery c.
Levin c.
Leycom volume conductance c.
Lifestream coronary dilation c.
long ACE fixed-wire
    balloon c.
Longdwel Teflon c.
Long Skinny over-the-wire
    balloon c.
Lo-Profile II c.
low-speed rotation
    angioplasty c.
Lumaguide c.
Lumelec pacing c.
c. manipulation
manometer-tipped c.
Mansfield Atri-Pace 1 c.
Mansfield orthogonal
    electrode c.
Mansfield Scientific dilatation
    balloon c.

C

NOTES

catheter *(continued)*
c. mapping
mapping/ablation c.
Marathon guiding c.
marker c.
Medi-Tech balloon c.
Medi-Tech steerable c.
memory c.
Metras c.
Mewissen infusion c.
Micor c.
Micro-Guide c.
micromanometer c.
Microsoftrac c.
Micross dilatation c.
Mikro-Tip micromanometer-tipped c.
Millar Doppler c.
Millar MPC-500 c.
Miller septostomy c.
Mini-Profile c.
Mirage over-the-wire balloon c.
Molina needle c.
monofoil c.
monometer-tipped c.
Monorail imaging c.
Monorail Piccolino c.
MS Classique balloon dilatation c.
MTC c.
multi-access c. (MAC)
multiflanged Portnoy c.
Multiflex c.
multilayer design c.
multiplex c.
multipolar c.
Multipurpose-SM c.
multisensor c.
MVP c.
Mylar c.
Namic c.
Nestor guiding c.
NIH cardiomarker c.
NIH marking c.
nonflotation c.
nonflow-directed c.
nontraumatizing c.
NoProfile balloon c.
Norton flow-directed Swan-Ganz thermodilution c.
Novoste c.
Numed intracoronary Doppler c.

Nycore pigtail c.
octapolar c.
Olbert balloon c.
Olympix II PTCA dilatation c.
Omniflex balloon c.
one-hole angiographic c.
Opta 5 c.
optical fiber c.
Opticath oximeter c.
Optiscope c.
Oracle Focus PTCA c.
Oracle Micro intravascular ultrasound c.
Oracle Micro Plus PTCA c.
Oreopoulos-Zellerman c.
OTW perfusion c.
over-the-wire PTCA balloon c.
Owens balloon c.
Owens Lo-Profile dilatation c.
oximetric c.
pacemaker c.
Paceport c.
Pacewedge dual-pressure bipolar pacing c.
pacing c.
Park blade septostomy c.
P.A.S. Port c.
c. patency
Pathfinder c.
PA Watch position-monitoring c.
pediatric pigtail c.
Peel-Away c.
PE-MT balloon dilatation c.
PentaCath c.
Pentalumen c.
PentaPace QRS c.
PE Plus II peripheral balloon c.
Percor-Stat-DL c.
percutaneous intra-aortic balloon counterpulsation c.
percutaneous rotational thrombectomy c.
perfusion balloon c. (PBC)
Periflow peripheral balloon angioplasty-infusion c.
peripherally-inserted c. (PIC)
Per-Q-Cath percutaneously inserted central venous c.
pervenous c.
Phantom V Plus c.
Piccolino Monorail c.

pigtail c.
Pilotip c.
Pinkerton .018 balloon c.
Polaris steerable diagnostic c.
Positrol II c.
Predator balloon c.
preshaped c.
probe balloon c.
Probing sheath exchange c.
Procath electrophysiology c.
Profile Plus balloon
  dilatation c.
Proflex 5 c.
Pro-Flo XT c.
Pruitt-Inahara balloon-tipped
  perfusion c.
pulmonary flotation c.
Q-cath c.
quadpolar w/Damato curve c.
quadripolar steerable
  electrode c.
Quanticor c.
QuickFlash arterial c.
Quinton PermCath c.
radiopaque calibrated c.
Rashkind septostomy balloon c.
recessed balloon septostomy c.
RediFurl TaperSeal IAB c.
Rentrop c.
reperfusion c.
RF Ablatr ablation c.
RF-generated thermal
  balloon c.
right coronary c.
right heart c.
right Judkins c.
Rigiflex TTS balloon c.
Ritchie c.
Rodriguez c.
Rodriguez-Alvarez c.
Rotablator c.
Rotacs motorized c.
rotational dynamic
  angioplasty c.
rove magnetic c.
Royal Flush c.
Rx perfusion c.

Rx Streak balloon c.
Safe-T-Coat heparin-coated
  thermodilution c.
SafTouch c.
Sarns wire-reinforced c.
SCA-EX ShortCutter c.
Schneider c.
Schoonmaker c.
Schwarten LP balloon c.
Scimed angioplasty c.
Scoop 1, 2 c.
Selecon coronary
  angiography c.
self-guiding c.
self-positioning balloon c.
Sensation intra-aortic balloon c.
Sentron pigtail angiographic
  micromanometer c.
Seroma-Cath c.
serrated c.
Shadow over-the-wire
  balloon c.
shaver c.
Sherpa guiding c.
Shiley c.
SHJR4 c.
ShortCutter c.
side-hole Judkins right, curve
  4 c.
sidewinder percutaneous intra-
  aortic balloon c.
Silastic c.
Silicore c.
Simmons II, III c.
Simmons-type sidewinder c.
Simplus PE/t dilatation c.
Simpson atherectomy c.
Simpson Coronary
  AtheroCath c.
Simpson-Robert c.
Simpson Ultra Lo-Profile II c.
Skinny dilatation c.
Skinny over-the-wire balloon c.
Sleek c.
Slider c.
sliding rail c.
Slinky balloon c.

NOTES

catheter *(continued)*
sliding rail c.
Slinky balloon c.
Slinky PTCA c.
Smart position-sensing c.
Smec balloon c.
snare c.
Softip c.
Softouch UHF cardiac
    pigtail c.
Softrac-PTA c.
Soft-Vu Omni flush c.
Solo c.
Sones Cardio-Marker c.
Sones coronary c.
Sones Hi-Flow c.
Sones Positrol c.
Sones woven Dacron c.
Sonicath imaging c.
Sorenson thermodilution c.
Spectra-Cath STP c.
Speedy balloon c.
Spring c.
Sprint c.
Stack perfusion c.
standard Lehman c.
steerable electrode c.
steerable guidewire c.
Steerocath c.
Steri-Cath c.
Stertzer brachial c.
Stertzer guiding c.
straight flush percutaneous c.
Sub-4 small vessel balloon
    dilatation c.
SULP II balloon c.
Superflow guiding c.
Super-9 guiding c.
Swan-Ganz balloon flotation c.
Swan-Ganz bipolar pacing c.
Swan-Ganz flow-directed c.
Swan-Ganz Pacing TD c.
TAC atherectomy c.
Teflon c.
TEGwire balloon dilatation c.
Tennis Racquet angiographic c.
Ten system balloon c.
Terumo SP coaxial c.
tetrapolar esophageal c.
thermistor thermodilution c.
thermodilution balloon c.
thin-walled c.
c. tip occluder

Torcon NB selective
    angiographic c.
Torktherm torque control c.
torque control balloon c.
Total Cross balloon c.
Tourguide guiding c.
TrachCare multi-access c.
Tracker-18 Soft Stream side-
    hole microinfusion c.
Trac Plus c.
Trakstar balloon c.
transcutaneous extraction c.
transluminal angioplasty c.
transluminal endarterectomy c.
    (TEC)
transluminal extraction c.
    (TEC)
transseptal c.
transtracheal oxygen c.
trefoil balloon c.
Triguide c.
triple-lumen balloon flotation
    thermistor c.
tripolar w/Damato curve c.
TTS c.
Tyshak c.
Uldall subclavian
    hemodialysis c.
ULP c.
ultra-low profile fixed-wire
    balloon dilatation c.
Ultra-Thin balloon c.
UMI c.
Uniweave c.
Uresil embolectomy
    thrombectomy c.
urinary c.
USCI c.
Van Andel c.
Van Tassel angled pigtail c.
Variflex catheter c.
Vas-Cath c.
vascular access c.
ventriculography c.
Ventureyra ventricular c.
Verbatim balloon c.
Viggo-Spectramed c.
Viper PTA c.
V. Mueller c.
Voda c.
waist of c.
Webster halo c.
Webster orthogonal electrode c.

wedge pressure balloon c.
Wexler c.
c. whip
c. whip artifact
Wilton-Webster coronary sinus
  thermodilution c.
X-Trode electrode c.
Zavod bronchospirometry c.
Z-Med c.
Zucker multipurpose bipolar c.
catheter-guided
  c.-g. biopsy
  c.-g. endoscopic intubation
    (CAGEIN)
catheter-induced thrombosis
catheterization
  bypass graft c.
  cardiac c.
  combined heart c.
  coronary sinus c.
  hepatic vein c.
  interventional cardiac c.
  left heart c.
  percutaneous transhepatic
    cardiac c.
  pulmonary artery c.
  retrograde c.
  right heart c.
  c. technique
  transseptal left heart c.
catheter-related peripheral vessel
  spasm
catheter-snare system
catheter-tip
  c.-t. micromanometer system
  c.-t. spasm
Cath-Finder
  C.-F. catheter
  C.-F. catheter tracking system
Cath-Lok catheter locking device
Cathlon IV catheter
Cathmark suction catheter
Cath-Secure
CATS
  Captopril and Thrombolysis Study
cat-scratch disease

cattaire
  frémissement c.
cauda equina syndrome
caudal
caudally-angled balloon occlusion
  aortography
caudocephalad
caudocranial hemiaxial view
causality assessment
CAV
  cardiac allograft vasculopathy
cava
  superior vena c. (SVC)
CAVB
  complete atrioventricular block
CAVEAT
  Coronary Angioplasty versus
  Excisional Atherectomy Trial
Caverject injection
cavernoma
cavernous
  c. rales
  c. respiration
  c. sinus thrombosis
  c. voice
Caves bioptome
cave sickness
Caves-Schultz bioptome
CAVH
  continuous arteriovenous
    hemofiltration
caviae
  Aeromonas c.
  Nocardia c.
cavitary
  c. lesion
cavitation
  pulmonary c.
cavitis
Cavitron ultrasonic surgical
  aspirator (CUSA)
cavocaval shunt
cavopulmonary
  c. anastomosis
  c. connection
CAZ beta-lactamase
C4B

C

NOTES

C-bar web-spacer
CBC
   complete blood count
CBF
   cerebral blood flow
   coronary blood flow
CBFV
   coronary blood flow velocity
CBG
   capillary blood gas
CB lead
CBS
   capillary blood sugar
C-C
   convexoconcave
   C-C heart valve
CCAIT
   Canadian Coronary Atherosclerosis
   Intervention Trial
CCAT
   Canadian Coronary Atherectomy
   Trial
CCE
   clubbing, cyanosis, and edema
CCPD
   continuous cyclical peritoneal
   dialysis
CCS
   Canadian Cardiovascular Society
      CCS endocardial pacing lead
CCU
   coronary care unit
Cd
   cadmium
CD4
      C. cell
CD4+
      C. cell
      C. measure
CD5 cell
CD8
      C. AIS CELLector
      C. cell
CD8+ T cell
CD18 antibodies
CD45
CDBR
   computerized diaphragmatic
   breathing retraining
      RFB System-I for CDBR
CDC
   Centers for Disease Control

CDE
   color Doppler energy
cDNA
   human cloned DNA
CEA
   carcinoembryonic antigen
Ceclor
cedar
   Western red c.
Cedars-Sinai classification
Cedax
Cedilanid-D
CEDIM
   L-Carnitine Ecocardiografia
   Digitalizzata Infarto Miocardico
Ceelen disease
CeeNU Oral
cefaclor
cefadroxil
   c. monohydrate
Cefadyl
cefamandole
   c. nafate
Cefanex
cefazolin sodium
cefixime
Cefizox
cefmenoxine
cefmetazole
   c. sodium
Cefobid
cefonicid sodium
cefoperazone
   c. sodium
ceforanide
Cefotan
cefotaxime
   c. sodium
cefotetan
   c. disodium
cefoxitin sodium
cefpiramide
cefpodoxime
   c. proxetil
cefprozil
ceftazidime
ceftibuten
Ceftin
   C. Oral
ceftizox
ceftizoxime
   c. sodium

ceftriaxone
   c. sodium
cefuroxime
Cefzil
Cegka sign
Celebenin
celer
   pulsus c.
Celermajer method
celerrimus
   pulsus c.
Celestin
   C. bougie
   C. esophageal tube
Celestone
   C. Soluspan
celiac
   c. artery
   c. disease
celiprolol
Cell
   C. Saver
   C. Saver autologous blood
      recovery system
   C. Saver Haemolite
   C. Saver Haemonetics
      Autotransfusion system
cell
   ameboid c.
   Aschoff c.
   B c.
   B1 c.
   bronchial epithelial c.
   c. button
   CD4+ c.
   CD4 c.
   CD5 c.
   CD8 c.
   CD8+ T c.
   chicken-wire myocardial c.
   ciliated epithelial c.
   Clara c.'s
   clear c.
   effector c.'s
   foam c.
   foamy myocardial c.
   giant c.

   goblet c.
   heart failure c.'s
   human aortic endothelial c.'s
      (HAEC)
   hyperplastic mucus-secreting
      goblet c.
   IgE-sensitized c.
   Kulchitsky c.
   Langerhans giant c.'s
   Langhans c.'s
   mast c.
   c. membrane
   c. membrane-bound adenylate
      cyclase
   mesangial c.
   mesenchymal intimal c.
   metaplastic mucus-secreting c.
   mononuclear c.
   multinucleated giant c.'s
   N c.
   oat c.
   P c.
   Pelger-Huet c.'s
   pi c.
   pup c.
   Purkinje c.'s
   RA c.
   Sala c.'s
   sensitized c.
   smooth muscle c. (SMC)
   c. sorter
   squamous c.
   T c.'s
   transitional c.
   c. type
   typical small c.
   vascular smooth muscle c.'s
      (VSMC)
CELLector
   CD8 AIS C.
cell-mediated immunity
Cellolite material
cellophane rales
celltrifuge
cellular embolism
cellulitis

C

NOTES

103

cellulose
    oxidized c.
celophlebitis
Celsa battery
Celsior
Cel-U-Jec
Cenafed
Cenflex central monitoring system
center
    cardioaccelerator c.
    cardioinhibitory c.
    cardiovascular excitatory c.'s
    cardiovascular inhibitory c.'s
    Chemetron HR-1 Humidity C.
    Kronecker c.
    pneumotaxic c.
    respiratory c.
    vasoconstrictor c.
    vasodilator c.
centerline method of wall motion analysis
Centers for Disease Control (CDC)
Centimist nebulizer
Centocor
CentoRx
central
    c. approach
    c. bradycardia
    c. core wire
    c. cyanosis
    c. fibrous body
    c. pneumonia
    c. respiration
    c. splanchnic venous thrombosis (CSVT)
    c. terminal electrode
    c. venous catheter (CVC)
    c. venous line
    c. venous pressure (CVP)
centriacinar emphysema
centrilobular emphysema
centripetal venous pulse
centronuclear myopathy
Centyl
CEP
    chronic eosinophilic pneumonia
cepacia
    Burkholderia c.
    Pseudomonas c.
cephalexin monohydrate
cephalic
    c. artery
    c. vein

cephalization of pulmonary flow pattern
cephalocaudad
cephalosporin
cephalothin
    c. sodium
cephapirin sodium
cephradine
Ceptaz
Cereblate catheter
cerebral
    c. aneurysm
    c. angiography
    c. anoxia
    c. apoplexy
    c. arteriosclerosis
    c. beriberi
    c. blood flow (CBF)
    c. edema
    c. embolus
    c. event
    c. infarct
    c. infarction
    c. ischemia
    c. perfusion
    c. perfusion pressure (CPP)
    c. pneumonia
    c. protective therapy
    c. respiration
    c. thrombosis
    c. tuberculosis
    c. vasculopathy
cerebritis
cerebrovascular
    c. accident (CVA)
    c. disease
    c. event
    c. insufficiency
    c. resistance (CVR)
    c. syncope
    c. thrombosis
cerebrum
Ceredase injection
cereolysin
Cerespan Oral
cereus
    Bacillus c.
Cerezyme
cervical
    c. aortic arch
    c. aortic knuckle
    c. disk
    c. heart

c. pleura
c. radiculitis
c. rib syndrome
c. spine deformity
c. venous hum
cervicalis
ansa c.
cervicothoracic
c. sympathectomy
cesium chloride
cessation
smoking c.
cestodic tuberculosis
Cetacaine
cetirizine
CF
cystic fibrosis
CF lead
CFA
cryptogenic fibrosing alveolitis
CFM-700
Vingmed C.
CFR
coronary flow reserve
CFTR
cystic fibrosis transmembrane
regulator
cGMP
cyclic guanosine monophosphate
Chagas heart disease
chagasic myocardiopathy
chagoma
chain
imaging c.
light c.
myosin heavy c.
myosin light c.
paratracheal c.
2-c. urokinase plasminogen
activator (tcu-PA)
challenge
Desferal Mesylate c.
ergonovine c.
histamine c.
methacholine
bronchoprovocation c.

chamber
anterior c.
atrialized c.
cardiac c.
Fisher-Paykel MR290 water-
feed c.
hyperbaric c.
c. rupture
c. stiffness
Chamberlain mediastinoscopy
Champ cardiac device
Chandler V-pacing probe
change
arteriovenous crossing c.'s
E to A c.'s
E to I c.'s
environmental c.
fibrinoid c.'s
Gerhardt c.
hyaline fatty c.
ischemic ECG c.'s
malignancy-associated c.'s
(MACs)
myxomatous c.
nonspecific climatic c.
rheologic c.
ST segment c.'s
ST-T wave c.'s
trophic c.'s
channel
calcium c.
fast c.
3-c. Holter monitor
ion c.
lymphatic c.
marker c.
membrane c.
receptor-operated calcium c.
sarcolemmal calcium c.
slow c.
sodium c.
thorough-fare c.
voltage-dependent calcium c.
chaotic
c. atrial tachycardia
c. heart

NOTES

Charcot
   C. sign
   C. syndrome
Charcot-Bouchard
   C.-B. aneurysm
   C.-B. microaneurysm
Charcot-Leyden crystals
Charcot-Marie-Tooth disease
Charcot-Weiss-Baker syndrome
Chardack-Greatbatch
   C.-G. implantable cardiac pulse
     generator
   C.-G. pacemaker
Chardack Medtronic pacemaker
CHARGE
   coloboma, heart anomaly, choanal
   atresia, retardation, and genital and
   ear anomalies
     CHARGE association
     CHARGE syndrome
charge-coupled device transducer
charge time
Charles procedure
Charlson comorbidity index
Charnley
   C. drain tube
   C. suction drain
Chasers
   Scot-Tussin DM Cough C.
Chassaignac axillary muscle
Chaussier tube
CHB
   complete heart block
CHC
   Canadian Heart Classification
CHD
   coronary heart disease
Chealamide
Check-Flo introducer
Checklist
   Hopkins symptom C.
check-valve sheath
cheese
   c. worker's lung
   c. worker's lung disease
cheesy
   c. bronchitis
   c. pneumonia
chelator
   iron c.
chelonae
   Mycobacterium c.
Chemetron HR-1 Humidity Center

chemical
   c. bronchiectasis
   c. cardioversion
   c. exposure
   c. pleurodesis
   c. pneumonitis
   c. stimulus
chemiluminescence
chemoattractant
chemodectoma
Chemo-Port
   C.-P. catheter
   C.-P. perivena catheter system
     device
chemoprophylaxis
   secondary c.
chemoreceptor reflex
chemosis
chemotactic cytokine
chemotaxis
   eosinophilic c.
chemotherapeutic
   c. agent
   c. index
chemotherapy
   antimycobacterial c.
   antituberculous c.
   tuberculous c.
chemotoxin
Cheracol
cherry angioma
cherry-picking procedure
chest
   alar c.
   barrel-shaped c.
   c. bellows
   blast c.
   c. cage
   cobbler's c.
   c. compression
   c. cuirass
   dirty c.
   dropsy c.
   emphysematous c.
   empyema of c.
   flail c.
   foveated c.
   funnel c.
   keeled c.
   c. leads
   c. and left arm (CL)
   noisy c.
   c. pain

paralytic c.
c. percussion
c. percussion and vibration
phthinoid c.
pigeon c.
c. port
c. PT
pterygoid c.
quiet c.
c. and right arm (CR)
c. roentgenogram
c. shield
tetrahedon c.
c. thump
c. tightness
c. tube
c. wall
c. x-ray
Chevalier
    C. Jackson bronchoscope
    C. Jackson tracheal tube
Cheyne-Stokes
    C.-S. asthma
    C.-S. breathing
    C.-S. respiration
    C.-S. sign
CHF
    congestive heart failure
Chiari
    C. network
    C. syndrome
Chiari-Budd syndrome
Chiba needle
chicken fat clot
chicken-wire myocardial cell
child-adult-mist (CAM)
Child classification
childhood tuberculosis
Children's
    C. Hold
    C. Motrin Suspension
    C. Silfedrine
Childs Cardio-Cuff
chimeric
    c. 7E3 Fab (c7E3 Fab)
Chinese restaurant syndrome
chi-square test

Chlamydia
    C. pneumonia
    C. pneumoniae
    C. psittaci
    C. trachomatis
chlamydial
Chlo-Amine Oral
chlorambucil
chloramine-T technique
chloramphenicol
Chlorate Oral
chlordiazepoxide
chloride
    ammonium c.
    Anectine C.
    bethanechol c.
    calcium c.
    cesium c.
    edrophonium c.
    c. ion
    methacholine c.
    polyvinyl c. (PVC)
    potassium c. (KCl)
    succinylcholine c.
    sweat c.
    triphenyl tetrazolium c. (TTC)
    tubocurarine c.
    vinyl c.
    xenon c. (XeCl)
chlorine
chloromethylether
Chloromycetin
Chloroptic Ophthalmic
chloroquine
    c. phosphate
chlorothiazide
    c. and methyldopa
    c. and reserpine
chlorotica
    aorta c.
chlorotic phlebitis
chlorpheniramine
    hydrocodone and c.
    c. maleate
Chlor-Pro injection
chlorpromazine
    c. hydrochloride

NOTES

chlorpropamide
chlortetracycline
    c. sensitivity
chlorthalidone
    atenolol and c.
    clonidine and c.
Chlor-Trimeton
    C.-T. injection
    C.-T. Oral
choc
    bruit de c.
choir
    vascular c.
cholangitis
    sclerosing c.
cholecystitis
Choledyl
cholelithiasis
cholera
    c. vaccine reaction
cholerae
    Vibrio c.
choleraesuis
    Salmonella c.
CholestaGel
Cholestech LDX system with TC and Glucose Panel
cholesterol
    c. cleft
    c. embolism
    c. embolization
    c. ester
    c. ester storage disease
    C. Lowering Atherosclerosis Study (CLAS)
    c. pericarditis
    c. pleurisy
    c. pneumonitis
    C. and Recurrent Events (CARE)
    c. thorax
Cholesterol-Saturated Fat Index (CSFI)
cholestyramine
    c. resin
cholinergic
    c. agent
    c. receptor
    c. response
cholinesterase inhibitor
Choloxin
chondral
chondralgia

chondrocostal
chondroitin sulfate
chondroma
chondrosarcoma
chondrosternal
chondrosternoplasty
chondroxiphoid
chorda, pl. chordae
    flail c.
    chordae tendinae cordis
    chordae tendineae
    c. tendineae rupture
chordal
    c. buckling
    c. length
    c. rupture
    c. transfer
chordalis
    endocarditis c.
chordoplasty
chorea
    amyotrophic c.
    c. cordis
    Huntington c.
    Sydenham c.
chorionic villus sampling
Chorus
    C. DDD pacemaker
    C. RM rate-responsive dual-chamber pacemaker
Christmas
    C. disease
    C. factor
chromaffin cell tumor
chromate
chromatography
    affinity c.
    gas c.
chromic catgut suture
chromium
chromogenic method
chronic
    c. aortic stenosis
    c. asthma
    c. asthmatic bronchitis
    c. atrial fibrillation
    c. catarrhal laryngitis
    c. catarrhal tonsillitis
    c. constrictive pericarditis
    c. endocarditis
    c. eosinophilic pneumonia (CEP)
    c. fibrous pneumonia

c. hemolytic anemia
c. hypertensive disease
c. hypertrophic emphysema
c. hyperventilation syndrome
c. idiopathic orthostatic hypotension
c. interstitial lung disease
c. lunger
c. lymphocytic thyroiditis
c. mucocutaneous moniliasis
c. myocarditis
c. obstructive airways disease
c. obstructive lung disease (COLD)
c. obstructive pulmonary disease (COPD)
c. obstructive pulmonary emphysema (COPE)
c. obstructive respiratory disease
c. passive congestion
c. pharyngitis
c. pleurisy
c. pulmonary cystic lymphangiectasis
c. pulmonary edema
c. pulmonary insufficiency of prematurity
c. renal failure
c. respiratory failure (CRF)
c. shock
c. stable angina
c. tamponade
c. thromboembolic pulmonary hypertension (CTEPH)
c. upper respiratory obstruction
c. valvulitis
chronicity
Chronocor IV external pacemaker
Chronos 04 pacemaker
chronotropic
c. incompetence
c. response
chronotropism
negative c.
positive c.
Church cardiovascular scissors

Churchill
C. cardiac suction cannula
C. sucker
Churchill-Cope reflex
Churg-Strauss
C.-S. angiitis
C.-S. syndrome (CSS)
chyliform
c. pleural effusion
c. pleurisy
chylomicron
c. remnant
c. remnant receptor
chylomicronemia
chylopericarditis
chylopericardium
chylothorax
chylous
c. hydrothorax
c. pericardial effusion
c. pleurisy
CI
cardiac index
CI-976
CI-981
Ciaglia percutaneous tracheostomy introducer
Ciba-Corning 2500 Co-Oximeter
cibenzoline
cicatricial stenosis
cidal effect
cifenline succinate
cigarette
c. cough
c. smoking
cilazapril
ciliary
c. beat frequency
c. movement
ciliated epithelial cell
ciliocytophthoria
Ciloxan Ophthalmic
cimetidine
Cimino arteriovenous shunt
Cimino-Brescia arteriovenous fistula
Cimochowski cardiac cannula
cinchonism

C

NOTES

cincinnatiensis
    Legionella c.
cine
    c. camera
    c. computed tomography
    c. gradient-echo MRI
    c. loop
cineangiocardiography
    radionuclide c.
cineangiogram
cineangiography
    conventional c.
cinearteriography
cinecamera
cinefilm
cinefluorography
cinefluoroscopy
cineloop recording
cine-pulse system
cineventriculogram
cineventriculography
CineView Plus Freeland system
C1-INH
cinnarizine
Cinobac Pulvules
cinoxacin
Cin-Quin
Cipralan
Cipro
    C. injection
    C. Oral
ciprofibrate
ciprofloxacin
    c. hydrochloride
ciprostene
Circadia dual-chamber rate-adaptive pacemaker
circadian
    c. event recorder
    c. pattern
    c. rhythm
    c. variation
circannual cycle
circaseptan cycle
circle
    DataVue calibrated reference c.
    c. of Vieussens
    c. of Willis
Circon videohydrothoracoscope
circuit
    aortoiliofemoral c.
    arrhythmia c.
    bypass c.

    Intertech anesthesia breathing c.
    Intertech Mapleson D nonrebreathing c.
    Intertech nonrebreathing modified Jackson-Rees c.
    macroreentrant c.
    reentrant c.
Circulaire aerosol drug delivery system
circulans
    Bacillus c.
circulating water blanket
circulation
    airway, breathing, and c. (ABC)
    allantoic c.
    assisted c.
    collateral c.
    compensatory c.
    coronary collateral c.
    derivative c.
    extracorporeal c.
    fetal c.
    left dominant coronary c.
    peripheral c.
    persistent fetal c.
    placental c.
    portal c.
    pulmonary c.
    systemic c.
    thebesian c.
    c. time
    c. volume
circulatory
    c. arrest
    c. collapse
    c. compromise
    c. congestion
    c. embarrassment
    c. failure
    c. hypoxemia
    c. hypoxia
    c. overload
    c. support system
circumferential
    c. fiber shortening
    c. wall stress (CWS)
circumflex (CX)
    c. aortic arch
    c. artery
circumoral cyanosis

circus-movement tachycardia
circus senilis
CIRF
   cocaine-induced respiratory failure
CirKuit-Gard device
CirKuit-Guard pressure relief valve
cirrhosis
   biliary c.
   cardiac c.
   congestive c.
   Laennec c.
   c. of liver
   stasis c.
cirrhotic
cirsoid
   c. aneurysm
   c. varix
cisapride
cisatracurium besylate
cisplatin
cisterna, pl. cisternae
   subsarcolemma c.
   terminal c.
citicoline
citrate
   diethylcarbamazine c.
   piperazine c.
   sufentanil c.
citrated
   c. caffeine
citric acid cycle
Citrobacter
   C. amalonaticus
   C. freundii
citrovorum rescue
CK
   creatine kinase
CK-MB
   myocardial muscle creatine kinase isoenzyme
CL
   chest and left arm
   CL lead
Cladosporium
Claforan
Clagett closure

clamp
   Acland microvascular c.
   Ahlquist-Durham embolism c.
   Alfred M. Large vena cava c.
   Allis c.
   aortic aneurysm c.
   Atlee c.
   Atra-grip c.
   Bahnson aortic c.
   Bailey aortic c.
   Beck miniature aortic c.
   Beck-Potts aortic and pulmonic c.
   Blalock-Niedner pulmonic stenosis c.
   Blalock pulmonary stenosis c.
   Bradshaw-O'Neill aorta c.
   bulldog c.
   Bunnell-Howard arthrodesis c.
   Calman carotid c.
   Calman ring c.
   cardiovascular c.
   Castaneda anastomosis c.
   Cooley anastomosis c.
   Cooley-Beck vessel c.
   Cooley bronchus c.
   Cooley-Derra anastomosis c.
   Cooley-Satinsky c.
   Cooley vena cava c.
   Crafoord coarctation c.
   Crile c.
   Crutchfield c.
   DeBakey-Bahnson c.
   DeBakey-Bainbridge c.
   DeBakey-Beck c.
   DeBakey-Derra anastomosis c.
   DeBakey-Harken auricle c.
   DeBakey-Howard aortic aneurysmal c.
   DeBakey-Kay aortic c.
   DeBakey-McQuigg-Mixter bronchial c.
   DeBakey-Satinsky vena cava c.
   DeBakey-Semb ligature-carrier c.
   Demos tibial artery c.
   Derra aortic c.

NOTES

clamp *(continued)*
Demos tibial artery c.
Derra aortic c.
Derra vena caval c.
DeWeese vena cava c.
Diethrich shunt c.
dreamer c.
Favaloro proximal
  anastomosis c.
Garcia aorta c.
Glassman c.
Glover auricular-appendage c.
Grant abdominal aortic
  aneurysmal c.
Gregory baby profunda c.
Grover c.
Gutgeman auricular
  appendage c.
Halsted c.
Hartmann c.
Hopkins aortic c.
Hufnagel ascending aortic c.
Hunter-Satinsky c.
Jacobson microbulldog c.
Jacobson modified vessel c.
Jacobson-Potts c.
Jahnke anastomosis c.
Javid carotid artery bypass c.
Juevenelle c.
Kantrowitz thoracic c.
Kelly c.
Lambert-Kay c.
Liddle aorta c.
microvascular c.
mosquito c.
Müller vena caval c.
mush c.
myocardial c.
Pilling microanastomosis c.
Rochester-Kocher c.
Rochester-Péan c.
Rumel c.
Sarnoff aortic c.
Sarot bronchus c.
Satinsky c.
Schumacher aorta c.
Subramanian c.
VascuClamp minibulldog
  vessel c.
VascuClamp vascular c.
vascular c.
vessel c.

clamshell
  c. device
  C. septal occluder
  C. septal umbrella
clandestine myocardial ischemia
clapotement
  bruit de c.
claquement
  bruit de c.
Clara cells
clarithromycin
Claritin
Clark
  C. classification of malignant
    melanoma
  C. expanding mesh catheter
  C. helix catheter
  C. oxygen electrode
  C. rotating cutter catheter
CLAS
  Cholesterol Lowering
  Atherosclerosis Study
classic angina
classification, class
  American Heart Association c.
  antiarrhythmic drug c. (Ia, Ib,
    Ic, II, III, IV)
  Astler-Coller c.
  Braunwald c. (I-IIIB)
  Canadian Cardiovascular
    Society c.
  Canadian Heart C. (CHC)
  Cedars-Sinai c.
  Child c.
  Clark c. of malignant
    melanoma
  Cohen-Rentrop c.
  congestive heart failure c. (I-
    IV)
  Croften c.
  DeBakey c.
  de Groot c.
  Dexter-Grossman c.
  Diamond c.
  Dukes c.
  Efron jackknife c.
  Forrester Therapeutic C. grades
    I through IV
  Fredrickson c.
  Fredrickson
    hyperlipoproteinemia c.
  Fredrickson, Levy and Lees c.

Hannover c.
Killip c. of heart disease
Killip-Kimball heart failure c.
KWB c.
Lev c.
Levine-Harvey c.
Loesche c.
Lown c.
Minnesota EKG c.
New York Heart
  Association c. (I-IV)
Rentrop c.
round-robin c.
Shaher-Puddu c.
Singh-Vaughan Williams
  antiarrhythmic drug c.
TIMI c.
TNM c.
Walter Reed c.
Yacoub and Radley-Smith c.
Classix pacemaker
claudication
  buttock c.
  calf c.
  intermittent c.
  one-block c.
  three-block c.
  two-block c.
  two-flights-of-stairs c.
Clauss assay
clavipectoral triangle
clear
  c. cell
  c. cell carcinoma
  c. cell tumor
  C. Tussin 30
clearance
  airway c.
  creatinine c.
  drug c.
  gas c.
  mucociliary c.
  c. technique
cleavage
  abnormal c. of cardiac valve
cleft
  c. anterior leaflet

cholesterol c.
c. mitral valve
Schmidt-Lanterman c.'s
clemastine
  c. fumarate
clenched fist sign
clentiazem
Cleocin
  C. HCl
  C. Pediatric
  C. Phosphate
click
  ejection c.
  Hamman c.
  metallic c.'s
  mitral c.
  c. murmur
  c. syndrome
  systolic c.
clicking
  c. pneumothorax
  c. rales
click-murmur syndrome
clindamycin
Clinitron air-fluidized therapy
Clinoril
clinostatic bradycardia
clip
  Adams-DeWeese vena caval
    serrated c.
  Astro-Trace Universal
    adapter c.
  Atrauclip hemostatic c.
  Autostat ligating and
    hemostatic c.
  Benjamin-Havas fiberoptic
    light c.
  cardiac retraction c.
  crankshaft c.
  Elgiloy-Heifitz aneurysm c.
  Horizon surgical ligating and
    marking c.
  ligation c.
  microbulldog c.
  Miles vena cava c.
  Moretz c.

NOTES

clip *(continued)*
    microbulldog c.
    Miles vena cava c.
    Moretz c.
    partial occlusion inferior vena
      cava c.
    vascular c.
    vena cava c.
Clip On torquer
ClipTip reusable sensor
CLM articulating laryngoscope
  blade
cloacae
    Enterobacter c.
clockwise
    c. rotation
    c. rotation of electrical axis
    c. torque
clofazimine
    c. palmitate
clofibrate
clofilium
clonidine
    c. and chlorthalidone
    c. hydrochloride
cloning
    DNA c.
clonogenic technique
clopidogrel
closed
    c. chest cardiac massage
    c. chest commissurotomy
    c. chest pneumothorax
    c. chest thoracostomy
    c. chest water-seal drainage
    c. transventricular mitral
      commissurotomy
closed-loop
    c.-l. delivery
    c.-l. device
closing snap
clostridial myocarditis
Clostridium
    C. perfringens
    C. septicum
closure
    Clagett c.
    clamshell c.
    double umbrella c.
    King ASD umbrella c.
    nonoperative c.
    percutaneous patent ductus
      arteriosus c.

    primary c.
    transcatheter c.
    umbrella c.
clot
    agonal c.
    agony c.
    antemortem c.
    autologous c.
    blood c.
    c. of blood
    chicken fat c.
    currant jelly c.
    fibrin c.
    laminated c.
    c. lysis
    passive c.
    postmortem c.
    c. retraction time
clot-bound thrombin
cloth
    Dacron c.
clotrimazole
Clot Stop drain
clotting
    c. abnormality
    c. disorder
clouded sensorium
clouding
    hilar c.
    mental c.
Cloverleaf catheter
cloxacillin
    c. sodium
Cloxapen
Clr deficiency
CLSE
    calf lung surfactant extract
clubbing
    digital c.
clubbing, cyanosis, and edema
  (CCE)
cluster-of-grapes appearance
CM3 cocktail
CMP-NANA
    cystidine monophospho-*N*-
      acetylneuraminic acid
CMS AccuProbe 450 system
CMV
    cytomegalovirus
      CMV IE-2 riboprobe
      CMV pneumonitis
CMV-IE-2

CNP
C-type natriuretic peptide
CO
carbon monoxide
cardiac output
CO oximetry
CO Sleuth
CO$_2$
carbon dioxide
arterial partial pressure of CO$_2$
(PaCO$_2$)
CO$_2$ oximetry
pulse oximeter/end tidal CO$_2$
(POET)
Coach incentive spirometer
Coag-A-mate coagulometer
coagulation
disseminated intravascular c.
(DIC)
c. factor
c. forceps
c. necrosis
c. protein
c. thrombosis
c. time
coagulative myocytolysis
coagulator
argon beam c.
Concept bipolar c.
coagulometer
Coag-A-mate c.
coagulopathy
consumption c.
disseminated intravascular c.
(DIC)
coagulum formation
coal
c. miner's lung
c. tar
c. workers' pneumoconiosis
coalescence
Coanda effect
coapt
coarctation
c. of aorta
aortic c.
juxtaductal c.

native c.
c. of pulmonary artery
reversed c.
coarctectomy
coarse
c. breath sounds
c. crackles
c. murmur
c. rales
c. thrill
CoA-set fibrin monomer assay
Coat-a-Count radioimmunoassay
coating
Pro/Pel c.
Teflon c.
coaxial pressure
cobalt
c. cardiomyopathy
c. in tungsten carbide
Cobas Fara centrifugal analyzer
cobbler's chest
cobblestoning
Cobe
C. cardiotomy reservoir
C. 2991 cell processor
C. double blood pump
C. gun
C. Optima hollow-fiber
membrane oxygenator
C. small vessel cannula
C. Spectra apheresis system
Cobe-Stockert heart-lung machine
cobra-head anastomosis
**Cobra over-the-wire balloon
catheter**
cocaine abuse
**cocaine-induced respiratory failure
(CIRF)**
cocci (*pl. of* coccus)
c. country
gram-negative c.
gram-positive c.
c. granuloma
coccidioidal
Coccidioides
C. immitis

NOTES

coccidioidomycosis
   primary c.
   pulmonary c.
coccobacillus
coccus, pl. **cocci**
Cochran test
Cockayne syndrome
Cockett procedure
cocktail
   Brompton c.
   cardiac c.
   CM3 c.
   scintillation c.
coctum
   sputum c.
code
   ICHD pacemaker c.
   Minnesota c.
   pacing c.
codeine
   guaifenesin and c.
   Guiatussin with C.
   Mallergan-VC with C.
   Phenergan VC with C.
   Pherazine with C.
   c. phosphate
   promethazine, phenylephrine,
      and c.
Codiclear DH
codominant system
coefficient
   capillary filtration c.
   damping c.
   c. of diffusion
   Pearson correlation c.
coenzyme
coenzyme A, Q, Q10
COER-24 delivery system
coeur en sabot
Coe virus
coexistent pathology
Cogan syndrome
Co-Gesic
cogwheel respiration
Cohen-Rentrop classification
cohort
   c. study
coil
   Cook retrievable
      embolization c.
   c. electrode
   c. embolization
   Gianturco wool-tufted wire c.

   c. stent
   tantalum balloon-expandable
      stent with helical c.
coil-tipped catheter
coin
   c. artifact
   c. lesion
   c. percussion
   c. sound
   c. test
coincidence detection
CO₂ject system
colchicine
COLD
   chronic obstructive lung disease
cold
   c. agglutinin pneumonia
   c. agglutinins
   c. blood cardioplegia
   c. crystalloid cardioplegia
   c. exposure
   c. gangrene
   c. ischemic arrest
   c. nodule
   c. potassium cardioplegia
   c. pressor test
   c. pressor testing maneuver
cold-induced angina
Coldloc
cold-mist humidifier
Cole
   C. pediatric tube
   C. polyethylene vein stripper
   C. uncuffed endotracheal tube
Cole-Cecil murmur
Colestid
colestipol
   c. hydrochloride
colfosceril palmitate
colic
   biliary c.
Colin ambulatory BP monitor
colistimethate sodium
colistin
collagen
   bovine biodegradable c.
   c. deposition
   endomysial c.
   c. plug
   c. (types I, II, III)
   c. vascular lung disease
collagenase

collagen-impregnated knitted Dacron velour graft
collagenolysis
collagenous pneumoconiosis
collapse
  cardiovascular c.
  circulatory c.
  hemodynamic c.
  massive c.
  c. rales
  respiratory c.
  right ventricular diastolic c.
  c. therapy
collapsed lung
collapsing pulse
collar
  c. incision
  c. prosthesis
  c. of Stokes
collateral
  aortopulmonary c.
  arcade c.
  bronchial c.
  c. circulation
  c. filling
  c. flow
  c. hyperemia
  jump c.'s
  rain of c.'s
  c. respiration
  systemic c.
  venous c.
  c. vessel
collateralization
  ventilation c.
collecting duct
collection
  expired air c.
collier's phthisis
collimation
collimator
  Picker Dyna Mo c.
  Sophy high-resolution c.
Collins
  C. bicycle ergometer
  C. Dry spirometer
  C. Eagle I spirometry unit

C. respiratometer
C. solution
C. Survey spirometer
C. SurveyTach with MicroTach assembly
colliquativa
  tuberculosis c.
Collis-Nissen fundoplication
colloid osmotic pressure
Collostat sponge
coloboma, heart anomaly, choanal atresia, retardation, and genital and ear anomalies (CHARGE)
colon
  angiodysplasia of c.
  marginal artery of c.
colonic ischemia
colonization
  airway bacterial c.
  atypical mycobacterial c.
Coloplast wafer
color
  c. Doppler energy (CDE)
  c. flow Doppler
  c.-flow mapping
  c. power angiography
color-coded flow mapping
Colorscan II
colorvascular Doppler ultrasound
ColorZone tape
Columbia S.K. virus
column
  plasma exchange c.
Coly-Mycin M Parenteral
coma
  apoplectic c.
  diabetic c.
combination beat
combined
  c. heart catheterization
  penicillin g benzathine and procaine c.
Combipres
Combitube airway
Command PS pacemaker
commissural
  c. bundle

C

NOTES

commissural *(continued)*
c. fusion
c. splitting
commissure
aortic c.
commissurotomy
balloon mitral c. (BMC)
Brockenbrough transseptal c.
closed chest c.
closed transventricular mitral c.
mitral balloon c.
percutaneous mitral c. (PMC)
percutaneous mitral balloon c.
(PMBC)
percutaneous transatrial
mitral c.
percutaneous transvenous
mitral c. (PTMC)
transventricular mitral valve c.
committed mode pacemaker
common
c. atrium
c. carotid artery
c. femoral artery
c. femoral vein
c. hepatic artery
c. iliac artery
Commucor A+V Patient monitor
communication
arteriovenous c.
interarterial c.
Communities
Atherosclerotic Risk in C.
(ARIC)
community-acquired
c.-a. infection
c.-a. pneumonia (CAP)
Compactin
compages thoracis
compartment
c. procedure
c. syndrome
Compazine
C. injection
C. Oral
compensated shock
compensating emphysema
compensation
cardiac c.
depth c.
electronic distance c.
time-gain c. (TGC)

compensatory
c. circulation
c. emphysema
c. hypertrophy
c. mechanism
c. pause
c. vessel enlargement
competence
cardiac c.
complement
c. system
complementary balloon angioplasty
complement-fixation test
complete
c. atrioventricular dissociation
c. A-V block
c. A-V dissociation
c. blood count (CBC)
c. heart block (CHB)
c. pacemaker patient testing
system (CPPTS)
c. transposition of great
arteries
completed
c. myocardial infarction
complex
aberrant QRS c.
Acinetobacter calcoaceticus-baumannii c.
amphotericin B lipid c.
(ABLC)
anisoylated plasminogen
streptokinase activator c.
(APSAC)
anomalous c.
anti-inhibitor coagulant c.
atrial premature c.'s
auricular c.
A-V junctional escape c.
Battey-avium c.
capture c.
diphasic c.
Eisenmenger c.
electrocardiographic wave c.
(QRS complex)
equiphasic c.
fusion c.
Ghon c.
HLA-DQ gene c.
HLA-DR gene c.
iron dextran c.
isodiphasic c.
junctional c.

LIP/PLH c.
Lutembacher c.
MAI c.
monophasic c.
multiform premature
 ventricular c.
Mycobacterium avium c.
 (MAC)
plasminogen-streptokinase c.
pleomorphic premature
 ventricular c.
polymorphic premature
 ventricular c.
polysaccharide-iron c.
premature atrial c.
premature atrioventricular
 junctional c.
premature ventricular c.
prothrombinase c.
QRS c.
 electrocardiographic wave
  complex
QRS-T c.
QS c.
Ranke c.
R-on-T premature ventricular c.
RS c.
Shone c.
sling ring c.
Steidele c.
streptokinase-plasminogen c.
thrombin-antithrombin III c.
transposition c.
TU c.
VATER c.
ventricular premature c. (VPC)
compliance
 aortic c.
 c. of heart
 left ventricular chamber c.
 left ventricular muscle c.
 patient c.
 c., rate, oxygenation, and
  pressure (CROP)
 c., rate, oxygenation, and
  pressure index
complicated myocardial infarction

complication
 cardiovascular c.
 groin c.'s
 c. rate
component
 bronchospastic c.
 elastic c.
 harmonic c.
 plasma thromboplastin c.
compound
 antimony c.
 c. cyst
 glycyl c.
 Hurler-Scheie c.
 Hycomine C.
 nitinol polymeric c.
compressed-air sickness
compressed Ivalon patch graft
compressible volume
compression
 c. atelectasis
 barrel-hooping c.
 c. boot
 cardiac c.
 chest c.
 c. cough
 FemoStop pneumatic c.
 c. gloves
 intermittent pneumatic c. (IPC)
 c. stockings
 c. thrombosis
 c. ultrasonography
Compression-Decompression
 Active C.-D. (ACD)
compressor
 Deschamps c.
 Freeway Lite portable
  aerosol c.
compromise
 circulatory c.
 side branch c.
 vascular c.
Compton
 C. effect
 C. scatter
Compu-Neb ultrasonic nebulizer

C

NOTES

Compuscan Hittman computerized electrocardioscanner
computed
  c. tomography (CT)
  c. tomography angiographic portography (CTAP)
  c. tomography scanner
computer
  CardioData Mark IV c.
  digital c.
  Inspiron Instromedix c.
computer-assisted diagnostics (CADs)
computerized
  c. axial tomography (CAT)
  c. diaphragmatic breathing retraining (CDBR)
Comtesse medical support stockings
conal septum
Concato disease
concealed
  c. bypass tract
  c. conduction
  c. entrainment
  c. rhythm
Concentraid Nasal
concentration
  hydrogen ion c. (pH)
  intracellular calcium c.
  minimum bactericidal c.
  minimum inhibitory c. (MIC)
  plasma endothelin c.
concentration-effect relation
concentrator
  NewLife oxygen c.
concentric
  c. hypertrophic cardiomyopathy
  c. left ventricular hypertrophy
  c. remodeling
concept
  C. bipolar coagulator
  leading circle c.
  solid angle c.
Conchapak
concordance
  atrioventricular situs c.
  ventriculoarterial c.
concordant
  c. alternans
  c. alternation
Concord line draw syringe

concretio
  c. cordis
  c. pericardii
concussion
  myocardial c.
condition
  isocapnic c.
  preexisting c.
conditio sine qua non
conductance
  c. catheter
  c. stroke volume
  c. vessel
conduction
  aberrant ventricular c.
  accelerated c.
  anisotropic c.
  anomalous c.
  antegrade c.
  anterograde c.
  atrioventricular c., A-V c. (AVC)
  A-V nodal c.
  c. block
  cardiac c.
  concealed c.
  decremental c.
  c. defect
  c. delay
  delayed c.
  c. disturbance
  forward c.
  His-Purkinje c.
  impulse c.
  internodal c.
  intra-atrial c.
  intraventricular c.
  orthograde c.
  c. pathway
  Purkinje c.
  c. ratio
  retrograde c.
  sinoventricular c.
  supranormal c.
  c. system
  c. time
  c. velocity
  ventricular c.
  ventriculoatrial c., V-A c. (VAC)
conductive coupling

conduit
    Rastelli c.
    respiratory syncytial virus c.
cone
    arterial c.
coned-down view
Conex
Conference
    Bethesda C.
configuration
    atrial sensing c.
    dome-and-dart c.
    doughnut c.
    horseshoe c.
    spadelike c.
    spike-and-dome c.
    ventricular sensing c.
confluent bronchopneumonia
congenita
    myotonia c.
congenital
    c. adrenal hyperplasia
    c. anomaly of mitral valve
    c. aortic aneurysm
    c. aortic stenosis
    c. aspiration pneumonia
    c. atelectasis
    c. central hypoventilation
      syndrome
    c. conotruncal anomaly
    c. heart block
    c. heart disease
    c. interrupted aortic arch
    c. laryngeal stridor
    c. lobar overinflation
    c. malformation
    c. mitral stenosis
    c. murmur
    c. pulmonary arteriovenous
      fistula
    c. single atrium
congenitale
    P c.
congenitally absent pericardium
Congess
Congestac
congested

congestion
    active c.
    chronic passive c.
    circulatory c.
    functional c.
    hypostatic c.
    passive c.
    physiologic c.
    venous c.
congestive
    c. cardiomyopathy
    c. cirrhosis
    c. edema
    c. heart failure (CHF)
    c. heart failure classification
      (I-IV)
    c. pulmonary disease
conjoined cusp
connection
    accessory arteriovenous c.
    anomalous pulmonary
      venous c.
    cavopulmonary c.
    Damus-Kaye-Stancel c.
    pulmonary venous c.
    systemic to pulmonary c.
    total anomalous pulmonary
      venous c. (TAPVC)
    total cavopulmonary c. (TCPC)
    univentricular atrioventricular c.
connective tissue
connector
    ACS angioplasty Y c.
    Biotronik lead c.
    Cordis c.
    Luer-Lok c.
    Medtronic c.
    unipolar c.
    Y c.
Connell airway
connexin 43
connori
    Nosema c.
Conn syndrome
conotruncal
    c. anomaly
conoventricular fold and groove

C

NOTES

Conradi-Hünermann syndrome
Conradi line
Conray
   C. contrast medium
consanguineous
consanguinity
consciousness
   loss of c.
CONSENSUS
   Cooperative North Scandinavian
   Enalapril Survival Study
consolidation
   airspace c.
   c. of lung
consolidative process
consonating rales
constant
   c. coupling
   empiric c.
   gas c. (R)
   Gorlin c.
   Hodgkin-Huxley c.
Constant-T
constellatus
   Peptococcus c.
constriction
   occult pericardial c.
constrictive
   c. endocarditis
   c. heart disease
   c. pericarditis
   c. physiology
constrictor muscle of pharynx
consumption
   c. coagulopathy
   maximum oxygen c. (VO_2 max)
   myocardial oxygen c. (MVO_2)
   oxygen c. (VO_2)
   peak exercise oxygen c. (VO_2)
   volume oxygen c. (VO_2)
Contac Cough Formula Liquid
contact metastasis
contagiosum
   molluscum c.
content
   harmonic c.
   oxygen c.
continuity equation
continuous
   c. albuterol nebulization (CAN)
   c. arrhythmia

c. arteriovenous hemofiltration (CAVH)
c. atrial fibrillation (CAF)
c. cyclical peritoneal dialysis (CCPD)
c. heart murmur
c. loop exercise echocardiogram
c. mandatory ventilation
c. pericardial lavage
c. positive air pressure
c. positive airway pressure (CPAP)
c. ramp protocol
c. venovenous hemofiltration (CVVH)
c. wave Doppler echocardiogram
continuous-flow ventilation
continuous-wave
   c.-w. Doppler
   c.-w. Doppler echocardiography
   c.-w. Doppler imaging
   c.-w. Doppler ultrasound
   c.-w. laser ablation
contour
   c. of heart
   Murgo pressure c.'s
   ventricular c.
contracta
   vena c.
contracted heart
contractile
   c. amplitude
   c. behavior
   c. element
   c. function
   c. protein
   c. ring dysphagia
   c. work index
contractility
   isovolumetric c.
   left ventricular c.
   myocardial c.
   ventricular c.
contraction
   anodal closure c.
   anodal opening c.
   atrial premature c. (APC)
   automatic ventricular c.
   c. band
   c. band necrosis
   cardiac c.

escape ventricular c.
Gowers c.
isometric c.
isotonic c.
nodal premature c.
c. pattern
premature atrial c. (PAC)
premature ventricular c. (PVC)
supraventricular premature c.
tertiary c.'s
ventricular premature c. (VPC)
contractor
  Bailey-Gibbon rib c.
  Graham rib c.
contracture
  ischemic c. of left ventricle
contraindication
contralateral
contrast
  c. agent
  angiographic c.
  c. echocardiography
  left atrial spontaneous echo c.
    (LASEC)
  c. material
  c. medium
  c. medium delivery
  negative c.
  Optiray c.
  c. ratio
  spontaneous echo c. (SEC)
  time-to-peak c.
  Ultravist c.
  c. venography
  c. ventriculography
contrast-enhanced echocardiogram
control
  axial c.
  Centers for Disease C. (CDC)
  damping c.
  gain c.
  quality c.
  reject c.
  time-gain c. (TGC)
  time-varied gain c. (TVGC)
  torque c.
  c. wire

controlled
  c. breathing
  c. coughing
  c. diaphragmatic respiration
  c. ventricular response
controller
  DOC-2000 demand oxygen c.
control-mode ventilation
ControlWire guidewire
contusion
  cardiac c.
  myocardial c.
  c. pneumonia
Contuss
conus
  c. arteriosus
  c. cordis
conventional cineangiography
conversion
  analog-to-digital c.
  pressure c.
converter
  scan c.
converting enzyme inhibitor
convex linear array
convexoconcave (C-C)
convulsion
cooing
  c. murmur
  c. sign
Cook
  C. arterial catheter
  C. County aspirator
  C. deflector
  C. flexible biopsy forceps
  C. FlexStent
  C. intracoronary stent
  C. pacemaker
  C. retrievable embolization coil
  C. TPN catheter
  C. yellow pigtail catheter
cookie
  Gelfoam c.
Cooley
  C. anastomosis clamp
  C. anemia
  C. aortic vent needle

C

NOTES

Cooley *(continued)*
    C. bronchus clamp
    C. cardiac tucker
    C. Dacron prosthesis
    C. dilator
    C. forceps
    C. intrapericardial anastomosis
    C. modification of Waterston anastomosis
    C. neonatal instruments
    C. retractor
    C. sump tube
    C. U sutures
    C. vena cava clamp
    C. Vital microvascular needle holder
    C. woven Dacron graft
Cooley-Baumgarten aortic forceps
Cooley-Beck vessel clamp
Cooley-Bloodwell-Cutter valve
Cooley-Bloodwell mitral valve prosthesis
Cooley-Cutter disk prosthetic valve
Cooley-Derra anastomosis clamp
Cooley-Merz sternum retractor
Cooley-Pontius sternal blade
Cooley-Satinsky clamp
cooling
    c. blanket
    cardioplegia c.
    core c.
    topical c.
cool mist
cool-tip laser
Cool-vapor vaporizer
Coombs
    C. murmur
    C. test
Coons Super Stiff long tip guidewire
Cooperative North Scandinavian Enalapril Survival Study (CONSENSUS)
Cooper ligament
Cooperman event probability
Cooper-Rand intraoral artificial larynx
coordinate system
Co-Oximeter
    Ciba-Corning 2500 C.-O.
    C.-O. module
co-oximetry

COPD
    chronic obstructive pulmonary disease
COPE
    chronic obstructive pulmonary emphysema
Cope
    C. method bronchography
    C. pleural biopsy needle
    C. thoracentesis needle
Copeland technique
Coping Strategies questionnaire
copious sputum
copolymer
    polyolefin c. (POC)
copper (CU)
    c. wire arteries
    c. wire effect
copper-62 (^{62}CU)
copper-wiring
cor
    c. adiposum
    c. arteriosum
    c. biloculare
    c. bovinum
    c. dextrum
    c. en cuirasse
    c. hirsutum
    c. mobile
    c. pendulum
    c. pseudotriloculare biatriatum
    c. pulmonale
    c. sinistrum
    c. taurinum
    c. triatriatum
    c. triatriatum dexter
    c. triloculare, c. triloculare biatriatum, c. triloculare biventriculare
    c. venosum
    c. villosum
coral thrombus
Coratomic
    C. implantable pulse generator
    C. prosthetic valve
    C. R wave inhibited pacemaker
Corazonix Predictor
Cordarone
Cordis
    C. Ancar pacing leads
    C. Atricor pacemaker
    C. bioptome

C. BriteTip guiding catheter
C. Chronocor IV pacemaker
C. connector
C. Ducor I, II, III catheter
C. Ducor pigtail catheter
C. Ectocor pacemaker
C. fixed-rate pacemaker
C. Gemini cardiac pacemaker
C. guiding catheter
C. Hakim pump
C. lead conversion kit
C. Lumelec catheter
C. Multicor pacemaker
C. Omni Stanicor Theta
transvenous pacemaker
C. Predator balloon catheter
C. radiopaque tantalum stent
C. Sentron transducer
C. Sequicor cardiac pacemaker
C. sheath
C. Son-II catheter
C. Stanicor unipolar ventricular
pacemaker
C. Synchrocor pacemaker
C. Theta Sequicor DDD pulse
generator
C. Titan balloon dilatation
catheter
C. Trakstar PTCA balloon
catheter
C. TransTaper tip catheter
C. Ventricor pacemaker
cordis
accretio c.
adipositas c.
angina c.
annuli fibrosi c.
apex c.
ataxia c.
atrium c.
bulbus c.
chordae tendinae c.
chorea c.
concretio c.
conus c.
crena c.
delirium c.

diastasis c.
ectasia c.
ectopia c.
hypodynamia c.
ictus c.
incisura apicis c.
malum c.
myasthenia c.
myofibrosis c.
myopathia c.
palpitatio cordis
pulsus c.
steatosis c.
trepidatio c.
tumultus c.
Cordis-Hakim shunt
cordy pulse
core
c. cooling
c. pneumonia
c. temperature
Coreg
Core-Vent implant
Cor-Flex
C.-F. guidewire
C.-F. wire guide
Corgard
Cori disease
corkscrew arteries
Corlon angiocatheter
Corlopam
Cormed ambulatory infusion pump
corneae
arcus c.
arcus lipoides c.
corneal arcus
cornealis
arcus c.
Cornelia de Lange syndrome
Cornell
C. exercise protocol
C. voltage
C. voltage-duration product
criteria
**Corometrics-Aloka echocardiograph
machine**
Corometrics Doppler scanner

NOTES

coronal
 c. cuts
 c. plane
 c. slice
coronarism
coronaritis
coronary
 c. anatomy
 c. aneurysm
 c. angiographic catheter
 c. angiography
 c. angioplasty
 C. Angioplasty versus Bypass
  Revascularization Investigation
  (CABRI)
 c. angioplasty versus excisional
  atherectomy
 C. Angioplasty versus
  Excisional Atherectomy Trial
  (CAVEAT)
 c. arterial reserve
 c. arteriography
 c. arteriosclerosis
 c. arteritis
 c. artery
 c. artery anomaly
 c. artery atherosclerosis
 c. artery bypass graft (CABG)
 c. artery bypass grafting
  surgery
 c. artery disease (CAD)
 c. artery dissection
 c. artery dominance
 c. artery ectasia
 c. artery lesion
 c. artery obstruction
 c. artery occlusion
 c. artery probe
 C. Artery Restenosis
  Prevention on Repeated
  Thromboxane Antagonism
  (CARPORT)
 c. artery-right ventricular
  fistula
 C. Artery Risk Development
  in Young Adults (CARDIA)
 c. artery spasm
 c. artery stenosis
 C. Artery Surgery Study
  (CASS)
 c. artery thrombosis
 c. atherectomy
 c. atheroma

 c. bifurcation
 c. blood flow (CBF)
 c. blood flow measurement
 c. blood flow velocity (CBFV)
 café c.
 c. care unit (CCU)
 c. collateral circulation
 c. cushion
 c. cusp
 c. embolism
 c. endarterectomy
 c. event
 c. failure
 c. flow reserve (CFR)
 c. flow reserve technique
 c. heart disease (CHD)
 c. insufficiency
 c. macroangiopathy
 c. microangiopathy
 c. microvascular disease
 c. nodal rhythm
 c. occlusive disease
 c. ostial dimple
 c. ostial stenosis
 c. ostium
 c. perfusion pressure
 C. Primary Prevention Trial
  (CPPT)
 c. prognostic index
 c. reflex
 c. resistance vessel
 c. revascularization
 c. ring
 c. roadmapping
 c. rotational ablation
 c. rotational atherectomy
  (CRA)
 c. seeking catheter
 c. sinus
 c. sinus blood flow (CSBF)
 c. sinus catheterization
 c. sinus electrogram
 c. sinus retroperfusion
 c. sinus rhythm
 c. sinus thermodilution
 c. spastic angina
 c. steal
 c. steal mechanism
 c. steal phenomenon
 c. stenting
 c. sulcus
 c. thrombolysis
 c. vascular reserve

c. vascular resistance
c. vascular turgor
c. vasodilation
c. vasodilator reserve
c. vasomotion
c. vasospasm
c. vein
c. venous pressure
Coronaviridae virus
COROSCOP C cardiac imaging system
corporeal
corpuscles
Donne c.
Drysdale c.
Hassall c.
corrected
c. dextrocardia
c. sinus node recovery time
c. transposition of the great vessels
correction
Bonferroni c.
Yates c.
correlation
Spearman nonparametric univariate c.
Correra line
corridor procedure
Corrigan
C. disease
C. pneumonia
C. pulse
C. respiration
C. sign
corrodens
Bacteroides c.
Eikenella c.
corrosive esophagitis
corset balloon catheter
Cortef
corticosteroid
corticotropin
cortisol
24-hour c.
cortisone acetate

Cortone
C. Acetate injection
C. Acetate Oral
Cortrosyn injection
Corvert
C. injection
Corvisart
C. disease
C. facies
Corwin
Coryllos
C. rib raspatory
C. thoracoscope
Coryllos-Bethune rib shears
Coryllos-Moure rib shears
Coryllos-Shoemaker rib shears
Corynebacterium
C. diphtheriae
coryza
coryzavirus
Corzide
Cosgrove
C. mitral valve replacement
C. retractor
Cosmegen
Cosmos
C. 283 DDD pacemaker
C. II DDD pacemaker
C. II pulse generator
C. pulse-generator pacemaker
Cosprin
cost
oxygen c.
costal
c. margin
c. pleurisy
c. respiration
costarum
arcus c.
costochondral
c. junction
c. syndrome
costochondritis
costoclavicular rib syndrome
costodiaphragmatic recess of pleura
costomediastinal recess of pleura

C

NOTES

costophrenic
  c. angle
  c. sulci
costosternal syndrome
costoversion thoracoplasty
costovertebral angle (CVA)
cosyntropin
Cotrim
co-trimoxazole
cottage-loaf appearance
cotton-dust asthma
cottonoid patty
cotton-wool
  c.-w. exudate
  c.-w. spot
cough
  aneurysmal c.
  Balme c.
  barking c.
  brassy c.
  cigarette c.
  compression c.
  c. CPR
  c. CPR technique
  croupy c.
  decubitus c.
  dog c.
  dry c.
  extrapulmonary c.
  c. fracture
  hacking c.
  mechanical c.
  minute-gun c.
  Morton c.
  paroxysmal c.
  privet c.
  productive c.
  reflex c.
  c. reflex
  c. resonance
  rhonchorous c.
  seal-bark c.
  smoker's c.
  stomach c.
  c. suppressant
  Sydenham c.
  c. syncope
  tea taster's c.
  c. threshold
  trigeminal c.
  wet c.
  whooping c.
  winter c.

coughing
  controlled c.
  expulsive c.
  paroxysm of c.
  quad c.
cough-thrill
Coulter counter
Coumadin
coumadinization
coumarin
  c. pulsed dye laser
Coumel tachycardia
count
  blood c.
  complete blood c. (CBC)
  differential blood c.
  end-diastolic c.
  end-systolic c.
  first shock c.
  c. rate
  second through fifth shock c.
  shock c.
  total patient shock c.
  touch shock c.
  white blood cell c.
counter
  Coulter c.
counterclockwise rotation
counteroccluder
counterpressor
  Acland-Buncke c.
counterpulsation
  balloon c.
  c. balloon
  enhanced external c. (EECP)
  intra-aortic balloon c.
  intra-arterial c.
  percutaneous intra-aortic
    balloon c.
countershock
  electrical c.
count-rate linearity
country
  cocci c.
coupled
  c. beats
  c. pulse
  c. rhythm
  c. suturing
couplet
  ventricular c.
coupling
  arterial c.

conductive c.
constant c.
electromechanical c.
excitation-contraction c.
fixed c.
intercellular c.
c. interval
variable c.
ventriculoarterial c.
Cournand
C. cardiac device
C. dip
C. needle
C. quadpolar catheter
Cournand-Grino angiography needle
Cournand-Potts needle
cove plane
cover
OxiLink oximeter probe c.
Covera-HS
Cover-Strip wound closure strips
coving of ST segments
Cox
C. organism
C. proportional hazards model
C. stepwise regression model
Co-Xan syrup
Coxiella burnetii
Coxsackie A, B, B3, B4 virus
coxsackievirus
c. carditis
c. myocarditis
Cozaar
CPAP
continuous positive airway pressure
nasal CPAP
NightBird nasal CPAP
Revitalizer Soft-Start nasal
CPAP
CPB
cardiopulmonary bypass
CPET
cardiopulmonary exercise test
CPI
Cardiac Pacemakers, Incorporated
CPI Astra pacemaker

CPI automatic implantable
defibrillator
CPI DDD pacemaker
CPI endocardial
defibrillation/rate-sensing/pacing
lead
CPI Endotak SQ electrode
lead
CPI Endotak transvenous
electrode
CPI Maxilith pacemaker
CPI Microthin DI, DII
lithium-powered programmable
pacemaker
CPI Minilith pacemaker
CPI porous tined-tip bipolar
pacing lead
CPI RPx implantable
cardioverter-defibrillator
CPI Sentra endocardial lead
CPI Sweet Tip lead
CPI tunneler
CPI Ultra II pacemaker
CPI Ventak AICD device
CPI Ventak PRx cardioverter-
defibrillator
CPI Vista-T pacemaker
CPI-PRx pulse generator
CPK
creatine phosphokinase
CPK isoenzymes
MB enzymes of CPK
myocardial band enzymes of
CPK (CPK-MB)
CPK-BB bands
CPK-MB
myocardial band enzymes of CPK
CPK-MB band
CPK-MB fraction
CPK-MM band
CPP
cerebral perfusion pressure
CPPT
Coronary Primary Prevention Trial
CPPTS
complete pacemaker patient testing
system

NOTES

CPR
    cardiopulmonary resuscitation
    cough CPR
    simultaneous compression-
      ventilation CPR (SCV-CPR)
CPS
    cardiopulmonary support
    CPS system
CPX
    CardioPulmonary eXercise
    CPX test
C1qR
CR
    chest and right arm
    CR lead
CR-10
    0 to 10 category ratio
CRA
    coronary rotational atherectomy
cracked-pot
    c.-p. resonance
    c.-p. sound
crackles
    bibasilar coarse c.
    coarse c.
    end-inspiratory c.
    pleural c.
crackling rales
cradle
    foot c.
Crafoord
    C. coarctation clamp
    C. lobectomy scissors
    C. pulmonary forceps
    C. tunneler
Crafoord-Cooley tucker
Crafoord-Sellor hemostatic forceps
Crafoord-Senning heart-lung
  machine
Cragg
    C. Convertible wire
    C. endoluminal graft
    C. Endopro system
    C. FX wire
    C. infusion wire
Craig test
Crampton test
cranial arteritis
craniocardiac reflex
craniocaudal view
craniopharyngeal duct tumor
crankshaft clip
Cranley-Grass phleborrheogram

craquement
    bruit de c.
crash technique
crassamentum
Crawford
    C. graft inclusion technique
    C. suture ring
C. R. Bard catheter
cream
    Synapse electrocardiographic c.
crease
    earlobe c.
creatine
    c. kinase (CK)
    c. phosphokinase (CPK)
creatinine
    c. clearance
Creech
    C. aortoiliac graft
    manner of C.
    C. technique
creeping thrombosis
Crego traction
crena, pl. crenae
    c. cordis
crenulated tantalum wire
creola bodies
Creo-Terpin
crepitance
crepitant rales
crepitation
crescendo
    c. angina
    c. murmur
    c. sleep
crescendo-decrescendo murmur
crest
    cardiac neural c.
    supraventricular c.
    vagal neural c.
CRF
    chronic respiratory failure
Cribier-Letac
    C.-L. aortic valvuloplasty
    balloon
    C.-L. catheter
Cribier method
Cricket
    C. pulse oximetry monitor
    C. recording pulse oximeter
cricopharyngeal achalasia syndrome
cricothyroid artery
cricotracheotomy

cri-du-chat syndrome
Crile
    C. clamp
    C. tip occluder
Crile-Duval lung-grasping forceps
crimper
crisis, pl. crises
    anaphylactic c.
    bronchial c.
    cardiac c.
    hypertensive c.
    laryngeal c.
    myasthenic c.
    pharyngeal c.
    sickle cell c.
    thoracic c.
Crisp aneurysm
crisscross
    c. atrioventricular valve
    c. heart
    c. heart malposition
crista
    c. supraventricularis
    c. terminalis
criteria, sing. criterion
    Airlie House c.
    Akaike information c.
    Allen-Brown c.
    Billingham c.
    Bogalusa c.
    Casale-Devereux c.
    Cornell voltage-duration
      product c.
    Dallas c.
    Eagle c.
    Estes EKG c.
    exclusion c.
    Gubner-Ungerleider voltage c.
    Heath-Edwards c.
    Jones c.
    12-lead voltage-duration
      product c.
    Penn Convention c.
    pseudodisappearance criterion
    Ratliff c. for c.
    Rautaharju ECG c.
    Romhilt-Estes point score c.

    Sokolow-Lyon voltage c.
    voltage c.
    Wilks lambda criterion
critical
    C. Care ventilator
    c. coupling interval
    c. flicker frequency
    c. flicker fusion
    c. rate
Criticare
    C. $ETCO_2$ multigas analyzer
    C. $ETCO_2/SpO_2$ monitor
    C. pulse oximeter
CritiCath thermodilution catheter
Critikon
    C. automated blood pressure
      cuff
    C. balloon temporary pacing
      catheter
    C. balloon thermodilution
      catheter
    C. balloon-tipped end-hole
      catheter
    C. balloon wedge pressure
      catheter
    C. guidewire
    C. pressure infuser
crochetage pattern
Crocq disease
Croften classification
Crolom Ophthalmic Solution
cromakalim
cromolyn
    c. sodium
Cronassial
CROP
    compliance, rate, oxygenation, and
    pressure
    CROP index
cross
    c. femoral-femoral bypass
    yellow c.
crossbridge
    actin-myosin c.
cross-clamp
    aortic c.-c.
    c.-c. time

NOTES

C

cross-clamping
crossed embolism
Cross-Jones
    C.-J. disk prosthetic valve
    C.-J. disk valve prosthesis
    C.-J. mitral valve
cross-linkage theory
crossover bypass
cross-reactive antibody
cross-sectional
    c.-s. echocardiography (CSE)
    c.-s. two-dimensional
      echocardiogram
crosstalk
cross-talk pacemaker
Cross Top replacement oxygen
  sensor
Crotalus
croup
    catarrhal c.
    diphtheritic c.
    false c.
    membranous c.
    pseudomembranous c.
    spasmodic c.
    c. tent
croup-associated (CA)
Croupette child tent
crouposa
    angina c.
croupous
    c. bronchitis
    c. laryngitis
    c. pharyngitis
    c. pneumonia
croupy
    c. cough
crowing
    c. breath sounds
    c. inspiration
Crown-Crisp index
Crown needle
cruces (*pl. of* crux)
crudum
    sputum c.
cruentum
    sputum c.
Crump vessel dilator
crunch
    Hamman c.
    Means-Lernan mediastinal c.
    mediastinal c.
crunching sound

cruris
    angina c.
crus, pl. crura
    c. dextrum fasciculi
    atrioventricularis
    c. sinistrum fasciculi
    atrioventricularis
crushing chest pain
Crutchfield clamp
Cruveilhier
    C. nodes
    C. sign
Cruveilhier-Baumgarten
    C.-B. murmur
    C.-B. sign
crux, pl. cruces
    c. dextrum fasciculi
    atrioventricularis
    c. of heart
    c. sinistrum fasciculi
    atrioventricularis
cruzi
    Trypanosoma c.
cryoablation
    encircling c.
cryocardioplegia
cryocrit
Cryo/Cuff pressure boot
Cryo-Cut microtome
cryofrigitronics
cryoglobulinemia
CryoLife
    C. Single Step dilution method
Cryolife valve graft
cryoprecipitate
cryopreservation
cryopreserved
    c. heart valve allograft
    c. homograft valve
    c. human aortic allograft
    c. vein
cryoprobe
    DATE c.
    ERBE c.
    MST c.
    Spembly c.
cryoprotectant
cryosurgical technique
CryoVein saphenous vein allograft
cryococcal
    c. myocarditis
cryptococcosis

Cryptococcus
    C. histolyticus
    C. neoformans
cryptogenic fibrosing alveolitis (CFA)
cryptophthalmos syndrome
cryptosporidiosis
Cryptosporidium
crystal
    asthma c.'s
    Charcot-Leyden c.'s
    LZT c.
    sonomicrometer
      piezoelectric c.'s
crystalloid
    c. cardioplegic solution
    c. fluid
    c. potassium cardioplegia
    c. prime
Crysticillin A.S. injection
Crystodigin   (\S-0\S)
CSBF
    coronary sinus blood flow
CSE
    cross-sectional echocardiography
CSFI
    Cholesterol-Saturated Fat Index
CSS
    Churg-Strauss syndrome
CSVT
    central splanchnic venous
      thrombosis
CT
    cardiothoracic ratio
    computed tomography
      high-resolution CT (HRCT)
      CT scan
      thin-section CT
CTAP
    computed tomography angiographic
      portography
CTEPH
    chronic thromboembolic pulmonary
      hypertension
cTn-I assay
CTR
    cardiothoracic ratio

CTS
    cardiothoracic surgery
C-type natriuretic peptide (CNP)
CU
    copper
^{62}CU
    copper-62
cuff
    antimicrobial catheter c.
    aortic c.
    Astropulse c.
    atrial c.
    blood pressure c.
    Critikon automated blood
      pressure c.
    Dinamap blood pressure c.
    Finapres finger c.
    finger c.
    Fome C.
    c. plethysmography
    pneumatic c.
    c. sign
    c. test
    tracheostomy c.
cuffed
    c. endotracheal tube
    c. hypertension
    c. tracheostomy tube
cuffing
    peribronchial c.
cuirass
    chest c.
    c. jacket
    c. respirator
    tabetic c.
    c. ventilator
cuirasse
    cor en c.
culbertsoni
    Acanthamoeba c.
culprit
    c. lesion
    c. lesion angioplasty
culture-negative endocarditis
Cunninghamella
cup
    Ster-O$_2$-Mist ultrasonic c.

NOTES

cupping artifact
cuprophane membrane
cupula
    c. of pleura
    pleural c.
curare
curette
Curosurf
Curracino-Silverman syndrome
currant
    c. jelly clot
    c. jelly sputum
    c. jelly thrombus
current
    alternating c. (AC)
    bioelectric c.
    diastolic c.
    direct c. (DC)
    fast sodium c.
    K c.
    low energy direct c. (LEDC)
    membrane c.
    pseudoalternating c.
    pump c.
    radiofrequency c. (RFC)
    range-alternating c.
    systolic c.
    toxin-insensitive c.
    transient inward c.
    transsarcolemmal calcium c.
Curretab Oral
Curry needle
Curschmann spirals
curse
    Ondine c.
curve
    actuarial survival c.
    A-H c.
    ascorbate dilution c.
    carbon dioxide dissociation c.
    dissociation c.
    dye-dilution c.
    Frank-Starling c.
    function c.
    green dye c.
    hemoglobin-oxygen
      dissociation c.
    indocyanine dilution c.
    intracardiac pressure c.
    J c.
    Kaplan-Meier event-free
      survival c.

    left ventricular pressure-
      volume c.
    length-active tension c.
    nitrogen c.
    oxygen dissociation c.
    oxyhemoglobin dissociation c.
    pressure-natriuresis c.
    pressure-volume c.
    pulse c.
    single-breath nitrogen c.
    Starling c.
    time-activity c.
    venous return c.
    venovenous dye dilution c.
    ventricular function c.
    volume-time c.
curved J-exchange wire
Curvularia
    C. lunata
CUSA
    Cavitron ultrasonic surgical aspirator
CUSALap device
Cushing
    C. forceps
    C. pressure response
    C. reflex
    C. syndrome
    C. triad
cushingoid
    c. facies
cushion
    atrioventricular canal c.
    cardiac c.
    coronary c.
    endocardial c.
cusp
    accessory c.
    aortic c.
    c. billowing
    conjoined c.
    coronary c.
    c. degeneration
    c. eversion
    c. fenestration
    fish-mouth c.
    c. motion
    noncoronary c.
cut
    coronal c.'s
    c. point
    sagittal c.'s
cutaneous
    c. asthma

c. hyperesthesia
c. thoracic patch electrode
cutdown
arterial c.
brachial artery c.
c. catheter
c. technique
venous c.
Cutinova Hydro dressing
cutis
c. laxa
c. laxa syndrome
tuberculosis c.
Cutler-Ederer method
cutpoint
Cutter aortic valve prosthesis
Cutter-Smeloff
C.-S. aortic valve prosthesis
C.-S. disk valve
C.-S. mitral valve
cuvette
dye c.
Cuvier
canal of C.
duct of C.
CVA
cerebrovascular accident
costovertebral angle
CVC
central venous catheter
CVD
cardiovascular disease
C-VEST radiation detector system
CVIS
CVIS imaging device
CVIS InterTherapy intravascular
ultrasound system
CVP
central venous pressure
CVP line
CVR
cerebrovascular resistance
c-v systolic wave
CVVH
continuous venovenous
hemofiltration
CV wave of jugular venous pulse

CWI
cardiac work index
CWS
circumferential wall stress
CX
circumflex
2-cyanoacrylate
isobutyl -c.
cyanochroic, cyanochrous
cyanogen bromide method
cyanosed
cyanosis
autotoxic c.
central c.
circumoral c.
edema, clubbing, and c. (ECC)
false c.
hereditary
methemoglobinemic c.
late c.
c. of nail beds
peripheral c.
pulmonary c.
c. retinae
shunt c.
tardive c.
cyanotic
c. asphyxia
c. atrophy of liver
c. atrophy of the liver
c. heart defect
cyanotica
asphyxia c.
Cyberlith
C. multiprogrammable pulse
generator
C. pacemaker
Cybertach
C. automatic-burst atrial
pacemaker
C. 60 bipolar pacemaker
Cybex isokinetic dynamometer
Cyclan
cyclandelate
cyclase
adenylate c.

C

NOTES

135

cyclase *(continued)*
 cell membrane-bound
  adenylate c.
 guanylate c.
cycle
 cardiac c.
 circannual c.
 circaseptan c.
 citric acid c.
 forced c.
 isometric period of cardiac c.
 Krebs c.
 c. length
 c. length alternans
 c. length alternation
 c. length window
 moiety-conserved c.
 restored c.
 returning c.
 RR c.
 short-long-short c.
 sound wave c.
 Wenckebach c.
cyclic
 c. adenosine monophosphate
  (cAMP)
 c. guanosine monophosphate
  (cGMP)
 c. nucleotide adenosine
  monophosphate
 c. respiration
cycloergometer
 Mijnhard electrical c.
cyclooxygenase
 c.-o. inhibitor
cyclooxygenase-lipoxygenase blocking
 agent BW755C
cyclopenthiazide
cyclophosphamide
cyclopropane
cycloserine
Cyclospasmol
cyclosporin A
cyclosporine
cyclothiazide
cyclotron
cyclotron-produced F-18
 fluorodeoxyglucose
Cycrin Oral
CYFRA 21-1 tumor marker
Cyklokapron
 C. injection
 C. Oral

cylindrical bronchiectasis
cylindroid aneurysm
Cynosar catheter
cyproheptadine
 c. hydrochloride
Cyriax syndrome
cyst
 aneurysmal bone c.
 apoplectic c.
 bronchial c.
 bronchogenic c.
 bronchopulmonary c.
 compound c.
 echinococcal c.
 hemorrhagic c.
 hydatid c.
 locular c.
 loculated c.
 mucoretention c.
 multilocular c.
 necrotic c.
 pericardial c.
 renal c.
 springwater c.
 thymic c.
 Tornwaldt c.
 true c.
 unilocular c.
cystathionine
 c. synthase deficiency
cysteine
cystic
 c. bronchiectasis
 c. disease of lung
 c. emphysema
 c. fibrosis (CF)
 c. fibrosis transmembrane
  regulator (CFTR)
 c. medial necrosis
cystica
 medionecrosis aortae
  idiopathica c.
cysticercosis
cystidine monophospho-*N*-
 acetylneuraminic acid (CMP-
 NANA)
Cytadren
cytarabine hydrochloride
cytobrush
cytocentrifugation
cytochalasin B

cytochrome
   c. c oxidase
   c. P450 system
CytoGam
cytokine
   chemotactic c.
cytological biopsy
cytology
   aspiration biopsy c. (ABC)
   sputum c.
cytomegalic inclusion disease
cytomegalovirus (CMV)
   c. immune globulin
     intravenous, human
   c. pneumonitis
cytometer
   Ortho Cytofluorograf 50-H
   flow c.

cytometric indirect
   immunofluorescence
Cytosar-U
cytosine arabinoside (CA)
cytosine-thymine-guanine
   trinucleotide
cytosolic protein
cytotoxic
cytotoxicity
Cytovene
Cytoxan
   C. injection
   C. Oral

NOTES

D

D to E amplitude
D to E slope
D gate
D loop
D point
D sleep
D wave

2-D

two-dimensional
2-D echocardiogram
2-D echocardiography
2-D TEE system Ultra-Neb 99

Daae disease
DaCosta syndrome
Dacron

D. catheter
D. cloth
D. intracardiac patch
D. onlay patch-graft
D. pledget
D. Sauvage graft
D. tube graft

dactinomycin
DAD

diffuse alveolar damage

dagger-shaped aortic envelope
DAH

disordered action of heart

Daig ESI-II or DSI-III screw-in lead pacemaker
d'airain

bruit d.

Dakin

D. biograft
D. solution

Dalalone
Dallas

D. Classification System
D. criteria

dalteparin

d. sodium

dalton
damage

diffuse alveolar d. (DAD)

D'Amato sign
Damian graft procedure
damping

Accudynamic adjustable d.
catheter d.

d. coefficient
d. control

Damus-Kaye-Stancel (DKS)

D.-K.-S. connection
D.-K.-S. operation
D.-K.-S. procedure
D.-K.-S. procedure for single ventricle physiology

Damus-Stancel-Kaye procedure
dance

brachial d.
hilar d.
St. Vitus d.

dander

animal d.

Dane particles
Danielson method
dantrolene sodium
dapsone (DDS)
Daranide
Daraprim
DAR breathing system
Dardik Biograft
darkfield microscopy
Darling disease
Darox cutaneous thoracic patch electrode
Dart pacemaker
Dash single-chamber rate-adaptic pacemaker
DASI

Duke Activity Status Index

Database

Duke Carcinoid D.

data base management
Datascope

D. balloon
D. DL-II percutaneous translucent balloon catheter
D. intra-aortic balloon pump
D. system 90 intra-aortic balloon pump

DataVue calibrated reference circle
DATE cryoprobe
Datex ETCO₂ multigas analyzer
DaunoXome
Davidson

D. pneumothorax apparatus
D. protocol exercise test

Davies
  D. disease
  D. endomyocardial fibrosis
  D. myocardial fibrosis
Davis
  D. bronchoscope
  D. rib spreader
  D. sign
Davol pacemaker introducer
Dazamide
dazoxiben
DBP
  diastolic blood pressure
DBPC
  dual balloon perfusion catheter
DC
  direct current
  dual-chamber
  DC electric shock
DCA
  directional coronary atherectomy
DCFM
  Doppler color flow mapping
DCI-S automated coronary analysis system
DCM
  dilated cardiomyopathy
DDAVP
  desmopressin acetate
  DDAVP injection
  DDAVP Nasal
ddC
  zalcitabine
DDD
  dual-mode, dual-pacing, dual-sensing
  DDD pacing
DDDR pacing
DD genotype
ddI
  didanosine
D-dimer
DDI pacing
DDIR pacing
DDS
  dapsone
DE
  dobutamine echocardiography
2DE
  two-dimensional echocardiography
3DE
  three-dimensional echocardiography

De
  De Martel scissors
  De Morgan spots
  De Vega prosthesis
de
  de Groot classification
  de la Camp sign
  de Lange syndrome
  de Musset sign (aortic aneurysm)
  de Mussy point
  de Mussy sign (pleurisy)
  de novo
  de novo atherosclerosis
  de novo lesion
  de Quervain thyroiditis
dead
  d. space:tidal volume ratio
  d. time
de-aired
de-airing procedure
deaminase
  adenosine d. (ADA)
Deane tube
dearterialization
  hepatic d.
death
  apoptotic cell d.
  brain d.
  cardiac d.
  ischemic sudden d.
  late d.
  sudden cardiac d. (SCD)
  voodoo d.
DeBakey
  D. Autraugrip forceps
  D. ball valve prosthesis
  D. chest retractor
  D. classification
  D. heart pump oxygenator
  D. rib spreader
  D. tissue forceps
  D. Vasculour-II vascular prosthesis
  D. Vital needle holder
DeBakey-Bahnson clamp
DeBakey-Bainbridge clamp
DeBakey-Beck clamp
DeBakey-Colovira-Rumel thoracic forceps
DeBakey-Creech
  D.-C. aneurysm repair
  manner of D.-C.
DeBakey-Derra anastomosis clamp

DeBakey-Harken auricle clamp
DeBakey-Howard aortic aneurysmal
  clamp
DeBakey-Kay aortic clamp
DeBakey-McQuigg-Mixter bronchial
  clamp
DeBakey-Mixter thoracic forceps
DeBakey-Péan cardiovascular
  forceps
DeBakey-Satinsky vena cava clamp
DeBakey-Semb ligature-carrier
  clamp
DeBakey-Surgitool prosthetic valve
DeBakey-type aortic dissection
debilis
  pulsus d.
debility
DeBove
  D. membrane
  D. treatment
debris
  calcific d.
  grumous d.
  pultaceous d.
  valve d.
debrisoquine sulfate
debt
  oxygen d.
debubbling procedure
debulking
  d. procedure
Decabid
Decadron
  D. Phosphate
Decaject
decamethonium
decapolar
  d. electrode catheter
  d. pacing catheter
decay
  pressure d.
deceleration
  early d.
  late d.
  d. time
  variable d.
decerebrate posturing

Decholin
declamping
  d. shock
  d. shock syndrome
Declomycin
Decofed Syrup
décollement
decompensate
decompensated shock
decompensation
  cardiac d.
decompression
  cardiac d.
  d. sickness
Deconamine
deconditioning
Deconsal II
decortication
  arterial d.
  d. of heart
  d. of lung
decreased
  d. breath sounds
  d. respiration
decrement
decremental
  d. atrial pacing
  d. conduction
decrescendo murmur
decrudescence
decrudescent arteriosclerosis
decubitus
  Andral d.
  d. angina
  angina pectoris d.
  d. cough
  d. ulcer
Dedo-Jako microlaryngoscope
Dedo-Pilling laryngoscope
deductive echocardiography
de-endothelialization
de-energization
  myocyte d.
deep
  d. chest therapy
  d. Doppler velocity
    interrogation

NOTES

deep *(continued)*
    d. hypothermia circulatory
      arrest (DHCA)
    d. sleep
    d. venous insufficiency (DVI)
    d. venous thrombosis (DVT)
de-epicardialization
deer-antler vascular pattern
Defares rebreathing method
defecation syncope
defect
    aorticopulmonary septal d.
    aortic septal d.
    atrial ostium primum d.
    atrial septal d. (ASD)
    atrioseptal d.
    atrioventricular canal d.
    atrioventricular conduction d.
    atrioventricular septal d.
    A-V conduction d.
    clamshell closure of atrial
      septal d.
    conduction d.
    cyanotic heart d.
    endocardial cushion d. (ECD)
    extrafusion d.
    filling d.
    fixed perfusion d.
    Gerbode d.
    humoral immune d.
    iatrogenic atrial septal d.
    infundibular septal d.
    lucent d.
    match d.
    napkin-ring d.
    nonuniform rotational d.
      (NURD)
    obstructive ventilatory d.
    ostium primum d.
    ostium secundum d.
    panconduction d.
    perfusion d.
    perimembranous ventricular
      septal d.
    primum atrial septal d.
    restrictive airways d.
    restrictive ventilatory d.
    reversible ischemic
      neurologic d. (RIND)
    scintigraphic perfusion d.
    secundum atrial septal d.
    septal d.
    sinus venosus atrial septal d.

    Swiss cheese d.
    T cell d.
    ventilation/perfusion d.
    ventricular septal d. (VSD)
    ventriculoseptal d. (VSD)
    V/Q d.
Defen-LA
deferoxamine mesylate
defervesce
defervescence
defibrillation
    cardiac d.
    d. paddles
    d. patch
    d. shock
    d. threshold
defibrillator
    Antiarrhythmics versus
      Implantable D.'s (AVID)
    automatic external d. (AED)
    automatic implantable d. (AID)
    automatic implantable
      cardioverter-d. (AICD)
    automatic internal d.
    automatic internal cardioverter-
      d. (AICD)
    automatic intracardiac d.
    Birtcher d.
    Cadence implantable
      cardioverter-d.
    Cadet V-115 implantable
      cardioverter-d.
    Cambridge d.
    Cardioserv d.
    cardioverter-d.
    CPI automatic implantable d.
    CPI RPx implantable
      cardioverter-d.
    CPI Ventak PRx cardioverter-
      d.
    Endotak nonthoracotomy
      implantable cardioverter-d.
    external d.
    external cardioverter-d. (ECD)
    Guardian ATP 4210
      implantable cardioverter-d.
    Heart Aid 80 d.
    Hewlett-Packard d.
    d. implant
    implantable cardioverter-d.
      (ICD)
    Intec implantable d.

Intermedics RES-Q implantable cardioverter-d.
IPCO-Partridge d.
Jewel pacer-cardioverter-d.
Lifepak d.
LT V-105 implantable cardioverter-d.
Marquette Responder 1500 multifunctional d.
Medtronic external cardioverter-d.
Medtronic PCD implantable cardioverter-d.
nonthoracotomy lead implantable cardioverter-d.
ODAM d.
pacer-cardioverter-d.
d. paddles
programmable cardioverter-d. (PCD)
Res-Q ACD implantable cardioverter-d.
Siemens Siecure implantable cardioverter-d.
smart d.
subpectoral implantation of cardioverter-d.
Telectronics ATP implantable cardioverter-d.
Transvene nonthoracotomy implantable cardioverter-d.
Ventak d.
Ventritex Cadence implantable cardioverter-d.
Zoll PD1200 external d.
deficiency
acetylcholinesterase d.
acid maltase d.
ADA d.
adenosine deaminase d.
alpha-1 antitrypsin d.
Apo A-1 d.
Clr d.
cystathionine synthase d.
dopamine beta-hydroxylase d.
galactosidase d.
glucosidase d.

hexosaminidase d.
homogentisic acid oxidase d.
HRF d.
hydroxylase d.
17-hydroxylase d.
maltase d.
Owren factor V d.
protein-calorie d.
protein S d.
selenium d.
surfactant d.
thiamine d.
vasopressor d.
deficit
pulse d.
definition
Lagrangian d.
deflated profile
deflazacort
deflectable quadripolar catheter
deflection
delta d.
intrinsic d.
intrinsicoid d.
QS d.
deflector
Cook d.
deformans
arteritis d.
endarteritis d.
deformity
buttonhole d.
cervical spine d.
gooseneck d.
hockey-stick d.
joint d.
parachute d.
pigeon-breast d.
shepherd's crook d.
degeneration
cusp d.
fibrinoid d.
glassy d.
Mönckeberg d.
mucoid medial d.
myxomatous d.

D

NOTES

degeneration *(continued)*
    Quain fatty d.
    spinocerebellar d.
DeGimard syndrome
deglutition
    d. apnea
    d. mechanism
    d. murmur
    d. pneumonia
    d. syncope
Degos disease
degranulation
    goblet cell d.
Dehio test
dehiscence
    annular d.
    bronchial d.
    sternal d.
dehydroemetine
dehydrogenase
    alpha-hydroxybutyrate d.
    branched chain alpha
      ketoacid d. (BCKD)
    glucose-6-phosphate d. (G6PD)
    hydroxybutyrate d. (HBDH)
    lactate d.
    lactic d. (LDH)
    lactic acid d.
    pyruvate d.
dehydromonocrotaline
DeKock two-way bronchial catheter
Delaborde tracheal dilator
delay
    conduction d.
    intraventricular conduction d.
delayed
    d. afterdepolarization
    d. conduction
Delbet sign
deletion
    22q11 d.
delimitation
delirium
    d. cordis
    toxic d.
delivery
    closed-loop d.
    contrast medium d.
    oxygen d.
    d. wire
Del Mar
    D. M. Avionics Scanner

    D. M. Avionics three-channel
      recorder
Delmege sign
Delorme thoracoplasty
Delphian node
Delrin
    D. frame of valve prosthesis
    D. heart valve
Delsym
Delta
    D. TRS pacemaker
delta
    d. deflection
    d. wave
Delta-Cortef Oral
Deltasone Oral
DeltaTrac II metabolic monitor
deltopectoral groove
Deltran disposable transducer
delux
    Ohio d.
Demadex
    D. injection
    D. Oral
demand
    myocardial oxygen d.
    d. pacemaker
    d. pulse generator
Demarquay sign
demeclocycline hydrochloride
dementia
    multi-infarct d.
Demerol
Demos tibial artery clamp
Demser
denatured homograft
dendritic lesion
denervated
dengue fever
Denhardt solution
denivelation
dense
    d. hemiplegia
    d. thrill
densitogram
    ear d.
densitometry
    video d.
density
    echo d.
    hydrogen d.
    proton d.
    spin d.

density-exposure relationship of film
dentocariosa
   Rothia d.
dentrificans
   Alcaligenes d.
Denucath
denudation
   endothelial d.
Denver
   D. Pak
   D. pleuroperitoneal shunt
2-deoxyglucose
   F-18 -d. (FDG)
deoxyribonuclease (DNase)
   human recombinant d.
deoxyribonucleic acid (DNA)
15-deoxyspergualin
dependence
   use d.
dependency
   ventilator d.
dependent
   d. beat
   d. edema
   d. rubor
depletion
   glycogen d.
   volume d.
deployment
   stent d.
depMedalone injection
Depoject injection
depolarization
   alternating, failure of response,
     mechanical, to electrical d.
     (AFORMED)
   atrial premature d.
   diastolic d.
   His bundle d.
   myocardial d.
   rapid d.
   transient d.
   ventricular premature d. (VPD)
Depo-Medrol
   D.-M. injection
Deponit
   D. Patch

Depopred injection
Depo-Provera injection
deposition
   calcium oxalate d.
   collagen d.
   mitochondrial calcium d.
depressant
   cardiac d.
depression
   aldosterone d.
   downhill ST segment d.
   downsloping ST segment d.
   junctional d.
   myocardial d.
   postdrive d.
   P-Q segment d.
   reciprocal ST d.
   ST segment d.
   x d.
depressor reflex
deprivation
   sleep d.
Depthalon
depth compensation
de Quervain thyroiditis
derivative
   d. circulation
   ergotamine d.'s
   hematoporphyrin d. (HPD)
   purified protein d. (PPD)
Dermaflex Gel
dermatan sulfate
dermatitidis
   Ajellomyces d.
   Blastomyces d.
dermatitis, pl. dermatitides
   exfoliative d.
   livedoid d.
   stasis d.
   weeping d.
dermatomyositis
dermonecrotic
Derra
   D. aortic clamp
   D. vena caval clamp
DES
   diethylstilbestrol

D

NOTES

desaturation
descendens
  aorta d.
descending
  d. aorta
  d. necrotizing mediastinitis
    (DNM)
  d. thoracic aneurysm
  d. thoracic aortofemoral-femoral
    bypass
descent
  rapid y d.
  x d.
  y d.
Deschamps compressor
Deseret
  D. angiocatheter
  D. flow-directed thermodilution
    catheter
  D. sump drain
deserpidine
  methyclothiazide and d.
desert fever
desethylamiodarone
Desferal
  D. Mesylate
  D. Mesylate challenge
desferrioxamine
desflurane
desiccation
  mucous d.
designed after natural anatomy
Desilets
  D. introducer
  D. introducer system
Desilets-Hoffman
  D.-H. catheter introducer
  D.-H. sheath
desipramine hydrochloride
desirudin
deslanoside
desmopressin acetate (DDAVP)
Desnos
  D. disease
  D. pneumonia
Desoxyn
d'Espine sign
desquamation
  peribronchial d.
desquamative
  d. alveolitis
  d. interstitial pneumonia (DIP)
  d. interstitial pneumonitis (DIP)

destruction
  plasmatic vascular d.
desulfatohirudin
  recombinant d.
desynchronized sleep
Desyrel
detection
  automated border d. (ABD)
  automated edge d.
  automatic boundary d. (ABD)
  coincidence d.
  echocardiographic automated
    border d.
  edge d.
  manual edge d.
  shunt d.
  single-photon d.
detective quantum efficiency
detector
  ambulatory nuclear d.
  Doppler blood flow d.
  TubeChek esophageal
    intubation d.
  VEST ambulatory nuclear d.
  VEST left ventricular
    function d.
detect time
detergent worker's lung
Determann syndrome
determination
  metabolic parameter d.
Detsky
  D. modified risk index
  D. score
DeVega tricuspid valve annuloplasty
Devereux-Reichek method
deviation
  abnormal left axis d. (ALAD)
  abnormal right axis d.
    (ARAD)
  axis d.
  left axis d. (LAD)
  right axis d. (RAD)
  standard d.'s
  ST-T d.
  tracheal d.
device
  abdominal aortic
    counterpulsation d. (AACD)
  abdominal left ventricular
    assist d. (ALVAD)
  Abiomed Cardiac d.
  ablative d.

Ablatr temperature control d.
Accutracker blood pressure d.
acute ventricular assist d.
(AVAD)
Adams-DeWeese d.
Aerochamber spacing d.
AICD plus Tachylog d.
A-mode echo-tracking d.
Ange-Med Sentinel ICD d.
Angio-Seal hemostatic puncture
closure d.
arrhythmia control d. (ACD)
Arrow-Clarke thoracentesis d.
ATL Ultramark 7
echocardiographic d.
atrial septal defect single disk
closure d.
Baim-Turi cardiac d.
battery-assisted heart assist d.
bioabsorbable closure d.
BIVAD centrifugal left and
right ventricular assist d.
biventricular assist d. (BVAD)
Block cardiac d.
bovine collagen plug d.
Brockenbrough cardiac d.
buttoned d.
BVM d.
cage catheter d.
CarboMedics valve d.
cardiac automatic
resuscitative d. (CARD)
Cardiomemo d.
Cath-Lok catheter locking d.
Champ cardiac d.
Chemo-Port perivena catheter
system d.
CirKuit-Gard d.
clamshell d.
closed-loop d.
Cournand cardiac d.
CPI Ventak AICD d.
CUSALap d.
CVIS imaging d.
DIASYS Novacor cardiac d.
Digiflator digital inflation d.
directional atherectomy d.

displacement sensing d.
double-umbrella d.
Durathane cardiac d.
Elecath circulatory support d.
El Gamal cardiac d.
Emergency Infusion D. (EID)
Encore inflation d.
Endo Grasp d.
esophageal detection d. (EDD)
extraction atherectomy d.
Femostop inflatable pneumatic
compression d.
Finesse cardiac d.
Flutter therapeutic d.
Gensini cardiac d.
Goetz cardiac d.
Goodale-Lubin cardiac d.
GRIP torque d.
HeartMate implantable
ventricular assist d.
hemostatic occlusive
leverage d. (HOLD)
hemostatic puncture closure d.
(HPCD)
Hi-Per cardiac d.
HSRA d.
ICD-ATP d.
Ideal cardiac d.
IMED infusion d.
In-Exsufflator respiratory d.
InspirEase d.
Insuflon d.
intra-aortic balloon d.
intracaval d.
Kendall Sequential
Compression d.
King cardiac d.
left ventricular assist d.
(LVAD)
Lehman cardiac d.
Light Talker d.
Linx-EZ cardiac d.
Linx guidewire extension
cardiac d.
locking d.
Mediflex-Bookler d.

D

NOTES

device *(continued)*

Medtronic defibrillator implant support d.
Medtronic External Tachyarrhythmia Control D.
Medtronic-Hall d.
Medtronic-Hancock d.
Medtronic Jewel 7219D and C d.
MicroDigitrapper-S apnea screening d.
Microsampler d.
Mullins cardiac d.
Multileaf collimator d.
NBIH cardiac d.
Needle-Pro needle protection d.
nonthoracotomy system antitachycardia d. (NTS-AICD)
Novacor DIASYS cardiac d.
Novacor left ventricular assist d.
Nycore cardiac d.
Omniscience valve d.
Oxymizer d.
Penn State ventricular assist d.
PET balloon atherectomy d.
phased array ultrasonographic d.
PhotoDerm VL d.
Pierce-Donachy Thoratec ventricular assist d.
Pleur-evac d.
PlexiPulse d.
POMS 20/50 oxygen conservation d.
Port-A-Cath d.
Portex Neo-Vac meconium suction d.
Positrol cardiac d.
Presto cardiac d.
Prima Total Occlusion D.
Probe cardiac d.
Pro/Pel coating cardiac d.
pulsatile assist d. (PAD)
pulse oximetry d.
radiant heat d. (RHD)
Rashkind cardiac d.
Rashkind double umbrella d.
rate-adaptive d.
Res-Q arrhythmia control d.
right ventricular assist d. (RVAD)

Rotablator atherectomy d.
Rotacs rotational atherectomy d.
rotary atherectomy d.
rotational atherectomy d.
Sarns ventricular assist d.
Sequential Compression D.
snare d.
Sofamor spinal instrumentation d.
SomaSensor d.
SomnoStar apnea testing d.
St. Jude cardiac d.
Stretch cardiac d.
subcutaneous tunneling d.
Sub-Q-Set subcutaneous continuous infusion d.
Sullivan III nasal continuous positive air pressure d.
Super-9 guiding cardiac d.
Swiss Kiss intrastent balloon inflation d.
Symbion cardiac d.
Tandem cardiac d.
Taperseal hemostatic d.
TEC atherectomy d.
tedding d.
Telectronics Guardian ATP 4210 d.
d. therapy
Thermedics cardiac d.
Thermedics HeartMate 10001P left anterior assist d.
Thermocardiosystems left ventricular assist d.
Thoratec cardiac d.
Thoratec ventricular assist d.
tiered-therapy antiarrhythmic d.
transvenous d.
Trapper catheter exchange d.
Unilink anastomotic d.
vascular hemostatic d. (VHD)
VasoSeal vascular hemostasis d.
ventricular assist d. (VAD)
Ventritex Cadence d.
Venture demand oxygen delivery d.
VeriFlex cardiac d.
Viringe vascular access flush d.
Vita-Stat automatic d.
Williams cardiac d.

Wizard cardiac d.
Wizard disposable inflation d.
XT cardiac d.
Zipper anti-disconnect d.
Zucker-Myler cardiac d.
Devices, Ltd. **pacemaker**
DeVilbiss nebulizer
devil's grip
DeWeese vena cava clamp
Dew sign
dexamethasone
    d. sodium phosphate (DSP)
    d. suppression test
Dexasone
Dexatrim
Dexchlor
dexchlorpheniramine maleate
Dexedrine
dexiocardia (*var. of* dextrocardia)
Dexone
Dexotic
dexrazoxane
dexter
    bronchus principalis d.
    cor triatriatum d.
Dexter-Grossman classification
dextran
    d. 1, 70
    high-molecular-weight d.
    low-molecular-weight d. (LOC)
    molecular-weight d.
dextroamphetamine
    d. sulfate
    d. toxicity
dextrocardia, dexiocardia
    corrected d.
    false d.
    isolated d.
    mirror-image d.
    secondary d.
    type 1, 2, 3, 4 d.
    d. with situs inversus
dextrocardiogram
dextrogastria
dextrogram
dextroisomer
dextroisomerism

dextromethorphan
    acetaminophen and d.
    guaifenesin and d.
    Phenergan with D.
    promethazine with d.
    pseudoephedrine and d.
dextroposition
    d. of hcart
dextropositioned aorta
dextrorotation
Dextrostat
Dextrostix
dextrothyroxine
    d. sodium
dextrotransposition
dextroversion
    d. of heart
dextrum
    atrium d.
    cor d.
Dey-Dose
    D.-D. isoproterenol
    D.-D. Metaproterenol
Dey-Lute Isoetharine
Dey-Pak
DFA
    direct fluorescent antibody
D/Flex
    D. filter
DFP
    diastolic filling pressure
3DFT
    three-dimensional Fourier transform
        3DFT magnetic resonance
            angiograph
DHCA
    deep hypothermia circulatory arrest
D.H.E. 45 injection
DHPG
    ganciclovir
DiaBeta
diabetes
    d. mellitus (DM)
**Diabetes Mellitus Insulin Glucose
    Infusion in Acute Myocardial
    Infarction (DIGAMI)**

D

NOTES

diabetic
    d. cardiomyopathy
    d. coma
    d. diet
    d. gangrene
    d. nephropathy
    d. neuropathy
    d. phthisis
    d. retinopathy
    d. ulcer
diabeticorum
    necrobiosis lipoidica d.
Diabinese
diable
    bruit de d.
diacylglycerate pathway
diacylglycerol
    d. lipase
diagnostics
    computer-assisted d. (CADs)
diagnostic ultrasound imaging catheter
diagonal artery
diagram
    Dieuaide d.
    ladder d.
    pressure-volume d.
Dialog pacemaker
dialysis
    continuous cyclical peritoneal d. (CCPD)
    peritoneal d.
    renal d.
dialyzer
    Terumo d.
diameter
    anteroposterior thoracic d.
    internal d.
    left ventricular internal diastolic d. (LVIDD)
    minimal luminal d. (MLD)
    stretched d.
    total end-diastolic d. (TEDD)
    total end-systolic d. (TESD)
diaminobenzidine tetrahydrochloride
Diamond
    D. classification
diamond-coated bur
diamond ejection murmur
Diamond-Forrester table
Diamond-Lite titanium instruments

diamond-shaped
    d.-s. murmur
    d.-s. tracing
Diamox
diaphoresis
diaphragm
    dome of d.
    eventration of d.
    d. phenomenon
    d. transducer
diaphragmalgia
diaphragmatic
    d. artery
    d. flutter
    d. hernia
    d. myocardial infarction
    d. pacing
    d. pericardium
    d. phenomenon
    d. pleurisy
    d. respiration
Diaqua
diary
    event d.
    Holter d.
Diasonics
    D. Cardiovue 3400 and 6400
    D. Cardiovue SectOR scanner
    D. catheter
    D. transducer
Diasonics/Sonotron Vingmed CFM 800 imaging system
diastasis
    d. cordis
diastatic
Diastat vascular access graft
diastole
    atrial d.
    cardiac d.
    electrical d.
    late d.
    ventricular d.
diastolic
    d. afterpotential
    d. blood pressure (DBP)
    d. blow
    d. closing velocity
    d. current
    d. current of injury
    d. depolarization
    d. doming
    d. dysfunction
    d. filling

d. filling period
d. filling pressure (DFP)
d. fluttering
d. fluttering aortic valve
d. function
d. gallop
d. gradient
d. grunt
d. heart disease
d. heart failure
d. hump
d. hypertension
d. motion
d. murmur
d. overload
d. pressure-time index (DPTI)
d. pressure-volume relation
d. relaxation
d. reserve
d. rumble
d. shock
d. stiffness
d. suction
d. thrill
d. upstroke
DIASYS Novacor cardiac device
DiaTAP vascular access button
diathermy
diathesis, pl. diatheses
allergic d.
bleeding d.
diatrizoate
sodium meglumine d.
diazepam
diazotrate
diazoxide
Dibenzyline
DIC
disseminated intravascular
coagulation
disseminated intravascular
coagulopathy
DIC tracheostomy tube
dichloroacetate
sodium d.

dichloroisoprenaline
dichloroisoproterenol
dichotomization
dichotomy
Dick cardiac valve dilator
dicloxacillin
d. sodium
dicrotic
d. notch
d. pulse
d. wave
dicrotism
dicumarol
didanosine (ddI)
didehydrodideoxythymidine
dideoxycytidine
dideoxyinosine
dideoxynucleoside
dielectrography
diet
American Heart Association d.
betaine d.
diabetic d.
high-fiber d.
Karell d.
Kempner d.
low-fat d.
low-methionine d.
low-salt d.
low-sodium d.
Ornish d.
prudent d.
renal d.
salt-free d.
Sauerbruch-Herrmannsdorfer-
Gerson d.
Step-One D.
dietary
d. fat
d. salt
d. sodium
Dieterle stain
Diethrich
D. coronary artery set
D. shunt clamp

D

NOTES

diethylcarbamazine
   d. citrate
diethylenetriamine pentaacetic acid (DPTA)
diethylstilbestrol (DES)
Dieuaide
   D. diagram
   D. sign
difference
   arterial-venous oxygen content d.
   arteriovenous oxygen d. (AVD O_2)
differens
   pulsus d.
differential
   d. blood count
   d. blood pressure
   d. bronchospirometry
differentiation
   echocardiographic d.
Diff-Quik stain
diffuse
   d. alveolar damage (DAD)
   d. arterial ectasia
   d. bronchopneumonia
   d. emphysema
   d. esophageal spasm
   d. infiltrative lung disease (DILD)
   d. interstitial lung disease (DILD)
   d. interstitial pulmonary fibrosis
   d. intimal thickening
   d. lung injury
   d. paroxysmal slowing
   d. pleurisy
   d. sclerosing alveolitis
diffusing
   d. capacity
   d. capacity of lung for carbon monoxide (DLCO)
diffusion
   d. capacity
   coefficient of d.
   single-breath d.
diffusum
   angiokeratoma corporis d.
Diflucan
   D. injection
   D. Oral
diflunisal

DIGAMI
   Diabetes Mellitus Insulin Glucose Infusion in Acute Myocardial Infarction
DiGeorge syndrome
digestive system vascular disease
Digibind
   D. digoxin immune Fab fragments
   D. pneumatonometer
Digidote digoxin immune Fab fragments
Digiflator digital inflation device
Digiflex high flow catheter
Digipate
digital
   d. averaging
   d. calipers
   d. clubbing
   d. computer
   d. constant-current pacing box
   d. endarteropathy
   d. fluoroscopic unit
   d. necrosis
   d. phase mapping (DPM)
   d. runoff
   d. smoothing
   d. subtraction
   d. subtraction angiography (DSA)
   d. subtraction arteriography
   d. subtraction echocardiography (DSE)
   d. subtraction imaging
   d. subtraction supravalvular aortogram
   d. subtraction supravalvular aortography
   d. subtraction technique
   d. vascular imaging
   d. videoangiography
digitalate pulse
Digitalis
   D. lanata
   D. purpurea
digitalis
   d. effect
   d. glycoside
   d. intoxication
   d. sensitivity
   d. toxicity
digitalis-specific antibody
digitalization

digitization
digitized subtraction angiography
digitizer
 Bitpad d.
digitoxicity
digitoxin
Digitrapper
 D. MKIII sleep monitor
digoxigenin-labeled DNA probe
digoxin
 d. effect
 d. level
 Prospective Randomized Study of Ventricular Failure and Efficacy of D. (PROVED)
 D. RIA Bead
 d. toxicity
digoxin-immune Fab
digoxin-specific Fab
dihydralazine
dihydrocodeine
dihydroergotamine
 d. mesylate
dihydropyridine
 d. calcium antagonist
dihydroxyphenylalanine
dihydroxypropyltheophylline
diisocyanate
 d. asthma
 toluene d. (TDI)
Dilacor
Dilantin
dilatable lesion
dilatancy
dilated cardiomyopathy (DCM)
dilation, dilatation
 aneurysmal d.
 balloon d.
 bootstrap d.
 cardiac d.
 catheter d.
 esophageal d.
 finger d.
 d. of heart
 idiopathic d.
 poststenotic d.
 reactive d.

 serial d.
 d. thrombosis
 ventricular d.
 Wirsung d.
dilator
 Amplatz d.
 argon vessel d.
 Bakes d.
 Beardsley aortic d.
 Brown-McHardy pneumatic d.
 Cooley d.
 Crump vessel d.
 Delaborde tracheal d.
 Dick cardiac valve d.
 Einhorn esophageal d.
 Encapsulon vessel d.
 Garrett d.
 Gohrbrand cardiac d.
 Hohn vessel d.
 Jackson-Trousseau d.
 Lucchese mitral valve d.
 Maloney mercury-filled esophageal d.
 Mullins d.
 Plummer water-filled pneumatic esophageal d.
 Savary-Gilliard esophageal d.
 Scanlan vessel d.
 d. and sheath technique
 Sippy esophageal d.
 Steele bronchial d.
 Tubbs d.
 vessel d.
 wire-guided oval intracostal d.
dilator-sheath system
DILD
 diffuse infiltrative lung disease
 diffuse interstitial lung disease
DILE
 drug-induced lupus erythematosus
dilevalol
Dilocaine
Dilor
diltiazem
 d. hydrochloride
dimenhydrinate

D

NOTES

dimension
    aortic root d.
    end-diastolic d.
    end-systolic d.
    left atrial d.
    left ventricular end-diastolic d.
    (LVEDD)
    left ventricular end-systolic d.
    (LVESD)
    left ventricular internal
    diastolic d.
    right ventricular d.
dimers
    excited d.
Dimetabs Oral
Dimetapp
    D. Sinus Caplets
dimethyl
    d. hydrazine
    d. sulfoxide
dimple
    blind coronary d.
    coronary ostial d.
DIMT
    Dutch Ibopamine Multicenter Trial
Dinamap
    D. blood pressure cuff
    D. blood pressure monitor
    D. system
    D. ultrasound blood pressure
    manometer
dinitrate
    isosorbide d.
dinitrile
    pyridazinone d.
dinucleotide
    nicotinamide adenine d. (NAD)
diode
    light-emitting d. (LED)
    Zener d.
DIOS
    distal intestinal obstruction
    syndrome
dioxide
    carbon d. (CO_2)
    end-tidal carbon d. ($ETCO_2$)
    fraction of expired carbon d.
    ($FECO_2$)
    fraction of inspired carbon d.
    ($FICO_2$)
    partial pressure of carbon d.
    (PCO_2)
    sulfur d. (SO_2)

DIP
    desquamative interstitial pneumonia
    desquamative interstitial pneumonitis
dip
    "a" d.
    Cournand d.
    midsystolic d.
    d. phenomenon
    septal d.
    type I, II d.
dipalmitoyl phosphatidylcholine
    (DPPC)
dip-and-plateau pattern
diphasic
    d. complex
    d. P wave
    d. T wave
diphenhydramine
    d. hydrochloride
diphenylhydantoin
diphosphate
    adenosine d. (ADP)
5'-diphosphate
2,3-diphosphoglycerate
diphosphonate
    methylene d. (MDP)
    technetium-99m methylene d.
diphtheria
    d. antitoxin
    d. and tetanus toxoid
    d., tetanus toxoids, and
    acellular pertussis vaccine
    d., tetanus toxoids, and whole-
    cell pertussis vaccine
    d., tetanus toxoids, and whole-
    cell pertussis vaccine and
    haemophilus b conjugate
    vaccine
diphtheriae
    Corynebacterium d.
diphtherial tonsillitis
diphtheric
    d. paralysis
    d. pharyngitis
diphtherin
diphtheritic
    d. croup
    d. laryngitis
    d. myocarditis
    d. paralysis
    d. pharyngitis
diphtheroid
diplocardia

diplococci
Diplococcus pneumoniae
diplodiotoxicosis
Diplos
    D. M 05 pacemaker
dipole theory
Diprivan
    D. injection
dipropionate
    beclomethasone d.
dipyridamole
    d. echocardiography
    d. handgrip test
    d. thallium-201 cardiac
      perfusion study
    d. thallium imaging
    d. thallium-201 scintigraphy
direct
    d. cardiac massage
    d. cardiac puncture
    d. current (DC)
    d. embolism
    d. excitation
    d. fluorescent antibody (DFA)
    d. Fourier transformation
      imaging
    d. insertion technique
    d. laryngoscopy
    d. lead
    d. mapping sequence
    d. mechanical ventricular
      actuation (DMVA)
    d. murmur
    d. respiration
direct-current
    d.-c. cardioversion
    d.-c. shock ablation
directional
    d. atherectomy device
    d. coronary atherectomy (DCA)
dirithromycin
Dirofilaria immitis
dirty
    d. chest
    d. film
    d. necrosis
dirty-lung appearance

Dirythmin
disability
    cardiovascular d.
Disalcid
disarticulation
    Burger technique for
      scapulothoracic d.
disc (*var. of* disk)
discission of pleura
discoid
discontinuity
    atrial-axis d.
discordance
    atrioventricular d.
    ventriculoarterial d.
discordant
    d. alternans
    d. alternation
discrete
    d. coronary lesion
    d. subvalvular aortic stenosis
disease
    Acosta d.
    acromegalic heart d.
    acyanotic heart d.
    Adams d.
    Adams-Stokes d.
    Addison d.
    airspace d.
    amyloid heart d.
    aortic aneurysmal d.
    aortic thromboembolic d.
    aortic valve d.
    aortoiliac obstructive d.
     (AIOD)
    aortoiliac occlusive d.
    apple picker's d.
    arrhythmogenic right
     ventricular d.
    arterial occlusive d. (AOD)
    arteriosclerotic cardiovascular d.
     (ASCVD)
    arteriosclerotic heart d.
     (ASHD)
    arteriosclerotic peripheral
     vascular d. (ASPVD)

D

NOTES

disease *(continued)*
arteriosclerotic vascular d.
(ASVD)
atherosclerotic aortic d.
atherosclerotic cardiovascular d.
(ASCVD)
atherosclerotic carotid artery d.
(ACAD)
atherosclerotic coronary
artery d. (ASCAD)
aviators' d.
Ayerza d.
Bamberger-Marie d.
Bannister d.
barometer-maker's d.
Bazin d.
Beau d.
Becker d.
Behçet d.
beryllium d.
biliary d.
Binswanger d.
black lung d.
blue d.
Boeck d.
Bornholm d.
Bostock d.
Bouillaud d.
Bouveret d.
Bright d.
Brill-Zinsser d.
Buerger d.
Bürger-Grütz d.
Buschke d.
Busse-Buschke d.
caisson d.
California d.
carcinoid heart d.
carcinoid valve d.
cardiovascular d. (CVD)
carotid artery d.
carotid occlusive d.
Castellani d.
Castleman d.
cat-scratch d.
Ceelen d.
celiac d.
cerebrovascular d.
Chagas heart d.
Charcot-Marie-Tooth d.
cheese worker's lung d.
cholesterol ester storage d.
Christmas d.

chronic hypertensive d.
chronic interstitial lung d.
chronic obstructive airways d.
chronic obstructive lung d.
(COLD)
chronic obstructive
pulmonary d. (COPD)
chronic obstructive
respiratory d.
collagen vascular lung d.
Concato d.
congenital heart d.
congestive pulmonary d.
constrictive heart d.
Cori d.
coronary artery d. (CAD)
coronary heart d. (CHD)
coronary microvascular d.
coronary occlusive d.
Corrigan d.
Corvisart d.
Crocq d.
cytomegalic inclusion d.
Daae d.
Darling d.
Davies d.
Degos d.
Desnos d.
diastolic heart d.
diffuse infiltrative lung d.
(DILD)
diffuse interstitial lung d.
(DILD)
digestive system vascular d.
Döhle d.
Duroziez d.
Ebstein d.
effusive-constrictive d.
Eisenmenger d.
electrical d.
elevator d.
Emery-Dreifuss d.
endomyocardial d.
end-stage liver d. (ESLD)
end-stage renal d.
environmental lung d.
eosinophilic endomyocardial d.
Epstein d.
Erb-Goldflam d.
Erdheim d.
extracranial cardiac d. (ECD)
extracranial carotid arterial d.
(ECAD)

Fabry d.
fibroplastic d.
fish meal lung d.
flax-dresser's d.
flint d.
Fothergill d.
Friedreich d.
functional cardiovascular d.
furrier's lung d.
Gairdner d.
gallbladder d.
gannister d.
gastroesophageal reflux d.
  (GERD)
Gaucher d.
glycogen storage d.
Goldflam d.
Goldflam-Erb d.
gonadal d.
granulomatous d.
Graves d.
Hamman d.
hand-foot-and-mouth d.
Hand-Schüller-Christian d.
hard metal d.
heart d.
Heller-Döhle d.
hematologic d.
hepatic d.
Hodgkin d.
Hodgson d.
Horton d.
Huchard d.
humeroperoneal
  neuromuscular d.
Hutinel d.
hyaline membrane d.
hypertensive arteriosclerotic
  heart d. (HASHD)
hypertensive pulmonary
  vascular d.
immune-mediated d.
inorganic dust d.
Inter-Society Commission for
  Heart D. (ICHD)
interstitial lung d. (ILD)
intrastent recurrent d.

iron storage d.
Isambert d.
ischemic heart d. (IHD)
Kawasaki d.
Keshan d.
Kikuchi d.
kinky-hair d.
Krishaber d.
Kugelberg-Welander d.
Kussmaul d.
Kussmaul-Maier d.
large-vessel d.
left main d. (LOC)
left main coronary artery d.
Legionnaire d.
Lemierre d.
Lenègre d.
Letterer-Siwe d.
Lev d.
Lewis upper limb
  cardiovascular d.
Little d.
Löffler d.
Long-Term Intervention with
  Pravastatin in Ischemic D.
  (LIPID)
Lucas-Championnière d.
luetic d.
lupus-associated valve d.
Lutz-Splendore-Almeida d.
Lyme d.
maple bark d.
McArdle d.
metastatic d.
Mikity-Wilson d.
Mondor d.
Monge d.
Morgagni d.
Morquio-Brailsford d.
Moschcowitz d.
moyamoya d.
multivalvular d.
multivessel d. (MVD)
myocardial d.
neoplastic d.
neurodegenerative d.
neuromuscular d.

D

NOTES

157

disease *(continued)*
Niemann-Pick d.
obstructive airway d. (OAD)
obstructive lung d.
occlusive d.
occupational lung d.
Osler-Weber-Rendu d.
Owren d.
Paget d.
Patella d.
pericardial d.
peripheral arterial d. (PAD)
peripheral atherosclerotic d.
peripheral vascular d. (PVD)
pigeon-breeder's d.
Plummer d.
polycystic kidney d.
polysaccharide storage d.
Pompe d.
Posadas-Wernicke d.
primary pulmonary
  parenchymal d.
pulmonary valve d.
pulmonary vascular
  obstructive d.
pulmonary veno-occlusive d.
  (PVOD)
pulseless d.
Quincke d.
radiation lung d.
ragpicker's d.
ragsorter's d.
Raynaud d.
reactive airways d. (RAD)
Refsum d.
Reiter d.
renal artery d.
renal parenchymal d.
Rendu-Osler-Weber d.
restrictive airways d.
restrictive heart d.
restrictive lung d.
reversible obstructive
  airways d. (ROAD)
rheumatic heart d. (RHD)
Roger d.
Rokitansky d.
Rosai-Dorfman d.
Rougnon-Heberden d.
Roussy-Lévy d.
Sandhoff d.
San Joaquin Valley d.
Schaumann d.

Shaver d.
Shoshin d.
shuttlemaker's d.
sickle cell d.
single-vessel d.
sinus node d.
slim d.
Sly d.
small airways d.
spirochetal d.
Steinert d.
Still d.
Stokes-Adams d.
Sylvest d.
Takayasu d.
Takayasu-Onishi d.
Tangier d.
Taussig-Bing d.
Tay-Sachs d.
Thomsen d.
thromboembolic d. (TED)
thyrocardiac d.
thyroid d.
thyrotoxic heart d.
transplant coronary artery d.
  (TCAD)
traumatic heart d.
tricuspid valve d.
TWAR d.
type I glycogen storage d.
Uhl d.
valvular heart d.
van den Bergh d.
Vaquez d.
veno-occlusive d.
vertebrobasilar occlusive d.
vibration d.
von Recklinghausen d.
von Willebrand d.
Weber-Christian d.
Weil d.
Werlhof d.
wheat weevil d.
Whipple d.
Wilkie d.
Wilson d.
Wilson-Kimmelsteil d.
Winiwarter-Buerger d.
winter vomiting d.
woven coronary artery d.
disintegration rate
disk, disc
  cervical d.

Eigon d.
intervertebral d.
Molnar d.
optic d.
d. oxygenation
d. oxygenator
d. spring
disk-cage valve
dismutase
superoxide d.
disodium
adenosine triphosphate d.
cefotetan d.
edetate d.
ticarcillin d.
disopyramide
d. phosphate
disorder
acid-base d.
autoimmune d.
clotting d.
endocrine d.
genetic d.
glycosphingolipid d.
iatrogenic d.
lymphocytic infiltrative d.
mendelian d.
movement d.
neurological d.
neuromuscular d.
neuromyopathic d.
panic d.
single-gene d.
disordered action of heart (DAH)
disorganization
segmental arterial d.
Disotate
dispersing electrode
dispersion
QT d.
QT/QTc d.
temporal d.
displacement
d. sensing device
display
liquid crystal d. (LCD)
Dispos-a-Med isoproterenol

Disprin
disruption
plaque d.
traumatic aortic d.
dissecans
pneumonia d.
dissected tissue arm
dissecting
d. aorta
d. aortic aneurysm
d. hematoma
dissection
d. of aorta
aortic d. (type A, type B)
arterial d.
coronary artery d.
DeBakey-type aortic d.
epiphenomena of d.
spiral d.
spontaneous coronary artery d.
(SCAD)
Stanford-type aortic d.
therapeutic d.
thoracic aortic d.
dissector
Spacemaker balloon d.
disseminata
tuberculosis miliaris d.
disseminated
d. intravascular coagulation
(DIC)
d. intravascular coagulopathy
(DIC)
d. lupus erythematosus
d. polyarteritis
d. tuberculosis
dissociation
atrial d.
atrioventricular d., A-V d.
(AVD)
complete atrioventricular d.,
complete A-V d.
d. curve
electromechanical d. (EMD)
electromyocardial d.
incomplete atrioventricular d.,
incomplete A-V d.

NOTES

dissociation *(continued)*
    interference d.
    d. by interference
    intracavitary pressure-
       electrogram d.
    isorhythmic d.
    longitudinal d.
dissolution
Distaflex balloon
distal
    d. anastomosis
    d. convoluted tubule
    d. ectasia
    d. intestinal obstruction
      syndrome (DIOS)
    d. runoff
    d. splenorenal shunt
    d. stenosis
distance
    half-power d.
    Mahalanobis d.
distant
    d. breath sounds
    d. heart sounds
distensibility
    ventricular d.
distention
    jugular venous d. (JVD)
distortion
    pincushion d.
distress
    respiratory d.
distribution
    blood volume d.
    Boltzmann d.
    stocking-glove d.
    volume of d.
distributive shock
disturbance
    conduction d.
    electrolytic d.
    rhythm d.
disulfide
    carbon d.
Dittrich
    D. plugs
    D. stenosis
Diucardin
Diulo
Diupres
diurese
diuresis
    loop d.

diuretic
    d. agent
    cardiac d.
    high-ceiling d.
    indirect d.
    loop d.
    osmotic d.
    potassium-sparing d.
    potassium-wasting d.
    thiazide d.
Diurexan
Diurigen
Diuril
diurnal
    d. rhythm
Diutensin
divergens
    Babesia d.
diversity
    antigen-binding d.
diver's syncope
diverticula
diverticulectomy
    Harrington esophageal d.
diverticulum, pl. **diverticula**
    Zenker d.
divided respiration
diving
    d. air embolism
    d. goiter
    d. reflex
division
    vascular ring d.
divisional heart block
Divistyramine
dizziness
DKS
    Damus-Kaye-Stancel
    DKS operation
DL
    double lumen
    QuickFurl DL
DLCO
    diffusing capacity of lung for carbon
    monoxide
D-looping
**D-loop transposition of the great
arteries**
DLP cardioplegic needle
DM
    diabetes mellitus
D-Med injection
DMI analyzer

DMVA
   direct mechanical ventricular
   actuation
DNA
   deoxyribonucleic acid
   DNA cloning
   DNA histogram
   human cloned DNA (cDNA)
   DNA probe
   DNA sequencing
   DNA switch
DNase
   deoxyribonuclease
DNM
   descending necrotizing mediastinitis
DNR
   do not resuscitate
dobutamine
   d. echocardiography (DE)
   d. holiday
   d. hydrochloride
   d. stress echocardiography
      (DSE)
   d. stress test
dobutamine-atropine stress
echocardiography
Dobutrex
   D. injection
DOC
   D. exchange technique
   D. guidewire extension
DOC-2000 demand oxygen
controller
Docke murmur
docosahexaenoic acid
Dodd perforating vein
dodecapeptide
Dodge area-length method
DOE
   dyspnea on exertion
Doesel-Huzly bronchoscopic tube
dofetilide
dog cough
dog-leg catheter
Döhle
   D. disease
   D. inclusion bodies

Döhle-Heller aortitis
Dolacet
dolens
   phlegmasia alba d.
   phlegmasia cerulea d.
dolichoectatic aneurysms
dolichol
dolichostenomelia
Dolobid
dolore
   angina pectoris sine d.
domain
   time d.
dome
   d. of diaphragm
   d. excursion
dome-and-dart configuration
dome-shaped
domestica
   Carinia d.
dominance
   coronary artery d.
doming
   diastolic d.
   d. of leaflets
   systolic d.
   tricuspid valve d.
domino procedure
domperidone
Donders pressure
Donne corpuscles
donor
   d. heart
   d. organ ischemic time
donor-specific transfusion
do not resuscitate (DNR)
L-dopa
dopamine
   d. beta-hydroxylase deficiency
   d. hydrochloride
dopaminergic agent
Dopastat
dopexamine
Doplette monitor
Doppler
   Aloka color D.
   D. auto-correlation technique

D

NOTES

Doppler *(continued)*
- D. blood flow detector
- D. cardiography
- Carolina color spectrum CW D.
- carotid D.
- D. catheter
- color flow D.
- D. color flow mapping (DCFM)
- D. color jet
- D. continuity equation
- continuous-wave D.
- D. echocardiography
- D. effect
- D. fetal heart monitor
- D. fetal stethoscope
- D. FloWire
- D. guidewire
- D. interrogation
- D. IntraDop
- D. measurement
- D. pressure gradient
- pulsed D. echocardiography
- quantitative D.
- D. recording
- D. shift
- D. signal
- D. spectral analysis
- D. study
- D. tissue imaging
- D. transducer
- D. transesophageal color flow imaging
- D. ultrasonography
- D. ultrasound
- D. velocimetry
- D. velocity probe
- D. waveform analysis

Doppler-Cavin monitor
dopplered
dopplergram
dopplergraphy
Doppler-tipped angioplasty guidewire
Dopplette
Dopram injection
Doptone monitoring
d'orange
- peau d.

Dorendorf sign
Dorian rib stripper
dormescent jerks

Dormin Oral
dornase alfa
Dorros
- D. brachial internal mammary guiding catheter
- D. infusion/probing catheter

dorsalis pedis pulse
dorsi
- latissimus d.

DORV
- double-outlet right ventricle

Doryx Oral
dosage regimen
dose
- nonpressor d.'s
- priming d.
- radiation absorbed d. (rad)

Dosepak
- Medrol D.

dosing
- trough d.

Dos Santos needle
Dotter
- D. caged-balloon catheter
- D. effect
- D. Intravascular Retrieval Set
- D. technique

dottering effect
Dotter-Judkins technique
double
- d. aortic arch
- d. aortic stenosis
- d. bubble flushing reservoir
- d.-disk occluder
- d. extrastimulus
- d.-J catheter
- d.-J stent
- d. lumen (DL)
- d. lung transplant
- d. pleurisy
- d. pneumonia
- d. product
- d. tachycardia
- d. triangular test
- d. umbrella
- d.-umbrella closure
- d. ventricular extrastimulus
- d. voice

double-balloon
- d.-b. catheter
- d.-b. valvotomy
- d.-b. valvuloplasty

double-barreled aorta

double-chain rt-PA
double-chip micromanometer
  catheter
double-dummy technique
double-flanged valve sewing ring
double-inlet ventricle
double-lumen
  d.-l. catheter
  d.-l. endobronchial tube
double-outlet
  d.-o. left ventricle
  d.-o. left ventricle malposition
  d.-o. right ventricle (DORV)
  d.-o. right ventricle malposition
double-sandwich IgM ELISA
double-sheath bronchial brushings
double-shock sound
double-thermistor coronary sinus
  catheter
double-umbrella device
double-wire technique
doubling time
doughnut
  d. configuration
  d. sign
Douglas
  D. bag
  D. bag collection method
  D. bag spirometer
  D. bag technique
Dow
  D. Corning tube
  D. method
down
  bradied d.
  D. flow generator
  D. syndrome
downgoing Babinski
downhill
  d. esophageal varices
  d. ST segment depression
down-regulation
downsloping ST segment depression
downstream
  d. sampling method
  d. venous pressure
doxapram hydrochloride

doxazosin
  d. mesylate
doxepin
  d. hydrochloride
doxofylline
doxorubicin
  d. cardiomyopathy
  d. cardiotoxicity
  d. hydrochloride
Doxychel
  D. injection
  D. Oral
doxycycline
  d. pleurodesis
Doxy Oral
Doyen
  D. elevator
  D. rib hook
Doyle vein stripper
DPAP interactive airway
  management system
dP/dt
  upstroke pattern on apexcardiogram
dP/dt$_{MAX}$-end-diastolic volume
D-penicillamine
D-Phe-L-Pro-L-Arg-chloromethyl
  ketone (PPACK)
DPM
  digital phase mapping
DPPC
  dipalmitoyl phosphatidylcholine
    DPPC test
DPTA
  diethylenetriamine pentaacetic acid
DPTI
  diastolic pressure-time index
DR
  dual-chamber rate-responsive
DR-70 tumor marker test
Drager Volumeter
drag forces
drain
  Charnley suction d.
  Clot Stop d.
  Deseret sump d.
  Relia-Vac d.

D

NOTES

drainage
anomalous pulmonary venous d. (APVD)
closed chest water-seal d.
partial anomalous pulmonary venous d. (PAPVD)
percussion and postural d. (P&PD)
postural d. (PD)
pulmonary venous d.
Snyder Surgivac d.
Thoracoseal d.
Thora-Drain III chest d.
total anomalous pulmonary venous d. (TAPVD)
underwater seal d.
water-seal d.
Dramamine Oral
Drapanas mesocaval shunt
drapeau
bruit de d.
dreamer clamp
dreaming sleep
dream pain
dressing
Cutinova Hydro d.
jacket-type chest d.
Kaltostat wound packing d.
Veingard d.
Dressler
D. beat
D. syndrome
Dr. Gibaud thermal health support
drift
drill-tip catheter
Drinker respirator
drip
heparin d.
Dripps-American Surgical Association score
Dristan Sinus Caplets
drive
d. cycle length
respiratory d.
d. trains
ventricular d.
Drixoral
D. Cough & Congestion Liquid Caps
D. Cough Liquid Caps
D. Cough & Sore Throat Liquid Caps
D. Non-Drowsy

Dromos pacemaker
dromotropic effect
dronabinol
droop
facial d.
drop
falling d.
d. heart
Rondec D.'s
droperidol
dropout
septal d.
dropped beat
dropsy
cardiac d.
d. chest
d. of pericardium
drowned
d. lung
d. newborn syndrome
drug
d. abuse
antituberculous d.
cardiotonic d.
d. clearance
pressor d.
sympathomimetic d.
vasoactive d.
drug-associated pericarditis
drug-induced
d.-i. cardiomyopathy
d.-i. lupus erythematosus (DILE)
d.-i. lupus syndrome
d.-i. pericarditis
drug-refractory tachycardia
Drummond
marginal arteries of D.
D. marginal artery
D. sign
dry
d. beriberi
d. bronchiectasis
d. bronchitis
d. cough
d. gangrene
d. pericarditis
d. pleurisy
d. rales
Drysdale corpuscles
DSA
digital subtraction angiography

DSE
> digital subtraction echocardiography
> dobutamine stress echocardiography

d-sotalol
> Survival with Oral d.-S.
> (SWORD)

DSP
> dexamethasone sodium phosphate

D-TGA
> D-transposition of great arteries

D-transposition of great arteries (D-TGA)

dual
> d. balloon perfusion catheter (DBPC)
> d. echophonocardiography

dual-chamber (DC)
> d.-c. pacemaker
> d.-c. pacing
> d.-c. rate-responsive (DR)

dual-demand pacemaker

duality

dual-mode, dual-pacing, dual-sensing (DDD)

dual-sensor micromanometric high-fidelity catheter

Dualtherm dual thermistor thermodilution catheter

Du Bois-Reymond law

DUCCS
> Duke University Clinical Cardiology Study

Duchenne
> D. muscular dystrophy
> D. sign

duckbill voice prosthesis

Duckworth phenomenon

Ducor
> D. balloon catheter
> D. HF catheter

Ducor-Cordis pigtail catheter

duct
> Botallo d.
> collecting d.
> d. of Cuvier
> medullary collecting d.
> thoracic d.

ductal cell carcinoma

ductus
> d. Arantii
> d. arteriosus
> d. bump
> d. thoracicus
> d. venosus

Duffield cardiovascular scissors

Duguet siphon

Duke
> D. Activity Status Index (DASI)
> D. bleeding time
> D. Carcinoid Database
> D. treadmill prognostic score
> D. University Clinical Cardiology Study (DUCCS)

Dukes classification

dullness
> absolute cardiac d. (ACD)
> area of cardiac d.
> border of cardiac d.
> cardiac border of d.
> percussion d.

dumoffii
> *Legionella d.*

Dumon
> D. bronchoscope
> D. tracheobronchial stent

Dumon-Harrell bronchoscope

Dumont thoracic scissors

Duncan
> D. multiple range test
> D. syndrome

Dunham fans

Dunlop thrombus stripper

Dunnett test

DuoCet

duodenal string test

Duo-Medihaler Aerosol

Duostat rotating hemostatic valve

Duo-Trach

Duotrate

DUPEL drug delivery system

duplex
> d. imaging

D

NOTES

duplex *(continued)*
d. pulsed-Doppler
ultrasonography
pulsus d.
d. scanning
d. ultrasound
dupp
Duracep biopsy forceps
Duraflow heart valve
Dura-Gest
Duralone injection
Duralutin injection
Duran annuloplasty ring
Durapulse pacemaker
Duraquin
Dura-Tabs
Quinaglute D.-T.
Durathane cardiac device
duration
action potential d. (APD)
d. of expiration (T_E)
half-amplitude pulse d.
d. of inspiration (T_I)
monophasic action potential d.
(MAPD)
pulse d.
Duratuss
Dura-Vent
Durham tube
Duricef
Duromedics
D. mitral valve
D. valve prosthesis
Duroziez
D. disease
D. murmur
D. sign
D. symptom
durus
pulsus d.
duskiness
dusky
dust
d. asthma
grain d.
mushroom d.
Dutch Ibopamine Multicenter Trial
(DIMT)
duteplase
duty factor
Duval-Coryllos rib shears
Duval-Crile lung forceps
Duval lung-grasping forceps

DVI
deep venous insufficiency
DVI pacing
DVT
deep venous thrombosis
dwarfism
aortic d.
Dyazide
Dycill
dye
Cardio-Green d.
d. cuvette
d. dilution technique
flashlamp excited pulsed d.
Fox green d.
indocyanine green d.
d. injection
d. laser
radiocontrast d.
Unisperse blue d.
dye-dilution
d.-d. curve
d.-d. method
Dymelor
Dymer
D. excimer delivery probe
D. excimer delivery system
Dynabac
Dynacin Oral
DynaCirc
dynamic
d. aorta
d. cardiomyoplasty
d. exercise
fluid d.'s
d. frequency response
funnel d.'s
d. intracavitary obstruction
left ventricular-left atrial
crossover d.'s
d. murmur
d. pressure
d. range
d. relaxation
D. Y stent
dynamite heart
dynamometer
bicycle d.
Cybex isokinetic d.
Dynapen
DynaPulse 5000 A
dyne
d. seconds

dyphylline
Dyrenium
dysarteriotony
dysarthria
dysautonomia
   familial d.
dysbetalipoproteinemia
dyscrasia
   blood d.
dysfibrinogenemia
dysfunction
   diastolic d.
   endothelial d.
   intellectual d.
   left ventricular d. (LVD)
   papillary muscle d.
   sinus node d.
   Studies of Left Ventricular D. (SOLVD)
   valvular d.
dysfunctional myocardium
dysgenesis
   gonadal d.
dysgeusia
dyskinesia
   d. intermittens
dyskinesis
   anterior wall d.
   anteroapical d.
   left ventricular d.
   posteroinferior d.
dyskinetic
dyslipidemia
   atherogenic d.
   Fredrickson d.
dyslipoproteinemia
dysmodulation
dysmotility
   esophageal d.
dysnystaxis
dyspeptica
   angina d.
dysphagia, dysphagy
   contractile ring d.
   d. inflammatoria
   d. lusoria
   d. nervosa

   d. paralytica
   sideropenic d.
   d. spastica
   vallecular d.
   d. valsalviana
dysphasia
dysphasic
dysplasia
   arrhythmogenic right ventricular d. (ARVD)
   atriodigital d.
   bronchopulmonary d. (BPD)
   ectodermal d.
   fibromuscular d.
   fibrous d.
   polyostotic fibrous d.
   right ventricular d.
   ventriculoradial d.
dysplastic
dyspnea
   cardiac d.
   effort d.
   episodic d.
   exertional d.
   expiratory d.
   functional d.
   inspiratory d.
   Monday d.
   nocturnal d.
   nonexpansional d.
   one-flight exertional d.
   d. on exertion (DOE)
   orthostatic d.
   paroxysmal nocturnal d. (PND)
   psychogenic d.
   renal d.
   rest d.
   d. scale
   sighing d.
   d. target
   Traube d.
   two-flight exertional d.
dyspneic
dysreflexia
   autonomic d.
dysrhythmia
   cardiac d.

D

NOTES

Dysshwannian syndrome
dyssynchronization
dyssynchrony
   thoracoabdominal d.
dyssynergic myocardial segment
dyssynergy
dystrophic calcification
dystrophin
dystrophinopathy
dystrophy
   asphyxiating thoracic d. (ATD)
   Becker-type tardive
   muscular d.

dZ/dt

Duchenne muscular d.
Emery-Dreifuss muscular d.
facioscapulohumeral d.
familial asphyxiant thoracic d.
Landouzy-Déjérine d.
limb-girdle muscular d.
muscular d.
myotonic muscular d.
reflex sympathetic d.
thoracic asphyxiant d.
thoracic-pelvic-phalangeal d.

E

E to A changes
E to F slope
E greater than A
E to I changes
E point
E point to septal separation (EPSS)
E sign
E wave
E wave to A wave (E/A)

E1

7E3

7E3 glycoprotein IIb/IIIa platelet antibody
7E3 monoclonal Fab antibody

E-4031

E-150 Breeze ventilator

E/A

E wave to A wave

EAC

expandable access catheter
EAC catheter

EAD

early afterdepolarization

EAE

effective arterial elastance

Eagle

E. criteria
E. equation
E. medium
E. spirometer

ear

e. densitogram
e. oximeter

earlobe crease

early

e. afterdepolarization (EAD)
e. deceleration
e. diastolic murmur
e. rapid repolarization

early-peaking systolic murmur

Easprin

EAST

Emory Angioplasty versus Surgery Trial
external rotation, abduction, stress test

EAT

ectopic atrial tachycardia

Eaton

E. agent
E. agent pneumonia

Eaton-Lambert syndrome

E:A wave ratio

EBCT

electron beam computed tomography

EBDA

effective balloon-dilated area

EBNA

Epstein-Barr nuclear antigen

Ebola virus

Ebstein

E. angle
E. cardiac anomaly
E. disease
E. sign

EBV

Epstein-Barr virus

E-CABG

endarterectomy and coronary artery bypass grafting

ECAD

extracranial carotid arterial disease

ECAT III positron tomograph

ECC

edema, clubbing, and cyanosis

eccentric

e. atrial activation
e. hypertrophy
e. ledge
E. locked rib shears
e. monocuspid tilting-disk prosthetic valve
e. narrowing
e. stenosis

eccentricity index

ecchymosis, pl. **ecchymoses**

ecchymotic mask

ECD

endocardial cushion defect
external cardioverter-defibrillator
extracranial cardiac disease
Ventak ECD

ECF-A

eosinophil chemotactic factors of anaphylaxis

ECG

electrocardiogram
electrocardiograph

E

ECG *(continued)*
  electrocardiography
    ambulatory ECG (AECG)
    Micro-Tracer portable ECG
    ECG signal-averaging technique
    ECG triggering unit
ECG-synchronized digital
  subtraction angiogram
echinococcal cyst
echinococcosis
Echinococcus
ECHO
  enterocytopathogenic human orphan
    ECHO virus
echo, pl. **echoes**
  amphoric e.
  atrial e.
  e. beat
  bright e.
  e. catheter
  e. delay time (TE)
  e. density
  e. guidance
  e. intensity
  metallic e.
  motion display e.
  nodus sinuatrialis e.
  NS e.
  pericardial e.
  e. ranging
  e. reverberation
  scattered e.
  e. score
  smokelike echoes
  specular e.
  transcutaneous e.
  transesophageal e.
  e. zone
echoaortography
echocardiogram
  apical five-chamber view e.
  apical four-chamber view e.
  apical two-chamber view e.
  continuous loop exercise e.
  continuous wave Doppler e.
  contrast-enhanced e.
  cross-sectional two-
    dimensional e.
  2-D e.
  Feigenbaum e.
  15-lead e.
  long-axis parasternal view e.
  meridian e.

  M-mode e.
  Ochsner-Mahorner e.
  parasternal long-axis view e.
  parasternal short-axis view e.
  signal-averaged e.
echocardiograph
  Acuson e.
  Biosound Surgiscan e.
echocardiographic
  e. assessment
  e. automated border detection
  e. automated boundary
    detection system
  e. differentiation
  e. scoring system
  e. transducer
echocardiography
  adenosine e.
  A-mode e.
  any-plane e.
  Assessment of Cardioversion
    Using Transesophageal E.
    (ACUTE)
  baseline e.
  bicycle e.
  B-mode e.
  continuous-wave Doppler e.
  contrast e.
  cross-sectional e. (CSE)
  2-D e.
  deductive e.
  digital subtraction e. (DSE)
  dipyridamole e.
  dobutamine e. (DE)
  dobutamine-atropine stress e.
  dobutamine stress e. (DSE)
  Doppler e.
  ergonovine e.
  esophageal e.
  exercise e.
  exercise stress e. (Ex-Echo)
  high-frequency epicardial e.
    (HFEE)
  interventional e.
  intrauterine e.
  meridian e.
  mitral valve e.
  M-mode e.
  myocardial contrast e. (MCE)
  paraplane e.
  pharmacologic stress e.
  pulmonary valve e.
  pulsed Doppler e.

quantitative two-dimensional e.
real-time three-dimensional e.
sector scan e.
signal-averaged e.
stress e.
stress-injected sestamibi-gated
SPECT with e.
supine bicycle stress e.
(SBSE)
three-dimensional e. (3DE)
transesophageal e. (TEE)
transesophageal contrast e.
transesophageal dobutamine
stress e.
transthoracic e. (TTE)
treadmill e.
two-dimensional e. (2DE)
echodense
e. mass
e. structure
echodensity
linear e.
superimposed e.
echo-Doppler cardiography
echoendoscope
Olympus GIF-EUM2 e.
echoes (*pl. of* echo)
echo-free space
EchoGen emulsion
echogenicity
echogenic plaque
echogram
echography
A-scan e.
echo-guided ultrasound
echolucent
e. plaque
EchoMark angiographic catheter
echophonocardiography
dual e.
echophony
echo-planar imaging
echoreflective
echoreflectivity
echoscanner
echoscope
echo-signal shape

echo-spared area
Echovar Doppler system
echovirus
e. myocarditis
Echovist
Eck fistula
eclampsia
ECLS
extracorporeal life support
ECMO
extracorporeal membrane
oxygenation
ECMO pump
EcoCheck oxygen monitor
Eco-Oxymax
Ecotrin
ECS
extracellular-like, calcium-free
solution
ECS cardioplegic solution
ECST
European Carotid Surgery Trial
ectasia, ectasis
alveolar e.
annuloaortic e.
aortoannular e.
artery e.
e. cordis
coronary artery e.
diffuse arterial e.
distal e.
vascular e.
Ectasule
ectatic
e. aneurysm
e. emphysema
ectocardia
ectocardiac, ectocardial
Ectocor pacemaker
ectodermal dysplasia
ectopia
e. cordis
e. lentis
ectopic
e. atrial tachycardia (EAT)
e. beat
e. impulse

E

NOTES

ectopic *(continued)*
 e. pacemaker
 e. rhythm
ectopy
 asymptomatic complex e.
 atrial e.
 supraventricular e.
 Survival and Ventricular E.
 (SAVE)
 ventricular e.
ECT pacemaker
EDA
 end-diastolic area
EDD
 esophageal detection device
eddy sounds
Edecrin
 E. Oral
 E. Sodium injection
edema
 acute cardiogenic pulmonary e.
 (ACPE)
 alveolar e.
 angioneurotic e.
 ankle e.
 bland e.
 boggy e.
 brawny e.
 brown e.
 cardiac e.
 cardiogenic pulmonary e.
 cerebral e.
 chronic pulmonary e.
 circumscribed e.
 clubbing, cyanosis, and e.
 (CCE)
 congestive e.
 dependent e.
 fingerprint e.
 flash pulmonary e.
 florid pulmonary e.
 focal e.
 hereditary angioneurotic e.
 (HANE)
 high-altitude pulmonary e.
 (HAPE)
 idiopathic cyclic e.
 interstitial pulmonary e.
 e. of lung
 lymphatic e.
 Milton e.
 mucosal e.
 myocardial e.

neurogenic pulmonary e.
nonpitting e.
paroxysmal pulmonary e.
passive e.
pedal e.
periodic e.
periorbital e.
peripheral e.
perivascular e.
pitting e.
postanesthesia pulmonary e.
postcardioversion pulmonary e.
presacral e.
pretibial e.
pulmonary interstitial e.
Quincke e.
sacral e.
stasis e.
subpleural e.
tense e.
terminal e.
vasogenic e.
woody e.
edema, clubbing, and cyanosis
 (ECC)
edematous
Eder-Hufford esophagoscope
Eder-Puestow wire
edetate disodium
edge
 e. detection
 leading e.
 trailing e.
edge-detection method
EDHF
 endothelium-derived hyperpolarizing
 factor
Edmark
 E. mitral valve
 E. monophasic waveform
EDM infusion catheter
EDP
 end-diastolic pressure
EDRF
 endothelium-derived relaxing factor
edrophonium
 e. chloride
EDTA
 ethylenediaminetetraacetic acid
EDV
 end-diastolic volume
EDVI
 end-diastolic volume index

Edwards
  E. catheter
  E. heart valve
  E. septectomy
  E. Teflon intracardiac patch
    prosthesis
  E. woven Teflon aortic
    bifurcation graft
**Edwards-Carpentier aortic valve
  brush**
**Edwards-Duromedics bileaflet heart
  valve**
Edwards-Tapp arterial graft
EECP
  enhanced external counterpulsation
EEG
  electroencephalogram
  electroencephalograph
  electroencephalography
E.E.S. Oral
EF
  ejection fraction
Efedron
efegatran
effect
  Anrep e.
  Bainbridge e.
  band saw e.
  blooming e.
  Bowditch staircase e.
  Brockenbrough e.
  cidal e.
  Coanda e.
  Compton e.
  copper wire e.
  digitalis e.
  digoxin e.
  Doppler e.
  Dotter e.
  dottering e.
  dromotropic e.
  erectile e.
  founder e.
  horse-race e.
  inotropic e.
  jet e.
  late proarrhythmic e.

  mille-feuilles e.
  neurotoxic e.
  nonhemodynamic e.
  Prinzmetal e.
  proarrhythmic e.
  proto-oncogenic e.
  Rivero-Carvallo e.
  silver-wire e.
  snowplow e.
  squeeze e.
  training e.
  Vaughan Williams class e.
  Venturi e.
  Wedensky e.
  Windkessel e.
effective
  e. arterial elastance (EAE)
  e. balloon-dilated area (EBDA)
  e. circulating blood volume
  e. refractory period (ERP)
  e. regurgitant orifice
  e. renal blood flow (ERBF)
effector cells
efferent
  e. arteriole
  e. artery
Efficacy
  Acute Infarction Ramipril E.
    (AIRE)
  Late Assessment of
    Thrombolytic E. (LATE)
efficiency
  detective quantum e.
Effler
  E. hiatal hernia repair
  E. tack
**Effler-Groves mode of Allison
  procedure**
effort
  e. angina
  e. dyspnea
  first e.
  e. syndrome
effort-induced thrombosis
effusion
  chyliform pleural e.
  chylous pericardial e.

E

NOTES

173

effusion *(continued)*
   exudative pleural e.
   malignant pleural e.
   parapneumonic e.
   pericardial e.
   pleural e.
   pulmonary e.
   silent pericardial e.
   transudative pleural e.
effusive-constrictive
   e.-c. disease
   e.-c. pericarditis
Efidac/24
eflornithine
Efron jackknife classification
Efudex Topical
eggcrate mattress
Eggleston method
egg-shaped heart
eggshell pattern
egg-yellow reaction
egg-yolk sputum
egobronchophony
egophony
Ehlers-Danlos syndrome
Ehret phenomenon
ehrlichiosis
EIA
   enzyme immunoassay
   exercise-induced asthma
Eicken method
eicosanoid excretion
eicosapentaenoic acid (EPA)
EID
   Emergency Infusion Device
   EID catheter
Eidemiller tunneler
eight-lumen manometry catheter
Eigon
   E. CardioLoop recorder
   E. disk
Eikenella
   E. corrodens
Einhorn esophageal dilator
Einthoven
   E. equation
   E. law
   E. lead
   E. string galvanometer
   E. triangle
E:I ratio
Eisenmenger
   E. complex

   E. disease
   E. reaction
   E. syndrome
   E. tetralogy
   E. VSD
ejection
   e. click
   e. fraction (EF)
   e. murmur
   e. period
   e. phase
   e. phase index
   e. rate
   e. shell image
   e. sounds (ES)
   e. time
   e. velocity
ejection-fraction image
Ejrup maneuver
EKG
   electrocardiogram
   baseline EKG
   borderline EKG
   EKG leads I, II, III; V1
      through V6; aVF, aVL, aVR
   Micro-Tracer portable EKG
   Minnesota classification of
      EKG
   EKG monitor strip
   EKG silence
   straight-line EKG
EKY
   electrokymogram
El
   E. Gamal cardiac device
   E. Gamal coronary bypass
      catheter
   E. Gamal guiding catheter
Ela
   E. Chorus DDD pacemaker
   E. ventricular pacing lead
E-LAM
   endothelium-leukocyte adhesion
      molecule
Elantan
elastance
   effective arterial e. (EAE)
   end-systolic e.
   maximum ventricular e.
      (Emax)
elastase
   leukocyte e.

neutrophil e.
Pseudomonas e.
elastic
    e. component
    e. fibers in sputum
    e. lamina
    e. pulse
    e. recoil
    e. recoil pressure
    e. resistance
    e. stiffness
    e. stockings
    e. tissue hyperplasia
elasticity
    lung e.
    sputum viscosity and e.
elasticum
    pseudoxanthoma e.
Elastorc catheter guidewire
Elavil
elbow flexion
ELCA
    excimer laser coronary angioplasty
    ELCA laser
Elderly
    Systolic Hypertension in
      the E.
Elecath
    E. circulatory support device
    E. pacemaker
    E. switch box
    E. thermodilution catheter
elective cardioversion
electrical
    e. activation abnormality
    e. alternans
    e. alternation of heart
    e. axis
    e. cardioversion
    e. catheter ablation
    e. countershock
    e. diastole
    e. disease
    e. failure
    e. fulguration
    e. heart position
    e. injury

e. potential
e. systole
electric cardiac pacemaker
electro-acuscope
electrocardiogram (ECG, EKG)
    Burdick e.
    His bundle e.
    3-lead e.
    6-lead e.
    12-lead e.
    16-lead e.
    orthogonal e.
    scalar e.
    signal-averaged e.
    stress MUGA e.
    thallium e.
    three-channel e.
    time domain signal-averaged e.
    treadmill e.
    unipolar e.
    vector e.
electrocardiograph (ECG)
    bioimpedance e.
    Cambridge e.
    Marquette e.
    Mingograf 62 6-channel e.
electrocardiographic
    e. leads
    e. transtelephonic monitor
    e. wave
    e. wave complex (QRS
      complex)
electrocardiography (ECG)
    ambulatory e.
    esophageal e.
    exercise e.
    exercise stress e. (Ex-ECG)
    fetal e.
    intracardiac e.
    12-lead e.
    precordial e.
    signal-averaged e.
electrocardiophonogram
electrocardiophonography
electrocardioscanner
    Compuscan Hittman
      computerized e.

E

NOTES

electrocautery
Bovie e.
needlepoint e.
electrochemical polarization
electroconvulsive therapy
electrode
AE-60-I-2 implantable pronged
unipolar e.
AE-85-I-2 implantable pronged
unipolar e.
AE-60-KB implantable unipolar
endocardial e.
AE-85-KB implantable unipolar
endocardial e.
AE-60-K-10 implantable
unipolar endocardial e.
AE-85-K-10 implantable
unipolar endocardial e.
AE-60-KS-10 implantable
unipolar endocardial e.
AE-85-KS-10 implantable
unipolar endocardial e.
anterior anodal patch e.
Arzco TAPSUL pill e.
Bard nonsteerable bipolar e.
Berkovits-Castellanos
hexapolar e.
Bioplus dispersive e.
bipolar myocardial e.
Bisping e.
button e.
Cambridge jelly e.
e. catheter
central terminal e.
Clark oxygen e.
coil e.
CPI Endotak transvenous e.
cutaneous thoracic patch e.
Darox cutaneous thoracic
patch e.
dispersing e.
EnGuard PFX lead e.
epicardial e.
esophageal pill e.
exploring e.
Fast-Patch disposable
defibrillation/electrocardi-
ographic e.
e. gel
Goetz bipolar e.
hydrogen e.'s
implantable cardioverter e.'s
indifferent e.

intravascular catheter e.
ion-selective e. (ISE)
e. jelly
J orthogonal e.
Josephson quadpolar
mapping e.
Laserdish e.
Lifeline e.
Mansfield Polaris e.
Medtronic Transvene e.
monopolar temporary e.
multipolar catheter e.
MVE-50 implantable
myocardial e.
Myowire II cardiac e.
Nyboer esophageal e.
Osypka Cereblate e.
pacemaker e.'s
e. pad
e. paddles
e. paste
PE-60-I-2 implantable pronged
unipolar e.
PE-85-I-2 implantable pronged
unipolar e.
PE-60-KB implantable unipolar
endocardial e.
PE-85-KB implantable unipolar
endocardial e.
PE-60-K-10 implantable
unipolar endocardial e.
PE-85-K-10 implantable
unipolar endocardial e.
PE-85-KS-10 implantable
unipolar endocardial e.
Polaris e.
QuadPolar e.
quadripolar Quad e.
reference e.
ring e.
scalp e.
screw-in epicardial e.
silent e.
silver bead e.
silver-silver chloride e.
Skylark surface e.
Soft-EZ reusable e.
stab-in epicardial e.
Stockert cardiac pacing e.
Surgicraft pacemaker e.
e. system
Tapcath esophageal e.
Tapsul pill e.

Transvene tripolar e.
transvenous e.
tripolar defibrillation coil e.
unipolar defibrillation coil e.
USCI Goetz bipolar e.
USCI NBIH bipolar e.
Vitatron catheter e.
electrodesiccation
electrode-skin interface
electrodispersive skin patch
electrodynogram
electroencephalogram (EEG)
electroencephalograph (EEG)
electroencephalography (EEG)
electrogram
coronary sinus e.
Furman Type II e.
His bundle e.
electrograph
Cardiotest portable e.
electrokymogram (EKY)
electrokymograph
electrokymography
electrolyte
e. imbalance
electrolytic disturbance
electromagnetic
interference/radiofrequency
interference (EMI/RFI)
electromanometer
electromechanical
e. artificial heart
e. coupling
e. dissociation (EMD)
e. interval
e. systole
electromyocardial dissociation
electromyogram (EMG)
electromyograph (EMG)
electromyography (EMG)
electron
e. beam computed tomography
(EBCT)
e. microscope
e. microscopy

e. paramagnetic resonance
spectroscopy
e. volt (eV)
electronic
e. distance compensation
e. fetal monitor
e. pacemaker
e. pacemaker load
e. scanning
electro-oculogram (EOG)
electro-oculograph (EOG)
electro-oculography (EOG)
electrophoresis
agarose gel e.
gradient gel e.
polyacrylamide gel e.
protein e.
sodium dodecylsulfate
polyacrylamide gel e.
electrophrenic respiration
electrophysiologic
e. mapping
e. study (EPS)
e. test
electrophysiology (EP)
intracardiac e.
E. Study versus
Electrocardiographic
Monitoring (ESVEM)
electrostethograph
electrosurgery
electrovectorcardiogram
electroversion
Elema
E. leads
E. pacemaker
Elema-Schonander pacemaker
element
contractile e.
series elastic e.
elephant-on-the-chest sensation
Elevath pacemaker
elevation
ST segment e.
elevator
Aufricht e.
Cameron-Haight e.

E

NOTES

elevator *(continued)*
  e. disease
  Doyen e.
  Friedrich rib e.
  Lemmon sternal e.
  Matson rib e.
  Phemister e.
eleventh cranial nerve
ELF
  epithelial lining fluid
  ELF levels
elfin
  e. facies
  e. facies syndrome
Elgiloy frame
Elgiloy-Heifitz aneurysm clip
elimination half-life
ELISA
  enzyme-linked immunosorbent assay
  double-sandwich IgM ELISA
ELISPOT test
Elite
  E. guide catheter
  E. pacemaker
Elixicon
Elixophyllin
Ellestad
  E. exercise stress test
  E. protocol
ellipse
  prolate e.
Ellipse compact spacer
elliptical loop
Ellis sign
Ellis-van Creveld syndrome
Eloesser flap
Elscint tomography system
Elsner asthma
Elspar
eluting stent
elution
Emax
  maximum ventricular elastance
EMB
  endomyocardial biopsy
embarrassment
  circulatory e.
  respiratory e.
embolectomy
  catheter e.
  e. catheter
  femoral e.
  pulmonary e.

emboli (*pl. of* embolus)
embolic
  e. abscess
  e. aneurysm
  e. event
  e. gangrene
  e. infarct
  e. phenomenon
  e. pneumonia
  e. shower
  e. stroke
  e. thrombosis
embolism
  acute pulmonary e.
  air pulmonary e.
  amniotic fluid e.
  aortic e.
  arterial e.
  atheromatous e.
  bacillary e.
  bland e.
  bone marrow e.
  capillary e.
  catheter e.
  cellular e.
  cholesterol e.
  coronary e.
  crossed e.
  direct e.
  diving air e.
  fat e.
  gas e.
  hematogenous e.
  infective e.
  miliary e.
  multiple e.
  myxomatous pulmonary e.
  obturating e.
  oil e.
  pantaloon e.
  paradoxical cerebral e.
  Plasmodium e.
  pulmonary e.
  pyemic e.
  retrograde e.
  riding e.
  saddle e.
  straddling e.
  submassive pulmonary e.
  tumor e.
  venous e.
embolization
  air e.

bronchial artery e. (BAE)
cholesterol e.
coil e.
paradoxical e.
pulmonary e.
septic e.
Silastic bead e.
e. therapy
transcatheter e.
embolized foreign material
embolomycotic aneurysm
embolotherapy
embolus, pl. **emboli**
air e.
catheter e.
cerebral e.
femoral e.
paradoxical e.
polyurethane foam e.
pulmonary e.
riding e.
saddle e.
threw an e.
embryocardia
jugular e.
e. rhythm
embryologic
embryology
embryoma
EMC virus
EMD
electromechanical dissociation
emergency
e. bailout stent
hypertensive e.
E. Infusion Device (EID)
e. reperfusion
Emerson
E. bronchoscope
E. cuirass respirator
E. Post-Op
Emery-Dreifuss
E.-D. disease
E.-D. muscular dystrophy
emesis
posttussive e.
emetine toxicity

EMG
electromyogram
electromyograph
electromyography
Eminase
EMIP
European Myocardial Infarction
Project
EMI/RFI
electromagnetic
interference/radiofrequency
interference
emission
single-photon e.
Emory Angioplasty versus Surgery Trial (EAST)
emotional stress
emphysema
alveolar duct e.
atrophic e.
bullous e.
centriacinar e.
centrilobular e.
chronic hypertrophic e.
chronic obstructive
pulmonary e. (COPE)
compensating e.
compensatory e.
cystic e.
diffuse e.
ectatic e.
false e.
focal-dust e.
gangrenous e.
glass blower's e.
hypertrophic e.
hypoplastic e.
idiopathic unilobar e.
infantile lobar e.
interlobular e.
interstitial e.
Jenner e.
lobar e.
localized obstructive e.
loculated e.
mediastinal e.
obstructive e.

NOTES

E

179

emphysema *(continued)*
    panacinar e.
    panlobular e.
    paracicatricial e.
    paraseptal e.
    predominant e.
    pulmonary interstitial e. (PIE)
    scar e.
    senile e.
    small-lunged e.
    subcutaneous e.
    surgical e.
    traumatic e.
    unilateral e.
    vesicular e.
emphysematous
    e. asthma
    e. bleb
    e. bulla
    e. chest
    e. gangrene
empiric
    e. constant
    e. therapy
Empirin
empyema
    anaerobic e.
    e. benignum
    e. of chest
    interlobar e.
    latent e.
    loculated e.
    metapneumonic e.
    e. necessitatis
    e. of pericardium
    pleural e.
    pneumococcal e.
    postpneumonectomy
      tuberculous e.
    pulsating e.
    putrid e.
    sacculated e.
    streptococcal e.
    synpneumonic e.
    thoracic e.
    tuberculous e.
empyesis
    tuberculous e.
EMS
    eosinophilia-myalgia syndrome
emulsion
    EchoGen e.
    fat e.

    intravascular
      perfluorochemical e.
E-Mycin Oral
en
    e. bloc
    e. bloc bilateral lung transplant
    e. bloc, no-touch technique
    e. face
enalapril
    e. and hydrochlorothiazide
    e. maleate
enalaprilat
enalaprilic acid
encainide
    e. hydrochloride
encapsulated organism
Encapsulon
    E. epidural catheter
    E. sheath introducer
    E. vessel dilator
encarditis
encased heart
Encephalitozoon
encephalomyelitis
encephalomyocarditis
    e. virus
encephalopathy
    hypertensive e.
    metabolic e.
encircling
    e. cryoablation
    e. endocardial ventriculotomy
encode
encoding
    respiratory ordered phase e.
    (ROPE)
Encor
    E. lead
    E. pacemaker
Encore inflation device
encroachment
    luminal e.
**encrustation theory of
atherosclerosis**
encysted pleurisy
Endal
endangiitis
endaortitis
endarterectomy
    blunt eversion carotid e.
    carotid e.
    coronary e.

e. and coronary artery bypass grafting (E-CABG)
femoral e.
gas e.
endarteritis
  e. deformans
  Heubner specific e.
  e. obliterans
  e. proliferans
  syphilitic e.
endarteropathy
  digital e.
endartery
end-diastole
end-diastolic
  e.-d. area (EDA)
  e.-d. count
  e.-d. dimension
  e.-d. left ventricular pressure
  e.-d. murmur
  e.-d. pressure (EDP)
  e.-d. velocity
  e.-d. volume (EDV)
  e.-d. volume index (EDVI)
endemic
  e. fungal infection
  e. influenza
end-hole
  e.-h. balloon-tipped catheter
  e.-h. #7 French catheter
end-inspiratory crackles
endless-loop tachycardia
endoaneurysmorrhaphy
  ventricular e.
endoaortitis
endoauscultation
Endo-Avitene
endobronchial
  e. brachytherapy
  e. tree
Endocam endoscope
endocardiac
endocardial
  e. balloon lead
  e. cushion
  e. cushion defect (ECD)
  e. fibroelastosis

e. fibrosis
e. flow
e. mapping
e. mapping of ventricular tachycardia
e. murmur
e. resection
e. sclerosis
e. stain
e. thickening
e. tube
e. vegetation
endocardiography
endocarditic
endocarditis
  abacterial thrombotic e.
  acute bacterial e. (ABE)
  acute infective e. (AIE)
  atypical verrucous e.
  bacteria-free stage of bacterial e.
  bacterial e. (BE)
  e. benigna
  cachectic e.
  e. chordalis
  chronic e.
  constrictive e.
  culture-negative e.
  enterococcal e.
  experimental enterococcal e.
  fungal e.
  gonococcal e.
  gram-negative e.
  green strep e.
  Haemophilus e.
  infectious e.
  infective e. (IE)
  isolated parietal e.
  e. lenta
  Libman-Sacks e.
  Löffler parietal fibroplastic e.
  malignant e.
  marantic e.
  methicillin-sensitive right-sided e.
  mitral valve e.
  mural e.

E

NOTES

endocarditis *(continued)*
    mycotic e.
    nonbacterial thrombotic e.
        (NBTE)
    nonbacterial verrucous e.
    nosocomial e.
    parietal e.
    e. parietalis fibroplastica
    plastic e.
    polypous e.
    prosthetic valve e.
    pulmonic e.
    rheumatic e.
    rickettsial e.
    septic e.
    staphylococcal e.
    streptococcal e.
    subacute bacterial e. (SBE)
    subacute infective e.
    syphilitic e.
    terminal e.
    thrombotic e.
    tuberculous e.
    ulcerative e.
    valvular e.
    vegetative e.
    verrucous e.
    viridans e.
endocardium
Endocoil stent
endocrine
    e. disorder
    e. system
endocytosis
end-of-life pacemaker
endogenous lipid
Endo Grasp device
Endoknot suture
endolumen enlargement
EndoLumina illuminated bougie
endoluminal
    e. stenting
endomyocardial
    e. biopsy (EMB)
    e. disease
    e. fibroelastosis
    e. fibrosis
endomyocarditis
endomysial collagen
endomysium
endonuclease
    restriction e.
EndoOctopus

endopeptidase
    e. inhibitor
endopericarditis
endoperimyocarditis
endoperoxide steal
endophthalmitis
endorphin
endoscope
    Endocam e.
    lung imaging fluorescence e.
        (LIFE)
    Messerklinger e.
    Sine-U-View nasal e.
    velolaryngeal e.
    Visicath e.
endoscopic biopsy
EndoSonics IVUS/balloon dilatation
    catheter
Endosound endoscopic ultrasound
    catheter
Endotak
    E. C lead transvenous catheter
    E. C tripolar
        pacing/sensing/defibrillation
        lead
    E. C tripolar transvenous lead
    E. lead system
    E. nonthoracotomy implantable
        cardioverter-defibrillator
endothelial
    e. denudation
    e. dysfunction
endothelialization
endothelin-1, -2, -3
    plasma e.
endothelin A, B receptors
endothelioma
endothelium
endothelium-dependent dilator
    response to substance P
endothelium-derived
    e.-d. hyperpolarizing factor
        (EDHF)
    e.-d. nitric oxide
    e.-d. relaxing factor (EDRF)
endothelium-leukocyte adhesion
    molecule (E-LAM)
endothelium-mediated relaxation
endotoxemia
endotracheal
    e. aspirate
    e. intubation
    e. tube

Endotrol
E. endotracheal tube
E. tracheal tube
endoventricular circular patch plasty
endpoint
Randomized Evaluation of Salvage Angioplasty with Combined Utilization of E.'s (RESCUE)
therapeutic e.
end-pressure artifact
endralazine
Endrate
end-stage
e.-s. heart failure
e.-s. liver disease (ESLD)
e.-s. renal disease
end-systole
end-systolic
e.-s. count
e.-s. dimension
e.-s. elastance
e.-s. force-velocity indices
e.-s. left ventricular pressure
e.-s. murmur
e.-s. pressure-volume relation
e.-s. stress-dimension relation
e.-s. volume (ESV)
e.-s. volume index (ESVI)
end-tidal
e.-t. carbon dioxide (ETCO$_2$)
end-to-end
end-to-side
e.-t.-s. suture
Enduron
Enduronyl
E. Forte
enema
barium e.
Kayexalate e.
sodium polystyrene sulfonate e.
energy
color Doppler e. (CDE)
e. production
e. resolution
e. supply

Enertrax 7100 pacemaker
enflurane
Englert forceps
engorgement
venous e.
Engstrom respirator
EnGuard
E. double-lead ICD system
E. pacing and defibrillation lead system
E. PFX lead electrode
enhanced
e. automaticity
e. external counterpulsation (EECP)
e. external counterpulsation unit
E. Torque 8F guiding catheter
enhancement
leading edge e.
mean contrast e.
Enhancer
Ace Cloud E.
Aerosol Cloud E.
enhancing lesion
Enkaid
enlargement
biatrial e.
cardiac e.
compensatory vessel e.
endolumen e.
left atrial e. (LAF)
panchamber e.
right atrial e. (RAE)
Enlon injection
Enomine
enoxacin
enoxaparin
e. sodium
enoximone
Enseals
Potassium Iodide E.
Entamoeba histolytica
entangling technique
enteric
e. cytopathogenic human orphan virus (ECHO virus)

E

NOTES

enteric *(continued)*
  e. fistula
    e. gram-negative bacilli
enteric-coated aspirin
enteroadherent
enteroaggregative
Enterobacter
    E. cloacae
enterococcal endocarditis
Enterococcus
    E. faecalis
    E. faecium
enterocolitica
    Yersinia e.
enterocolitis
enterocytopathogenic human orphan
  (ECHO)
enterohemorrhagic
enteroinvasive
enterotoxin
    Escherichia coli e.
enteroviral
enterovirus
Entex
entoptic pulse
entrained beat
entrainment
    concealed e.
    epicardial e.
    e. of tachycardia
    e. with concealed fusion
entrance
    e. block
    e. wound
EnTre guidewire
entry
    air e.
    e. site
enucleation of subaortic stenosis
envelope
    aortic e.
    dagger-shaped aortic e.
    flow e.
    spectral e.
env gene
environmental
    e. allergen
    e. change
    e. lung disease
    e. survey
Enzygnost
    E. F1+2 ELISA kit

E. TAT complex kit
E. TAT ELISA assay
enzyme
    allosteric modification of e.
    angiotensin-converting e. (ACE)
    angiotensin-I converting e.
    Bacillus subtilis e.'s
    cardiac e.
    glycolytic e.'s
    e. immunoassay (EIA)
    lysosomal e.
    mitochondrial e.'s
    phosphodiesterase e.
    proteolytic e.
    Randomized Assessment of
      Digoxin on Inhibitors of
      Angiotensin Converting E.
      (RADIANCE)
    sarcoplasmic reticulum-
      associated glycolytic e.'s
enzyme-linked immunosorbent assay
  (ELISA)
Enzymun-Test System ES22
  analyzer
EOG
    electro-oculogram
    electro-oculograph
    electro-oculography
eosin
    hematoxylin and e. (H&E)
eosinophil
    e. by-products
    e. cationic protein
    e. chemotactic factors of
      anaphylaxis (ECF-A)
eosinophilia
    peripheral blood e.
    pulmonary infiltration with e.
      (PIE)
    tropical pulmonary e.
eosinophilia-myalgia syndrome
  (EMS)
eosinophilic
    e. chemotaxis
    e. endomyocardial disease
    e. granuloma
    e. lung
    e. pneumonia
    e. pneumonitis
    e. pneumonopathy
    e. pulmonary syndrome

EP
    electrophysiology
    EP mapping
EPA
    eicosapentaenoic acid
Epanutin
EPAP
    expiratory positive airway pressure
ephedrine
    aminophylline, amobarbital,
        and e.
    e. sulfate
Ephedsol
ephelides
    nevi, atrial myxoma, myxoid
        neurofibromas, and e.
        (NAME)
ephemeral pneumonia
**epibronchial right pulmonary artery
    syndrome**
epicardial
    e. defibrillator patch
    e. electrode
    e. entrainment
    e. fat
    e. fat tag
    e. flow
    e. lead
    e. vessel patency
epicardium
epidemic capillary bronchitis
epidermal growth factor
epidermidis
    Staphylococcus e.
epidermoid
    e. carcinoma
EpiE-ZPen
Epifrin
epigastric bruit
epiglottiditis
    petiolous e.
epiglottoplasty
epilepsy
epilepticus
    status e.
epimyocarditis
epimysium

epinephrine
    racemic e.
EpiPen
epiphenomena of dissection
episode
    presyncopal e.
episodic dyspnea
Epistat double balloon
epistaxis
epistenocardica
    pericarditis e.
epithelial
    e. lining fluid (ELF)
    e. 5'-nucleotide receptor
epithelium
    sloughed bronchial e.
Epivir
epoprostenol sodium
Eppendorf
    E. angiocatheter
    E. catheter
EPS
    electrophysiologic study
EPS-410
    Venodyne external pneumatic
        compression System E.
EPSS
    E point to septal separation
Epstein-Barr
    E.-B. nuclear antigen (EBNA)
    E.-B. virus (EBV)
Epstein disease
EPT-1000 cardiac ablation system
EPTFE, ePTFE
    expanded polytetrafluoroethylene
        EPTFE graft
        EPTFE vascular sutures
equation
    Bernoulli e.
    Bloch e.
    Carter e.
    continuity e.
    Doppler continuity e.
    Eagle e.
    Einthoven e.
    Fick e.
    Ford e.

E

NOTES

equation *(continued)*
Ford e.
Friedewald e.
Gorlin e.
Hagenbach extension of
Poiseuille e.
Henderson-Hesselbalch e.
Holen-Hatle e.
Krovetz-Gessner e.
Navier-Stokes e.
Nernst e.
regression e.
Riley-Cournand e.
Rodrigo e.
Starling e.
Torricelli orifice e.
Equen magnet
equi
Rhodococcus e.
equilibration
equilibrium
e. image
e. multigated radionuclide
ventriculography
e. radionuclide angiography
(ERNA)
voltage e.
equilibrium-gated blood pool study
equiphasic complex
equipment
equivalency
left main e.
equivalent
Abell-Kendall e.
anginal e.
metabolic e. of task (MET,
METs)
right anterior oblique e.
ventilation e.
ventilatory e.
equuli
Actinobacillus e.
Erb
E. area
E. atrophy
E. point
ERBE cryoprobe
Erben reflex
ERBF
effective renal blood flow
Erb-Goldflam disease
erbium:YAG laser

erbumine
perindopril e.
Ercaf
Erdheim
E. cystic medial necrosis
E. disease
erectile effect
Ergamisol
Ergoline bicycle ergometer
Ergomar
ergometer
Bosch ERG 500 e.
Collins bicycle e.
Ergoline bicycle e.
Gauthier bicycle e.
Monark bicycle e.
pedal-mode e.
Siemens-Albis bicycle e.
Siemens-Elema AG bicycle e.
Tunturi EL400 bicycle e.
ergometry
bicycle e.
ergonomic vascular access needle
(EVAN)
ergonovine
e. challenge
e. echocardiography
e. maleate
e. maleate provocation angina
e. provocation test
ergonovine-induced
e.-i. spasm
e.-i. vasospasm
Ergos O$_2$ dual-chamber rate-
responsive pacemaker
Ergostat
ergot alkaloid
ergotamine
e. derivatives
Medihaler E.
Erie System
ERIG serum
Erlanger sphygmomanometer
ERNA
equilibrium radionuclide
angiography
Erni sign
erosion
spark e.
erosive
e. esophagitis
e. reflux

ERV
  expiratory reserve volume
Erwinia
Erwiniar
Eryc Oral
EryPed Oral
Erysipelothrix
Ery-Tab Oral
erythema
  e. marginatum
  e. migrans
  e. multiforme
  e. nodosum
  palmar e.
erythematosus
  disseminated lupus e.
  drug-induced lupus e. (DILE)
  lupus e. (LE)
  systemic lupus e. (SLE)
erythematous, maculopapular rash
erythrityl tetranitrate
Erythrocin Oral
erythrocyte sedimentation rate
  (ESR)
erythrocytosis
erythroderma
Erythroflex hydromer-coated central
  venous catheter
erythrogenin
erythromelalgia
erythromycin
  e. and sulfisoxazole
erythropheresis
erythropoietin
  plasma e.
Eryzole Oral
ES
  ejection sounds
ESAT-6 protein
escape
  e. beat
  e. impulse
  e. interval
  junctional e.
  nodal e.
  e. pacemaker
  e. rhythm

  vagal e.
  ventricular e.
  e. ventricular contraction
escape-capture bigeminy
Escherichia coli **enterotoxin**
Escherich test
E-selectin
Esidrix
Esimil
ESLD
  end-stage liver disease
Esmarch tourniquet
esmolol hydrochloride
EsophaCoil self-expanding
  esophageal stent
esophagagram
esophagalgia
esophageal
  e. achalasia
  e. adventitia
  e. angina
  e. A-ring
  e. artery
  e. atresia
  e. bougienage
  e. B-ring
  e. cardiogram
  e. contraction ring
  e. detection device (EDD)
  e. dilation
  e. dysmotility
  e. echocardiography
  e. electrocardiography
  e. hiatus
  e. lead
  e. lumen
  e. lung
  e. manometry
  e. motility
  e. obturator airway
  e. pill electrode
  e. prosthesis
  e. reflux
  e. rupture
  e. sling procedure
  e. sound
  e. spasm

NOTES

187

esophageal *(continued)*
 e. speech
 e. sphincter
 e. stricture
 e. tamponade
 e. temperature probe
 e. transit time
 e. varices
 e. web
esophagectomy
esophagism
 hiatal e.
esophagismus
esophagitis
 corrosive e.
 e. dissecans superficialis
 erosive e.
 infectious e.
 monilial e.
 peptic e.
 reflux e.
esophagogastric tamponade
esophagomyotomy
 Heller e.
esophagoplasty
 Belsey e.
 Grondahl e.
esophagoplication
esophagosalivary reflex
esophagoscope
 Boros e.
 Eder-Hufford e.
 Foregger rigid e.
 Jesberg e.
 Lell e.
 Moure e.
 Schindler e.
esophagoscopy
 fiberoptic e.
esophagospasm
esophagotracheal
esophagus
 Barrett e.
 brusque dilatation of e.
 nutcracker e.
 thoracic e.
ESP radiation reduction
 examination gloves
ESR
 erythrocyte sedimentation rate
essential
 e. asthma
 e. bradycardia

 e. brown induration of lung
 e. hypertension
 e. pulmonary hemosiderosis
 e. tachycardia
EST
 exercise stress test
estazolam
ester
 cholesterol e.
Estes
 E. EKG criteria
 E. point system
 E. score
Estes-Romhilt EKG point-score
 system
estimated Fick method
Estlander operation
estrogen
 e. & medroxyprogesterone
Estrovis
ESV
 end-systolic volume
ESVEM
 Electrophysiology Study versus
 Electrocardiographic Monitoring
ESVI
 end-systolic volume index
ETCO$_2$
 end-tidal carbon dioxide
 ETCO$_2$ multigas analyzer
E-test
ethacrynic acid
Ethalloy needle
ethambutol
 e. hydrochloride
Ethamolin injection
ethanol (EtOH)
ethanolamine
 aminoethyl e.
 e. oleate
Ethaquin
Ethatab
ethaverine hydrochloride
Ethavex-100
ether
 bis(chloromethyl) e.
 e. bronchitis
 e. pneumonia
 e. test
Ethibond suture
ethidium bromide
ethionamide
ethmozin

Ethmozine
ethoxysclerol
ethyl alcohol
ethylenediaminetetraacetic
    e. acid (EDTA)
    e. acid disodium salt
ethylnorepinephrine
    e. hydrochloride
etiennei
    Octomyces e.
etilefrine
EtOH
    ethanol
etomidate
etoposide
ETO Sleuth
ETT
    exercise tolerance test
    exercise treadmill test
Eudal-SR
euglobulin clot lysis time
eunuchoid voice
Euro-Collins multiorgan perfusion
  kit
European
    E. Carotid Surgery Trial
    (ECST)
    E. Coronary Surgery Study
    E. Myocardial Infarction
    Project (EMIP)
Eustace Smith murmur
eustachian valve
eusystole
eusystolic
euthyroid
    e. sick syndrome
Eutron
euvolemic
eV
    electron volt
evagination
evaluation
    acute physiologic assessment
    and chronic health e.
    (APACHE)
    Angioplasty Compared to
    Medicine E. (ACME)

    anthropometric e.
    noninvasive e.
    Prospective Randomized
    Milrinone Survival E.
    (PROMISE)
    Survival of Myocardial
    Infarction Long-Term E.
    (SMILE)
    Trandolapril Cardiac E.
    (TRACE)
EVAN
    ergonomic vascular access needle
Evans blue powder
Eve method
event
    cardiac e.
    cerebral e.
    cerebrovascular e.
    Cholesterol and Recurrent E.'s
    (CARE)
    coronary e.
    e. diary
    embolic e.
    intracardiac e.
    e. monitor
    e. recorder
    soft e.
eventration of diaphragm
eversion
    blunt e.
    cusp e.
everting mattress suture
evolutus
    Peptostreptococcus e.
evolving myocardial infarction
Ewald tube
Ewart sign
Ewing sign
ex
    e. vivo
    e. vivo gene transfer
ExacTech blood glucose meter
examination
    cardiac e.
    funduscopic e.
    neurologic e.
    parasternal e.

E

NOTES

examination *(continued)*
    supraclavicular e.
    suprasternal e.
excavatum
    pectus e.
Excedrin IB
EXCEL
    Expanded Clinical Evaluation of
    Lovastatin Study
exchange
    air e.
    catheter e.
    gas e.
    e. guidewire
    pulmonary gas e.
    respiratory e.
    sodium-potassium e.
    e. technique
    e. transfusion
exchanger
    heat/moisture e. (HME)
    Portex ThermoVent heat and
    moisture e.
    ThermoVent heat and
    moisture e.
excimer
    e. cool laser
    e. gas laser
    e. laser coronary angioplasty
    (ELCA)
    e. vascular recanalization
excision
    wedge e.
excisional
    e. biopsy
    e. cardiac surgery
excitability
    supranormal e.
excitable gap
excitation
    anomalous atrioventricular e.
    direct e.
    premature e.
    supranormal e.
excitation-contraction coupling
excited dimers
exclusion criteria
excrescence
    Lambl e.'s
excretion
    eicosanoid e.

excursion
    dome e.
    respiratory e.
Ex-ECG
    exercise stress electrocardiography
Ex-Echo
    exercise stress echocardiography
eXercise
    CardioPulmonary e. (CPX)
exercise
    ankle e.
    Buerger-Allen e.
    e. capacity
    dynamic e.
    e. echocardiography
    e. electrocardiography
    e. factor
    e. imaging
    e. index
    International Multicenter
    Angina E. (IMAGE)
    e. intolerance
    isometric e.
    isotonic e.
    e. load
    peak e.
    e. prescription
    e. regimen
    strenuous e.
    e. stress echocardiography (Ex-
    Echo)
    e. stress electrocardiography
    (Ex-ECG)
    e. stress test (EST)
    e. study
    supine e.
    e. thallium-201 scintigraphy
    e. tolerance test (ETT)
    e. treadmill
    e. treadmill test (ETT)
    upright e.
exercise-induced
    e.-i. angina
    e.-i. arrhythmia
    e.-i. asthma (EIA)
    e.-i. bronchospasm
    e.-i. silent myocardial ischemia
    e.-i. ventricular tachycardia
exerciser
    Resistex expiratory
    resistance e.
exertion
    dyspnea on e. (DOE)

perceived e.
ratings of perceived e. (RPE)
exertional
  e. angina
  e. dyspnea
  e. syncope
exfoliative dermatitis
Exirel
exit
  e. block
  e. block murmur
  e. point
  e. wound
Exna
exocardia
exocardial murmur
exogenous
  e. lipid
  e. obesity
exon
exophthalmica
  tachycardia traumosa e.
exophthalmos
exophytic
exopneumopexy
exopolysaccharide
  mucoid e.
Exorcist technique
Exosurf
  E. Neonatal
  E. Pediatric
exotoxin
  Pseudomonas e.
expandable access catheter (EAC)
expanded
  E. Clinical Evaluation of Lovastatin Study (EXCEL)
  e. polytetrafluoroethylene (EPTFE, ePTFE)
  e. polytetrafluoroethylene vascular graft
expander
  blood e.
  Hespan plasma volume e.
  hetastarch plasma e.
  plasma volume e.

PMT AccuSpan tissue e.
Ruiz-Cohen round e.
expansion
  infarct e.
  stent e.
expectorant
  Benylin E.
  Fedahist E.
  Genamin E.
  liquifying e.
  Myminic E.
  Silaminic E.
  Stokes e.
  Theramin E.
  Triaminic E.
  Tri-Clear E.
  Triphenyl E.
expectoration
Expedited Recovery Program
experiment
  Müller e.
  Weber e.
experimental enterococcal endocarditis
expiration
  duration of e. (T_E)
  prolongation of e.
expiratory
  e. dyspnea
  e. flow rate
  e. grunt
  e. murmur
  e. positive airway pressure (EPAP)
  e. reserve volume (ERV)
  e. retard
  e. rhonchi
  e. trapping of air
  e. wheezing
expired air collection
expirograph
  Godart e.
explant
explanted heart
Explorer
  E. 360-degree rotational diagnostic EP catheter

NOTES

191

Explorer *(continued)*
   E. pre-curved diagnostic EP
     catheter
exploring electrode
exposure
   allergen e.
   chemical e.
   cold e.
   toxin e.
Express
   E. balloon
   E. over-the-wire balloon
     catheter
expression
   gene e.
expressive aphasia
expulsive coughing
exsanguination protocol
exsanguinotransfusion
EXS femoropopliteal bypass graft
extender
   Taq e.
extension
   DOC guidewire e.
   infarct e.
   knee e.
   Linx guidewire e.
   LOC guidewire e.
Extentabs
   Quinidex E.
external
   e. cardiac massage
   e. cardioverter-defibrillator
     (ECD)
   e. carotid artery
   e. defibrillator
   e. grid
   e. jugular vein
   e. mammary artery
   e. pacemaker
   e. respiration
   e. rotation, abduction, stress
     test (EAST)
externum
   pericardium e.
Extra
   E. Action Cough Syrup
   E. Strength Bayer Enteric 500
     Aspirin
extracardiac
   e. murmur
   e. shunt

extracellular
   e. lipid
   e. matrix
extracellular-like, calcium-free
   solution (ECS)
extracoronary
extracorporeal
   e. circulation
   e. exchange hypothermia
   e. heart
   e. life support (ECLS)
   e. membrane oxygenation
     (ECMO)
   e. membrane oxygenator
   e. pump oxygenator
extracranial
   e. cardiac disease (ECD)
   e. carotid arterial disease
     (ECAD)
extract
   calf lung surfactant e. (CLSE)
   pancreatic e.
   Rauwolfia e.
   shiitake mushroom e.
   thyroid e.
extraction
   e. atherectomy device
   lactate e.
   e. reserve
Extractor three-lumen retrieval
   balloon
eXtract specimen bag
extraesophageal reflux
extrafusion defect
extralobar
extrapleural
   e. air
   e. apicolysis
   e. pneumothorax
   e. space
extrapulmonary
   e. cough
   e. site
   e. tuberculosis
extrarenal azotemia
extrastimulation
   single premature e.
extrastimulus, pl. extrastimuli
   double e.
   double ventricular e.
   e. test
extra-support guidewire

extrasystole
  atrial e.
  atrioventricular e., A-V e. (AVE)
  atrioventricular nodal e., A-V nodal e.
  auricular e.
  auriculoventricular e.
  A-V junctional e.
  infranodal e.
  interpolated e.
  junctional e.
  lower nodal e.
  midnodal e.
  nodal e.
  return e.
  supraventricular e.
  upper nodal e.
  ventricular e.
extrasystolic beat
extrathoracic
  e. neoplasm
  e. rales
  e. tumor
extravascular
  e. granulomatous features
  e. lung water

extremitas
extremities
  mottling of e.
extremity ischemia
extrinsic
  e. allergic alveolitis
  e. asthma
  e. factors
exudate
  cotton-wool e.
  fibrinous e.
  fluffy cotton-wool e.
exudativa
  bronchiolitis e.
exudative
  e. bronchitis
  e. pleural effusion
  e. pleurisy
  e. tuberculosis
eyeball compression reflex
eyeball-heart reflex
eyeless needle
EZ-3
Ezide

NOTES

E

F

F gate
F point of cardiac apex pulse

f

f wave
f wave of jugular venous
pulse

F-18 2-deoxyglucose (FDG)

Fab

c7E3 Fab
chimeric 7E3 Fab
chimeric 7E3 Fab (c7E3 Fab)
digoxin-immune Fab
digoxin-specific Fab
Fab fragment
m7E3 Fab
murine-derived monoclonal
antibody 7E3 Fab

fabric baffle
Fabry disease
face

en f.
moon f.
f. shield

facial

f. droop
f. vein

facies, pl. facies

aortic f.
Corvisart f.
cushingoid f.
elfin f.
mitral f.
f. mitralis

facilitated angioplasty
facioscapulohumeral

f. dystrophy
f. dystrophy of Landouzy-
Déjérine

**FACT coronary balloon angioplasty
catheter**
factor

acidic fibroblast growth f.
(aFGF)
active-site inhibited f. VIIa
antihemophilic f. (recombinant)
atrial natriuretic f. (ANF)
f. B
basic fibroblast growth f.
(bFGF)

behavioral f.
blood coagulation f. (I-XIII)
cardiac risk f.
Christmas f.
coagulation f.
f. D
duty f.
endothelium-derived
hyperpolarizing f. (EDHF)
endothelium-derived relaxing f.
(EDRF)
epidermal growth f.
exercise f.
extrinsic f.'s
fibrin-stabilizing blood
coagulation f.
fibroblast growth f. (FGF)
Fletcher f.
granulocyte/macrophage colony-
stimulating f. (GM-CSF)
gravitation f.
growth f.
f. H
Hageman f.
f. I (fibrinogen)
f. III (thromboplastin)
f. II (prothrombin)
insulin-like growth f. (IGF)
f. IV (calcium ions)
f. IX (Christmas f.)
f. IX complex (human)
myocardial depressant f.
(MDF)
necrosis f.
neurohumoral f.'s
N-terminal proatrial
natriuretic f.
f. P
platelet f. 4
platelet activating f. (PAF)
platelet-aggregating f.
platelet-derived growth f.
(PDGF)
proatrial natriuretic f.
(proANF)
psychological f.
psychosocial f.
Rh f.
rheumatoid f.
risk f.

F

factor *(continued)*
    Stuart-Prower f.
    tissue f.
    transforming growth f. (TGF)
    tumor necrosis f. (TNF)
    vascular endothelial growth f. (VEGF)
    f. VI (factor VI - cannot be identified)
    f. VIII (antihemophilic f.)
    f. viii:c (porcine)
    f. VIII:C (von Willebrand f.)
    f. VII (proconvertin)
    von Willebrand f.
    f. V (proaccelerin)
    f. Xa
    f. XII (Hageman f.)
    f. XIII (fibrin stabilizing f.)
    f. XI (plasma thromboplastin antecedent f.)
    f. X (Stuart f. or Stuart-Prower f.)
facultative bacteria
faecalis
    Alcaligenes f.
    Enterococcus f.
    Streptococcus f.
faecium
    Enterococcus f.
faeni
    Micropolyspora f.
Faget sign
failing lung sign
failure
    acute renal f.
    acute respiratory f. (ARF)
    backward heart f.
    cardiac f.
    chronic renal f.
    chronic respiratory f. (CRF)
    circulatory f.
    cocaine-induced respiratory f. (CIRF)
    congestive heart f. (CHF)
    coronary f.
    diastolic heart f.
    electrical f.
    end-stage heart f.
    florid congestive heart f.
    forward heart f.
    heart f.
    hepatic f.
    high-output heart f.

    impending respiratory f.
    left-sided heart f.
    left ventricular f.
    Living with Heart F.
    low-output heart f.
    multisystem organ f. (MSOF)
    myocardial f.
    pacemaker f.
    pulmonary f.
    pump f.
    renal f.
    respiratory f.
    right heart f.
    right-sided heart f.
    right ventricular f.
    systolic heart f.
    Veterans Heart F. (VeHF)
fainting
    hysterical f.
faintness
Falcon single-operator exchange balloon catheter
falling drop
Fallot
    F. pentalogy
    pentalogy of F.
    pink tetralogy of F.
    F. pink tetralogy
    F. tetrad
    tetralogy of F.
    F. triad
    trilogy of F.
    F. trilogy
false
    f. angina
    f. aortic aneurysm
    f. bruit
    f. cardiomegaly
    f. cardiomyopathy
    f. combined hyperlipidemia
    f. croup
    f. cyanosis
    f. dextrocardia
    f. emphysema
    f. hypercholesterolemia
    f. tendon
false-negative
false-positive
FAMA
    fluorescent antimembrane antibody
famciclovir
familial
    f. abetalipoproteinemia

f. amyloidosis
f. asphyxiant thoracic
dystrophy
F. Atherosclerosis Treatment
Study (FATS)
f. cholestasis syndrome
f. dysautonomia
f. dyslipidemic hypertension
f. hypercholesterolemia (FH)
f. hypertrophic obstructive
cardiomyopathy
f. hypocalciuric hypercalcemia
f. nephritis
f. pulmonary fibrosis
Famvir
fan
Dunham f.'s
Fansidar
Fansimef
far field
farmer's lung
Farr test
FAS
fetal alcohol syndrome
fascia
Scarpa f.
fascial layer
fascicular
f. beat
f. heart block
fasciculation
fasciculoventricular Mahaim fiber
fasciotomy
fashion
stoichiometric f.
string of pearls f.
FAST
flow-assisted, short-term
FAST balloon flotation catheter
FAST right heart
cardiovascular catheter
fast
f. channel
f. low-angle shot (FLASH)
f. pathway
f. sodium current
f. wave sleep

Fast-Fit vascular stockings
fast Fourier
f.F. spectral analysis
f.F. transform
Fast-Pass endocardial lead
Fast-Patch disposable
defibrillation/electrocardiographic
electrode
fast-pathway radiofrequency ablation
FasTrac
F. guidewire
F. hydrophilic-coated guidewire
F. introducer
fat
body f.
dietary f.
f. embolism
f. embolism syndrome (FES)
f. emulsion
epicardial f.
trans f.
fat-laden microphages
FATS
Familial Atherosclerosis Treatment
Study
fatty
f. acid
f. degeneration of heart
f. heart
f. streak
faucium
Mycoplasma f.
Faught sphygmomanometer
Fauvel granules
Favaloro
F. proximal anastomosis clamp
F. saphenous vein bypass graft
Favaloro-Morse rib spreader
FB
fiberoptic bronchoscopy
Fc receptors
FDG
F-18 2-deoxyglucose
2-fluoro-2-deoxyglucose
FE
Slow FE

F

NOTES

features
>   extravascular granulomatous f.

FEC
>   forced expiratory capacity

FECO$_2$
>   fraction of expired carbon dioxide

Fedahist
>   F. Expectorant
>   F. Expectorant Pediatric

Federici sign
feedback
>   mechanoelectrical f.
>   respiratory f. (RFb)

feeder vessel
feeleii
>   *Legionella f.*

FEF
>   forced expiratory flow

FEF$_{25-75\%}$
>   mean midexpiratory flow rate

FEFmax
>   maximal forced expiratory flow

Feiba VH Immuno
Feigenbaum echocardiogram
felé
>   bruit de pot f.

Fell-O'Dwyer apparatus
felodipine
female hormone
fem-fem bypass
Femiron
femoral
>   f. approach
>   f. arteriography
>   f. artery
>   f. artery occlusion
>   f. artery thrombosis
>   f. canal
>   f. embolectomy
>   f. embolus
>   f. endarterectomy
>   f. perfusion cannula
>   f. vascular injury
>   f. vein
>   f. vein occlusion
>   f. venous thrombosis
>   f. vessel

femoral-femoral bypass
femoral-popliteal bypass
femoral-tibial bypass
femoral-tibial-peroneal bypass
femoroaxillary bypass
femorofemoral crossover bypass

femoropopliteal bypass
femorotibial
>   f. bypass

FemoStop
>   F. femoral artery compression arch
>   F. inflatable pneumatic compression device
>   F. pneumatic compression

fem-pop bypass
femtoliter (fL)
fenbufen
fence
>   Kirklin f.

Fenesin DM
fenestrated
>   f. Fontan operation
>   f. tracheostomy tube

fenestration
>   aortopulmonary f.
>   baffle f.
>   cusp f.

fenfluramine hydrochloride
Fenico
fenofibrate
fenoldopam mesylate
fenoprofen calcium
fenoterol
fentanyl
Feosol
Feostat
FEP-ringed Gore-Tex vascular graft
Ferancee
Feratab
Fergie needle
Fergon
Ferguson needle
Fergus percutaneous introducer kit
Fer-In-Sol
Fer-Iron
Fernandez reaction
Fero-Grad 500
Fero-Gradumet
Ferospace
Ferralet
Ferralyn Lanacaps
Ferra-TD
Ferretts
ferritin
Ferromar
Ferro-Sequels
ferrous
>   f. fumarate

f. gluconate
f. salt and ascorbic acid
f. sulfate
f. sulfate, ascorbic acid, and vitamin B-complex
f. sulfate, ascorbic acid, vitamin B-complex, and folic acid
ferruginous bodies
FES
fat embolism syndrome
flame emission spectroscopy
forced expiratory spirogram
FET
forced expiratory time
fetal
f. alcohol syndrome (FAS)
f. bradycardia
f. circulation
f. electrocardiography
f. heart rate
f. souffle
f. tachycardia
FEV
forced expiratory volume
FEV₁
forced expiratory volume in 1 second
fever
acute rheumatic f.
Australian Q f.
dengue f.
desert f.
hay f.
hemorrhagic f.
Jaccoud dissociated f.
Lassa f.
lung f.
Monday f.
Omsk hemorrhagic f.
parrot f.
pharyngoconjunctival f.
pneumonic f.
Pontiac f.
pulmonary f.
Q f.
Queensland f.

query f.
relapsing f.
rheumatic f. (RF)
Rocky Mountain spotted f.
San Joaquin Valley f.
scarlet f.
septic f.
shoddy f.
sthenic f.
thermic f.
threshing f.
typhoid f.
Valley f.
yellow f.
zinc fume f.
FEV/FVC
forced expiratory volume timed to forced vital capacity ratio
FEV₁/FVC
forced expiratory volume in 1 second to forced vital capacity ratio
FF
fibrillation-flutter
FFA
free fatty acids
FFA-labeled scintigraphy
FFB
flexible fiberoptic bronchoscopy
f-f interval
FFP
fresh frozen plasma
FGF
fibroblast growth factor
FH
familial hypercholesterolemia
fiber
afferent nerve f.'s
atrio-Hisian f.
blocking vagal afferent f.'s
blocking vagal efferent f.'s
Brechenmacher f.
fasciculoventricular Mahaim f.
His-Purkinje f.'s
James f.'s
Kent f.'s
Mahaim f.'s

F

NOTES

fiber *(continued)*
>nodoventricular f.
>parasympathetic nerve f.'s
>pseudo-Mahaim f.
>Purkinje f.'s
>f. shortening
>terminal Purkinje f.'s
>wavy f.

Fiberlase system
fiberoptic
>f. bronchoscope
>f. bronchoscopy (FB, FOB)
>f. catheter delivery system
>f. esophagoscopy
>f. oximeter catheter
>f. pressure catheter

fibric acid
fibrillar collagen network
fibrillary waves
fibrillation
>atrial f., auricular f. (AF)
>cardiac f.
>chronic atrial f.
>continuous atrial f. (CAF)
>idiopathic ventricular f.
>lone atrial f.
>paroxysmal atrial f. (PAF)
>f. potential
>f. rhythm
>Stroke Prevention in Atrial F. (SPAF)
>f. threshold
>ventricular f. (VF)
>ventricular tachycardia/ventricular f. (VT/VF)

fibrillation-flutter (FF)
>atrial f.-f. (AFF)

fibrillatory wave
fibrilloflutter
fibrin
>f. bodies of pleura
>f. clot
>f. glue
>f. split product
>f. thrombus

fibrinogen
>f. degradation product
>plasma f.
>radiolabeled f.

fibrinogen-fibrin
>f.-f. conversion syndrome
>f.-f. degradation product

fibrinogenolysis
fibrinohematic material
fibrinoid
>f. arteritis
>f. changes
>f. degeneration
>f. necrosis

fibrinolysis
fibrinolytic
>f. reaction
>f. system
>f. therapy

fibrinopeptide A
fibrinous
>f. acute lobar pneumonia
>f. acute pleuritis
>f. adhesion
>f. bronchitis
>f. exudate
>f. pericarditis
>f. pleurisy

fibrin-specific antibody
fibrin-stabilizing blood coagulation factor
Fibriscint
fibroblast growth factor (FGF)
fibrobronchoscope
fibrobullous
fibrocalcification
fibrocalcific lesion
fibrocystic sarcoidosis
fibroelastoma
>papillary f.

fibroelastosis
>endocardial f.
>endomyocardial f.

fibrofatty plaque
fibrogenesis
fibroid
>f. heart
>f. lung
>f. phthisis

fibroma
fibromuscular dysplasia
fibromusculoelastic lesion
fibronectin
fibroplastic
>f. cardiomyopathy
>f. disease

fibroplastica
>endocarditis parietalis f.

fibroproliferative
fibrosarcoma

fibrosing alveolitis
fibrosis
    African endomyocardial f.
    amiodarone pulmonary f.
    biventricular endomyocardial f.
    bundle-branch f.
    cystic f. (CF)
    Davies endomyocardial f.
    Davies myocardial f.
    diffuse interstitial pulmonary f.
    endocardial f.
    endomyocardial f.
    familial pulmonary f.
    idiopathic pulmonary f. (IPF)
    interstitial pulmonary f.
    myocardial f.
    parenchymal f.
    partial intermixed f.
    peribronchial f.
    perielectrode f.
    perivascular f.
    progressive interstitial
      pulmonary f.
    pulmonary f.
    rejection-associated
      pulmonary f.
    tropical endomyocardial f.
fibrosum
    pericardium f.
fibrosus
    annulus a.
fibrothorax
fibrotic
fibrous
    f. body
    f. dysplasia
    f. dysplasia of bone
    f. mediastinitis
    f. pericarditis
    f. pericardium
    f. plaque
    f. pneumonia
    f. skeleton
    f. subaortic stenosis
FIC
    forced inspiratory capacity

Fick
    F. cardiac output
    F. equation
    F. oxygen method
    F. principle
    F. technique
$FICO_2$
    fraction of inspired carbon dioxide
Fiedler myocarditis
field
    far f.
    near f.
    f. of view (FOV)
FIF
    forced inspiratory flow
fight-or-flight
    f.-o.-f. reaction
    f.-o.-f. response
figure 8 heart
figure-of-8 abnormality
figure-of-eight suture
filariasis
Filcard vena cava filter
filiformis
    pulsus f.
filiform pulse
filling
    collateral f.
    f. defect
    diastolic f.
    f. fraction
    f. gallop
    f. rumble
    ventricular f.
film
    density-exposure relationship
      of f.
    dirty f.
    f. fixer bath
    f. oxygenation
    f. processing
    scout f.
    serial cut f.'s
    f. wash bath
filming
    serialographic f.

F

NOTES

Filmtab
> Biaxin F.'s
> Rondec F.

Filoviridae virus

filter
> arterial f.
> bandpass f.
> bidirectional four-pole
> Butterworth high-pass
> digital f.
> bird's nest vena cava f.
> BTF-37 arterial blood f.
> Butterworth bidirectional f.
> D/Flex f.
> Filcard vena cava f.
> Gianturco-Roehm bird's nest
> vena cava f.
> Greenfield f.
> Greenfield IVC f.
> Greenfield vena cava f.
> Hamming-Hahn f.
> heparin arterial f.
> Interface arterial blood f.
> Jostra arterial blood f.
> Kim-Ray Greenfield
> antiembolus f.
> K-37 pediatric arterial blood f.
> LeukoNet F.
> mediastinal sump f.
> Millipore f.
> Mobin-Uddin vena cava f.
> Re/Flex f.
> Simon nitinol inferior vena
> cava f.
> Simon nitinol IVC f.
> Swank high-flow arterial
> blood f.
> triple-bandpass f.
> umbrella f.
> Vena Tech LGM f.
> Wiener f.
> William Harvey arterial
> blood f.

filtragometry

filtration
> x-ray beam f.

final
> f. common pathway
> f. rapid repolarization

Finapres
> F. blood pressure monitor
> F. finger cuff

fine-needle
> f.-n. aspiration (FNA)
> f.-n. aspiration biopsy

Finesse
> F. cardiac device
> F. guiding catheter

finger
> f. cuff
> f. dilation
> f. oximetry
> F. Phantom pulse oximeter
> testing system

finger-in-glove appearance

fingernail
> watch-crystal f.

fingerprint edema

finned pacemaker lead

Finney mask

Finochietto-Geissendorfer rib retractor

Finochietto retractor

FIO$_2$
> fraction of inspired oxygen

firing
> laser f.

first
> F. American Study of Infarct
> Survival (ASIS-1)
> f. effort
> f. heart sound (S$_1$)
> f. obtuse marginal artery (OM-
> 1)
> F. Response manual
> resuscitator
> f. shock count

first-degree
> f.-d. A-V block
> f.-d. heart block

first-effort angina

first-order kinetics

first-pass
> f.-p. radionuclide
> angiocardiography
> f.-p. technique

first-third filling fraction

Fischer
> F. pneumothoracic needle
> F. sign
> F. symptom

FISH
> fluorescent in situ hybridization

fish
> f. meal lung

f. meal lung disease
f. oil
Fisher
F. exact tesι
F. murmur
**Fisher-Paykel MR290 water-feed
chamber**
fishhook lead
fish-mouth
f.-m. cusp
f.-m. incision
f.-m. mitral stenosis
fishnet pattern
fissuring
plaque f.
fist percussion
fistula, pl. **fistulae, fistulas**
aortocaval f.
arteriovenous f. (AVF)
A-V Gore-Tex f.
brachioaxillary bridge graft f.
Brescia-Cimino A-V f.
bronchopleural f.
bronchopulmonary f.
cameral f.
carotid-cavernous f.
Cimino-Brescia arteriovenous f.
congenital pulmonary
arteriovenous f.
coronary artery-right
ventricular f.
Eck f.
enteric f.
Gore-Tex AF f.
Gross tracheoesophageal f.
pleuroesophageal f.
pulmonary arteriovenous f.
renal f.
solitary pulmonary
arteriovenous f.
subclavian arteriovenous f.
traumatic f.
Fitch obturator
fitness
biological f.
cardiovascular f.
Fitzgerald forceps

FIVC
forced inspiratory vital capacity
five-chamber view
**five-view chest x-ray with AP, PA,
lateral, and both oblique views**
fixative
Saccomanno f.
fixed
f. airflow obstruction
f. coupling
f. perfusion defect
fixed-rate
f.-r. mode
f.-r. pacemaker
f.-r. pulse generator
fixed-wire balloon dilatation system
fixer bath
FK-506
fL
femtoliter
FL4 guide
flabby airway
Flack node
Flagyl
F. Oral
flail
f. chest
f. chordae
f. leaflet
f. mitral valve
f. segments
flair valve
flame emission spectroscopy (FES)
flame-shaped hemorrhages
Flantadin
flap
Abbe f.
Eloesser f.
intimal f.
Linton f.
liver f.
microvascular free f.
pericardial f.
f. tracheostomy
flapping
f. sound

NOTES

F

flapping *(continued)*
  f. tremor
  f. valve syndrome
flare
  asthma f.
  wheal and f.
flaring
  alar f.
  nasal f.
FLASH
  fast low-angle shot
  FLASH MRI
  FLASH sequences
flash
  F. portable spirometer
  f. pulmonary edema
flashlamp excited pulsed dye
flashlamp-pulsed Nd:YAG laser
flask-shaped heart
flattening
  T wave f.
flavus
  Aspergillus f.
flax-dresser's disease
Flaxedil
flea-bitten kidney
flecainide
Fleischner syndrome
Fleisch pneumotachograph
Fletcher factor
Flex
  F. stent
  F. Tip guidewire
Flexguard Tip catheter
Flexguide intubation guide
flexibility
flexible
  f. fiberoptic bronchoscope
  f. fiberoptic bronchoscopy
    (FFB)
  f. guidewire
Flexicath silicone subclavian
  cannula
flexion
  elbow f.
  hip f.
  shoulder horizontal f.
  trunk forward f.
FlexStent
  Cook F.
FlexStent
  Cook F.
Flexxicon Blue dialysis catheter
flicker fusion threshold

flint
  f. disease
  F. murmur
flip
  f. angle
  LDH f.
flipped T wave
floating wall motion study
Flolan
  F. injection
FloMap
  F. guidewire
  F. velocimeter
Flonase
flooding
  alveolar f.
floppy
  f. mitral valve (FMV)
  f. valve syndrome
floppy-tipped guidewire
flora
  mixed f.
  respiratory f.
Flo-Rester vascular occluder
Florex medical compression
  stockings
florid
  f. congestive heart failure
  f. pulmonary edema
Florinef Acetate
flosequinan
flow
  f. across orifice
  anterograde f.
  arterial blood f.
  f. artifact
  blood f.
  cerebral blood f. (CBF)
  collateral f.
  f. convergence method
  coronary blood f. (CBF)
  coronary sinus blood f.
    (CSBF)
  effective renal blood f.
    (ERBF)
  endocardial f.
  f. envelope
  epicardial f.
  forced expiratory f. (FEF)
  forced inspiratory f. (FIF)
  forced midexpiratory f. (FMF)
  hepatofugal f.
  hepatopetal f.

high f. (HF)
f. injector
laminar blood f.
f. mapping
f. mapping technique
maximal forced expiratory f.
  (FEFmax)
maximal midexpiratory f.
  (MMEF)
mean forced midexpiratory f.
myocardial blood f. (MBF)
pansystolic f.
peak expiratory f. (PEF)
peak inspiratory f. (PIF)
peak tidal inspiratory f. (PTIF)
petal-fugal f.
pulmonary blood f.
pulsatile f.
f. rate
f. ratio (Qp/Qs)
regional myocardial blood f.
  (RMBF)
splanchnic blood f.
systemic blood f. (SBF)
transvalvular f.
tricuspid valve f.
f. velocity
f. wire
Wright peak f.
flow-assisted, short-term (FAST)
flow-directed balloon cardiovascular
  catheter
FloWire
Doppler F.
F. guidewire
flow-limiting stenosis
flowmeter (*See also* meter)
Gould electromagnetic f.
Narcomatic f.
peak f.
Transonic f.
flowmetry
magnetic resonance f. (MRF)
pulsed Doppler f.
Flowtron
F. DVT pump
F. DVT pump system

flow-volume loop
Floxin
F. injection
F. Oral
Floyd loop cannula
fluconazole
flucytosine
fludrocortisone
f. acetate
fluens
pulsus f.
FLUENT
Fluvastatin Long-Term Extension
  Trial
fluffy
f. alveolar infiltrate
f. cotton-wool exudate
fluffy-cuffed tube
Flu-Glow strip
fluid
f. aspiration
bronchoalveolar lavage f.
  (BALF)
crystalloid f.
f. dynamics
epithelial lining f. (ELF)
f. mechanics
pericardial f.
pleural f.
retained lung f. (RLF)
f. therapy
fluid-filled
f.-f. balloon-tipped flow-directed
  catheter
f.-f. pigtail catheter
f.-f. pressure monitoring
  guidewire
Flu-Imune
Fluitran
fluke
lung f.
Flumadine
F. Oral
flumazenil
flunarizine
flunisolide
flunitrazepam

F

NOTES

Fluogen
fluorescein angiography
fluorescence
    laser-induced arterial f. (LIAF)
    f. polarization
    f. spectroscopy
fluorescence-guided smart laser
fluorescent
    f. antimembrane antibody
      (FAMA)
    f. in situ hybridization (FISH)
    f. treponemal antibody
      absorption (FTA-ABS)
fluoride
    hydrogen f.
    f. toxicity
fluorine-18
    f. fluorodeoxyglucose
fluorocarbon poisoning
5-fluorocytosine
fluorodeoxyglucose
    cyclotron-produced F-18 f.
    fluorine-18 f.
2-fluoro-2-deoxyglucose (FDG)
fluorodopamine positron emission
    tomographic scanning
Fluoro-Free
    P.A.S. Port F.-F.
fluorography
    spot-film f.
fluorohydrocortisone
Fluoroplex Topical
fluoroquinolone
fluoroscopic
    f. guidance
    f. visualization
fluoroscopy
    biplane f.
    C-arm f.
    kV f.
Fluoro Tip cannula
fluorouracil
5-fluorouracil (5-FU)
Fluosol
    F. artificial blood
Fluotec vaporizer
fluoxetine
    f. hydrochloride
flurazepam
flush
    f. aortogram
    f. aortography
    f. and bathe technique

    heparin f.
    mahogany f.
    malar f.
flushed
    aspirated and f.
flushing
    f. time
fluticasone propionate
flutter
    atrial f., auricular f.
    f. cycle length
    diaphragmatic f.
    impure f.
    mediastinal f.
    pure f.
    f. R interval
    ventricular f.
flutter-fibrillation
    f.-f. waves
Flutter therapeutic device
Fluvastatin
    F. Long-Term Extension Trial
    (FLUENT)
fluvastatin
    f. sodium
flux
    soldering f.
    transmembrane calcium f.
fluxionary hyperemia
Fluzone
flying W sign
Flynt needle
FMA cardiovascular imaging system
FMF
    forced midexpiratory flow
FMIV
    forced mandatory intermittent
      ventilation
FMV
    floppy mitral valve
FNA
    fine-needle aspiration
foam
    f. cell
    polyurethane f.
    f. stability test
foamy
    f. macrophage
    f. myocardial cell
FOB
    fiberoptic bronchoscopy
focal
    f. block

f. bronchopneumonia
f. eccentric stenosis
f. edema
focal-dust emphysema
focus, pl. **foci**
    arrhythmia f.
    Assman f.
    Ghon f.
    Simon foci
Foerger airway
Foerster forceps
Fogarty
    F. adherent clot catheter
    F. calibrator
    F. embolectomy catheter
    F. graft thrombectomy catheter
Fogarty-Chin extrusion balloon
  catheter
fold
    bulboventricular f.
    Marshall f.
    vestigial f.
Folex PFS
folic acid
follicular
    f. bronchiectasis
    f. bronchiolitis
    f. pharyngitis
Foltz-Overton cardiac catheter
Fome-Cuf tracheostomy tube
Fontan
    F. atriopulmonary anastomosis
    F. modification of Norwood
      procedure
    F. operation
    F. repair
Fontan-Baudet procedure
Fontan-Kreutzer procedure
food
    f. angina
    f. asthma
foot
    f. cradle
    trash f.
    f. ulcer
Foradil
foramen, pl. **foramina**

bulboventricular f.
Galen f.
interventricular f.
f. of Monro
f. of Morgagni
f. ovale, oval f.
f. secundum
thebesian foramina
f. venae cavae
force
    atrial ejection f.
    drag f.'s
    left ventricular f.'s
    peak twitch f.
    P terminal f.
    shear f.
    Starling f.
    Venturi f.'s
forced
    f. beat
    f. cycle
    f. expiratory capacity (FEC)
    f. expiratory flow (FEF)
    f. expiratory spirogram (FES)
    f. expiratory time (FET)
    f. expiratory volume (FEV)
    f. expiratory volume in 1
      second (FEV_1)
    f. expiratory volume in 1
      second to forced vital
      capacity ratio (FEV_1/FVC)
    f. expiratory volume timed to
      forced vital capacity ratio
      (FEV/FVC)
    f. inspiratory capacity (FIC)
    f. inspiratory flow (FIF)
    f. inspiratory vital capacity
      (FIVC)
    f. ischemia-reperfusion
      transition
    f. mandatory intermittent
      ventilation (FMIV)
    f. midexpiratory flow (FMF)
    f. oscillation technique (FOT)
    f. respiration
    f. vital capacity (FVC)

F

NOTES

forced *(continued)*
  f. vital capacity analysis
    (FVCA)
force-frequency relation
force-length relation
forceps
  Adson f.
  Babcock thoracic tissue-
    holding f.
  Barraya f.
  Bengolea f.
  biopsy f.
  Bloodwell f.
  Boettcher f.
  bronchus-grasping f.
  Brown-Adson f.
  Bycep biopsy f.
  Carmalt f.
  coagulation f.
  Cook flexible biopsy f.
  Cooley f.
  Cooley-Baumgarten aortic f.
  Crafoord pulmonary f.
  Crafoord-Sellor hemostatic f.
  Crile-Duval lung-grasping f.
  Cushing f.
  DeBakey Autraugrip f.
  DeBakey-Colovira-Rumel
    thoracic f.
  DeBakey-Mixter thoracic f.
  DeBakey-Péan cardiovascular f.
  DeBakey tissue f.
  Duracep biopsy f.
  Duval-Crile lung f.
  Duval lung-grasping f.
  Englert f.
  Fitzgerald f.
  Foerster f.
  Foss cardiovascular f.
  Fraenkel f.
  Gerald f.
  Harken f.
  Hopkins f.
  Iselin f.
  Julian thoracic f.
  Kahler bronchial biopsy f.
  McQuigg-Mixter bronchial f.
  Potts bronchial f.
  Price-Thomas bronchial f.
  Ruel f.
  Rumel thoracic f.
  Sam Roberts bronchial
    biopsy f.

Scheinmann laryngeal f.
Scholten endomyocardial
  bioptome and biopsy f.
Tuttle thoracic f.
Varco thoracic f.
force-velocity-length relation
force-velocity relation
force-velocity-volume relation
Ford equation
Foregger
  F. laryngoscope
  F. rigid esophagoscope
Forerunner coronary sinus guiding
  catheter
Forlanini treatment
form
  myocardial infarction in
    dumbbell f.
  pentamidine in aerosol f.
formaldehyde
format
  quad screen f.
  scanning f.
formation
  aspergilloma f.
  coagulum f.
  impulse f.
  rouleaux f.
forme fruste
formicans
  pulsus f.
formicant pulse
formoterol
formula, pl. **formulas, formulae**
  Bayer Select Pain Relief F.
  Bazett f.
  biplane f.
  Bohr f.
  Brozek f.
  Cannon f.
  Friedewald f.
  Ganz f.
  geometric cube f.
  Gorlin f.
  Gorlin hydraulic f.
  Hakki f.
  Hamilton-Stewart f.
  Impact specialized feeding f.
  Janz f.
  f. of Mirsky
  Poiseuille resistance f.
  Sramek f.
  Teichholz f.

Triaminic AM Decongestant F.
Yeager f.
Forney syndrome
Forrester
F. syndrome
F. Therapeutic Classification
grades I through IV
forskolin
adenylate cyclase stimulator f.
Fortaz
Forte
Aristocort F.
Enduronyl F.
Robinul F.
fortis
pulsus f.
fortuitum
Mycobacterium f.
forward
f. conduction
f. heart failure
f. triangle method
f. triangle technique
foscarnet
Foscavir injection
fosinoprilat
fosinoprilic acid
fosinopril sodium
fossa, pl. **fossae**
antecubital f.
f. ovalis
supraclavicular f.
Foss cardiovascular forceps
FOT
forced oscillation technique
Fothergill disease
founder effect
four-beam laser Doppler probe
four-chamber view
four-day syndrome
Fourier
F. series analysis
F. transform
F. transform analysis
F. two-dimensional imaging
four-legged cage valve
Fourmentin thoracic index

Fournier gangrene
fourth heart sound (S_4)
**four-view chest x-ray with PA and
lateral, and both oblique views**
FOV
field of view
foveated chest
Fowler
F. single-breath test
F. thoracoplasty
Fox green dye
FPV
FR139317
fractal
fraction
CPK-MB f.
ejection f. (EF)
f. of expired carbon dioxide
($FECO_2$)
filling f.
first-third filling f.
global left ventricular
ejection f.
f. of inspired carbon dioxide
($FICO_2$)
f. of inspired oxygen (FIO_2)
left ventricular ejection f.
(LVEF)
light pen-determined ejection f.
MB f.
regurgitant f.
rest ejection f.
right ventricular ejection f.
(RVEF)
shortening f.
Teichholz ejection f.
fractional myocardial shortening
fracture
cough f.
outlet strut f. (OSF)
pacemaker lead f.
plaque f.
Fraenkel
F. forceps
F. nodes
fragment
f. antigen-binding

F

NOTES

fragment *(continued)*
   antimyosin monoclonal antibody
     with Fab f. (AMA-Fab)
   catheter f.
   Digibind digoxin immune
     Fab f.'s
   Digidote digoxin immune
     Fab f.'s
   Fab f.
fragmentation
   f. myocarditis
   f. of myocardium
Fragmin
frame
   B-scan f.
   Elgiloy f.
Framingham Heart study
Francisella tularensis
Frank
   F. EKG lead placement system
   F. XYZ orthogonal lead
   F. XYZ orthogonal lead
     system
Frankel treatment
Frank-Starling
   F.-S. curve
   F.-S. mechanism
   F.-S. reserve
Frank-Straub-Wiggers-Starling
   principle
Fräntzel murmur
Franzen needle guide
Franz monophasic action potential
   catheter
frappage
Fraser Harlake respirometer
Frater
   F. intracardiac retractor
   F. suture
Fraunhofer zone
FRC
   functional residual capacity
Frederick pneumothorax needle
Fredrickson
   F. classification
   F. dyslipidemia
   F. hyperlipoproteinemia
     classification
Fredrickson, Levy and Lees
   classification
free
   f. fatty acids (FFA)
   f. thyrotoxin index

free-beam laser
Freedom
   Accu-Chek II F.
FreeDop
   F. portable Doppler unit
Freestyle aortic root bioprosthesis
Freeway Lite portable aerosol
   compressor
Freitag stent
frémissement cattaire
fremitus
   auditory f.
   bronchial f.
   friction f.
   hydatid f.
   pectoral f.
   pericardial f.
   pleural f.
   rhonchal f.
   subjective f.
   tactile f.
   tussive f.
   vocal f.
French
   F. double-lumen catheter
   F. JR4 Schneider catheter
   F. paradox
   F. SAL catheter
   F. scale
   F. shaft catheter
   F. sheath
   F. size
   F. sizing of catheter
frequency
   ciliary beat f.
   critical flicker f.
   f. domain imaging
   dynamic f. response
   fundamental f.
   natural f.
   pulse repetition f. (PRF)
   resonant f.
   f. response
   f. shifter
   f. tracer
frequency-domain analysis
frequens
   pulsus f.
fresh frozen plasma (FFP)
Fresnel zone
Freund
   F. anomaly
   F. operation

freundii
  Citrobacter f.
Frey-Sauerbruch rib shears
friction
  f. fremitus
  f. murmur
  f. rub
  f. sound
Friedewald
  F. approximation
  F. equation
  F. formula
Friedländer
  F. bacillus pneumonia
  F. pneumobacillus
Friedman
  Friedman Splint brace
  Friedman test
Friedreich
  F. ataxia
  F. disease
  F. sign
Friedrich rib elevator
frog breathing
froissement
  bruit de f.
fronds
  sea f.
front wall needle
frosted heart
frosting heart
frothy sputum
frottement
  bruit de f.
Frouin
  quadrangulation of F.
frozen thorax
FRP
  functional refractory period
fructosamine
Frumil
fruste
  forme f.
frustrate systole

FTA-ABS
  fluorescent treponemal antibody
  absorption
  FTA-ABS test
5-FU
  5-fluorouracil
fucosidosis
fugax
  amaurosis partialis f.
Fujinon
  F. flexible bronchoscope
  F. variceal injector
**Fukunaga-Hayes unbiased jackknife
  classification**
fulguration
  electrical f.
Fuller bivalve trach tube
fully automatic pacemaker
fulminans
  purpura f.
fumagillin
fumarate
  bisoprolol f.
  clemastine f.
  ferrous f.
  ibutilide f.
Fumasorb
Fumerin
fumes
  cadmium f.
  soldering f.
fumigatus
  Aspergillus f.
function
  atrial transport f.
  cardiac f.
  cardiovascular f.
  contractile f.
  f. curve
  diastolic f.
  hepatic f.
  left ventricular f.
  lung f.
  mitochondrial f.
  myocardial f.
  neurohormonal f.
  parasympathetic f.

F

NOTES

function *(continued)*
    perturbed autonomic nervous
      system f.
    phagocytic f.
    probability density f. (PDF)
    pulmonary f. (PF)
    pump f.
    renal f.
    respiratory f.
    right ventricular f.
    sigh f.
    sinus node f.
    systolic f.
    ventricular f.
functional
    f. assessment
    f. block
    f. capacity classification
    f. cardiovascular disease
    f. congestion
    f. dyspnea
    f. image
    f. imaging
    f. murmur
    f. pain
    f. refractory period (FRP)
    f. residual capacity (FRC)
    f. subtraction
fundamental frequency
fundoplication
    Belsey Mark II, IV f.
    Belsey two-thirds wrap f.
    Collis-Nissen f.
    Nissen 360-degree wrap f.
    Rossetti modification of
      Nissen f.
fundus, pl. **fundi**
funduscopic examination
fungal
    f. endocarditis
    f. infection
fungating mass
fungi (*pl. of* fungus)

Fungizone
    F. Intravenous
fungoides
    mycosis f.
fungus, pl. **fungi**
    f. ball
funic
    f. pulse
    f. souffle
funnel
    f. chest
    f. dynamics
    mitral f.
    vascular f.
Furadantin
Furalan
Furan
Furanite
furifosmin
Furman Type II electrogram
furosemide
furrier's
    f. lung
    f. lung disease
furrow
    atrioventricular f.
    Schmorl f.
fusidic acid
fusiform
    f. aortic aneurysm
    f. bronchiectasis
fusion
    f. beat
    commissural f.
    f. complex
    critical flicker f.
    entrainment with concealed f.
Fusobacterium
    F. nucleatum
FVC
    forced vital capacity
FVCA
    forced vital capacity analysis

3G4
G5
G5 massage and percussion
machine
G5 Neocussor percussor
Ga
gallium
⁶⁸Ga
gallium-68
GABI
German Angioplasty Bypass Surgery
Investigation
Gabriel Tucker tube
Gad hypothesis
gadolinium-diethylenetriamine
pentaacetic acid (Gd-DTPA)
gadolinium-DTPA
gag
g. gene
g. reflex
Gailliard syndrome
gain
g. control
time compensation g. (TCG)
time-varied g. (TVG)
Gairdner disease
Gaisböck syndrome
gait
ataxic g.
gaiter perforators
galactose
galactosidase deficiency
Galanti-Giusti colorimetric method
Galaxy pacemaker
Galen foramen
Gallagher bipolar mapping probe
gallamine triethiodide
Gallavardin
G. murmur
G. phenomenon
gallinatum
pectus g.
gallium (Ga)
g. scan
gallium-67
g. imaging
g. scintigraphy
gallium-68 (⁶⁸Ga)
gallop
atrial diastolic g.

diastolic g.
filling g.
presystolic g.
protodiastolic g.
g. rhythm
S₄ g.
S₇ g.
S₃ g.
g. sound
summation g. (S₇)
systolic g.
gallopamil
galop
bruit de g.
galvanometer
Einthoven string g.
gambiense
Trypanosoma g.
Gambro
G. Lundia Minor hemodialyzer
G. oxygenator
Gamimune N
gamma
g. globulin
g. hydroxybutyrate (GHB)
g. knife
g. ray
g. scintillation camera
gamma-aminobutyric acid
gamma-1b
interferon g.
Gammagard S/D
gammopathy
polyclonal g.
Gamna-Gandy bodies
ganciclovir (DHPG)
ganglion
Bock g.
stellate g.
Wrisberg g.
ganglionic blocker
gangliosidosis
gangrene
angiosclerotic g.
cold g.
diabetic g.
dry g.
embolic g.
emphysematous g.
Fournier g.

G

213

gangrene *(continued)*
  gas g.
  hot g.
gangrenosa
  angina g.
gangrenous
  g. emphysema
  g. pharyngitis
  g. pneumonia
gannister disease
Gantanol
gantry
Ganz-Edwards coronary infusion catheter
Ganz formula
gap
  anion g.
  auscultatory g.
  g. conduction phenomenon
  excitable g.
  g. junction
  silent g.
Garamycin
  G. injection
Garcia aorta clamp
Garfield-Holinger laryngoscope
gargoylism
garment
  antishock g.
  Jobst pressure g.
  pneumatic antishock g. (PASG)
garnet
  yttrium-aluminum-g. (YAG)
Garrett dilator
Gärtner
  G. method
  G. tonometer
  G. vein phenomenon
gas, pl. gases
  arterial blood g. (ABG)
  blood g.
  capillary blood g. (CBG)
  g. chromatography
  g. clearance
  g. clearance measurement
  g. clearance method
  g. constant (R)
  g. embolism
  g. endarterectomy
  g. exchange
  g. gangrene

  partial pressure of CO g. (PCO)
  partial pressure of CO_2 g.
gaseous pulse
gasp reflex
gastric lung
gastrocardiac syndrome
gastroepiploic artery (GEA)
gastroesophageal
  g. reflux (GER)
  g. reflux disease (GERD)
  g. sphincter
gastrointestinal
  g. symptom
  g. therapeutic system (GITS)
  g. tract
gate
  acquisition g.
  D g.
  F g.
  H g.
  M g.
gated
  g. blood-pool angiography
  g. blood-pool imaging
  g. blood-pool scanning
  g. blood-pool scintigraphy
  g. blood-pool study (GBPS)
  g. cardiac scan
  g. computed tomography
  g. equilibrium ventriculography, frame-mode acquisition
  g. equilibrium ventriculography, list-mode acquisition
  g. list mode
  g. nuclear angiogram
  g. radionuclide angiography
  g. sweep magnetic resonance imaging
  g. system
  g. technique
GateWay Y-adapter rotating hemostatic valve
gating
  cardiac g.
  in-memory g.
  g. mechanism
  R wave g.
  g. signal
Gaucher disease
gauge
  mercury-in-Silastic strain g.

pounds per square inch g. (psig)
Silastic strain g.
strain g.
gaussian
Gauthier bicycle ergometer
gauze
Teletrast g.
Xeroform g.
GBPS
gated blood-pool study
Gc protein
GCS
graduated compression stockings
Gd-DTPA
gadolinium-diethylenetriamine pentaacetic acid
Gd-DTPA-enhanced MRI
GDP
guanosine 5′-diphosphate
GEA
gastroepiploic artery
GEA graft
Gehan statistic
gel
aluminum hydroxide g.
Cann-Ease moisturizing nasal g.
Dermaflex G.
electrode g.
H.P. Acthar G.
gelatin
absorbable g.
g. compression body
g. compression boot
g. sponge slurry
zinc g.
gelatinous acute pneumonia
Gelfilm Ophthalmic
gelfiltration
Gelfoam
G. cookie
thrombin-soaked G.
G. Topical
Gelpi retractor
gelsolin
Gemcor

gemfibrozil
Gemini DDD pacemaker
Gen2 pacemaker
Genabid Oral
Genahist Oral
Genamin Expectorant
Genatuss DM
gene
angiotensinogen g.
beta-myosin heavy-chain g.
env g.
g. expression
gag g.
human preproendothelin-1 g.
g. secretor
g. transcription
tuple-1 g.
zinc finger g.
General
G. Electric Advantx system
G. Electric Pass-C echocardiograph machine
G. Well-Being Index
generation
thrombin g.
generator
asynchronous pulse g.
atrial synchronous pulse g.
atrial triggered pulse g.
Aurora pulse g.
Bird neonatal CPAP g.
Chardack-Greatbatch implantable cardiac pulse g.
Coratomic implantable pulse g.
Cordis Theta Sequicor DDD pulse g.
Cosmos II pulse g.
CPI-PRx pulse g.
Cyberlith multiprogrammable pulse g.
demand pulse g.
Down flow g.
fixed-rate pulse g.
Intec AID cardioverter-defibrillator g.
Itrel 1 unipolar pulse g.
Maxilith pacemaker pulse g.

G

NOTES

generator *(continued)*
   Medtronic pulse g.
   Microlith pacemaker pulse g.
   Minilith pacemaker pulse g.
   Programalith III pulse g.
   pulse g.
   quadripolar Itrel 2 pulse g.
   standby pulse g.
   Stilith implantable cardiac
     pulse g.
   tantalum-178 g.
   Trilogy DC, DR, SR pulse g.
   unipolar Itrel 1 pulse g.
   ventricular inhibited pulse g.
   ventricular synchronous
     pulse g.
   ventricular triggered pulse g.
   Vivalith II pulse g.
   x-ray g.
GenESA closed-loop delivery system
genetic
   g. disorder
   g. heterogeneity
   g. hypertrophic cardiomyopathy
   g. locus
   g. transmission
Genisis pacemaker
GenJect
genotype
   DD g.
Genpril
Gensan
Gensini
   G. cardiac device
   G. coronary arteriography
     catheter
   G. index
   G. score
   G. Teflon catheter
Gentab-LA
gentamicin
   g. sulfate
Gentle-Flo suction catheter
Gentran
Geocillin
geometric cube formula
geometry
   normal g.
   g. of stenosis
   ventricular g.
Geopen

George
   G. Lewis technique
   G. Washington strut
geotrichosis
GER
   gastroesophageal reflux
Gerald forceps
Gerbode
   G. annuloplasty
   G. defect
   G. sternal retractor
GERD
   gastroesophageal reflux disease
Gerdy intra-auricular loop
Gerhardt
   G. change
   G. syndrome
   G. triangle
German Angioplasty Bypass
   Surgery Investigation (GABI)
germ cell tumor
gerontology
gestational hypertension
Gesterol injection
Gey solution
GHB
   gamma hydroxybutyrate
Ghon
   G. complex
   G. focus
   G. primary lesion
ghost vessel
giant
   g. cell
   g. cell aortitis
   g. cell arteritis
   g. cell carcinoma
   g. cell myocarditis
   g. cell pneumonia
   g. v wave
   g. a wave
Gianturco
   G. wool-tufted wire coil
   G. Z stent
Gianturco-Roehm bird's nest vena
   cava filter
Gianturco-Roubin stent
Gibbon-Landis test
Gibson
   G. circularity index
   G. murmur
   G. rule
Giertz rib guillotine

Giertz-Shoemaker rib shears
GIK
 glucose, insulin, and potassium
Gill I respirator
Gill-Jonas modification of Norwood procedure
GISSI
 Gruppo Italiano Per lo Studio Della Streptokinase Nell'Infarto Miocardio
gitalin
GITS
 gastrointestinal therapeutic system
giving-up/given-up response
glabrata
 Candida g.
 Torulopsis g.
glandular pharyngitis
glare
 veiling g.
Glasgow
 G. Coma Scale
 G. sign
glass blower's emphysema
Glassman clamp
glassy degeneration
Glattelast compression pantyhose
Glaucon
glebae
 Acanthamoeba g.
Glenn
 G. anastomosis
 G. operation
 G. procedure
 G. shunt
glibenclamide
Glidecath hydrophilic coated catheter
Glidewire
 G. Gold surgical guidewire
glipizide
Glisson capsule
glissonitis
global
 g. amnesia
 g. aphasia
 g. hypokinesis

 g. left ventricular ejection fraction
 G. Utilization of Streptokinase and t-PA for Occluded Coronary Arteries (GUSTO)
 G. Utilization of Streptokinase and t-PA for Occluded Coronary Arteries protocol
globoid heart
globular
 g. heart
 g. sputum
 g. thrombus
globulin
 antithymocyte g.
 gamma g.
 lymphocyte immune g. (Atgam)
 rabbit antithymocyte g.
 respiratory syncytial virus IV immune g.
 Rho(D) immune g.
globus
 g. hystericus
 g. pharyngis
glomerulonephritis
 acute g. (AGN)
glossopharyngeal
 g. breathing
 g. neuralgia
glottic atresia
glove
 compression g.'s
 ESP radiation reduction examination g.'s
gloved fist technique
Glover auricular-appendage clamp
glucagon
gluceptate
 calcium g.
Gluck rib shears
glucocorticoid
glucocorticoid-induced hypertension
glucocorticosteroid
glucometer
gluconate
 calcium g.

NOTES

217

gluconate *(continued)*
  ferrous g.
  potassium g.
  quinidine g.
Glucophage
glucose
  g. intolerance
  g. metabolism
  g. uptake
glucose-6-phosphate dehydrogenase (G6PD)
glucose, insulin, and potassium (GIK)
glucose-6-phosphatase
glucosidase deficiency
Glucotrol
GlucoWatch
glucuronate
  trimetrexate g.
glue
  fibrin g.
glu-plasminogen
glutamate
glutamic-oxaloacetic transaminase (GOT)
glutamic oxalotransaminase
glutaraldehyde-tanned
  g.-t. bovine collagen tube
  g.-t. bovine heart valve
  g.-t. porcine heart valve
glutathione
glutethimide
Glutose
glyburide
glyceraldehyde 3-phosphate
glycerin
glycerol
  G.-T
glyceryl trinitrate
glycocalicin
  plasma g.
glycocalicine index
Glycofed
glycogen
  g. cardiomegaly
  g. depletion
  g. loading
  g. phosphorylase
  g. storage disease
  g. synthase
glycogenosis
  cardiac g.
glycolysis

glycolytic enzymes
glycopeptide teicoplanin
glycoprotein
  g. IIb/IIIa receptor
  platelet receptor g.
glycopyrrolate
glycoside
  cardiac g.
  digitalis g.
glycosis
glycosphingolipid disorder
glycosylated hemoglobin
glycosylation of intracellular proteins
Glycotuss-dM
glycyl compound
glycyrrhizinic acid
Glydeine
Glynase PresTab
Glyrol
GM-CSF
  granulocyte/macrophage colony-stimulating factor
GMP
  guanosine monophosphate
GNB
  gram-negative bacilli
goblet
  g. cell
  g. cell degranulation
  g. cell metaplasia
Godart expirograph
Goeltec catheter
Goethlin test
Goetz
  G. bipolar electrode
  G. cardiac device
Gohrbrand cardiac dilator
goiter
  diving g.
  plunging g.
  suffocative g.
  wandering g.
Golaski knitted Dacron graft
Golaski-UMI vascular prosthesis
gold (Au)
  g. marker
  g. salt
Goldberg-MPC mediastinoscope
Goldblatt
  G. hypertension
  G. phenomenon

Golden
S sign of G.
Goldenhar syndrome
Goldflam disease
Goldflam-Erb disease
gold-195m
g. radionuclide
Goldman
G. cardiac risk index score
G. index of risk
G. risk-factor index
Goldscheider percussion
Goldsmith operation
Goldstein hemoptysis
Golgi tendon organs
Golub EKG lead
Gomco thoracic drainage pump
Gomori methenamine silver stain
gondii
Toxoplasma g.
gonococcal endocarditis
Goodale-Lubin
G.-L. cardiac device
G.-L. catheter
Goodpasture syndrome
goose-honk murmur
gooseneck deformity
Goosen vascular punch
gordonae
Mycobacterium g.
Gordon elementary body
Gore-Tex
G.-T. AF fistula
G.-T. baffle
G.-T. cardiovascular patch
G.-T. jump graft
G.-T. surgical membrane
G.-T. tube
G.-T. vascular graft
Goris background subtraction technique
Gorlin
G. catheter
G. constant
G. equation
G. formula

G. hydraulic formula
G. syndrome
gormanii
Legionella g.
GOT
glutamic oxaloacetic transaminase
Gott
G. butterfly heart valve
G. shunt
Gott-Daggett heart valve prosthesis
Gould
G. electromagnetic flowmeter
G. PentaCath 5-lumen thermodilution catheter
G. Statham pressure transducer
gout
gouty phlebitis
Gowers
G. contraction
G. sign
G. syndrome
G6PD
glucose-6-phosphate dehydrogenase
G proteins
grabbing technique
gracile habitus
Gradational Step exercise stress test
grade
thrombus g.
g. 1 through 6 murmur
Graded Exercise exercise stress test
gradient
alveolar-arterial oxygen tension g., alveoloarterial oxygen tension g.
alveolocapillary partial pressure g.
aortic pressure g.
aortic valve g. (AVG)
arm-leg g.
atrioventricular g.
diastolic g.
Doppler pressure g.
g. gel electrophoresis
hemodynamic g.
intracavitary pressure g.

G

gradient *(continued)*
    mitral valve g. (MVG)
    peak instantaneous g.
    peak systolic g. (PSG)
    peak transaortic valve g.
    pressure g.
    pulmonary valve g.
    g. reduction
    residual g.
    systolic g.
    transaortic valve g.
    transvalvular aortic g.
    ventricular g.
gradient-recalled acquisition in the
    steady state (GRASS)
grading
    Canadian Cardiovascular
      Society g.
graduated compression stockings
    (GCS)
graft
    albumin-coated vascular g.
    albuminized woven Dacron
      tube g.
    aldehyde-tanned bovine carotid
      artery g.
    aortic tube g.
    aortocoronary bypass g.
      (ACBG)
    aortocoronary snake g.
    aortofemoral bypass g. (AFBG)
    aortoiliac bypass g.
    araldehyde-tanned bovine
      carotid artery g.
    autogenic g.
    autologous fat g.
    Biograft g.
    Bionit vascular g.
    BioPolyMeric vascular g.
    Björk-Shiley g.
    bypass g.
    Carbo-Seal cardiovascular
      composite g.
    collagen-impregnated knitted
      Dacron velour g.
    compressed Ivalon patch g.
    Cooley woven Dacron g.
    coronary artery bypass g.
      (CABG)
    Cragg endoluminal g.
    Creech aortoiliac g.
    Cryolife valve g.
    Dacron Sauvage g.

    Dacron tube g.
    Diastat vascular access g.
    Edwards-Tapp arterial g.
    Edwards woven Teflon aortic
      bifurcation g.
    EPTFE g.
    expanded polytetrafluoroethylene
      vascular g.
    EXS femoropopliteal bypass g.
    Favaloro saphenous vein
      bypass g.
    FEP-ringed Gore-Tex
      vascular g.
    GEA g.
    Golaski knitted Dacron g.
    Gore-Tex jump g.
    Gore-Tex vascular g.
    Hancock pericardial valve g.
    Hancock vascular g.
    HUV bypass g.
    IEA g.
    Impra bypass g.
    Impra-Graft microporous PTFE
      vascular g.
    Ionescu-Shiley vascular g.
    ITA g.
    jump g.
    Kimura cartilage g.
    lower extremity bypass g.
    mammary artery g.
    mandrel g.
    Meadox g.
    mesenteric bypass g.
    Microknit patch g.
    Microvel double velour g.
    pedicle g.
    Perma-Flow coronary g.
    Poly-Plus Dacron vascular g.
    portacaval H g.
    g. rejection
    renal artery bypass g.
    reversed saphenous vein g.
    saphenous vein g.
    SCA-EX 7F g.
    Shiley Tetraflex vascular g.
    skip g.
    snake g.
    subclavian artery bypass g.
    Teflon g.
    Varivas R denatured
      homologous vein g.
    g. vasculopathy
    Vascutek gelseal vascular g.

Vascutek knitted vascular g.
Vascutek woven vascular g.
vein g.
Velex woven Dacron
vascular g.
velour collar g.
vertebral artery bypass g.
Vitagraft vascular g.
Weavenit patch g.
woven Dacron tube g.
GraftAssist vein-graft holder
grafting
endarterectomy and coronary
artery bypass g. (E-CABG)
port-access coronary artery
bypass g.
graft-seeking catheter
Graham
G. rib contractor
G. Steell murmur
grain dust
gram-negative
g.-n. bacilli (GNB)
g.-n. cocci
g.-n. endocarditis
g.-n. organism
g.-n. pericarditis
Grampian Region Early
Anistreplase Trial (GREAT)
gram-positive
g.-p. bacilli
g.-p. cocci
g.-p. organism
Gram stain
Grancher
G. sign
G. triad
Grant abdominal aortic aneurysmal
clamp
granular
g. cell tumor
g. pharyngitis
g. respiration
granulation
Bayle g.'s
g. stenosis

granule
azurophil g.
Fauvel g.'s
Much g.'s
Granulex
granulocyte/macrophage colony-
stimulating factor (GM-CSF)
granulocytopenia
granuloma
cocci g.
eosinophilic g.
sarcoid g.
granulomatosis
allergic g.
bronchocentric g. (BCG)
lymphomatoid g.
Wegener g.
granulomatous
g. arteritis
g. disease
g. hepatitis
g. pneumonitis
grapes
Carswell g.
Graphtec
GRASS
gradient-recalled acquisition in the
steady state
GRASS MRI
Grass S88 muscle stimulator
gratus
Strophanthus g.
Gräupner method
Graves disease
gravis
myalgia g.
myasthenia g.
gravitation factor
gray scale
gray-scale ultrasound
GREAT
Grampian Region Early Anistreplase
Trial
great
g. artery
G. Ormond Street tracheostomy
g. vessel

G

NOTES

green
 g. coffee bean
 g. dye curve
 g. sputum
 g. strep endocarditis
Greene sign
Greenfield
 G. filter
 G. IVC filter
 G. vena cava filter
Gregg
 G. cannula
 G. phenomenon
Gregory baby profunda clamp
grelot
 bruit de g.
greyout spell
grid
 external g.
Griesinger sign
grinders'
 g. asthma
 g. phthisis
grip
 devil's g.
GRIP torque device
griseofulvin
groaning murmur
Grocco sign
Grocott methenamine silver
groin complications
Grollman pulmonary artery-seeking catheter
Grönblad-Strandberg syndrome
Grondahl esophagoplasty
Grondahl-Finney operation
Groningen voice prosthesis
groove
 arterial g.
 atrioventricular g.
 auriculoventricular g.
 A-V g.
 bulboventricular g.
 conoventricular fold and g.
 deltopectoral g.
 Harrison g.
 terminal g.
 vascular g.
 venous g.'s
 Waterston g.
Groshong double-lumen catheter

Gross
 G. tracheoesophageal atresia
 G. tracheoesophageal fistula
Grossman
 G. scale
 G. sign
Gross-Pomeranz-Watkins retractor
ground-glass
 g.-g. appearance
 g.-g. opacification
 g.-g. opacity
 g.-g. pattern
group
 Multicenter Postinfarction
  Research G. (MPRG)
 pseudomallei g.
 Toronto Lung Transplant G.
Grover clamp
growth
 g. factor
 g. hormone
grumous
 g. debris
grunt
 diastolic g.
 expiratory g.
Grüntzig
 G. catheter
 G. femoral stiffening cannula
 G. technique
Gruppo Italiano Per lo Studio Della Streptokinase Nell'Infarto Miocardio (GISSI)
G-strophanthin
G-suit
GTP
 guanosine triphosphate
 guanosine 5′-triphosphate
Guaifed
guaifenesin
 g. and codeine
 g. and dextromethorphan
 hydrocodone and g.
 g. and phenylpropanolamine
 g., phenylpropanolamine, and
  phenylephrine (ULR)
 g. and pseudoephedrine
 theophylline and g.
Guaifenex
 G. DM
 G. PSE
GuaiMax-D
Guaipax

Guaitab
Guaituss AC
Guai-Vent/PSE
guanabenz
    g. acetate
guanadrel
    g. sulfate
guanethidine
    g. monosulfate
    g. sulfate
guanfacine
    g. acetate
    g. hydrochloride
Guangzhou GD-1 prosthetic valve
guanine nucleotide modulatable
  binding
guanosine
    g. monophosphate (GMP)
    g. triphosphate (GTP)
guanosine 5′-diphosphate (GDP)
guanosine 5′-triphosphate (GTP)
guanylate cyclase
Guardian
    G. AICD
    G. ATP 4210 implantable
      cardioverter-defibrillator
    G. ICD
    G. pacemaker
guar gum
Gubner-Ungerleider
    G.-U. voltage
    G.-U. voltage criteria
Guedel airway
Guéneau de Mussy point
GuiaCough
Guiatex
Guiatuss DM
Guiatussin with Codeine
guidance
    echo g.
    fluoroscopic g.
Guidant TRIAD three-electrode
  energy defibrillation system
guide
    Amplatz tube g.
    Cor-Flex wire g.
    FL4 g.

    Flexguide intubation g.
    Franzen needle g.
    movable core straight safety
      wire g.
    Pilotip catheter g.
    Slick stylette endotracheal
      tube g.
    Slidewire extension g.
    tapered movable core curved
      wire g.
    Tefcor movable core straight
      wire g.
    TEGwire g.
    TrueTorque wire g.
    wire g.
guidelines
    McGoon g.
guider
    NL3 g.
guidewire, guide wire
    ACS Amplatz g.
    ACS extra-support g.
    ACS LIMA g.
    Amplatz Super Stiff g.
    Amplex g.
    atherolytic reperfusion g.
    Becton-Dickinson g.
    Bentson exchange straight g.
    Bentson floppy-tip g.
    catheter g.
    ControlWire g.
    Coons Super Stiff long tip g.
    Cor-Flex g.
    Critikon g.
    Doppler-tipped angioplasty g.
    Elastorc catheter g.
    EnTre g.
    exchange g.
    extra-support g.
    FasTrac g.
    FasTrac hydrophilic-coated g.
    flexible g.
    Flex Tip g.
    FloMap g.
    floppy-tipped g.
    FloWire g.

G

NOTES

guidewire *(continued)*
fluid-filled pressure
  monitoring g.
Glidewire Gold surgical g.
heparin-coated g.
Hi-Torque Flex-T g.
Hi-Torque Floppy exchange g.
Hi-Torque Floppy II g.
Hi-Torque Floppy
  intermediate g.
Hi-Torque Standard g.
hydrophilic coated g.
J g.
J Rosen g.
J-tip g.
g. loop
Magic Torque g.
Magnum g.
Medi-Tech g.
Newton g.
PDT g.
g. perforation
Phantom cardiac g.
Platinum PLUS g.
Preceder interventional g.
Premo g.
Pressure guide g.
Radifocus catheter g.
Redifocus g.
g. reflection
Reflex SuperSoft steerable g.
Roadrunner PC g.
Rotacs g.
safety g.
Schwarten LP g.
Seeker g.
silk g.
SOF-T g.
Sones g.
Sos g.
stainless steel g.
steerable angioplastic g.
Superselector Y-K g.
TAD g.
Taper g.
Tapered Torque g.
g. technique

Teflon-coated g.
Terumo g.
Ultra-Select nitinol PTCA g.
USCI Hyperflex g.
VeriFlex g.
Wholey Hi-Torque Floppy g.
Wholey Hi-Torque modified
  J g.
Wholey Hi-Torque standard g.
guiding catheter
Guillain-Barré syndrome
guilliermondii
  Candida g.
guillotine
Giertz rib g.
Sauerbruch rib g.
Guisez tube
Gulf War syndrome
gum
g. acacia
g. elastic bougie introducer
guar g.
Nicorette DS G.
polacrilex chewing g.
Stay Trim Diet G.
gun
Cobe g.
skin g.
Gunn crossing sign
gunshot wound
gurgling rales
Gurvich biphasic waveform
GUSTO
Global Utilization of Streptokinase
  and t-PA for Occluded Coronary
  Arteries
GUSTO protocol
Gutgeman auricular appendage
  clamp
guttural
g. pulse
g. rales
Gyroscan
ACS G.
G. HP Philips 15S whole-body
  system

H
- H gate
- H space
- H spike
- H wave
- H zone

h
- h peak
- h plateau

H1 receptor
Haake water bath
Haber-Weiss reaction
Habitrol
- H. Patch

habitus
- gracile h.

HACEK
- *Haemophilus aphrophilus, Actinobacillus actinomycetemcomitans, Cardiobacterium hominis, Eikenella corrodens, and Kingella kingae*

hacking cough
Hadow balloon
HAEC
- human aortic endothelial cells

H-Ae interval
Haemolite
- H. autologous blood recovery system
- Cell Saver H.

haemolyticus
- *Haemophilus h.*

Haemonetics
- H. Cell Saver
- H. Cell Saver system

Haemophilus
- *H. aphrophilus*
- *H. aphrophilus, Actinobacillus actinomycetemcomitans, Cardiobacterium hominis, Eikenella corrodens, and Kingella kingae* (HACEK)
- *H. haemolyticus*
- *H. influenzae*
- *H. parahaemolyticus*
- *H. parainfluenzae*
- *H. pertussis*

haemophilus
- h. b conjugate vaccine
- h. endocarditis

Hagar probe
Hageman factor
Hagenbach extension of Poiseuille equation
Haight-Finochietto rib retractor
Haimovici arteriotomy scissors
hair-matrix carcinoma
hairy heart
Hakim-Cordis pump
Hakki formula
Hakko Dwellcath catheter
Halbrecht syndrome
Haldane-Priestley tube
Haldrone
Hales piesimeter
half-amplitude pulse duration
half-life
- biological h.-l.
- elimination h.-l.

half-power distance
Halfprin
half-time
- h.-t. method
- pressure h.-t.

half-value layer
Hall
- H. prosthetic heart valve
- H. sign
- H. valvulotome

Hallion test
Hall-Kaster prosthetic valve
hallucination
- hypnagogic h.'s

Halo
- H. catheter

halofantrine
halogenated
- h. hydrocarbon
- h. hydrocarbon propellant

haloperidol
Haloscale respirometer
halo sheathing
halothane
Halotussin AC
Halsted clamp
Haltran

H

225

hamartoma
  myocardial h.
  pulmonary h.
Hamburger test
Hamilton-Stewart formula
Hamilton ventilator
Hamman
  H. click
  H. crunch
  H. disease
  H. murmur
  H. sign
Hamman-Rich syndrome
Hammersmith mitral prosthesis
Hamming-Hahn filter
hammocking of posterior mitral leaflet
Hampton hump
Ham test
Hancock
  H. bipolar balloon pacemaker
  H. embolectomy catheter
  H. fiberoptic catheter
  H. hydrogen detection catheter
  H. luminal electrophysiologic recording catheter
  H. mitral valve prosthesis
  H. modified orifice valve
  H. M.O. II porcine bioprosthesis
  H. pericardial valve graft
  H. porcine heterograft
  H. porcine valve
  H. temporary cardiac pacing wire
  H. vascular graft
  H. wedge-pressure catheter
Hand-E-Vent
hand-foot-and-mouth disease
handgrip
  isometric h.
hand-held nebulizer
Hand-Schüller-Christian disease
HANE
  hereditary angioneurotic edema
hanging heart
hangout interval
Hank balanced salt solution
Hanley-McNeil method
Hanning window
Hannover classification
hANP
  human atrial natriuretic peptide

Hans
  H. Rudolph nonbreathing valve
  H. Rudolph three-way valve
Hantaan virus
Hantavirus
  H. pulmonary syndrome (HPS)
HAPE
  high-altitude pulmonary edema
haplotype
  HLA-DQA1 gene h.
  HLA-DQB1 gene h.
hard
  h. metal disease
  h. metal pneumoconiosis
  h. pulse
Hare syndrome
Harken
  H. ball valve
  H. forceps
  H. rib spreader
harmonic
  h. component
  h. content
harness
  Heart Hugger sternum support h.
HARP
  Harvard Atherosclerosis Reversibility Project
Harpoon suture anchor
Harrington esophageal diverticulectomy
Harris adapter
Harrison groove
harsh
  h. murmur
  h. respiration
HART
  Heparin Aspirin Reperfusion Trial
Hartmann
  H. clamp
  H. solution
HARTS
  heat-activated recoverable temporary stent
Hartzler
  H. ACX II catheter
  H. balloon catheter
  H. dilatation catheter
  H. Excel catheter
  H. LPS dilatation catheter
  H. Micro-600 catheter
  H. Micro II catheter

H. Micro XT catheter
H. rib retractor
H. RX-014 balloon catheter
Harvard
H. Atherosclerosis Reversibility
Project (HARP)
H. pump
harvester's lung
HASHD
hypertensive arteriosclerotic heart
disease
Hashimoto thyroiditis
Hassall corpuscles
HAST
high-altitude simulation test
hat
bishop's h.
**Hatafuku fundus onlay patch
esophageal repair**
hatchetti
Acanthamoeba h.
Hatle method
**Hawksley random zero mercury
sphygmomanometer**
Hayek oscillator
hay fever
Haynes 25 material
haze
hilar h.
hazy
h. appearance
h. infiltrate
Hb
hemoglobin
Hb oximetry
HbCO
carboxyhemoglobin
HbCO oximetry
HBDH
hydroxybutyrate dehydrogenase
HbO$_2$
oxyhemoglobin
HbO$_2$ oximetry
HbOC vaccine
HBT Sleuth
HBW 023

HCl
hydrochloride
HCM
hypertrophic cardiomyopathy
HCO$_3$
bicarbonate
HCTZ
hydrochlorothiazide
HDFP
Hypertension Detection and Follow-
Up Program
HDL
high-density lipoprotein
H&E
hematoxylin and eosin
H&E stain
headache
migraine h.
syncopal migraine h.
head-down tilt test
headhunter angiography catheter
head-out water immersion
Head paradoxical reflex
head-tilt method
head-up
h.-u. tilt-table test (HUTTT)
h.-u. tilt test
Heaf test
healing
H. and Early Afterload
Reducing Therapy (HEART)
per primam h.
per secondam h.
health
h. level seven (HL7)
H. Locus of Control Scale
HEART
Healing and Early Afterload
Reducing Therapy
heart
abdominal h.
H. Aid 80 defibrillator
air-driven artificial h.
Akutsu III total artificial h.
ALVAD artificial h.
armored h.
h. arrest

NOTES

H

227

heart *(continued)*
artificial h. (AH)
athlete's h.
athletic h.
atrium of h.
h. attack
baggy h.
balloon-shaped h.
Baylor total artificial h.
h. beat
beer h.
beriberi h.
Berlin total artificial h.
h. block
3:1 h. block
3:2 h. block
boat-shaped h.
bony h.
booster h.
boot-shaped h.
bovine h.
CardioWest total artificial h.
cervical h.
chaotic h.
compliance of h.
contour of h.
contracted h.
crisscross h.
crux of h.
decortication of h.
dextroposition of h.
dextroversion of h.
dilation of h.
h. disease
disordered action of h. (DAH)
donor h.
drop h.
dynamite h.
egg-shaped h.
electrical alternation of h.
electromechanical artificial h.
encased h.
explanted h.
extracorporeal h.
h. failure
h. failure cells
fatty h.
fatty degeneration of h.
fibroid h.
figure 8 h.
flask-shaped h.
frosted h.
frosting h.

globoid h.
globular h.
hairy h.
h. and hand syndrome
hanging h.
Hershey total artificial h.
holiday h.
Holmes h.
horizontal h.
H. Hugger sternum support
    harness
hyperthyroid h.
hypoplastic left h.
icing h.
intermediate h.
intracorporeal h.
irritable h.
Jarvik 7 and 8 artificial h.
Jarvik 7-70 artificial h.
Jarvik 2000 artificial h.
Kolff-Jarvik artificial h.
h. laser revascularization
H. Laser for TMR
law of the h.
left h.
Liotta total artificial h.
h. loop
luxus h.
h. massage
mechanical h.
mechanical alternation of h.
movable h.
h. murmur
myocytolysis of h.
myxedema h.
one-ventricle h.
orthotopic biventricular
    artificial h.
orthotopic univentricular
    artificial h.
ox h.
paracorporeal h.
parchment h.
pear-shaped h.
pectoral h.
pendulous h.
Penn State total artificial h.
Phoenix total artificial h.
h. position
postischemic h.
pulmonary h.
h. pump
Quain fatty h.

h. rate (HR)
H. Rate 1-2-3 monitor
h. rate reserve (HRR)
h. rate variability (HRV)
recipient h.
h. reflex
rheumatism of h.
right h.
round h.
RTV total artificial h.
sabot h.
semihorizontal h.
semivertical h.
senescent h.
septation of h.
skin h.
snowman h.
soldier's h.
h. sounds S1, S2, S3, S4
stiff h.
stone h.
h. stroke
superoinferior h.
suspended h.
swinging h.
Symbion/CardioWest 100 mL
   total artificial h.
Symbion Jarvik-7 artificial h.
Symbion J-7 70-mL ventricle
   total artificial h.
systemic h.
tabby cat h.
h. tamponade
Taussig-Bing h.
teardrop h.
H. Technology Rotablator
three-chambered h.
thrush breast h.
tiger h.
tiger lily h.
tobacco h.
h. tones
total artificial h. (TAH)
h. transplant
transverse section of h.
Traube h.

triatrial h.
trilocular h.
univentricular h.
University of Akron
   artificial h.
upstairs-downstairs h.
Utah total artificial h.
h. valve
h. valve prosthesis
venous h.
vertical h.
Vienna total artificial h.
waist of h.
wandering h.
water-bottle h.
wooden-shoe h.
heartbeat
HeartCard
   H. monitor
heart-hand syndrome
HeartLine service
heart-lung
   h.-l. bloc
   h.-l. bypass
   h.-l. machine
   h.-l. resuscitation
   h.-l. transplant (HLT)
HeartMate
   H. implantable pneumatic left
      ventricular assist system
   H. implantable ventricular
      assist device
   H. LVAD
   H. pump
HEARTrac I Cardiac Monitoring
   system
Heartwire
   H. lead
heat
   h. load
   h. shock protein (HSP)
   h. stroke
heat-activated recoverable temporary
   stent (HARTS)
heat-expandable stent
Heath-Edwards criteria

NOTES

H

heating
  ohmic h.
  resistive h.
heat/moisture exchanger (HME)
Heat-Treated
  Profilnine H.-T.
heave
  parasternal h.
  precordial h.
  right ventricular h.
heavy metal
Heberden
  H. angina
  H. asthma
  H. nodes
Hecht pneumonia
Hegglin syndrome
Heim-Kreysig sign
Heimlich
  H. chest drainage valve
  H. heart valve
  H. maneuver
  H. sign
Heinecke method
Heiner syndrome
Heinz body
helical coil stent
helical-tip Halo catheter
helices (*pl. of* helix)
heliox
  helium-oxygen mixture
Helistat
helium
  h. dilution method
  h. washout
helium-cadmium diagnostic laser
helium-filled balloon catheter
helium-oxygen mixture (heliox)
helix, pl. **helices**
  amphipathic h.
  H. balloon
  H. PTCA dilatation catheter
Heller-Belsey operation
Heller-Döhle disease
Heller esophagomyotomy
Heller-Nissen operation
helminth
helminthic
  h. myocarditis
Helminthosporium
HELP
  heparin-induced extracorporeal low-
  density lipoprotein precipitation

Helsinki Heart Study
hemadostenosis
Hemaflex
  H. PTCA sheath with
  obturator
  H. sheath
hemagglutinin
hemangioendothelioma
hemangioma
  sclerosing h.
hemangioma-thrombocytopenia
  syndrome
hemangiomatosis
hemangiosarcoma
Hemaquet
  H. introducer
  H. PTCA sheath with
  obturator
  H. sheath
Hemashield
hematocrit
hematogenous
  h. embolism
  h. tuberculosis
hematologic disease
hematology rocker
hematoma
  aneurysmal h.
  aortic intramural h.
  dissecting h.
hematopoiesis
hematopoietic system
hematoporphyrin derivative (HPD)
hematoxylin-eosin
  h.-e. stain
hematoxylin and eosin (H&E)
hematuria
hemautogram
Hemex prosthetic valve
hemiaxial view
hemiazygos vein
hemiblock
  left anterior h. (LAH)
  left middle h.
  left posterior h.
  left septal h.
hemic
  h. murmur
  h. systole
hemicardia
hemidiaphragm
  tenting of h.

hemi-Fontan
    h.-F. operation
    h.-F. procedure
hemifundoplication
    Toupet h.
hemin
hemiplegia
    dense h.
hemisystole
hemithorax
hemitruncus
hemizygosity
hemizygous
hemochromatosis
Hemochron high-dose thrombin time assay
hemoclip
hemoconcentrator
    Biofilter cardiovascular h.
HemoCue photometer
hemocyanin
    keyhole-limpet h.
Hemocyte
hemocytometer
hemodialysis
hemodialyzer
    Gambro Lundia Minor h.
hemodilution
hemodynamic
    h. abnormality
    h. assessment
    h. collapse
    h. gradient
    intraoperative h.'s
    h. maneuver
    h. measurement
    h. principle
    systemic h.'s
    h. tolerance
    h. vise
hemodynamically significant stenosis
hemodynamic-angiographic study
Hemofil M
hemofiltration
    continuous arteriovenous h. (CAVH)

    continuous venovenous h. (CVVH)
hemoglobin (Hb)
    glycosylated h.
    pyridoxilated stroma-free h. (SFHb)
hemoglobinemia
hemoglobin-oxygen dissociation curve
hemoglobinuria
    paroxysmal nocturnal h. (PNH)
hemolysis
hemolytic anemia
hemoperfusion
hemopericardium
Hemophilus
hemopneumopericardium
hemoptysis
    cardiac h.
    Goldstein h.
    oriental h.
hemopump
    Johnson & Johnson h.
    Nimbus h.
hemorheology
hemorrhage
    flame-shaped h.'s
    pulmonary alveolar h.
    reperfusion-induced h.
    splinter h.'s
hemorrhagic
    h. bronchitis
    h. bronchopneumonia
    h. cyst
    h. fever
    h. pericarditis
    h. pleurisy
    h. sputum
    h. telangiectasia
hemosiderin
hemosiderin-laden macrophage
hemosiderosis
    essential pulmonary h.
    idiopathic pulmonary h.
    pulmonary h.
    transfusional h.
hemostasis valve

NOTES

H

231

hemostat
  Kelly h.
  Mayo h.
  microfibrillar collagen h.
  mosquito h.
  straight h.
hemostatic
  h. occlusive leverage device
  (HOLD)
  h. puncture closure device
  (HPCD)
HemoTec activated clotting time
  monitor
Hemotene
hemothorax, pl. **hemothoraces**
  catamenial h.
Hemovac
  Arbrook H.
hen-cluck stertor
Henderson-Haggard inhaler
Henderson-Hasselbalch equation
Henle
  ascending loop of H.
  H. elastic membrane
  H. fenestrated membrane
  H. loop
Henle-Coenen test
Henoch-Schönlein
  H.-S. purpura
  H.-S. syndrome
  H.-S. vasculitis
Henry-Gauer response
HEPA
  high-efficiency particulate air
heparin
  h. arterial filter
  H. Aspirin Reperfusion Trial
  (HART)
  beef-lung h.
  h. block
  h. drip
  h. flush
  h. injection
  h. lock
  low-molecular-weight h.
  (LMWH)
heparin-coated guidewire
heparin-dihydroergotamine
heparin-induced extracorporeal low-
  density lipoprotein precipitation
  (HELP)
heparinization
heparinized saline

hepatic
  h. artery
  h. dearterialization
  h. disease
  h. failure
  h. function
  h. hydrothorax
  h. lipase
  h. sphincter
  h. vein
  h. vein catheterization
hepatis
  porta h.
hepatitis
  h. A, B, C, D, E
  granulomatous h.
  viral h.
hepatization
hepatofugal flow
hepatojugular
  h. reflex
  h. reflux (HJR)
  h. reflux test
hepatomegaly
hepatopetal flow
hepatosplenomegaly
hepatotoxicity
Hep-Lock
  H.-L. injection
heptahydrate
  magnesium sulfate h.
heptanol
heptapeptide
hereditary
  h. angioneurotic edema
  (HANE)
  h. ataxia
  h. hemorrhagic telangiectasia
  h. methemoglobinemic cyanosis
heredopathia atactica
  polyneuritiformis
Hering
  nerve of H.
  H. phenomenon
Hering-Breuer reflex
Hermansky-Pudlak syndrome
Herner syndrome
hernia
  Beclard h.
  Bochdalek h.
  diaphragmatic h.
  hiatal h.
  Larrey h.

Morgagni h.
paraesophageal h.
rolling h.
Serafini h.
sliding hiatal h.
Velpeau h.
herniation
cardiac h.
heroin
herpangina pharyngitis
herpes
h. pneumonia
h. simplex
h. simplex pneumonitis
h. simplex virus (HSV)
h. zoster
herpetic
Hershey total artificial heart
herzstoss
Hespan
H. plasma volume expander
Hess capillary test
hetastarch plasma expander
heterochronicus
pulsus h.
heterogeneity
genetic h.
heterogeneous attenuation
heterograft
bovine h.
Hancock porcine h.
porcine h.
heterologous cardiac transplant
heterometric autoregulation
heterophyiasis
heteroscedastic
heterotaxia
cardiac h.
heterotaxy
h. syndrome
visceral h.
heterotopic
h. cardiac transplant
h. heart transplant (HHT)
h. stimulus
heterozygosity
heterozygote

heterozygous familial
hypercholesterolemia (hFH)
Hetzel forward triangle method
Heubner specific endarteritis
Hewlett
Hewlett-Packard
H.-P. 78720 A SDN monitor
H.-P. defibrillator
H.-P. ear oximeter
H.-P. 5 MHz phased-array
TEE system
H.-P. Sonos 1000, 1500
ultrasound system
Hexabrix
H. contrast material
Hexadrol
H. Phosphate
hexafluoride
sulphur h.
hexamethylmelamine
hexapolar catheter
Hexastat
hexaxial reference system
Hexlixate
hexokinase reaction
Hexonate
hexosaminidase deficiency
HF
high flow
HF infrared laser
HFEE
high-frequency epicardial
echocardiography
hFH
heterozygous familial
hypercholesterolemia
HFJV
high-frequency jet ventilation
HFO
high-frequency oscillation
HFPPV
high-frequency positive pressure
ventilation
HFV
high-frequency ventilation
Hg
mercury

NOTES

H

^{195m}Hg
  mercury-195m
H₁-H₂ interval
H.H.R.
HHT
  heterotopic heart transplant
hiatal
  h. esophagism
  h. hernia
hiatus
  aortic h.
  esophageal h.
hibernating myocardium
hibernation
  myocardial h.
HibTITER
Hib-VAX
hiccough, hiccup
high
  h. blood pressure
  h. flow (HF)
  h. lung volume
  H. Oxygen PRM resuscitator
  h. resolution computed
    tomography (HRCT)
  h. resolution thin section
    computed tomographic
  h. right atrium
high-altitude
  h.-a. pulmonary edema (HAPE)
  h.-a. simulation test (HAST)
high-ceiling diuretic
high-density lipoprotein (HDL)
high-dose steroid
high-efficiency particulate air
  (HEPA)
high-energy
  h.-e. laser
  h.-e. transthoracic shock
high-fiber diet
high-flow catheter
high-frequency
  h.-f. epicardial
    echocardiography (HFEE)
  h.-f. jet ventilation (HFJV)
  h.-f. jet ventilator
  h.-f. murmur
  h.-f. oscillation (HFO)
  h.-f. oscillation ventilator
  h.-f. oscillatory ventilation
  h.-f. positive pressure
    ventilation (HFPPV)
  h.-f. ventilation (HFV)

high-grade stenosis
high-molecular-weight dextran
high-output heart failure
high-pitched murmur
high-resolution
  h.-r. B-mode ultrasonography
  h.-r. CT (HRCT)
high-risk
  h.-r. angioplasty
  h.-r. phenotype
high-speed
  h.-s. rotational atherectomy
    (HSRA)
  h.-s. rotation dynamic
    angioplasty catheter
  h.-s. volumetric imaging
high-torque wire
Hilal modified headhunter catheter
hilar
  h. adenopathy
  h. clouding
  h. dance
  h. haze
  h. lymphadenopathy
Hill
  H. phenomenon
  H. sign
Hillis-Müller maneuver
Hi-Lo Jet tracheal tube
Hilton sac
hilum
  h. convergence sign
  h. overlay sign
hilus tuberculosis
Hines-Brown test
hinge
  annulocuspid h.
Hi-Per
  H.-P. cardiac device
  H.-P. Flex exchange wire
hip flexion
hippocratic
  h. angina
  h. sound
  h. succussion
hirsutum
  cor h.
Hirtz rales
hirudin
  recombinant h. (r-hirudin)
  H. in Thrombolysis (HIT)
Hirudo medicinalis
Hirulog

His
　　H. bundle, H. of His
　　bundle of H. (*var. of*
　　　His H.)
　　H. bundle ablation
　　H. bundle depolarization
　　H. bundle electrocardiogram
　　H. bundle electrogram
　　H. bundle heart block
　　H. canal
　　H. catheter
　　H. perivascular space
　　H. spindle
His-Hass procedure
Hismanal
His-Purkinje
　　H.-P. conduction
　　H.-P. fibers
　　H.-P. system
　　H.-P. tissue
Histalet X
histaminase
histamine
　　h. challenge
His-Tawara node
histiocyte
　　palisading h.
histiocytoma
histiocytosis
　　primary pulmonary h. X
histocompatibility agent B27
Histocryl Blue tissue adhesive
histogram
　　DNA h.
　　h. mode
histologic
histolytica
　　Entamoeba h.
　　Torula h.
histolyticus
　　Cryptococcus h.
histopathology
Histoplasma
　　H. capsulatum
　　H. myocarditis
histoplasmic pericarditis

histoplasmosis
　　African h.
history
　　pack-year smoking h.
　　smoking h.
HIT
　　Hirudin in Thrombolysis
Hitachi U-2000 spectrophotometer
Hi-Torque
　　H.-T. Flex-T guidewire
　　H.-T. Floppy exchange
　　　guidewire
　　H.-T. Floppy II guidewire
　　H.-T. Floppy Intermediate
　　　guidewire
　　H.-T. Floppy with Pro/Pel
　　H.-T. Standard guidewire
Hitzenberg test
HIV
　　human immunodeficiency virus
　　　HIV cardiomyopathy
HIV-1 riboprobe
HIVAGEN test
Hivid
Hixson-Vernier protocol
HJR
　　hepatojugular reflux
HL7
　　health level seven
HLA
　　human leukocyte antigen
　　human lymphocyte antigen
HLA-129
HLA-A11
HLA-DQA1 gene haplotype
HLA-DQB1 gene haplotype
HLA-DQ gene complex
HLA-DR gene complex
HLHS
　　hypoplastic left heart syndrome
HLT
　　heart-lung transplant
HME
　　heat/moisture exchanger
　　Tracheolife HME
HMG-CoA
　　hydroxymethylglutaryl coenzyme A

NOTES

H

235

HMG-CoA *(continued)*
3-hydroxy-3-methylglutaryl
coenzyme A
HMG-CoA reductase inhibitor
hoarseness
hockey-stick
h.-s. catheter
h.-s. deformity
h.-s. tricuspid valve
HOCM
hypertrophic obstructive
cardiomyopathy
Hodgkin disease
Hodgkin-Huxley
H.-H. constant
H.-H. model
Hodgkin-Key murmur
Hodgson disease
Hoffman reflex
Hoffrel transesophageal probe
Hohn vessel dilator
hoist
Temco h.
HOLD
hemostatic occlusive leverage device
Hold
Children's H.
holder
Ayers cardiovascular needle h.
Berry sternal needle h.
Björk-Shiley heart valve h.
blade control wire h.
Castroviejo needle h.
catheter guide h.
Cooley Vital microvascular
needle h.
DeBakey Vital needle h.
GraftAssist vein-graft h.
Lewy chest h.
Marquette 3-channel laser h.
needle h.
Vital-Cooley microvascular
needle h.
Vital-Ryder microvascular
needle h.
Watson heart valve h.
wire h.
Holen-Hatle equation
holiday
dobutamine h.
h. heart
h. heart syndrome

Holinger anterior commissure
laryngoscope
holism
Hollenberg treadmill score
Hollenhorst plaques
Holmes heart
Holmes-Rahe scale
holmium laser
holmium:yttrium-aluminum-garnet
(Ho:YAG)
holodiastolic
h. murmur
holography
ultrasound h.
holosystolic
h. murmur
Holter
H. diary
Marquette 3-channel laser H.
H. monitor
H. tube
Holt-Oram syndrome
Holzknecht space
Homans sign
homatropine
hydrocodone and h.
Hombach
H. lead placement system
H. placement of leads
homeometric autoregulation
homeostasis
hominis
Actinobacillus h.
Cardiobacterium h.
Mycoplasma h.
Pentatrichomonas h.
Homochron monitor
homocollateral reconstitution
homocysteine
homocystinemia
homocystinuria syndrome
homodimer
alpha-alpha h.
beta-beta h.
homogentisic acid oxidase deficiency
homograft
aortic h.
denatured h.
homologous cardiac transplant
homoscedastic
homozygosity
homozygote

honeycomb
    h. lesion
    h. lung
honeycombing
    h. of lung
Hong Kong influenza
honk
    precordial h.
    systolic h.
honking murmur
hood
    h. O_2
    H. stoma stent
Hood-Westaby T-Y stent
hook
    barbed h.
    Bryant mitral h.
    Doyen rib h.
Hooke law
Hoover sign
Hope
    H. bag
    H. resuscitator
    H. sign
Hopkins
    H. aortic clamp
    H. forceps
    H. symptom checklist
Horder spots
horehound lozenge
Horizon
    H. AutoAdjust CPAP system
    H. nasal CPAP system
    H. surgical ligating and
        marking clip
horizontal
    h. heart
    h. long-axis view
hormone
    adrenocorticotropic h. (ACTH)
    antidiuretic h. (ADH)
    female h.
    growth h.
    mineralocorticoid h.
    natriuretic h.
    parathyroid h.

    syndrome of inappropriate
        antidiuretic h. (SIADH)
    thyroid-stimulating h. (TSH)
Horner syndrome
horripilation
horse asthma
horse-race effect
horseshoe
    h. configuration
    h. lung
Horton
    H. arteritis
    H. disease
hose
    Juzo h.
hospital-acquired infection
host
    humoral h.
    immunocompetent h.
    nonimmunocompromised h.
host-generated neutrophils
  recruitment
HOT
    hypertension optimal treatment
    HOT study
hot
    h. gangrene
    h. potato voice
    h. spot
Hotelling T2 test
hot-tipped laser probe
hot-wire pneumotachometer
Hounsfield unit
24-hour
    -h. ambulatory
        electrocardiographic recorder
    -h. cortisol
hourglass
    h. murmur
    h. pattern
    h. stenosis
Howard method
Howel-Evans syndrome
Howell test
Ho:YAG
    holmium:yttrium-aluminum-garnet

NOTES

H

Ho:YAG *(continued)*
   Ho:YAG laser
   Ho:YAG laser angioplasty
HP
   hypersensitivity pneumonitis
H.P. Acthar Gel
HPCD
   hemostatic puncture closure device
HPD
   hematoporphyrin derivative
H′P interval
H-proline
HPS
   Hantavirus pulmonary syndrome
HPV
   human papillomavirus
   hypoxic pulmonary vasoconstriction
H-Q interval
H-QRS interval
HR
   heart rate
H-R conduction time
HRCT
   high resolution computed
   tomography
   high-resolution CT
     HRCT scan
HRF deficiency
HRR
   heart rate reserve
HRV
   heart rate variability
HSP
   heat shock protein
HSRA
   high-speed rotational atherectomy
     HSRA device
HSS
   hypertrophic subaortic stenosis
HSV
   herpes simplex virus
     Mollaret HSV
5HT
   5-hydroxytryptamine
HTLV
   human T-cell leukemia/lymphoma
   virus
   human T-cell lymphotropic virus
     HTLV-I, II
HTN
   hypertension
hub
   catheter h.

Huchard
   H. disease
   H. sign
Hudson
   H. Lifesaver resuscitator
   H. Multi-Vent
Hufnagel
   H. ascending aortic clamp
   H. prosthetic valve
Hugenholtz method
Hugger
   Bair H.
Hughes-Stovin syndrome
Hull triad
hum
   cervical venous h.
   venous h.
human
   antihemophilic factor (h.)
   h. aortic endothelial cells
   (HAEC)
   h. atrial natriuretic peptide
   (hANP)
   h. cloned DNA (cDNA)
   cytomegalovirus immune
   globulin intravenous, h.
   factor IX complex (h.)
   h. immunodeficiency virus
   (HIV)
   h. leukocyte antigen (HLA)
   h. lymphocyte antigen (HLA)
   h. lymphocyte antigen typing
   h. menopausal gonadotropin
   coenzyme A reductase
   inhibitor
   h. papillomavirus (HPV)
   h. pooled AAT
   h. preproendothelin-1 gene
   h. recombinant
   deoxyribonuclease
   H. Surf
   h. T-cell leukemia/lymphoma
   virus (HTLV)
   h. T-cell lymphotropic virus
   (HTLV)
   h. umbilical vein (HUV)
   Velosulin H.
Humate-P
Humatin
humeroperoneal neuromuscular
   disease
Humibid DM
humid asthma

humidification
humidified oxygen
humidifier
>Bard-Parker U-Mid/Lo h.
>Bennett Cascade II Servo
>Controlled Heated H.
>bubble h.
>cold-mist h.
>jet h.
>h. lung
>Mistogen passover h.
>MRT Tidal H.
>OEM 503 h.
>Ohio Bubble h.
>passover h.
>Whisper Mist h.

humidity
humming murmur
humming-top murmur
humoral
>h. host
>h. immune defect

hump
>Hampton h.

Humulin L, N, R, U insulin
hunger
>air h.

Hunter
>H. canal
>H. detachable balloon occluder
>H. operation
>H. syndrome

Hunter-Hurler syndrome
Hunter-Satinsky clamp
Hunter-Sessions balloon
Huntington chorea
Hurler-Scheie compound
Hurler syndrome
Hurricaine spray
Hürthle
>H. cell tumor
>H. manometer

Hurwitz thoracic trocar
Hustead needle
Hutinel disease
HUTTT
>head-up tilt-table test

HUV
>human umbilical vein
>HUV bypass graft

Huygens principle
H-V
>H-V conduction time
>H-V interval

hyaline
>h. arterionecrosis
>h. arteriosclerosis
>h. fatty change
>h. membrane disease
>h. thrombus

hyalinosis
>arteriolar h.

hyaloserositis
>progressive multiple h.

Hyate:C
hybridization
>fluorescent in situ h. (FISH)
>in situ h.

hybrid unit
Hybritech immunoradiometric assay
HycoClear Tuss
Hycodan
Hycomine Compound
Hycotuss Expectorant Liquid
hydatid
>h. cyst
>h. fremitus

Hydeltrasol injection
Hydeltra-T.B.A. injection
hydralazine
>h. hydrochloride
>h. and hydrochlorothiazide
>h., hydrochlorothiazide, and
>reserpine

Hydramyn Syrup
Hydrap-ES
hydraulic
>h. resistance
>h. vein stripper

Hydrazide
hydrazine
>dimethyl h.

Hydrea
Hydrenox

NOTES

H

hydrobromide
    hydroxyamphetamine h.
hydrocarbon
    halogenated h.
    h. toxicity
HydroCath catheter
Hydrocet
hydrochloric acid
hydrochloride (HCl)
    acebutolol h.
    acecainide h.
    alfentanil h.
    amantadine h.
    amiloride h.
    amiodarone h.
    amprolium h.
    bacampicillin h.
    benazepril h.
    bepridil h.
    betaxolol h.
    carteolol h.
    chlorpromazine h.
    ciprofloxacin h.
    clonidine h.
    colestipol h.
    cyproheptadine h.
    cytarabine h.
    demeclocycline h.
    desipramine h.
    diltiazem h.
    diphenhydramine h.
    dobutamine h.
    dopamine h.
    doxapram h.
    doxepin h.
    doxorubicin h.
    encainide h.
    esmolol h.
    ethambutol h.
    ethaverine h.
    ethylnorepinephrine h.
    fenfluramine h.
    fluoxetine h.
    guanfacine h.
    hydralazine h.
    idarubicin h.
    isoxsuprine h.
    labetalol h.
    levamisole h.
    lidocaine h.
    lincomycin h.
    lomefloxacin h.
    mecamylamine h.

    mechlorethamine h.
    mefloquine h.
    meperidine h.
    mepivacaine h.
    methamphetamine h.
    methoxamine h.
    metoclopramide h.
    mexiletine h.
    minocycline h.
    mitoxantrone h.
    moexipril h.
    Mustargen H.
    nalmefene h.
    naloxone h.
    nicardipine h.
    nortriptyline h.
    oxytetracycline h.
    papaverine h.
    phenoxybenzamine h.
    phentolamine h.
    phenylephrine h.
    phenylpropanolamine h.
    prazosin h.
    prenalterol h.
    procainamide h.
    procaine h.
    promethazine h.
    propafenone h.
    propranolol h.
    protriptyline h.
    pyridoxine h.
    quinapril h.
    rimantadine h.
    sematilide h.
    sertraline h.
    sotalol h.
    spirapril h.
    terazosin h.
    tetracaine h.
    thioridazine h.
    ticlopidine h.
    tocainide h.
    tolazoline h.
    trazodone h.
    vancomycin h.
    verapamil h.
    yohimbine h.
hydrochlorothiazide (HCTZ)
    amiloride and h.
    bisoprolol and h.
    captopril and h.
    enalapril and h.
    hydralazine and h.

losartan and h.
methyldopa and h.
propranolol and h.
h. and reserpine
h. and spironolactone
h. and triamterene
hydrocodone
h. and acetaminophen
h. bitartrate
h. and chlorpheniramine
h. and guaifenesin
h. and homatropine
Hydrocort
hydrocortisone
h. sodium succinate
Hydrocortone
H. Acetate
H. Phosphate
hydrocyanic acid
HydroDIURIL
hydroflumethiazide
h. and reserpine
Hydro-Fluserpine
Hydrogel-coated PTCA balloon catheter
hydrogen
h. density
h. electrodes
h. fluoride
h. inhalation technique
h. ion concentration (pH)
h. peroxide
h. sulfide
hydrogen-3 mazindol
Hydrogesic
hydrolases
lysosomal h.
Hydrolyser
hydrolysis
ATP h.
h. of surfactant
Hydromet
hydromorphone
Hydromox
hydronephrosis
Hydropane
Hydro-Par

hydropericarditis
hydropericardium
Hydrophen
hydrophilic coated guidewire
hydropneumopericardium
Hydropres
hydrops pericardii
hydroquinidine
Hydro-Serp
Hydroserpine
hydrosphygmograph
Hydro-Splint II
Hydro-T
hydrothorax
chylous h.
hepatic h.
Hydrotropine
hydroxephedrine
C-11 h.
hydroxide
potassium h. (KOH)
hydroxyamphetamine hydrobromide
hydroxyapatite
hydroxybutyrate
h. dehydrogenase (HBDH)
gamma h. (GHB)
hydroxychloroquine
h. sulfate
18-hydroxycorticosterone
hydroxyephedrine
carbon-11 h.
hydroxyethyl starch
hydroxylase
h. deficiency
17-h. deficiency
hydroxyl radical
hydroxymethylglutaryl
h. coenzyme A (HMG-CoA)
h. coenzyme A reductase inhibitor
3-hydroxy-3-methylglutaryl
3-h.-3-m. coenzyme A (HMG-CoA)
3-h.-3-m. coenzyme A reductase
3-h.-3-m. coenzyme A reductase inhibitor

NOTES

H

hydroxyprogesterone caproate
hydroxyproline
  h. analysis
5-hydroxytryptamine (5HT)
hydroxyurea
hydroxyzine
  theophylline, ephedrine, and h.
  (T.E.H.)
Hy-Gestrone injection
Hygroton
Hylorel
Hylutin injection
Hynes pharyngoplasty
Hypaque
hyperabduction syndrome
hyperaldosteronism
hyperalimentation
hyperalphalipoproteinemia
hyperammonemia
hyperapobetalipoproteinemia
hyperapolipoprotein B syndrome
hyperbaric
  h. chamber
  h. oxygen
  h. oxygenation
  h. pressure
hypercalcemia
  familial hypocalciuric h.
hypercalciuria
hypercapnia
  permissive h.
hypercapnic acidosis
hypercarbia
hypercardia
hyperchloremic acidosis
hypercholesterolemia
  false h.
  familial h. (FH)
  heterozygous familial h. (hFH)
  polygenic h.
  h. (types IIa and IIb)
hypercholesterolemic
hyperchylomicronemia
hypercoagulable state
hypercontractile
hypercontractility
hypercyanotic
  h. angina
  h. spell
hyperdiastole
hyperdicrotic
hyperdicrotism
hyperdynamic state

hyperemia
  active h.
  arterial h.
  collateral h.
  fluxionary h.
  passive h.
  peristatic h.
  reactive h.
  venous h.
hyperemic
hypereosinophilia
  h. syndrome
hypereosinophilic syndrome
hyperesthesia
  cutaneous h.
hyperestrogenemia
Hyperflex tracheostomy tube
hypergammaglobulinemia
hyperglycemia
hyperhomocystinemia
hyperinflated
hyperinflation
hyperinsulinemia
hyperirritability
hyperkalemia
hyperkalemic cardioplegia
hyperkinemia
hyperkinesia
hyperkinesis
hyperkinetic
  h. heart syndrome
  h. pulse
  h. state
hyperlipidemia
  false combined h.
  multiple lipoprotein-type h.
  polygenic h.
  Program on the Surgical
    Control of H.'s (POSCH)
hyperlipoproteinemia
hyperlucent
  h. lung
  h. lung syndrome
hypermagnesemia
hypernatremia
hypernephroma
hyperoxaluria
hyperparathyroidism
hyperphosphatemia
hyperpiesis, hyperpiesia
hyperpietic
hyperpigmentation

hyperplasia
    adrenal h.
    bilateral adrenal h.
    congenital adrenal h.
    elastic tissue h.
    intimal h.
    lymphoid h.
hyperplastica
    arteritis h.
hyperplastic mucus-secreting goblet cell
hyperpnea
    isocapnic h.
hyperreactivity
    bronchial h.
hyperreflexia
    autonomic h.
hyperreninemia
hyperresonance
hyperresonant
hyperresponsiveness
hypersecretion
    mucus h.
hypersensitive carotid sinus syndrome
hypersensitivity
    aminosalicylic acid h.
    carotid sinus h.
    h. myocarditis
    h. pneumonia
    h. pneumonitis (HP)
    h. vasculitis
hyperserotonemia
    vasculocardiac syndrome of h.
hypersomnolence
hypersphyxia
Hyperstat
    H. I.V.
hypersystole
hypersystolic
hypertension (HTN)
    accelerated h.
    adrenal h.
    alveolar h.
    arterial h.
    benign intracranial h.
    borderline h.

chronic thromboembolic
    pulmonary h. (CTEPH)
cuffed h.
H. Detection and Follow-Up
    Program (HDFP)
diastolic h.
essential h.
familial dyslipidemic h.
gestational h.
glucocorticoid-induced h.
Goldblatt h.
hypoxic pulmonary h.
idiopathic h.
intracranial h.
kidney Goldblatt h.
labile h.
left atrial h.
malignant h.
masked h.
mineralocorticoid-induced h.
neuromuscular h.
office h.
h. optimal treatment (HOT)
h. optimal treatment study
oral contraceptive-induced h.
orthostatic h.
Page episodic h.
pale h.
pediatric h.
portal h.
postpartum h.
pregnancy-induced h. (PIH)
pulmonary h.
recalcitrant h.
red h.
renal h.
renoprival h.
renovascular h.
resistant h.
salt-and-water dependent h.
secondary h.
splenoportal h.
stress-related h.
systemic vascular h.
systemic venous h.
systolic h.
thromboembolic pulmonary h.

NOTES

H

hypertension *(continued)*
  venous h.
  white-coat h.
hypertensive
  h. arteriopathy
  h. arteriosclerosis
  h. arteriosclerotic heart disease
    (HASHD)
  h. crisis
  h. emergency
  h. encephalopathy
  h. hypertrophic cardiomyopathy
  h. nephropathy
  h. pulmonary vascular disease
  h. retinopathy
  h. urgency
  h. vasculopathy
hyperthermia
  whole body h.
hyperthyroid heart
hyperthyroidism
  amiodarone-induced h.
  apathetic h.
hypertonica
  polycythemia h.
hypertriglyceridemia
hypertrophic
  h. adenoids
  h. cardiomyopathy (HCM)
  h. catarrh
  h. emphysema
  h. obstructive cardiomyopathy
    (HOCM)
  h. pulmonary osteoarthropathy
  h. smooth muscle layer
  h. subaortic stenosis (HSS)
hypertrophy
  asymmetric septal h. (ASH)
  basal-septal h.
  cardiac h.
  compensatory h.
  concentric left ventricular h.
  eccentric h.
  isolated septal h. (ISH)
  left ventricular h. (LVH)
  lipomatous h.
  myocardial h.
  myocyte h.
  right ventricular h. (RVH)
  septal h.
  submucosal gland h.
  trabecular h.

  ventricular h.
  volume load h.
hyperuricemia
hyperuricemic nephropathy
hyperventilation
  alveolar h.
  h. maneuver
  h. syndrome
hyperviscosity syndrome
hypervitaminosis
hypervolemia
hypervolemic
hypha, pl. hyphae
hyphemia
Hy-Phen
hypnagogic hallucinations
hypnagogue
hypnalgia
hypnesthesia
hypnic
hypnology
hypnopompic
hypnosis
hypnotic
hypoadrenalism
hypoaeration
hypoalbuminemia
hypoaldosteronism
  hyporeninemic h.
hypoalphalipoproteinemia
hypobaric hypoxia
hypocalcemia
hypocapnia
hypocholesterolemia
hypochondrial reflex
hypochondriasis
hypodynamia
  h. cordis
hypoechoic
hypofunction
hypoglossal nerve
hypoglycemia
hypoglycemic
  h. agent
  h. syncope
hypokalemia
hypokalemia-induced arrhythmia
hypokinemia
hypokinesis, hypokinesia
  anteromesial h.
  cardiac wall h.
  global h.
hypokinetic pulse

hypomagnesemia
hyponatremia
hypoparathyroidism
hypoperfusion
hypophosphatemia
hypophyscal-pituitary adrenal axis
hypopiesis
    orthostatic h.
hypoplasia
    mitral valve h.
    h. of right ventricle
    right ventricular h.
hypoplastic
    h. emphysema
    h. left heart
    h. left heart syndrome (HLHS)
hypopnea
hypopneic
hyporeninemia
hyporeninemic hypoaldosteronism
hyposphyxia
hypostasis
hypostatic
    h. bronchopneumonia
    h. congestion
    h. pneumonia
hyposystole
hypotension
    acute severe h.
    arterial h.
    chronic idiopathic orthostatic h.
    idiopathic orthostatic h.
    orthostatic h.
    postural h.
    vasovagal h.
hypotensive
hypothermia
    h. blanket
    extracorporeal exchange h.
    h. mattress
    topical h.
hypothermic fibrillating arrest
hypothesis, pl. hypotheses
    Gad h.
    leading circle h.
    lipid h.
    Lyon h.

    monoclonal h.
    null h.
    premature ventricular complex-
      trigger h.
    response-to-injury h.
    sulfhydryl depletion h.
    Wu-Hoak h.
hypothyroidism
hypotonia
hypotonicity
hypotonus, hypotony
Hypovase
hypoventilation
    alveolar h.
hypovolemia
hypovolemic
    h. shock
hypoxanthine
hypoxemia
    arterial h.
    circulatory h.
    REM sleep-related h.
    rest h.
    h. test
hypoxia
    altitude h.
    alveolar h.
    anemic h.
    circulatory h.
    hypobaric h.
    hypoxic h.
    ischemic h.
    sleep h.
    stagnant h.
hypoxic
    h. hypoxia
    h. lap swimming
    h. pulmonary hypertension
    h. pulmonary vasoconstriction
    (HPV)
    h. response study
    h. spell
    h. syncope
hypoxidosis
HypRho-D
    H.-D. Mini-Dose
Hyprogest injection

NOTES

H

hysteresis
 pacemaker h.
 pacing h.
 rate h.
hysterical
 h. fainting
 h. syncope
hysteric angina

hystericus
 globus h.
hysterosystole
Hy-Tape
Hytinic
Hytrin
Hyzaar
Hy-Zide

I-123
iodine-123
I-123 metaiodobenzylguanidine
I-123 MIBG
I-123 MIBG uptake
I-125
I-125 metaiodobenzylguanidine
(I-125 MIBG)
I-125 MIBG
I-124 IPPA
IAB
intra-aortic balloon
IAB catheter
IAIA
immune adherence immunosorbent
assay
iatrogenic
i. atrial septal defect
i. disorder
i. pneumothorax
I band
Iberet-Folic-500
ibopamine
Ibuprin
ibuprofen
Arthritis Foundation I.
pseudoephedrine and i.
Ibuprohm
Ibu-Tab
ibutilide
i. fumarate
IC
inspiratory capacity
ICA
internal carotid artery
ICAM-1
intercellular adhesion molecule-1
ICD
implantable cardioverter-defibrillator
Cadence biphasic ICD
Guardian ICD
Telectronics Guardian ATP II
ICD
Ventritex Cadence ICD
Vitatron Diamond ICD
ICD-ATP
implantable cardioverter-
defibrillator/atrial tachycardia
pacing
ICD-ATP device

ice
i. mapping
i. slush
slushed i.
iced saline
ice-pick view
ICEUS
intracaval endovascular
ultrasonography
ICHD
Inter-Society Commission for Heart
Disease
ICHD pacemaker code
ichorous pleurisy
icing heart
Icorel
ICS
intracellular-like, calcium-bearing
crystalloid solution
ICS cardioplegic solution
icteric sputum
ictometer
ICTP
type I collagen telopeptide
ictus
i. cordis
i. sanguinis
ICUS
intracoronary ultrasound
ICV-10 ventilator
ICXA
intermediate circumflex artery
Idamycin
idarubicin hydrochloride
IDC
idiopathic dilated cardiomyopathy
IDDM
insulin-dependent diabetes mellitus
Ideal cardiac device
idiojunctional rhythm
idionodal
i. rhythm
idiopathic
i. acute eosinophilic pneumonia
i. arteritis of Takayasu
i. bradycardia
i. brown induration
i. cardiomegaly
i. cyclic edema

idiopathic *(continued)*
 i. dilated cardiomyopathy
  (IDC)
 i. dilation
 i. hypereosinophilic syndrome
  (IHES)
 i. hypertension
 i. hypertrophic subaortic
  stenosis (IHSS)
 i. interstitial pneumonia
 i. long Q-T interval syndrome
 i. myocarditis
 i. orthostatic hypotension
 i. pericarditis
 i. pulmonary fibrosis (IPF)
 i. pulmonary hemosiderosis
 i. restrictive cardiomyopathy
 i. thrombocytopenic purpura
  (ITP)
 i. unilobar emphysema
 i. ventricular fibrillation
 i. ventricular tachycardia (IVT)
idioventricular
 i. bradycardia
 i. kick
 i. rhythm
 i. tachycardia
IDIS
 intraoperative digital subtraction
  IDIS system
idoxuridine
IDSA
 intraoperative digital subtraction
  angiography
IDV
 intermittent demand ventilation
IE
 infective endocarditis
I:E
 inspiratory to expiratory ratio
  I:E ratio
IE-2 riboprobe
IEA
 inferior epigastric artery
  IEA graft
IEL
 internal elastic lamina
IgE
 serum I.
IgE-sensitized cell
IGF
 insulin-like growth factor
IgG avidity test

IHD
 ischemic heart disease
IHES
 idiopathic hypereosinophilic
  syndrome
IHSS
 idiopathic hypertrophic subaortic
  stenosis
Ikorel
IL-8
 interleukin-8
ILD
 interstitial lung disease
ileus
 meconium i.
iliac
 i. artery
 i. artery occlusion
 i. steal
 i. vein
 i. vein thrombosis
iliopopliteal bypass
Illumen-8 guiding catheter
Iloprost
Ilosone Oral
ILUS
 intraluminal ultrasound
  ILUS catheter
IMA
 internal mammary artery
IMAGE
 International Multicenter Angina
  Exercise
image
 i. aliasing
 amplitude i.
 i. bundle
 ejection-fraction i.
 ejection shell i.
 equilibrium i.
 functional i.
 i. intensifier
 paradox i.
 parametric i.
 phase i.
 phase-encoded velocity i.
 SE i.
 stress washout myocardial
  perfusion i.
 supine rest gated equilibrium i.
 T1, T2 weighted i.
Imagecath rapid exchange
angioscope

**Image-Measure morphometry
software**
imager
  Sonos 2000 ultrasound i.
Imager Torque selective catheter
Image-View system
imaging
  acoustic i.
  adenosine radionuclide
    perfusion i.
  i. agent
  Aloka color Doppler system
    for blood flow i.
  antifibrin antibody i.
  antimyosin antibody i.
  biplane i.
  blood-pool i.
  cardiac blood-pool i.
  i. chain
  continuous-wave Doppler i.
  digital subtraction i.
  digital vascular i.
  dipyridamole-thallium i.
  direct Fourier transformation i.
  Doppler tissue i.
  Doppler transesophageal color
    flow i.
  duplex i.
  echo-planar i.
  exercise i.
  Fourier two-dimensional i.
  frequency domain i.
  functional i.
  gallium-67 i.
  gated blood-pool i.
  gated sweep magnetic
    resonance i.
  high-speed volumetric i.
  indium-111-labeled
    lymphocyte i.
  infarct-avid i.
  INTEGRIS cardiovascular i.
  krypton-8lm ventilation i.
  magnetic resonance i. (MRI)
  magnetic source i. (MSI)
  mask-mode cardiac i.
  myocardial perfusion i.

  nuclear magnetic resonance i.
    (NMRI)
  parametric i.
  pharmacologic stress
    perfusion i.
  phase i.
  planar myocardial i.
  platelet i.
  PYP i.
  pyrophosphate i.
  radionuclide i.
  redistribution i.
  rest-redistribution thallium-
    201 i.
  rubidium-82 i.
  sestamibi i.
  single-photon emission
    tomography i. (SPET imaging)
  SPET i.
    single-photon emission
      tomography imaging
  spin-echo i.
  stress-redistribution-reinjection
    thallium-201 i.
  stress thallium-201 myocardial
    perfusion i.
  i. study
  teboroxime i.
  technetium-99m i.
  technetium-99m MIBI i.
  thallium perfusion i.
  tissue Doppler i.
  transient response i. (TRI)
  velocity-encoded cine-magnetic
    resonance i. (VE-cMRI)
  ventilation/perfusion i.
  video i.
  i. window
  xenon lung ventilation i.
imaging-angioplasty balloon catheter
Imatron
  I. C-100 system
  I. C-100 tomographic scanner
  I. Ultrafast CT scanner
imazodan
imbalance
  acid-base i.

NOTES

imbalance *(continued)*
 electrolyte i.
 protease-antiprotease i.
 sympathovagal i.
imciromab pentetate
Imdur
IMED
 I. infusion device
 I. infusion pump
I-Methasone
imglucerase
I-123-MIBG
 iodine-123 metaiodobenzylguanidine
imipenem/cilastatin
imipramine
immersion
 head-out water i.
immitis
 Coccidioides i.
 Dirofilaria i.
immotile cilia syndrome
immune
 i. adherence immunosorbent
 assay (IAIA)
 i. globulin, intravenous
immune-mediated
 i.-m. disease
 i.-m. membranous nephritis
immunity
 cell-mediated i.
Immuno
 Feiba VH I.
immunoassay
 enzyme i. (EIA)
 nifedipine enzyme i.
 Thrombus Precursor Protein i.
immunochemical abnormalities
immunocompetent host
immunocompromised
immunodeficiency
immunofluorescence
 cytometric indirect i.
immunoglobulin
 varicella-zoster i. (VZIG)
immunological theory
immunology
immunometric sandwich method
immunonephelometry
 rate i.
immunoperoxidase stain
immunoprecipitin analysis
immunoradiometric assay (IRMA)
immunoseparation

immunostaining technique
immunosuppressant
immunosuppression
 i. therapy
immunotherapy
immunoturbidimetric assay
Imovax vaccine
IMPACT
 Integrelin to Manage Platelet
 Aggregation to Prevent Coronary
 Thrombosis
Impact specialized feeding formula
impairment
 restrictive functional i.
IMP-Capello arm support
impedance
 i. aggregometry
 aortic i.
 arterial i.
 atrial lead i.
 i. catheter
 lead i.
 i. modulus
 pacemaker i.
 i. plethysmography (IPG)
 thoracic i.
 i. variables
 vascular i.
impending respiratory failure
imperfecta
 osteogenesis i.
implant
 Biocell RTV i.
 Biomatrix ocular i.
 bioresorbable i.
 Core-Vent i.
 defibrillator i.
implantable
 i. cardioverter-defibrillator
 (ICD)
 i. cardioverter-defibrillator/atrial
 tachycardia pacing (ICD-ATP)
 i. cardioverter electrodes
 i. left ventricular assist system
 (IPLVAS)
Implantaid Di-Lock cardiac lead
 introducer
implantation
 i. metastasis
 i. response
 stent i.
impotence
 vasculogenic i.

Impra bypass graft
Impra-Graft microporous PTFE
   vascular graft
impulse
   afferent i.
   apex i.
   apical i. (AI)
   cardiac i.
   i. conduction
   ectopic i.
   escape i.
   i. formation
   paradoxic rocking i.
   point of maximum i. (PMI)
   i. propagation
   right parasternal i.
   i. summation
   systolic apical i.
impure flutter
IMREG-1
IMT
   intimal-medial thickness
Imulyse t-PA ELISA kit
IMV
   intermittent mandatory ventilation
IMVbird
¹¹¹In
   indium-111
in
   in situ hybridization
   in vitro
   in vivo
   in vivo gene transfer
inactivated
   i. poliovirus vaccine
inactivity
   physical i.
inaequalis
   pulsus i.
INCA
   infant nasal cannula assembly
   INCA system
Incenti-neb nebulizer
incentive
   i. spirometer
   i. spirometry
incessant tachycardia

inch
   pounds per square i. (psi)
incidence
   peak i.
incident
   vascular i.
incidental murmur
incision
   collar i.
   fish-mouth i.
   ladder i.'s
   median sternotomy i.
   racquet i.
   stab i.
   sternal-splitting i.
   stocking-seam i.
   thoracotomy i.
   transverse i.
incisura
   i. apicis cordis
   cardiac i.
   i. pulse
incisure
   thoracic i.
inclusion
   Rocha-Lima i.
   i. technique of Bentall
incognitus
   Mycoplasma i.
incompetence, incompetency
   aortic i.
   cardiac valvular i.
   chronotropic i.
   mitral i.
   muscular i.
   pulmonary i., pulmonic i.
   pyloric i.
   relative i.
   tricuspid i.
   valvular i.
incomplete
   i. atrioventricular block
   i. atrioventricular dissociation
   i. A-V dissociation
incongruens
   pulsus i.
incontinentia pigmenti syndrome

NOTES

incremental
   i. atrial pacing
   i. ventricular pacing
incrementing response
Indacrinone
indanyl carbenicillin
indapamide
indecainide
Indeflator
   ACS I.
   I. Plus 20
Inderal
Inderide
index, pl. **indices, indexes**
   airway reactivity i. (ARI)
   ankle-arm i.
   ankle-brachial i. (ABI)
   apnea-hypopnea i. (AHI)
   arm-ankle indices
   asynchrony i.
   atherectomy i.
   atherogenicity i.
   atrial stasis i.
   Barthel i.
   body mass i. (BMI)
   brachial-ankle i.
   Broders i.
   cardiac i. (CI)
   cardiac output i.
   cardiac risk i.
   cardiac work i. (CWI)
   Charlson comorbidity i.
   chemotherapeutic i.
   Cholesterol-Saturated Fat I.
    (CSFI)
   compliance, rate, oxygenation,
    and pressure i.
   contractile work i.
   coronary prognostic i.
   CROP i.
   Crown-Crisp i.
   Detsky modified risk i.
   diastolic pressure-time i.
    (DPTI)
   Duke Activity Status I.
    (DASI)
   eccentricity i.
   ejection phase i.
   end-diastolic volume i. (EDVI)
   end-systolic force-velocity
    indices
   end-systolic volume i. (ESVI)

   exercise i.
   Fourmentin thoracic i.
   free thyrotoxin i.
   General Well-Being I.
   Gensini i.
   Gibson circularity i.
   glycocalicine i.
   Goldman i. of risk
   Goldman risk-factor i.
   isovolumetric phase i.
   isovolumic i.
   ITPA i.
   left atrial emptying i.
   left ventricular diastolic
    phase i.
   Lewis i.
   mitral valve closure i.
   myocardial jeopardy i.
   oxygen consumption i.
   penile-brachial pressure i.
   ponderal i.
   Pourcelot i.
   pulmonary vascular
    resistance i. (PVRI)
   Quality of Well-Being I.
   Quetelet i.
   Reid i.
   relaxation time i.
   respiratory disturbance i. (RDI)
   risk i.
   Robinson i.
   saturation i.
   Schneider i.
   segmental pressure i.
   shock i.
   Sokolow electrocardiographic i.
   sphericity i.
   stiffness i.
   stroke volume i. (SVI)
   stroke work i. (SWI)
   systemic vascular resistance i.
    (SVRI)
   systolic pressure time i. (SPTI)
   tension-time i.
   total peripheral resistance i.
    (TPRI)
   i. value
   vascular resistance i.
   volume thickness i. (VTI)
   wall motion score i. (WMSI)
   Wood units i.
   Youden i.

indicator
  i. dilution technique
  xylol pulse i.
indifferent electrode
indirect
  i. diuretic
  i. lead
  i. murmur
indium-111 (^{111}In)
  i. scintigraphy
indium-111-labeled lymphocyte
  imaging
Indocin
  I. I.V. injection
  I. Oral
indocyanine
  i. dilution curve
  i. green
  i. green angiography
  i. green dye
  i. green indicator dilution
    technique
  i. green method
indomethacin
indoramin
induced pneumothorax
inducibility
inducible
  i. arrhythmia
  i. polymorphic ventricular
    tachycardia
induction
  rapid sequence i. (RSI)
  sputum i.
induration
  idiopathic brown i.
indurativa
  tuberculosis i.
indurative
  i. myocarditis
  i. pleurisy
  i. pneumonia
industrial anthrax
indux
  rale i.
indwelling line
inertia

In-Exsufflator respiratory device
infant
  i. Ambu resuscitator
  i. nasal cannula assembly
    (INCA)
  i. respiratory distress syndrome
    (IRDS)
infantile
  i. arteritis
  i. beriberi
  i. lobar emphysema
infarct
  brain i.
  i. bulging
  cerebral i.
  embolic i.
  i. expansion
  i. extension
  lacunar i.
  pulmonary i.
  red i.
  i. scar
  i. thinning
  watershed i.
infarct-avid
  i.-a. hot-spot scintigraphy
  i.-a. imaging
  i.-a. myocardial scintigraphy
infarction
  acute myocardial i. (AMI)
  age-undetermined myocardial i.
  anterior myocardial i. (AMI)
  anterior wall myocardial i.
  anteroinferior myocardial i.
  anterolateral myocardial i.
  anteroseptal myocardial i.
    (ASMI)
  atrial i.
  atrial myocardial i.
  cardiac i.
  cerebral i.
  completed myocardial i.
  complicated myocardial i.
  Diabetes Mellitus Insulin
    Glucose Infusion in Acute
    Myocardial I. (DIGAMI)
  diaphragmatic myocardial i.

NOTES

infarction *(continued)*
  evolving myocardial i.
  inferior wall myocardial i.
  (IWMI)
  inferolateral myocardial i.
  ischemic cerebral i.
  lacunar i.
  lateral myocardial i.
  MITI Classification of
    Terminal Events in Patients
    with Acute Myocardial I.
  myocardial i. (MI)
  myocardial i. in H-form
  National Registry of
    Myocardial I. (NRMI)
  non-Q-wave myocardial i.
  (NQWMI)
  nontransmural myocardial i.
  (NTMI)
  posterior myocardial i.
  postmyocardial i.
  Primary Angioplasty in
    Myocardial I. (PAMI)
  Prourokinase in Myocardial I.
  (PRIMI)
  pulmonary i.
  Q wave myocardial i.
  recurrent myocardial i.
  right ventricular i.
  Roesler-Bressler i.
  rule out myocardial i. (ROMI)
  silent myocardial i. (SMI)
  stuttering myocardial i.
  subacute myocardial i.
  subendocardial myocardial i.
  Thrombolysis and Angioplasty
    in Myocardial I. (TAMI)
  Thrombolysis in Myocardial I.
  (TIMI)
  Thrombolytic Trial of Eminase
    in Acute Myocardial I.
  (TEAM)
  through-and-through
    myocardial i.
  transmural myocardial i.
  watershed i.
infarct-related vessel
Infasurf
infected
  i. aneurysm
  i. myxoma
infection
  adenoviral type 40/41 i.

  bacterial i.
  community-acquired i.
  endemic fungal i.
  fungal i.
  hospital-acquired i.
  laryngeal i.
  MAC i.
  MAI i.
  Mycobacterium avium
    complex i.
  Mycobacterium avium-
    intracellulare i.
  mycotic i.
  nosocomial i.
  opportunistic i.
  respiratory i.
  rhinocerebral i.
  secondary i.
  spirochetal i.
  staphylococcal i.
  streptococcal i.
  systemic i.
  upper respiratory i. (URI)
  viral respiratory i.
infectious
  i. asthmatic bronchitis
  i. endocarditis
  i. esophagitis
  i. mononucleosis
infective
  i. asthma
  i. embolism
  i. endocarditis (IE)
  i. pericarditis
  i. thrombosis
  i. thrombus
InFed injection
inferior
  i. epigastric artery (IEA)
  i. mesenteric artery
  i. mesenteric vascular occlusion
  i. vena cava (IVC)
  i. vena cava occlusion
  i. wall myocardial infarction
    (IWMI)
inferoapical
inferobasal wall
inferobasilar
inferolateral myocardial infarction
infestans
  Triatoma i.
infestation
  parasitic i.

infiltrate
    Assmann tuberculous i.
    bronchopneumonic i.
    fluffy alveolar i.
    hazy i.
    interstitial i.
    migratory pulmonary i.
    patchy i.
    perivascular eosinophilic i.'s
    strandy i.
    streaky i.
    Wasserman-positive
        pulmonary i.
infiltrating lobular carcinoma
infiltration
    patchy i.
infiltrative cardiomyopathy
Infiniti
    I. catheter
    I. catheter introducer system
inflammatoria
    dysphagia i.
inflammatory
    i. pericarditis
    i. reaction
inflation
    balloon i.
    i. reflex
inflow
    i. tract
    turbulent diastolic mitral i.
influenza, pl. **influenzae**
    i. A, B, C
    Asian i.
    endemic i.
    Hong Kong i.
    Russian i.
    Texas i.
    i. virus pneumonia
    i. virus vaccine
    yuppie i.
influenzae
    Haemophilus i.
influenzal pneumonia
infraclavicular triangle
infracristal
infracubital bypass

infradiaphragmatic portion
infra-Hisian
    i.-H. block
    i.-H. conduction system
infranodal extrasystole
infrared-pulsed laser
infrared thermography
infrarenal abdominal aortic
    aneurysm
Infrasonics ventilator
infrequens
    pulsus i.
infundibular
    i. obstruction
    i. septal defect
    i. wedge resection
infundibulectomy
    Brock i.
infundibulum
Infusaid infusion pump
Infus-a-port pump
InfusaSleeve
    Kaplan-Simpson I.
    LocalMed I.
Infuse-A-Port pump
infuser
    Critikon pressure i.
infusion
    brain-heart i.
    nitroprusside i.
ingravescent apoplexy
INH
    isoniazid
inhalant
    antifoaming i.
    i. antigen
inhalation
    i. agent
    Atrovent Aerosol I.
    i. bronchography
    isoproterenol sulfate i.
    NebuPent I.
    oxygen i.
    i. pneumonia
    i. tuberculosis
inhaled bronchodilator

NOTES

inhaler
　　AeroBid Oral Aerosol I.
　　albuterol i.
　　AREx i.
　　Beclovent Oral I.
　　Beconase AQ Nasal I.
　　Henderson-Haggard i.
　　Intal Oral I.
　　ipratropium i.
　　Junker i.
　　metered-dose i. (MDI)
　　Spiral Mark V portable
　　　ultrasonic drug i.
　　Tilade i.
　　Vancenase AQ I.
　　Vanceril Oral I.
Inhibace
inhibited
　　atrial demand-i. (AAI)
　　i. pacing
inhibition
　　leukotriene i.
　　potassium i.
inhibitor
　　ACE i.
　　acyl-CoA:cholesterol
　　　acyltransferase i.
　　alpha-1 proteinase i.
　　angiotensin-converting
　　　enzyme i. (ACEI)
　　beta-lactamase i.
　　bronchial mucus i.
　　carbonic anhydrase i.
　　cholinesterase i.
　　converting enzyme i.
　　cyclooxygenase i.
　　endopeptidase i.
　　HMG-CoA reductase i.
　　human menopausal
　　　gonadotropin coenzyme A
　　　reductase i.
　　hydroxymethylglutaryl coenzyme
　　　A reductase i.
　　3-hydroxy-3-methylglutaryl
　　　coenzyme A reductase i.
　　lipoprotein-associated
　　　coagulation i. (LACI)
　　MAO i.
　　　monoamine oxidase inhibitor
　　mast cell i.
　　monoamine oxidase i. (MAO
　　　inhibitor, MAOI)
　　mucus i.

oxysterol i.
PDE isoenzyme i.
phosphodiesterase i. (PDE)
phosphodiesterase
　isoenzyme i.'s
α_2-plasmin i.
plasminogen activator i. (PAI)
protease i.
α_1-proteinase i. (α_1-AT)
renin i.
secretory leukoproteinase i.
thromboxane synthetase i.
inhibitor-1
　plasminogen activator i. (PAI-
　　1)
inhomogeneity
initial apnea
Injectable
　Cardizem I.
injection
　Abbokinase i.
　Activase i.
　Adenocard i.
　Adlone i.
　Adrucil i.
　A-methaPred i.
　Amikin i.
　Apresoline i.
　AquaMEPHYTON i.
　Arfonad i.
　Articulose-50 i.
　Baci-IM i.
　Bactocill i.
　Bena-D i.
　Benadryl i.
　Benahist i.
　Benoject i.
　Bicillin L-A i.
　blood patch i.
　bolus i.
　Brethine i.
　Brevibloc i.
　Bricanyl i.
　Bronkephrine i.
　Caverject i.
　Ceredase i.
　Chlor-Pro i.
　Chlor-Trimeton i.
　Cipro i.
　Compazine i.
　Cortone Acetate i.
　Cortrosyn i.
　Corvert i.

Crysticillin A.S. i.
Cyklokapron i.
Cytoxan i.
DDAVP i.
Demadex i.
depMedalone i.
Depoject i.
Depo-Medrol i.
Depopred i.
Depo-Provera i.
D.H.E. 45 i.
Diflucan i.
Diprivan i.
D-Med i.
Dobutrex i.
Dopram i.
Doxychel i.
Duralone i.
Duralutin i.
dye i.
Edecrin Sodium i.
Enlon i.
Ethamolin i.
Flolan i.
Floxin i.
Foscavir i.
Garamycin i.
Gesterol i.
heparin i.
Hep-Lock i.
Hydeltrasol i.
Hydeltra-T.B.A. i.
Hy-Gestrone i.
Hylutin i.
Hyprogest i.
Indocin I.V. i.
InFed i.
Intropin i.
iopromide i.
Jenamicin i.
Keflin i.
Kefurox i.
Kenalog i.
Key-Pred-SP i.
Konakion i.
Lasix i.
Levophed i.

Lincocin i.
Lincorex i.
Liquaemin i.
Lovenox i.
Lyphocin i.
Medralone i.
Metro I.V. i.
Minocin I.V. i.
M-Prednisol i.
Nafcil i.
Nallpen i.
Narcan i.
Nebcin i.
Neosar i.
Netromycin i.
Neutrexin i.
Nitro-Bid I.V. i.
Normodyne i.
Nydrazid i.
Oncovin i.
Osmitrol i.
Pentacarinat i.
Pentam-300 i.
Permapen i.
Pfizerpen-AS i.
Phenazine i.
Phenergan i.
Pitressin i.
Predaject i.
Predalone i.
Predcor i.
Predicort-50 i.
Prednisol TBA i.
Priscoline i.
Pro-Depo i.
Prodrox i.
Prometh i.
Prorex i.
Prostaphlin i.
Prostin VR Pediatric i.
Prothazine i.
Retrovir i.
Reversol i.
Rifadin i.
root i.
Solu-Medrol i.
Sotradecol i.

NOTES

257

injection *(continued)*
    Tensilon i.
    Terramycin I.M. i.
    Toposar i.
    Trandate i.
    Tridil i.
    Ultravist i.
    Unipen i.
    Vancocin i.
    Vancoled i.
    VePesid i.
    V-Gan i.
    Vibramycin i.
    Vumon i.
    Wycillin i.
    Zinacef i.
injector
    flow i.
    Fujinon variceal i.
    Medrad Mark IV
      angiographic i.
    Mill-Rose esophageal i.
    modified Mark IV R-wave-
      triggered power i.
    power i.
    pressure i.
    Viamonte-Hobbs dye i.
injury
    blunt i.
    diastolic current of i.
    diffuse lung i.
    electrical i.
    femoral vascular i.
    median nerve i.
    mesangial immune i.
    myocardial i.
    penetrating i.
    reperfusion i.
    systolic current of i.
    vascular i.
inlet
    thoracic i.
in-memory gating
innervation
    autonomic sensory i.
innocent
    i. heart murmur
    i. murmur of elderly
innominate
    i. aneurysm
    i. artery
    i. vein
Innovace

Innovar
Innovator Holter system
Inocor
inoculation
Inokucki vascular stapler
inorganic
    i. dust disease
    i. murmur
inosine
inositol triphosphate
inotrope
    negative i.
inotropic
    i. agent
    i. arrhythmia
    i. effect
    i. support
inotropy
Inoue
    I. balloon catheter
    I. balloon mitral valvotomy
    I. self-guiding balloon
INR
    international normalized ratio
insertion
    percutaneous catheter i.
    retrograde catheter i.
    route of i.
    wire i.
insipidus
    nephrogenic diabetes i.
insomnia
insomniac
inspiration
    crowing i.
    duration of i. (T_1)
inspirator
inspiratory
    i. capacity (IC)
    i. dyspnea
    i. to expiratory ratio (I:E)
    i. flow rate
    i. positive airway pressure
      (IPAP)
    i. rales
    i. reserve capacity (IRC)
    i. reserve volume (IRV)
    i. stridor
    i. vital capacity (IVC)
InspirEase
    I. device
inspirometer

Inspiron
    I. AccurOx Mask
    I. Instromedix computer
Inspirx incentive spirometer
inspissated
instability
    catheter i.
instantaneous
    i. electrical axis
    i. spectral peak velocity
    i. vector
Insta-Pulse heart rate monitor
InStent CarotidCoil stent
instillation
    lavage i.
Institute
    Cardiopulmonary Research I.
    (CAPRI)
    National Heart, Lung, and
    Blood I. (NHLBI)
instrument
    arterial oscillator
    endarterectomy i.
    Cooley neonatal i.'s
    Diamond-Lite titanium i.'s
    KinetiX i.'s
    Matsuda titanium surgical i.'s
    NeoKnife electrosurgical i.
    Neuro-Trace i.
    OPG-Gee i.
    Pneumo-Needle reusable i.
    Wolvek sternal approximation
    fixation i.
instrumentation
    angiographic i.
    MIDA CoroNet i.
insudate
insufficiency
    aortic valvular i.
    arterial i.
    atrioventricular valve i.
    cardiac i.
    cerebrovascular i.
    coronary i.
    deep venous i. (DVI)
    mitral i.

    multivalve i.
    myocardial i.
    pulmonary i.
    pulmonic i.
    renal i.
    respiratory i.
    rheumatic mitral i.
    Sternberg myocardial i.
    tricuspid i.
    valvular i.
    velopharyngeal i.
    venous valvular i.
insufflation
    thoracoscopic talc i.
insufflator
    Venturi i.
Insuflon device
insulin
    beef i.
    NPH Iletin i.
    pork i.
    i. preparation
    regular purified pork i.
    i. shock
insulin-dependent diabetes mellitus
    (IDDM)
insulin-like growth factor (IGF)
insult
    cardiac i.
    vascular i.
Intal
    I. Nebulizer Solution
    I. Oral Inhaler
Intec
    I. AID cardioverter-defibrillator
    generator
    I. implantable defibrillator
Integra
    I. catheter
    I. II balloon
integrated
    i. bipolar sensing
    i. lead system
Integrelin to Manage Platelet
    Aggregation to Prevent Coronary
    Thrombosis (IMPACT)

NOTES

259

INTEGRIS
  I. cardiac imaging system
  I. cardiovascular imaging
intellectual dysfunction
Intellicath pulmonary artery
  catheter
intensifier
  image i.
intensity
  echo i.
  spatial i.
intentionem
  per primam i.
  per secondam i.
interaction
  adhesin-receptor i.
interarterial
  i. communication
  i. septum
  i. shunt
interatrial septum
intercadence
intercadent
intercalary
intercellular
  i. adhesion molecule-1 (ICAM-1)
  i. coupling
intercept angle
intercidens
  pulsus i.
intercostal
  i. space
intercurrens
  pulsus i.
interdependence
  ventricular i.
interdigitating coil stent
interectopic interval
interface
  I. arterial blood filter
  electrode-skin i.
  Monarch Mini Mask nasal i.
interfascicular fibrous tissue
interference
  i. beat
  dissociation by i.
  i. dissociation
  electromagnetic
    interference/radiofrequency i.
  (EMI/RFI)
α-interferon

interferon
  i. alfa-2a
  i. alfa-2b
  i. alpha
  i. gamma-1b
interlaced scanning
interleukin-2
  PEG i.
interleukin-3
interleukin-4
interleukin-5
interleukin-6
interleukin-7
interleukin-8 (IL-8)
interleukin-9
interleukin-10
interleukin-11
interlobar
  i. empyema
  i. pleurisy
interlobular
  i. emphysema
  i. pleurisy
  i. septa
intermediary vesicle
intermediate
  i. circumflex artery (ICXA)
  i. coronary syndrome
  i. heart
intermediate-density lipoprotein
Intermedics
  I. RES-Q implantable
    cardioverter-defibrillator
  I. Stride pacemaker
intermedius
  bronchus i.
  ramus i.
intermittence, intermittency
intermittens
  dyskinesia i.
  pulsus respiratione i.
intermittent
  i. claudication
  i. coronary sinus occlusion
  i. demand ventilation (IDV)
  i. mandatory ventilation (IMV)
  i. pneumatic compression (IPC)
  i. positive pressure (IPP)
  i. positive pressure breathing
  (IPPB)
  i. positive pressure ventilation
  (IPPV)

i. pulse
i. sinus arrest
interna
lamina elastica i.
internal
i. adhesive pericarditis
i. carotid artery (ICA)
i. diameter
i. elastic lamina (IEL)
i. jugular vein
i. mammary artery (IMA)
i. mammary artery bypass
i. mammary artery catheter
i. mammary artery graft
angiography
i. respiration
i. thoracic artery (ITA)
international
I. Multicenter Angina Exercise (IMAGE)
i. normalized ratio (INR)
I. Society for Heart and Lung Transplant (ISHLT)
I. Standards Organization (ISO)
internodal
i. conduction
i. pathways
i. tract of Bachmann
internum
pericardium i.
interpolated
i. beat
i. extrasystole
Interpret ultrasound catheter
interquartile range
interrogation
deep Doppler velocity i.
Doppler i.
stereoscopic i.
interrupted
i. aortic arch
i. pledgeted suture
i. respiration
interruption
aortic arch i.
azygoportal i.
intersegmental arteries

Intersept cardiotomy reservoir
Inter-Society Commission for Heart Disease (ICHD)
Interspec XL ultrasound
interstitial
i. emphyscma
i. infiltrate
i. lung disease (ILD)
i. markings
i. and perivascular collagen network
i. plasma cell pneumonia
i. pneumonitis
i. pulmonary edema
i. pulmonary fibrosis
i. space
interstitium
cardiac i.
intersystole
intersystolic period
Intertach
I. II pacer
I. pacemaker
Intertech
I. anesthesia breathing circuit
I. Mapleson D nonrebreathing circuit
I. nonrebreathing modified Jackson-Rees circuit
I. Perkin-Elmer gas sampling line
Intertherapy intravascular ultrasound
interval
A-A i.
A_1-A_2 i.
A-C i.
Ae-H i.
A-H i.
A-N i.
A2 to opening snap i.
atrial escape i.
atriocarotid i.
atrio-Hisian i.
atrioventricular i.
auriculoventricular i.
A-V delay i.

NOTES

261

interval *(continued)*
Bazett corrected QT i.
B-H i.
cardioarterial i., c-a i.
coupling i.
critical coupling i.
electromechanical i.
escape i.
f-f i.
flutter R i.
H-Ae i.
hangout i.
H_1-H_2 i.
H'P i.
H-Q i.
H-QRS i.
H-V i.
interectopic i.
isoelectric i.
isometric i.
isovolumic i.
JT i.
magnet pacing i.
P-A i.
pacemaker escape i.
passive i.
P-H i.
P-J i.
postsphygmic i.
P-P i.
P-Q i.
P-R i.
presphygmic i.
Q-H i.
Q-M i.
Q-R i.
Q-RB i.
QRS i.
QRS-T i.
Q-S_2 i.
Q-T i.
QTc i.
Q-U i.
right ventricular systolic
time i.
R-P i.
R-R i.
R-R prime i.
RS-T i.
sphygmic i.
S-QRS i.
ST i.
symptom-free i.

systolic time i. (STI)
TP i.
V-A i.
V-H i.
interval-strength relation
intervention
Myocardial Infarction Triage
and I. (MITI)
vagomimetic i.
interventional
i. cardiac catheterization
i. echocardiography
i. study
interventricular
i. foramen
i. septal motion
i. septal rupture
i. septum
i. septum aneurysm
i. sulcus
i. veins
intervertebral disk
Interview
Alexithymia Provoked
Response I.
intestinal
i. ischemia
i. lipodystrophy
intima
aortic tunica i.
intimal
i. flap
i. hyperplasia
i. tear
i. thickening
intimal-medial thickness (IMT)
Intimax vascular catheter
intolerance
carbohydrate i.
exercise i.
glucose i.
intoxication
alcohol i.
digitalis i.
intra-aortic
i.-a. balloon (IAB)
i.-a. balloon catheter
i.-a. balloon counterpulsation
i.-a. balloon device
intra-arterial
i.-a. counterpulsation
intra-atrial
i.-a. activation sequence

i.-a. baffle
i.-a. block
i.-a. conduction
i.-a. conduction time
i.-a. reentrant tachycardia
intracardiac
  i. atrial activation sequence
  i. catheter
  i. electrocardiography
  i. electrophysiologic study
  i. electrophysiology
  i. event
  i. lead
  i. mapping
  i. mass
  i. pacing
  i. pressure
  i. pressure curve
  i. shunt
  i. sucker
  i. thrombus
intracaval
  i. device
  i. endovascular ultrasonography
    (ICEUS)
intracavitary
  i. pressure-electrogram
    dissociation
  i. pressure gradient
intracellular
  i. calcium concentration
  i. lipid
intracellulare
  Mycobacterium i.
intracellular-like, calcium-bearing
  crystalloid solution (ICS)
intracoronary
  i. sonicated meglumine
  i. thrombolysis balloon
    valvuloplasty
  i. ultrasound (ICUS)
intracorporeal heart
intracranial
  i. aneurysm
  i. hypertension
IntraDop
  Doppler I.

intra-Hisian block
Intralipid
intralobar
intraluminal
  i. plaque
  i. ultrasound (ILUS)
intramural
  i. coronary arteries
  i. thrombi
  i. thrombosis
intramyocardial
  i. prearteriolar vessel
  i. pressure
Intra-Op autotransfusion system
intraoperative
  i. digital subtraction (IDIS)
  i. digital subtraction
    angiography (IDSA)
  i. hemodynamics
  i. mapping
  i. vascular angiography (IVA)
intrapericardial pressure
intraperitoneal rupture
intrapleural
  i. rupture
  i. sealed drainage unit
intrapulmonic
intrastent
  i. recurrent disease
  i. restenosis
intrathoracic
  i. pressure
  i. thyroid
intrauterine
  i. echocardiography
  i. pneumonia
  i. respiration
intravascular
  i. catheter electrode
  i. fetal air sign
  i. foreign body retrieval
  i. oxygenator (IVOX)
  i. perfluorochemical emulsion
  i. pressure
  i. stent
  i. thrombus
  i. ultrasound (IVUS)

I

NOTES

intravascular *(continued)*
  i. ultrasound catheter
  i. volume
intravenous (I.V.)
  i. digital subtraction
    angiography (IVDSA)
  Fungizone I.
  immune globulin, i.
  Saventrine I.
Intravenous Streptokinase in Acute
Myocardial Infarction Study
(ISAM)
intraventricular
  i. aberration
  i. block (IVB)
  i. conduction
  i. conduction delay
  i. conduction pattern
Intrepid balloon catheter
intrinsic
  i. asthma
  i. deflection
  i. sympathomimetic activity
intrinsicoid deflection
introducer
  Angestat hemostasis i.
  Angetear tearaway i.
  aortic assist balloon i.
  Avanti i.
  Cardak percutaneous catheter i.
  Check-Flo i.
  Ciaglia percutaneous
    tracheostomy i.
  Davol pacemaker i.
  Desilets i.
  Desilets-Hoffman catheter i.
  Encapsulon sheath i.
  FasTrac i.
  gum elastic bougie i.
  Hemaquet i.
  Implantaid Di-Lock cardiac
    lead i.
  LPS Peel-Away i.
  Micropuncture Peel-Away i.
  Nottingham i.
  Razi cannula i.
  i. sheath
  888 i. sheath
  split-sheath i.
  Tuohy-Borst i.
  UMI transseptal Cath-Seal
    catheter i.
  USCI i.

intron
  i. 16
  I. A
Intropin injection
intubation
  catheter-guided endoscopic i.
    (CAGEIN)
  endotracheal i.
  nasotracheal i.
  O'Dwyer i.
  RSI orotracheal i.
  tracheal i.
intussusception
invasive
  i. assessment
  i. pressure measurement
  i. pulmonary aspergillosis
Inventory
  Beck Depression I.
  State Trait Anxiety I.
inverse-ratio ventilation (IRV)
Inversine
inversion
  U wave i.
  ventricular i.
inversus
  dextrocardia with situs i.
  levocardia with situs i.
  situs i.
inverted T wave
Investigation
  Bypass Angioplasty
    Revascularization I. (BARI)
  Coronary Angioplasty versus
    Bypass Revascularization I.
    (CABRI)
  German Angioplasty Bypass
    Surgery I. (GABI)
Invirase
inward-going rectification
Iobid DM
iodide
  metocurine i.
  potassium i.
  saturated solution of
    potassium i. (SSKI)
iodine
  radiolabeled i.
iodine-123 (I-123)
  i. heptadecanoic acid
    radioactive tracer
  i. metaiodobenzylguanidine (I-
    123-MIBG)

I

i. metaiodobenzylguanidine
uptake (I-123 MIBG uptake)
iodine-125 isotope
iodine-131 MIBG scintigraphy
iodoquinol
iohexol
ion
calcium i.
i. channel
chloride i.
potassium i.
i. pump
sodium i.
Ionescu-Shiley
I.-S. pericardial patch
I.-S. pericardial valve
I.-S. valve prosthesis
I.-S. vascular graft
Ionescu trileaflet valve
ionizing radiation (IR)
ion-selective electrode (ISE)
Ionyx lead
iopamidol
Iopamiro
iopromide
i. injection
**iothalamate meglumine contrast
medium**
ioversol
ioxaglate
i. meglumine
i. meglumine contrast medium
i. sodium
sodium meglumine i.
IPAP
inspiratory positive airway pressure
IPC
intermittent pneumatic compression
IPC boots
IPCO-Partridge defibrillator
IPF
idiopathic pulmonary fibrosis
IPG
impedance plethysmography
IPLVAS
implantable left ventricular assist
system

IPOL
IPP
intermittent positive pressure
IPPA
I-124 I.
IPPB
intermittent positive pressure
breathing
IPPV
intermittent positive pressure
ventilation
Iprafen
ipratropium
i. bromide
i. inhaler
ipsilateral
IR
ionizing radiation
IRC
inspiratory reserve capacity
Ircon
IRDS
infant respiratory distress syndrome
Irex Exemplar ultrasound
iridium strand
IRMA
immunoradiometric assay
iron
i. chelator
i. dextran complex
i. lung
serum i.
i. storage disease
irradiation
total axial node i. (TANI)
total lymphoid i. (TLI)
irregularly
i. irregular pulse
i. irregular rhythm
irregular rhythm
irreversible
i. airway obstruction
i. shock
Irri-Cath suction system
irritable heart
irritant receptor

NOTES

265

IRV
  inspiratory reserve volume
  inverse-ratio ventilation
Irvine viable organ-tissue transport system (IVOTTS)
ISAM
  Intravenous Streptokinase in Acute
  Myocardial Infarction Study
Isambert disease
ischemia
  asymptomatic cardiac i. (ACI)
  brachiocephalic i.
  Canadian Amlodipine/Atenolol
    in Silent I. (CASIS)
  cardiac i.
  cerebral i.
  clandestine myocardial i.
  colonic i.
  exercise-induced silent
    myocardial i.
  extremity i.
  intestinal i.
  limb i.
  manifest i.
  mesenteric i.
  myocardial i. (MI)
  nonocclusive mesenteric i.
  recurrent mesenteric i.
  silent myocardial i.
  subendocardial i.
  transient i.
  transient mesenteric i.
ischemia-guided medical therapy
ischemic
  i. burden
  i. cardiomyopathy
  i. cerebral infarction
  i. contracture of left ventricle
  i. contracture of the left
    ventricle
  i. ECG changes
  i. heart disease (IHD)
  i. hypoxia
  i. mitral regurgitation
  i. myocardium
  i. paralysis
  i. pericarditis
  i. rest angina
  i. sudden death
  i. threshold
ISE
  ion-selective electrode
Iselin forceps

isethionate
  pentamidine i.
ISH
  isolated septal hypertrophy
ISHLT
  International Society for Heart and
  Lung Transplant
ISIS-2
  Second International Study of Infarct
  Survival
Ismelin
IS-5-MN
  isosorbide-5-mononitrate
Ismo
ISO
  International Standards Organization
isoactin switch
isobutyl 2-cyanoacrylate
isocapnia
isocapnic, isocapneic
  i. condition
  i. hyperpnea
isocenter system
isochoric
isocyanate
  methyl i.
isocyanate-induced asthma
isodiametric bipolar screw-in lead
isodiphasic complex
isoechoic
isoelectric
  i. interval
  i. line
  i. period
  i. point
isoenzyme
  CPK i.'s
  myocardial muscle creatine
    kinase i. (CK-MB)
isoetharine
  Arm-a-Med I.
  Dey-Lute I.
isoflurane
isoform
  Apo E3 i.
isolated
  i. dextrocardia
  i. heat perfusion
  i. parietal endocarditis
  i. septal hypertrophy (ISH)
isomer
  dextro i.
  levo i.

I

isomerism
isometric
  i. contraction
  i. contraction period
  i. exercise
  i. handgrip
  i. handgrip test
  i. interval
  i. period of cardiac cycle
  i. relaxation period
isomyosin switch
isoniazid (INH)
  rifampin and i.
isonitrile
  carbomethoxyisopropyl i.
  methoxyisobutyl i. (MIBI)
  technetium-99m
    methoxyisobutyl i.
Isopaque
isoprenaline
isoproterenol
  Arm-a-Med i.
  Dey-Dose i.
  Dispos-a-Med i.
  i. and phenylephrine
  i. stress test
  i. sulfate inhalation
  i. tilt-table test
Isoptin
isorhythmic dissociation
isosorbide
  i. dinitrate
  i. mononitrate
isosorbide-5-mononitrate (IS-5-MN)
Isospora belli
isotonic
  i. contraction
  i. exercise
isotope
  iodine-125 i.
isotypic
Isovex
isovolume
isovolumetric
  i. contractility
  i. phase index

  i. relaxation
  i. relaxation period (IVRP)
isovolumic
  i. index
  i. interval
  i. relaxation
  i. relaxation period
  i. relaxation time (IVRT)
  i. systole
Isovue contrast medium
isoxsuprine hydrochloride
isradipine
Israel Benzedrine vaporizer
israelii
  Actinomyces i.
  Nocardia i.
isthmectomy
isthmus, pl. **isthmi**
  aortic i.
  Krönig i.
  thyroid i.
Isuprel
ITA
  internal thoracic artery
  ITA graft
ITC balloon catheter
ITP
  idiopathic thrombocytopenic purpura
ITPA index
itraconazole
Itrel 1 unipolar pulse generator
IV
  IV block
  intraventricular
I.V.
  intravenous
IVA
  intraoperative vascular angiography
IVAC
  I. electronic thermometer
  I. ventilator
  I. volumetric infusion pump
Ivalon
  I. plug
  I. sponge
IVA-S2000

NOTES

IVCD intraventricular conduction delay

IVB
intraventricular block
IVC
inferior vena cava
inspiratory vital capacity
IVDSA
intravenous digital subtraction
angiography
Ivemark syndrome
ivermectin
IVOTTS
Irvine viable organ-tissue transport
system
IVOX
intravascular oxygenator

IVRP
isovolumetric relaxation period
IVRT
isovolumic relaxation time
IVT
idiopathic ventricular tachycardia
IVT percutaneous catheter
introducer sheath
IVUS
intravascular ultrasound
Ivy bleeding time
IWMI
inferior wall myocardial infarction

J

joule
J curve
J exchange wire
J guidewire
J junction
J loop technique
J orthogonal electrode
J point
J point electrical axis
J point treadmill test
J Rosen guidewire
J wave
J wire
J5 lipopolysaccharidase
Jabaley-Stille Super Cut Scissors
Jaccoud
    J. dissociated fever
    J. sign
jacket
    Bonchek-Shiley cardiac j.
    cardiac cooling j.
    cuirass j.
    Medtronic cardiac cooling j.
    Willock respiratory j.
jacket-type chest dressing
Jackman
    J. coronary sinus electrode catheter
    J. orthogonal catheter
Jackson
    J. bistoury
    J. cane-shaped tracheal tube
    J. safety triangle
    J. sign
    J. syndrome
Jackson-Trousseau dilator
Jacobaeus
    J. procedure
    J. thoracoscope
Jacobaeus-Unverricht thoracoscope
Jacobson
    J. microbulldog clamp
    J. modified vessel clamp
Jacobson-Potts clamp
Jacquet apparatus
Jahnke anastomosis clamp
Jahnke-Barron heart support net
Jako laryngoscope

James
    J. accessory tracts
    J. bundlc
    J. exercise protocol
    J. fibers
Jamshidi needle
Janeway
    J. lesion
    J. sphygmomanometer
Janus syndrome
Janz formula
Jarvik
    J. 7 and 8 artificial heart
    J. 7-70 artificial heart
    J. 2000 artificial heart
Jatene
    J. arterial switch procedure
Jatene-Macchi prosthetic valve
Javid
    J. carotid artery bypass clamp
    J. shunt
jaw thrust maneuver
jejunal artery
jelly
    cardiac j.
    electrode j.
Jenamicin injection
Jenkins Activity Survey
Jenner emphysema
jeopardized myocardium
jeopardy score
jerkin plethysmograph
jerks
    dormescent j.
jerky
    j. pulse
    j. respiration
Jervell and Lange-Nielsen syndrome
Jesberg esophagoscope
JET
    junctional ectopic tachycardia
jet
    anteriorly-directed j.
    aortic stenosis j.
    Doppler color j.
    j. effect
    j. humidifier
    j. lesion
    mitral regurgitant j.
    mosaic j.

jet *(continued)*
    j. nebulizer
    regurgitant j.
    residual j.
    turbulent j.
Jeune syndrome
Jewel
    J. pacer-cardioverter-defibrillator
    J. PCD
Jinotti closed suctioning system
JL4
    Judkins left 4
Jobst
    J. extremity pump
    J. pressure garment
    J. VPGS stockings
Jobst-Stride support stockings
Jobst-Stridette support stockings
Job syndrome
Johnson & Johnson hemopump
joint
    j. deformity
    tuberculosis of bones and j.'s
Joklik medium
Jonas modification of Norwood procedure
Jones criteria
Jonnson maneuver
Jopamiro 370
jordanis
    Legionella j.
Jorgenson thoracic scissors
josamycin
Josephson
    J. quadpolar mapping electrode
    J. quadripolar catheter
Jostra
    J. arterial blood filter
    J. cardiotomy reservoir
    J. catheter
joule (J)
JR4, JR5 catheter
J-shaped tube
JT
    junctional tachycardia
    JT interval
JTc value
J-tip
    J.-t. guidewire
Judkins
    J. coronary catheter
    J. curve LAD catheter
    J. curve LCX catheter

    J. curve STD catheter
    J. guiding catheter
    J. technique
    J. torque control catheter
Judkins left 4 (JL4)
Judkins-Sones technique of cardiac catheterization
Juevenelle clamp
jugular
    j. bulb catheter placement assessment
    j. embryocardia
    j. vein
    j. venous arch
    j. venous catechol spillover
    j. venous distention (JVD)
    j. venous pressure (JVP)
    j. venous pulse
    j. venous pulse tracing
Julian thoracic forceps
jump
    j. collaterals
    j. graft
jumping thrombosis
junction
    atrioventricular j.
    A-V j.
    cardioesophageal j.
    costochondral j.
    gap j.
    J j.
    loose j.
    QRS-ST j.
    saphenofemoral j.
    sino-tubular j.
    ST j.
    sternochondral j.
    tight j.
    tracheoesophageal j.
    triadic j.
junctional
    j. axis
    j. bigeminy
    j. bradycardia
    j. complex
    j. depression
    j. ectopic tachycardia (JET)
    j. escape
    j. escape beat
    j. escape rhythm
    j. extrasystole
    j. reciprocating tachycardia
    j. tachycardia (JT)

Junker inhaler
Junod procedure
Jürgensen sign
jute workers' lung
juvenile
    j. arrhythmia
    j. pattern
    j. rheumatoid arthritis
juxtacapillary receptor
juxtacardiac pleural pressure
juxtaductal
    j. coarctation

Juzo
    J. hose
    J. shrinker
    J. stockings
J-Vac
JVD
    jugular venous distention
JVP
    jugular venous pressure

J

NOTES

K
potassium
K current
K-37 pediatric arterial blood filter
KAAT II Plus intra-aortic balloon
pump
Kabikinase
KabiVitrum
Kahler bronchial biopsy forceps
Kalcinate
kallidinogenase inactivator unit
kallikrein
    k. inactivating units (KIU)
kallikrein-bradykinin system
kallikrein-kinin (KK)
Kallmann syndrome
Kalos pacemaker
Kaltostat
    K. wound packing dressing
    K. wound packing material
kanamycin
Kangaroo pump
kansasii
    Mycobacterium k.
Kantor-Berci video laryngoscope
Kantrowitz
    K. pacemaker
    K. thoracic clamp
kaolin pneumoconiosis
Kaon
Kaopectate
Kaplan-Meier
    K.-M. event-free survival curve
    K.-M. life table
    K.-M. method
Kaplan-Simpson InfusaSleeve
Kaposi sarcoma (KS)
Kardegic
Karell diet
Karhunen-Loeve procedure
Karmen units
Karmody venous scissors
Karnovsky rating scale
Karplus sign
Kartagener
    K. syndrome
    K. triad
Kasabach-Merritt syndrome
Kasser-Kennedy method
Kaster mitral valve prosthesis

Kattus
    K. exercise stress test
    K. treadmill protocol
Katzen
    K. infusion wire
    K. long balloon dilatation
      catheter
Katz-Wachtel phenomenon
Kaufman pneumonia
Kawai bioptome
Kawasaki
    K. disease
    K. syndrome
Kawashima intraventricular tunnel
Kay balloon
Kayexalate enema
Kay-Shiley caged-disk valve
KCl
    potassium chloride
kd
    kilodalton
Kearns-Sayre syndrome
Kearns syndrome
keel
    McNaught k.
keeled chest
Keflex
Keflin
    K. injection
Keftab
Kefurox
    K. injection
Kefzol
Keith
    K. bundle
    K. node
Keith-Flack node
Keith-Wagener-Barker (KWB)
Kellner questionnaire
Kellock sign
Kelly
    K. clamp
    K. hemostat
Kelly-Wick vascular tunneler
keloidal
Kelvin Sensor pacemaker
Kempner diet
Kenacort
    K. Syrup
    K. Tablet**

Kenalog injection
Kendall
  K. compression stockings
  K. Sequential Compression
    device
Kennedy area-length method
Kenonel
Kensey atherectomy catheter
Kent
  K. bundle
  K. bundle ablation
  bundle of Stanley K.
  K. fibers
  K. pathway
  K. potential
Kent-His bundle
Keofeed feeding tube
Kerley A, B, C lines
Kerlone
  K. Oral
Kernan-Jackson bronchoscope
Kern technique
kerosene pneumonitis
Keshan disease
ketamine
ketanserin
ketoconazole
ketone
  D-Phe-L-Pro-L-Arg-
    chloromethyl k. (PPACK)
ketoprofen
ketorolac
ketotifen
Kety-Schmidt method
keV
  kiloelectron volt
Key
  ResCue K.
  Walking with Angina-Learning
    is K. (WALK)
keyhole-limpet hemocyanin
keyhole surgery
Key-Pred-SP injection
kg/m2
  kilogram per meter squared
KI antigen
kick
  atrial k.
  idioventricular k.
kidney
  Ask-Upmark k.
  flea-bitten k.

  k. Goldblatt hypertension
  polycystic k.
Kiel classification of lymphoma
Kienbock phenomenon
Kiethly-DAS series 500 data-
  acquisition system
Kifa catheter material
Kikuchi disease
Killian-Lynch laryngoscope
Killip
  K. classification of heart
    disease
  K. wire
Killip-Kimball heart failure
  classification
kilodalton (kd)
45-kilodalton protein
kiloelectron volt (keV)
kilogram
  milligrams per k. (mg/kg)
  milliliter per k. (mL/kg)
  k. per meter squared (kg/m2)
kilohm
kilopascal (kPa)
kilopond (KP)
  k. meters (KPM)
kilovolt (kV)
Kimmelstiel-Wilson syndrome
Kim-Ray
  K.-R. Greenfield antiembolus
    filter
  K.-R. thermodilution
Kimura cartilage graft
kinase
  creatine k. (CK)
  phosphorylase k.
  protein k.
  serum creatine k.
kinetics
  first-order k.
  zero-order k.
KinetiX
  K. instruments
  K. ventilation monitor
kinetocardiogram
kinetocardiograph
King
  K. ASD umbrella closure
  K. biopsy method
  K. bioptome
  K. cardiac device
  K. double umbrella closure
    system

K. guiding catheter
K. of Hearts event recorder
K. of Hearts Holter monitor
K. multipurpose catheter
kingae
*Haemophilus aphrophilus,
Actinobacillus
actinomycetemcomitans,
Cardiobacterium hominis,
Eikenella corrodens, and
Kingella k.* (HACEK)
Kingella k.
Kingella kingae
kinin
kininogen
kinked aorta
kinky-hair disease
Kinsey
K. atherectomy
K. atherectomy catheter
K. rotation atherectomy
extrusion angioplasty
Kinyoun stain
Kirklin fence
Kirstein method
Kisch reflex
kissing
k. balloon angioplasty
k. balloon technique
Kistner tracheal button
kit
Alatest Latex-specific IgE
allergen test k.
Arrow pneumothorax k.
BiPort hemostasis introducer
sheath k.
Cordis lead conversion k.
Enzygnost F1+2 ELISA k.
Enzygnost TAT complex k.
Euro-Collins multiorgan
perfusion k.
Fergus percutaneous
introducer k.
Imulyse t-PA ELISA k.
neonatal internal jugular
puncture k.

No Pour Pak suction
catheter k.
percutaneous access k. (PAK)
percutaneous catheter
introducer k.
Per-fit percutaneous
tracheostomy k.
Portex Per-Fit tracheostomy k.
Pro-Vent arterial blood gas k.
Pro-Vent arterial blood
sampling k.
Pulsator dry heparin arterial
blood gas k.
Sub-4 Platinum Plus wire k.
thermodilution catheter
introducer k.
TintElize PAI-1 ELISA k.
TriPort hemostasis introducer
sheath k.
UniPort hemostasis introducer
sheath k.
Yamasa assay k.
KIU
kallikrein inactivating units
KK
kallikrein-kinin
KK system
Klebsiella
K. oxytoca
K. pneumonia
K. pneumoniae
Klebs-Löffler bacillus
Kleihauer-Betke test
Kleihauer test
Klein transseptal introducer sheath
Klein-Waardenburg syndrome
Klinefelter syndrome
Klippel-Feil syndrome
Klippel-Trenaunay-Weber syndrome
knee extension
knife, pl. **knives**
A-K diamond k.
A-OK ShortCut k.
Bailey-Glover-O'Neill
commissurotomy k.
Bosher commissurotomy k.
gamma k.

NOTES

275

knife *(continued)*
    Lebsche sternal k.
    Neoflex bendable k.
    roentgen k.
    UltraCision ultrasonic k.
    valvotomy k.
    k. wound
knitted
    k. sewing ring
    k. vascular prosthesis
knob
    aortic k.
knock
    pericardial k.
knuckle
    aortic k.
    b k.
    cervical aortic k.
    k. sign
Ko-Airan bleeding control procedure
Koate-HP
Koch
    K. node
    K. phenomenon
    triangle of K.
    K. triangle
    K. tuberculin
Kocher-Cushing reflex
Koga treatment
KoGENate
KOH
    potassium hydroxide
Kohn pores
Kolephrin GG/DM
Kolff-Jarvik artificial heart
Kolmogorov-Smirnov
    K.-S. goodness-of-fit test
    K.-S. procedure
Konakion injection
Kondoleon-Sistrunk elephantiasis procedure
Konigsberg catheter
Konno
    K. biopsy method
    K. bioptome
    K. operation
    K. procedure
Kontron
    K. balloon
    K. balloon catheter
    K. intra-aortic balloon pump
Konyne 80

Kopp asthma
Korányi
    K. auscultation
    K. sign
Korotkoff
    K. phase
    K. sound
Kostmann syndrome
Kotonkan virus
KP
    kilopond
kPa
    kilopascal
KPM
    kilopond meters
^{81m}Kr
    krypton-81m
Krebs
    K. cycle
    K. solution
Krebs-Henseleit
    K.-H. buffer
    K.-H. solution
Kredex
Kreiselman unit
Kreysig sign
kringle
Krishaber disease
KRM-1648/Isoniazid
Krogh apparatus spirometer
Kronecker center
Krönig
    K. area
    K. isthmus
    K. steps
Krovetz-Gessner equation
Kruskal-Wallis test
krypton-81m ventilation imaging
krypton-81m (^{81m}Kr)
KS
    Kaposi sarcoma
k-space segmentation
K-Sponge
Kugel
    K. anastomosis
    K. anastomotic artery
Kugelberg-Welander
    K.-W. disease
    K.-W. syndrome
Kuhn
    K. mask
    K. tube
Kulchitsky cell

Kuntz
    nerve of K.
Kurten vein stripper
Kussmaul
    K. breathing
    K. disease
    K. paradoxical pulse
    K. respiration
    K. sign
    K. symptom
Kussmaul-Kien respiration
Kussmaul-Maier disease
kV
    kilovolt
    kV fluoroscopy

Kveim
    K. antigen skin test
    K. reaction
Kveim-Stilzbach test
KWB
    Keith-Wagener-Barker
    KWB classification
Kwelcof
kymogram
kymograph
kymography
kymoscope
kyphoscoliosis

NOTES

LA
    left atrium
LAA
    left atrial appendage
    LAA thrombi
La:A
    left atrial to aortic
    La:A ratio
LABA
    laser-assisted balloon angioplasty
labeled FFA scintigraphy
labetalol
    l. hydrochloride
labile
    l. blood pressure
    l. hypertension
    l. pulse
Laboratories
    Venereal Disease Research L.
    (VDRL)
Laborde method
labored respiration
LACI
    lipoprotein-associated coagulation
    inhibitor
lacidipine
Lacipil
lactamase
    beta l.
lactate
    amrinone l.
    l. dehydrogenase
    l. extraction
    milrinone l.
    Ringer l.
    l. threshold
lactea
    macula l.
lactic
    l. acid
    l. acid dehydrogenase
    l. acidosis
    l. dehydrogenase (LDH)
LactiCare-HC
Lactobacillus
lacunar
    l. angina
    l. infarct
    l. infarction
    l. stroke

LAD
    left anterior descending artery
    left axis deviation
ladder
    l. diagram
    l. incisions
Laennec
    L. catarrh
    L. cirrhosis
    L. pearls
    L. sign
Laerdal
    L. infant resuscitator
    L. Resusci Folding Bag II
Laevovist
LAF
    left atrial enlargement
Lagrangian
    L. definition
    L. strain
LAH
    left anterior hemiblock
laid-back
    l.-b. balloon occlusion
    aortography
    l.-b. view
laidlawii
    Acholeplasma l.
LAIS laser
laiteuse
    tache l.
lakes
    venous l.
LAMA
    laser-assisted microanastomosis
LAMB
    lentigines, atrial myxoma, and blue
    nevi
    LAMB syndrome
Lambert
    canals of L.
Lambert-Kay clamp
Lambl excrescences
lamina
    elastic l.
    l. elastica interna
    internal elastic l. (IEL)
laminar blood flow

L

laminated
l. clot
l. thrombus
laminin
lamivudine
lamp
Wood l.
Lamprene
Lam procedure
LAN
local area network
Lanacaps
Ferralyn L.
lanata
Digitalis l.
lanatoside C
Lancisi sign
Landolfi sign
Landouzy-Déjérine
L.-D. dystrophy
facioscapulohumeral dystrophy
of L.-D.
L.-D. syndrome
Landry-Guillain-Barre syndrome
Landry Vein Light Venoscope
Lange calipers
Langendorff
L. apparatus
L. heart preparation
Langer axillary arch
Langerhans giant cells
Langevin updating procedure
Langhans cells
Laniazid Oral
Lanophyllin-GG
Lanoxicaps
Lanoxin
lansingensis
Legionella l.
Lanz low-pressure cuff endotracheal tube
LAO
left anterior oblique
LAO position
LAPIS
Late Potential Italian Study
Laplace
L. law
L. relationship
Laplacian mapping
lapping murmur
Lap Sac

large
l. cell carcinoma
l. cell undifferentiated carcinoma
large-bore
l.-b. catheter
l.-b. slotted aspirating needle
large-vessel disease
L-arginine
Lariam
Larrey
L. hernia
L. spaces
larva migrans
laryngalgia
laryngea
angina l.
laryngeal
l. atresia
l. crisis
l. infection
l. nerve
l. pouch
l. rales
l. reflex
l. stridor
l. syncope
l. vertigo
l. web
laryngectomee
laryngis
phlebectasia l.
laryngismus
l. paralyticus
l. stridulus
laryngitis
atrophic l.
catarrhal l.
chronic catarrhal l.
croupous l.
diphtheritic l.
membranous l.
phlegmonous l.
l. sicca
l. stridulosa
subglottic l.
syphilitic l.
tuberculous l.
vestibular l.
Laryngoflex reinforced endotracheal tube
laryngomalacia

laryngoscope
  Benjamin binocular slimline l.
  Benjamin pediatric l.
  Bizzari-Guiffrida l.
  Broyles anterior commissure l.
  Bullard intubating l.
  Dedo-Pilling l.
  Foregger l.
  Garfield-Holinger l.
  Holinger anterior commissure l.
  Jako l.
  Kantor-Berci video l.
  Killian-Lynch l.
  Lindholm operating l.
  Machida fiberoptic l.
  MacIntosh l.
  Magill l.
  Ossoff-Karlan l.
  Sanders intubation l.
  shadow-free l.
  Shapshay-Healy l.
  Storz-Hopkins l.
laryngoscopy
  direct l.
  mirror-image l.
  suspension l.
laryngotracheitis
laryngotracheobronchitis
larynx
  artificial l.
  Cooper-Rand intraoral
    artificial l.
  Nu-Vois artificial l.
  tuberculosis of l.
LASEC
  left atrial spontaneous echo contrast
laser
  l. ablation
  alexandrite l.
  ArF excimer l.
  argon ion l.
  atheroblation l.
  balloon-centered argon l.
  cool-tip l.
  coumarin pulsed dye l.
  dye l.
  ELCA l.

  erbium:YAG l.
  excimer cool l.
  excimer gas l.
  l. firing
  flashlamp-pulsed Nd:YAG l.
  fluorescence-guided smart l.
  free-beam l.
  helium-cadmium diagnostic l.
  HF infrared l.
  high-energy l.
  holmium l.
  Ho:YAG l.
  infrared-pulsed l.
  LAIS l.
  low-energy l.
  Lumonics YAG l.
  MCM smart l.
  microsecond pulsed flashlamp
    pumped dye l.
  mid-infrared pulsed l.
  Nd:YAG l.
    neodymium:yttrium-
      aluminum-garnet laser
  neodymium:yttrium-aluminum-
    garnet l. (Nd:YAG laser)
  pulsed dye l.
  Q-switched Nd:YAG l.
  rotational ablation l.
  ruby l.
  Spectranetics l.
  spectroscopy-directed l.
  Surgica K6 l.
  Surgilase 150 l.
  THC:YAG l.
  ultraviolet l.
  XeCl excimer l.
  xenon chloride excimer l.
  YAG l.
laser-assisted
  l.-a. balloon angioplasty
    (LABA)
  l.-a. microanastomosis (LAMA)
  l.-a. uvulopalatoplasty (LAUP)
Laserdish
  L. electrode
  L. pacing lead

L

NOTES

laser-induced
  l.-i. arterial fluorescence
     (LIAF)
  l.-i. thrombosis
Laserpor pacing lead
laserprobe catheter
Lasix
  L. injection
  L. Oral
Lassa
  L. fever
  L. virus
LATE
  Late Assessment of Thrombolytic
     Efficacy
  LATE study
late
  l. apical systolic murmur
  l. apnea
  L. Assessment of Thrombolytic
     Efficacy (LATE)
  l. cyanosis
  l. death
  l. deceleration
  l. diastole
  l. diastolic murmur
  L. Potential Italian Study
     (LAPIS)
  l. proarrhythmic effect
  l. reperfusion
  l. systole
latent
  l. empyema
  l. pleurisy
late-peaking systolic murmur
lateral
  l. myocardial infarction
  l. sac
  l. thrombus
  l. wall (LW)
laterosporus
  Bacillus l.
latex balloon
Lathyrus odoratus
latissimus
  l. dorsi
  l. dorsi muscle
  l. dorsi procedure
Latrodectus
Laubry-Soulle syndrome
LAUP
  laser-assisted uvulopalatoplasty
Laurell method

Laurence-Moon-Bardet-Biedl
  syndrome
Laurence-Moon-Biedl syndrome
Lautier test
lavage
  bronchial l.
  bronchoalveolar l. (BAL)
  continuous pericardial l.
  l. instillation
  pericardial l.
  pleural l.
  tracheobronchial l.
law
  all-or-none l.
  Bowditch l.
  Du Bois-Reymond l.
  Einthoven l.
  l. of the heart
  Hooke l.
  Laplace l.
  Louis l.
  Marey l.
  Ohm l.
  Poiseuille l.
  Starling l.
  Sutton l.
  Torricelli l.
LAX
  long axis
laxa
  cutis l.
layer
  adventitial l.
  fascial l.
  half-value l.
  hypertrophic smooth muscle l.
  subendocardial l.
LBBB
  left bundle-branch block
LBNP
  lower body negative pressure
LCA
  left coronary artery
L-Carnitine Ecocardiografia
  Digitalizzata Infarto Miocardico
  (CEDIM)
LCAT
  lecithin-cholesterol acyltransferase
LCD
  liquid crystal display
LCL
  Levinthal-Coles-Lillie
  LCL bodies

LCX
    left circumflex artery
LDH
    lactic dehydrogenase
        LDH flip
LDL
    low-density lipoprotein
        LDL Direct blood test
LE
    lupus erythematosus
lead
    ABC l.'s
    Accufix pacemaker l.
    aVF, aVL, aVR l.'s
    barbed epicardial pacing l.
    barb-tip l.
    bifurcated J-shaped tined atrial
        pacing and defibrillation l.
    bipolar limb l.'s
    Cadence TVL
        nonthoracotomy l.
    capped l.
    CapSure cardiac pacing l.
    CB l.
    CCS endocardial pacing l.
    CF l.
    chest l.'s
    CL l.
    Cordis Ancar pacing l.'s
    CPI endocardial
        defibrillation/rate-
        sensing/pacing l.
    CPI Endotak SQ electrode l.
    CPI porous tined-tip bipolar
        pacing l.
    CPI Sentra endocardial l.
    CPI Sweet Tip l.
    CR l.
    direct l.
    Einthoven l.
    Ela ventricular pacing l.
    electrocardiographic l.'s
    Elema l.'s
    Encor l.
    endocardial balloon l.
    Endotak C tripolar
        pacing/sensing/defibrillation l.

    Endotak C tripolar
        transvenous l.
    epicardial l.
    esophageal l.
    Fast-Pass endocardial l.
    finned pacemaker l.
    fishhook l.
    Frank XYZ orthogonal l.
    Golub EKG l.
    Heartwire l.
    Hombach placement of l.'s
    l. impedance
    indirect l.
    intracardiac l.
    Ionyx l.
    isodiametric bipolar screw-in l.
    Laserdish pacing l.
    Laserpor pacing l.
    Lewis l.
    limb l.
    Mason-Likar placement of
        EKG l.'s
    Medtronic l.'s
    monitor l.'s
    myocardial l.
    Myopore l.
    Nehb D l.
    nonintegrated transvenous
        defibrillation l.
    nonintegrated tripolar l.
    Oscor atrial l.
    Oscor pacing l.'s
    Osypka atrial l.
    pacemaker l.'s
    permanent cardiac pacing l.
    Permathane l.
    l. placement
    l. poisoning
    Precept l.
    precordial l.'s
    l. reversal
    reversed arm l.'s
    scalar l.'s
    screw-in l.
    screw-on l.
    segmented ring tripolar l.
    semidirect l.'s

L

NOTES

lead *(continued)*
    single-pass l.
    standard limb l.
    Stela electrode l.
    steroid-eluting pacemaker l.
    Sweet Tip l.
    l. system
    Target Tip l.
    Telectronics l.'s
    temporary pervenous l.
    three-turn epicardial l.
    l. threshold
    Transvene-RV l.
    transvenous defibrillator l.
    tripolar l.
    two-turn epicardial l.
    Unipass endocardial pacing l.
    unipolar limb l.'s
    unipolar precordial l.
    V l.
    Vitatron l.'s
    V-Pace transluminal pacing l.
    V_1 to V_6 l.'s
    Wilson l.
3-lead electrocardiogram
6-lead electrocardiogram
12-lead
    12-l. electrocardiogram
    12-l. electrocardiography
    12-l. voltage-duration product
    criteria
15-lead echocardiogram
16-lead electrocardiogram
leading
    l. circle concept
    l. circle hypothesis
    l. edge
    l. edge enhancement
lead-letter marker
lead/zirconium/titanium (LZT)
leaflet
    anterior l.
    aortic valve l.
    bowing of mitral valve l.
    calcified mitral l.
    cleft anterior l.
    doming of l.'s
    flail l.
    hammocking of posterior
    mitral l.
    mitral valve l.
    posterior l.
    l. thickening

    tricuspid valvular l.
    l. vegetation
leak
    alveolar l.
    baffle l.
    perivalvular l.
leakage
    spectral l.
least-squares
    l.-s. method
    l.-s. regression
Lebsche sternal knife
lecithin
lecithin-cholesterol acyltransferase
    (LCAT)
lecithin/sphingomyelin (L/S)
Lecompte maneuver
LED
    light-emitting diode
LEDC
    low energy direct current
Ledercillin VK Oral
ledge
    eccentric l.
    limbic l.
Lee-Desu
    L.-D. log rank test
    L.-D. statistic
Lee-White method
left
    l. anterior descending artery
    (LAD)
    l. anterior hemiblock (LAH)
    l. anterior oblique (LAO)
    l. anterior oblique position
    l. anterior oblique projection
    l. aortic angiography
    l. atrial angiography
    l. atrial to aortic (La:A)
    l. atrial appendage (LAA)
    l. atrial dimension
    l. atrial emptying index
    l. atrial enlargement (LAF)
    l. atrial hypertension
    l. atrial isolation procedure
    l. atrial myxoma
    l. atrial partitioning
    l. atrial pressure
    l. atrial spontaneous echo
    contrast (LASEC)
    l. atrium (LA)
    l. axis deviation (LAD)
    l. bundle-branch block (LBBB)

l. circumflex artery (LCX)
l. common carotid artery
l. coronary artery (LCA)
l. coronary catheter
l. dominant coronary circulation
l. heart
l. heart bypass
l. heart catheter
l. heart catheterization
l. internal jugular vein
l. internal mammary artery (LIMA)
l. Judkins catheter
l. lateral projection
l. main coronary artery (LMCA)
l. main coronary artery disease
l. main coronary stenosis
l. main disease (LOC)
l. main equivalency
l. middle hemiblock
l. posterior hemiblock
l. septal hemiblock
l. subclavian artery (LSCA)
l. ventricle (LV)
l. ventricular aneurysm
l. ventricular angiography
l. ventricular apex
l. ventricular assist device (LVAD)
l. ventricular assist system (LVAS)
l. ventricular bypass pump
l. ventricular chamber compliance
l. ventricular contractility
l. ventricular diastolic phase index
l. ventricular diastolic pressure
l. ventricular diastolic relaxation
l. ventricular dysfunction (LVD)
l. ventricular dyskinesis
l. ventricular ejection fraction (LVEF)

l. ventricular ejection time (LVET)
l. ventricular end-diastolic dimension (LVEDD)
l. ventricular end-diastolic pressure (LVEDP)
l. ventricular end-diastolic volume
l. ventricular end-systolic dimension (LVESD)
l. ventricular end-systolic stress
l. ventricular failure
l. ventricular filling pressure
l. ventricular forces
l. ventricular function
l. ventricular hypertrophy (LVH)
l. ventricular inflow tract obstruction
l. ventricular internal diastolic diameter (LVIDD)
l. ventricular internal diastolic dimension
l. ventricular-left atrial crossover dynamics
l. ventricular mass
l. ventricular muscle compliance
l. ventricular myxoma
l. ventricular outflow tract (LVOT)
l. ventricular outflow tract obstruction
l. ventricular outflow tract velocity
l. ventricular output
l. ventricular power
l. ventricular pressure-volume curve
l. ventricular puncture
l. ventricular-right atrial communication murmur
l. ventricular stroke volume
l. ventricular sump catheter
l. ventricular systolic performance
l. ventricular systolic pressure

L

NOTES

left *(continued)*
    l. ventricular tension
    l. ventricular wall
    l. ventricular wall motion
      abnormality
    l. ventricular wall stress
    l. ventriculography
left-sided heart failure
left-to-right shunt
Legend pacemaker
Legionella
    L. anisa
    L. birminghamensis
    L. bozemanii
    L. cincinnatiensis
    L. dumoffii
    L. feeleii
    L. gormanii
    L. jordanis
    L. lansingensis
    L. longbeachae
    L. micdadei
    L. oakridgensis
    L. pneumonia
    L. pneumophila
legionellosis
Legionnaire
    L. disease
    L. pneumonia
Legroux remission
Lehman
    L. cardiac device
    L. ventriculography catheter
**Leicester Intravenous Magnesium
    Intervention Trial (LIMIT)**
leiomyoma, pl. **leiomyomata**
leiomyosarcoma
Leishmania
leishmaniasis
Leitner syndrome
Lell esophagoscope
Lemakalim
Lemierre disease
Lemmon sternal elevator
lemon squeezer
Lenègre
    L. disease
    L. syndrome
length
    antegrade block cycle l.
    atrial-paced cycle l.
    basic cycle l. (BCL)
    basic drive cycle l.

block cycle l.
chordal l.
cycle l.
drive cycle l.
flutter cycle l.
paced cycle l.
pacing cycle l.
sinus cycle l.
tachycardia cycle l.
ventricular tachycardia cycle l.
    (VTCL)
length-active tension curve
length-dependent activation
length-resting tension relation
length-tension relation
LENI
    lower extremity noninvasive
Lennarson tube
**lensed fiber-tip laser delivery
    catheter**
lenta
    endocarditis l.
Lente Iletin I, L insulin
lentiginosis
lentigo, pl. **lentigines**
    lentigines, atrial myxoma, and
      blue nevi (LAMB)
    lentigines, electrocardiographic
      abnormalities, ocular
      hypertelorism, pulmonary
      stenosis, abnormalities of
      genitalia, retardation of
      growth, and deafness
      (LEOPARD)
lentis
    ectopia l.
Lenz syndrome
Leocor hemoperfusion system
LEOPARD
    lentigines, electrocardiographic
      abnormalities, ocular
      hypertelorism, pulmonary stenosis,
      abnormalities of genitalia,
      retardation of growth, and deafness
    LEOPARD syndrome
Lepley-Ernst tracheal tube
leprae
    Mycobacterium l.
lepromin test
leptospirosis
Leptotrichia buccalis
Leredde syndrome
Leriche syndrome

Lerman-Means scratch
Lescol
lesion
    aorto-ostial l.
    bifurcation l.
    bird's nest l.
    Blumenthal l.
    Bracht-Wachter l.
    braid-like l.
    branch l.
    calcified l.
    cavitary l.
    coin l.
    coronary artery l.
    culprit l.
    dendritic l.
    de novo l.
    dilatable l.
    discrete coronary l.
    enhancing l.
    fibrocalcific l.
    fibromusculoelastic l.
    Ghon primary l.
    honeycomb l.
    Janeway l.
    jet l.
    Libman-Sacks l.
    Lohlein-Baehr l.
    long l.
    macrovascular coronary l.
    monotypic l.
    nonbacterial thrombotic
      endocardial l.
    onion scale l.
    ostial l.
    plexiform l.
    polypoidal l.
    restenosis l.
    satellite l.
    space-occupying l.
    stenotic l.
    synchronous airway l.'s
    tandem l.
    target l.
    vegetative l.
    wire-loop l.
lesser resection

lethal arrhythmia
Letterer-Siwe disease
leucine
leucovorin
leukemia
Leukeran
leukocidin
leukocyte
    l. elastase
    polymorphonuclear l.
leukocytoblastic vasculitis
leukocytoclastic angiitis
leukocytosis
    transient l.
leukoencephalopathy
    progressive multifocal l. (PML)
LeukoNet Filter
Leukos pacemaker
Leukotrap red cell storage system
leukotriene
    l. B4 (LTB4)
    l. inhibition
leukotriene C, E
Leutrol
Lev
    L. classification
    L. disease
    L. syndrome
levamisole
    l. hydrochloride
Levatol
LeVeen
    L. peritoneovenous shunt
    L. plaque-cracker
level
    air-fluid l.
    blood oxygen l.
    digoxin l.
    ELF l.'s
    malondialdehyde l.
    multiple shunt l.'s
    myofibrillar calcium l.
    peak and trough l.'s
    predose l.
    reflecting l.
    sarcolemmal l.
    serum renin l.

L

NOTES

level *(continued)*
> triglyceride l.
> trough l.
> trough-and-peak l.'s

Levenberg-Marquardt algorithm
Levin catheter
Levine
> L. gradation 1 through 6 of cardiac murmurs
> L. sign

Levine-Harvey classification
Levinson-Durbin recursion
Levinthal-Coles-Lillie (LCL)
levoatriocardinal vein
levocardia
> l. malposition
> mixed l.
> l. with situs inversus

levocardiogram
levodopa
levogram
levo isomer
levoisomerism
Levophed
> L. injection

levosimendan
levo-transposed position
levotransposition
levoversion
Levovist
Levy Chimeric Faces Test
Lewis
> L. index
> L. lead
> L. lines
> L. thoracotomy
> L. upper limb cardiovascular disease

Lewis-Pickering test
Lewis-Tanner procedure
Lewy chest holder
Lewy-Rubin needle
Leycom volume conductance catheter
LFT
> liver function test

LGV
> lymphogranuloma venereum

LIAF
> laser-induced arterial fluorescence

Libman-Sacks
> L.-S. endocarditis

> L.-S. lesion
> L.-S. syndrome

licheniformis
> *Bacillus l.*

lichenoides
> tuberculosis l.

licorice
Liddle aorta clamp
lidocaine
> l. hydrochloride

lidoflazine
Lido-Pen Auto-Injector
Liebermann-Burchard test
Liebermeister rule
lienis
> porta l.

LIFE
> lung imaging fluorescence endoscope

life
> L. Care Pump
> l. change unit
> Study of Economics and Quality of L. (SEQOL)
> L. Suit

Lifeline electrode
Lifepak
> L. 7 monitor/defibrillator

Lifesaver disposable resuscitator bag
Lifescan
Lifestream coronary dilation catheter
lifestyle
> sedentary l.

lift
> parasternal systolic l.

ligament
> Cooper l.
> Marshall l.
> pericardiosternal l.

ligamentum
> l. arteriosum
> l. teres cardiopexy

ligand
> macromolecular l.

ligation
> Bardenheurer l.
> l. clip
> variceal l.
> varicose vein stripping and l.

ligature
> Stannius l.

light
　　l. chain
　　l. microscopy
　　l. pen
　　l. pen-determined ejection
　　　fraction
　　Questran L.
　　L. Talker device
light-emitting diode (LED)
lightwire
Lignieres test
lignocaine
　　M l.
Lillehei-Cruz-Kaster prosthesis
Lillehei-Kaster
　　L.-K. cardiac valve prosthesis
　　L.-K. mitral valve prosthesis
　　L.-K. pivoting-disk prosthetic
　　　valve
Lilliput oxygenator
LIMA
　　left internal mammary artery
limb
　　anacrotic l.
　　l. ischemia
　　l. lead
　　l. salvage
　　thoracic l.
limb-girdle muscular dystrophy
limbic ledge
lime
　　bruit de l.
LIMIT
　　Leicester Intravenous Magnesium
　　　Intervention Trial
limit
　　Nyquist l.
LIMITS
　　Liquaemin in Myocardial Infarction
　　　during Thrombolysis with
　　　Saruplase
Lincocin
　　L. injection
　　L. Oral
lincomycin
　　l. hydrochloride
Lincorex injection

lincosamide
Lindbergh pump
Lindesmith operation
Linde Walker Oxygen Program
Lindholm
　　L. operating laryngoscope
　　L. tracheal tube
line
　　anterior axillary l. (AAL)
　　arterial mean l.
　　Cantlie l.
　　central venous l.
　　Conradi l.
　　Correra l.
　　CVP l.
　　indwelling l.
　　Intertech Perkin-Elmer gas
　　　sampling l.
　　isoelectric l.
　　Kerley A, B, C l.'s
　　Lewis l.'s
　　Linton l.
　　M l.'s
　　midclavicular l. (MCL)
　　tram l.'s
　　Z l.
　　Zahn l.'s
linear
　　l. echodensity
　　l. phonocardiograph
　　l. regression
linearity
　　amplitude l.
　　count-rate l.
lingoscope
lingual
　　l. quinsy
　　l. thyroid
lingula
lingular
　　l. bronchus
　　l. pneumonia
linoleic acid
linsidomine
Linton
　　L. elastic stockings

L

NOTES

Linton *(continued)*
 L. flap
 L. line
Linx
 L. extension wire
 L. guidewire extension
 L. guidewire extension cardiac
  device
Linx-EZ cardiac device
Liotta-BioImplant LPB prosthetic
 valve
Liotta total artificial heart
LIP
 lymphocytic interstitial pneumonitis
lipase
 diacylglycerol l.
 hepatic l.
 lipoprotein l. (LPL)
lipedema
LIPID
 Long-Term Intervention with
  Pravastatin in Ischemic Disease
lipid
 l. accumulation
 endogenous l.
 exogenous l.
 extracellular l.
 l. hypothesis
 intracellular l.
 l. panel
 l. peroxidation product
 l. pneumonia
 renomedullary l.
 sarcolemma l.
 l. solubility
lipid-A
Lipidil
lipidosis, pl. lipidoses
lipid-rich plaque
lipocardiac
lipodystrophy
 intestinal l.
lipofuscinosis
 neuronal ceroid l.
lipogenic theory of atherosclerosis
lipohyalinosis
lipoid pneumonia
lipoma, pl. lipomata
lipomatous hypertrophy
lipoparticle
lipoperoxide
lipophilicity
 properties of l.

lipopolysaccharidase
 J5 l.
lipopolysaccharide
 l. vaccine
lipoprotein
 alpha l.
 beta l.
 high-density l. (HDL)
 intermediate-density l.
 l. lipase (LPL)
 low-density l. (LDL)
 pre-beta l.
 triglyceride-rich l.'s (TRL)
 very-low-density l. (VLDL)
lipoprotein-associated coagulation
 inhibitor (LACI)
lipoproteinemia
liposarcoma
Liposorber LA-15 system
Liposyn
lipothymia
Lipovnik virus
lipoxygenase
5-lipoxygenase
LIP/PLH complex
lip pursing
Liquaemin
 L. injection
 L. in Myocardial Infarction
  during Thrombolysis with
  Saruplase (LIMITS)
liquefaciens
 Serratia l.
Liqui-Caps
 Vicks 44 Non-Drowsy Cold &
  Cough L.-C.
liquid
 Brontex L.
 Contac Cough Formula L.
 l. crystal display (LCD)
 Hycotuss Expectorant L.
 oxygen-carrying
  perfluorochemical l.
 L. Pred Oral
 l. scintillation spectrophotometer
liquifying expectorant
Liqui-Gels
 Robitussin Severe
  Congestion L.-G.
LiquiVent
LIS
 lung injury score
lisinopril

Lissajou loop
Listeria
    L. monocytogenes
list mode
Lite Blade
Liteguard mini-defibrillator
liter
    millimoles per l. (mmol/L)
    l.'s per minute (lpm)
    l.'s per minute per meter
        squared
lithium
    l. battery
    l. pacemaker
Litten
    L. diaphragm sign
    L. phenomenon
Little disease
Littman defibrillation pad
Litwak
    L. left atrial-aortic bypass
Live
    Bacillus Calmette-Guérin L.
livedo
    l. reticularis
    l. vasculitis
livedoid dermatitis
liver
    cardiac l.
    cirrhosis of l.
    cyanotic atrophy of the l.
    l. flap
    l. function test (LFT)
    l. palm
livida
    asphyxia l.
Livierato
    L. reflex
    L. sign
    L. test
Living with Heart Failure
LIZ-88 ablation unit
L loop
L-looping of the ventricle
LMCA
    left main coronary artery
LMD

LMWH
    low-molecular-weight heparin
L-NMMA
    L-N-monomethylarginine
L-N-monomethylarginine (L-NMMA)
load
    electronic pacemaker l.
    exercise l.
    heat l.
    peak work l.
loading
    glycogen l.
    methionine l.
    relaxation l.
    saline l.
    volume l.
lobar
    l. atelectasis
    l. bronchus
    l. emphysema
    l. pneumonia
lobe
    side l.
lobectomize
lobectomy
    sleeve l.
lobular pneumonia
lobule
LOC
    left main disease
    low-molecular-weight dextran
    LOC guidewire extension
local
    l. area network (LAN)
    l. asphyxia
    l. syncope
localization
    anatomic l.
localized
    l. obstructive emphysema
    l. pericarditis
    l. sacculation
LocalMed
    L. catheter infusion sleeve
    L. InfusaSleeve
loci (*pl. of* locus)

NOTES

lock
  heparin l.
locking device
LOCM
  low-osmolality contrast material
locular cyst
loculated
  l. cyst
  l. emphysema
  l. empyema
loculation
locus, pl. loci
  genetic l.
Loeffler (var. of Löffler)
Loesche classification
lofexidine
Löffler, Loeffler
  L. bacillus
  L. disease
  L. parietal fibroplastic
    endocarditis
  L. pneumonia
  L. syndrome
logarithmic
  l. dynamic range
  l. phonocardiograph
log-rank test
Lohlein-Baehr lesion
Lombardi sign
lomefloxacin
  l. hydrochloride
lomustine
lone atrial fibrillation
long
  l. ACE fixed-wire balloon
    catheter
  l. axial oblique view
  l. axis (LAX)
  l. lesion
  l. pulse
  l. Q-T syndrome (LQTS)
  l. Q-TU syndrome
  L. Skinny over-the-wire
    balloon catheter
long-acting nitrate
long-axis
  l.-a. parasternal view
    echocardiogram
  l.-a. view
longbeachae
  Legionella l.
Longdwel Teflon catheter
longitudinal dissociation

Longmire valvotomy
Long-Term
  L.-T. Intervention with
    Pravastatin in Ischemic
    Disease (LIPID)
  L.-T. oxygen therapy (LTOT)
Loniten
loop
  atrial vector l.
  bulboventricular l.
  Cannon endartereçtomy l.
  cine l.
  D l.
  l. diuresis
  l. diuretic
  elliptical l.
  flow-volume l.
  Gerdy intra-auricular l.
  guidewire l.
  heart l.
  Henle l.
  L l.
  Lissajou l.
  maxi-vessel l.'s
  memory l.
  P l.
  QRS l.
  reentrant l.
  sewing ring l.
  T l.
  U l.
  Uresil radiopaque silicone band
    vessel l.'s
  U-shaped catheter l.
  vector l.
  ventricular pressure-volume l.
  video l.
loose junction
Lopid
Lopressor
Lo-Profile II catheter
Lo-Pro tracheal tube
Lorabid
loracarbef
loratadine
lorazepam
lorcainide
Lorcet
  L. Plus
Lore-Lawrence trachea tube
Lorelco
Lortat-Jacob approach

losartan
 l. and hydrochlorothiazide
 l. potassium
 l. potassium/HCTZ
 l. potassium/hydrochlorothiazide
loss of consciousness
Lotensin
Lotrel
Louis
 L. angle
 L. law
Louisiana pneumonia
loupe magnification
lovastatin
Lovenox
 L. injection
Loven reflex
loversol
low
 l. energy direct current (LEDC)
 l. flow rate
 l.'s Profile Port vascular access
 l. septal atrium
low-density lipoprotein (LDL)
Lowell pleural needle
Löwenberg cuff sign
low-energy
 l.-e. laser
 l.-e. synchronized cardioversion
lower
 l. body negative pressure (LBNP)
 l. extremity bypass graft
 l. extremity noninvasive (LENI)
 l. lobe bronchus
 l. nodal extrasystole
 l. nodal rhythm
Lower rings
Lower-Shumway cardiac transplant
low-fat diet
low-frequency murmur
low-methionine diet

low-molecular-weight
 l.-m.-w. dextran (LOC)
 l.-m.-w. heparin (LMWH)
Lown
 L. arrhythmia
 L. class 4a or b ventricular ectopic beats
 L. classification
 L. technique
 L. and Woolf method
Lown-Edmark waveform
Lown-Ganong-Levine syndrome
low-osmolality contrast material (LOCM)
low-output heart failure
low-pitched murmur
low-pressure tamponade
low-salt
 l.-s. diet
 l.-s. syndrome
low-sodium
 l.-s. diet
 l.-s. syndrome
low-speed rotation angioplasty catheter
lozenge
 horehound l.
Lozol
L-phenylalinine mustard
LPL
 lipoprotein lipase
lpm
 liters per minute
LPS Peel-Away introducer
LQTS
 long Q-T syndrome
L/S
 lecithin/sphingomyelin
 L/S ratio
LSCA
 left subclavian artery
L-selectin
LTB4
 leukotriene B4
LTOT
 long-term oxygen therapy

L

NOTES

LT V-105 implantable cardioverter-
defibrillator
LTx
   lung transplant
lubb-dupp
lubricity
Lucas-Championnière disease
Lucchese mitral valve dilator
lucency
lucent defect
Luciani-Wenckebach atrioventricular
   block
lucigenin
Ludiomil
Ludwig
   L. angina
   L. angle
Luer-Lok
   L.-L. connector
   L.-L. needle
   L.-L. needle tip
   L.-L. port
Luer tracheal tube
lues
luetic
   l. aneurysm
   l. aortitis
   l. disease
Lufyllin
Lugol solution
Lukens thymus retractor
Luke procedure
Lumaguide catheter
lumbar sympathectomy
Lumelec pacing catheter
lumen, pl. lumina
   bronchial l.
   double l. (DL)
   esophageal l.
   single l.
   ThruLumen l.
   vessel l.
lumina
luminal
   l. encroachment
   l. narrowing
luminescence
Lumonics YAG laser
lunata
   Curvularia l.
lung
   l. abscess
   l. acinus

l. architecture
arc-welder l.
artificial l.
atrium of l.'s
bible printer's l.
l. biopsy
bird-breeder's l.
black l.
blast l.
brown induration of l.
l. capacity
l. carcinoma
cardiac l.
cheese worker's l.
coal miner's l.
collapsed l.
consolidation of l.
cystic disease of l.
decortication of l.
detergent worker's l.
drowned l.
edema of l.
l. elasticity
eosinophilic l.
esophageal l.
essential brown induration
   of l.
farmer's l.
l. fever
fibroid l.
fish meal l.
l. fluke
l. function
furrier's l.
gastric l.
harvester's l.
honeycomb l.
honeycombing of l.
horseshoe l.
humidifier l.
hyperlucent l.
l. imaging fluorescence
   endoscope (LIFE)
l. injury score (LIS)
iron l.
jute workers' l.
l. markings
mason's l.
l. mechanics
mushroom worker's l.
pigeon-breeder's l.
polycystic l.
postperfusion l.

pump l.
respirator l.
rheumatoid l.
l. scan
l. scanning
scleroderma l.
shock l.
silo-filler's l.
stiff l.
l. stone
thresher's l.
l. transplant (LTx)
trench l.
tuberculosis of l.'s
unilateral hyperlucency of the l.
unilateral nonfunctioning l.
l. uptake
vanishing l.
vernal edema of l.
l. volume
l. volume reduction surgery (LVRS)
l. washings
wet l.
white l.
wood pulp worker's l.

lunger
chronic l.
lungmotor
lungworm
lunula, pl. **lunulae**
lupoid
lupus
l. anticoagulant
l. erythematosus (LE)
l. pernio
l. pleuritis
lupus-associated valve disease
Lurselle
lusitaniae
Candida l.
lusitropic
l. abnormality
lusitropy
lusoria
dysphagia l.

Lutembacher
L. complex
L. syndrome
Lutz-Splendore-Almeida disease
Luxtec fiberoptic system
luxus heart
LV
left ventricle
LVAD
left ventricular assist device
HeartMate LVAD
Novacor LVAD
vented-electric HeartMate LVAD
LVAS
left ventricular assist system
LVD
left ventricular dysfunction
LVEDD
left ventricular end-diastolic dimension
LVEDP
left ventricular end-diastolic pressure
LVEF
left ventricular ejection fraction
LVESD
left ventricular end-systolic dimension
LVET
left ventricular ejection time
LVH
left ventricular hypertrophy
LVIDD
left ventricular internal diastolic diameter
LVOT
left ventricular outflow tract
LVRS
lung volume reduction surgery
LW
lateral wall
lwoffi
Acinetobacter l.
Lyme
L. borreliosis
L. disease
L. titer

L

NOTES

lymphadenitis
lymphadenopathy
    hilar l.
lymphangiectasis
    chronic pulmonary cystic l.
lymphangioendothelioma
lymphangioleiomyomatosis
lymphangioma
lymphangiomyomatosis
lymphangitic
    l. carcinoma
    l. spread
lymphangitis
    l. carcinomatosa
Lymphapress compression therapy
lymphatic
    l. channel
    l. edema
    obtuse marginal l.
    subclavian l.
lymphedema
    l. praecox
lymph node
lymphocyte
    l. immune globulin (Atgam)
lymphocytic
    l. infiltrative disorder
    l. interstitial pneumonitis (LIP)
lymphogranuloma venereum (LGV)
lymphoid
    l. alveolitis
    l. hyperplasia
    l. interstitial pneumonia
lymphokines
lymphoma
    African Burkitt l.

    B cell l.
    Burkitt l.
    Kiel classification of l.
    noncleaved cell l.
    non-Hodgkin l.
    pulmonary l.
lymphomatoid granulomatosis
lymphosarcoma
lymphotoxin
Lyo-Ject
    Cardizem L.-J.
Lyon-Horgan procedure
Lyon hypothesis
lyophilize
lyophilized powder
Lyphocin injection
lysine
lysine-acetylsalicylate
lysis
    clot l.
    l. time
lysophosphatidylcholine
    l. scavenger
lysophospholipase
lysosomal
    l. enzyme
    l. hydrolases
lysosome
lysozyme
lys-plasminogen
    recombinant l.-p.
Lyssavirus
LZT
    lead/zirconium/titanium
    LZT crystal

M

M gate
M lignocaine
M lines
M protein
M₂
mitral second sound
M₁
mitral first sound
m7E3 Fab
mA
milliampere
MAAS
Multicenter Anti-Atheroma Study
MABP
mean arterial blood pressure
MAC
multi-access catheter
Mycobacterium avium complex
MAC infection
MacCallum patch
Macewen sign
Machado-Guerreiro test
Machida fiberoptic laryngoscope
machine
Aloka echocardiograph m.
Apogee CX 100 Interspec
ultrasound m.
Bird m.
Burdick EKG m.
bypass m.
Cobe-Stockert heart-lung m.
Corometrics-Aloka
echocardiograph m.
Crafoord-Senning heart-lung m.
General Electric Pass-C
echocardiograph m.
G5 massage and percussion m.
heart-lung m.
Mayo-Gibbon heart-lung m.
Respironics CPAP m.
Respitrace m.
Toshiba electrocardiography m.
machinery murmur
MacIntosh
M. blade anesthesia
M. laryngoscope
Mackenzie polygraph
Mackler tube
Macleod syndrome

macroangiopathy
coronary m.
Macrobid
macrocardia
Macrodantin
Macrodex
macroglobulin
alpha-2 m.
macroglobulinemia
Waldenström m.
macrolide
m. antibiotics
m. antimicrobial
m. antimicrobial agent
macromolecular ligand
macrophage
foamy m.
hemosiderin-laden m.
macroreentrant
m. atrial tachycardia
m. circuit
macrovascular coronary lesion
MACs
malignancy-associated changes
macula, pl. **maculae**
m. albida
m. lactea
m. tendinea
maculopapular
m. rash
**Maestro implantable cardiac
pacemaker**
Magellan monitor
Magic Torque guidewire
Magill
M. laryngoscope
M. Safety Clear Plus
endotracheal tube
magna
arteria anastomotica
auricularis m.
Magnascanner
Picker M.
magnesium
m. oxide
m. sulfate
m. sulfate heptahydrate
magnet
bronchoscopic m.
Equen m.

M

magnet *(continued)*
    m. pacing interval
    m. rate
    m. wire
magnetic
    m. moment
    m. relaxation time
    m. resonance flowmetry (MRF)
    m. resonance imaging (MRI)
    m. resonance signal
    m. resonance spectography
    m. resonance spectroscopy
    m. source imaging (MSI)
magnetocardiogram (MCG)
magnetocardiograph
magnetocardiography
magnet rate
Magnevist
magnification
    loupe m.
magnitude
    average pulse m.
    peak m.
Magnum guidewire
Magnum-Meier system
magnus
    pulsus m.
Magovern-Cromie ball-cage
  prosthetic valve
Mag-Ox 400
Mahaim
    M. bundle
    M. fibers
Mahaim-type tachycardia
Mahalanobis distance
Mahler sign
mahogany flush
MAI
    Mycobacterium avium-intracellulare
    MAI complex
    MAI infection
Maigret-50
main
    m. bundle
    m. pulmonary artery (MPA)
    m. stem bronchus
mainstem coronary artery
major
    Babesia m.
    pectoralis m.
Makin murmur
malabsorption

maladie
    m. de Roger
malaise
malar flush
malaria
malarial pneumonitis
malayi
    Brugia m.
maleate
    azatadine m.
    chlorpheniramine m.
    dexchlorpheniramine m.
    enalapril m.
    ergonovine m.
    methysergide m.
    nomifensine m.
    timolol m.
    trimipramine m.
malformation
    angiographically occult
      intracranial vascular m.
      (AOIVM)
    arteriovenous m. (AVM)
    atrioventricular m. (AVM)
    congenital m.
    Mondini pulmonary
      arteriovenous m.
    neural crest m.
    pulmonary arteriovenous m.
      (PAVM)
    Uhl m.
malfunction
    pacemaker m.
malignancy-associated changes
  (MACs)
malignant
    m. beat
    m. carcinoid syndrome
    m. endocarditis
    m. hypertension
    m. mesothelioma
    m. pleural effusion
    m. ventricular arrhythmia
      (MVA)
    m. ventricular tachycardia
malingering
Mallergan-VC with Codeine
Mallinckrodt radioimmunoassay
Mallory
    M. RM-1 cell pacemaker
    M. stain

Mallory-Weiss
    M.-W. syndrome
    M.-W. tear
malnutrition
    alcoholic m.
    myocardial m.
    protein-calorie m.
malondialdehyde
    m. level
Maloney mercury-filled esophageal dilator
malonylcoenzyme A, malonyl-CoA
malposition
    crisscross heart m.
    double-outlet left ventricle m.
    double-outlet right ventricle m.
    m. of great arteries (MGA)
    levocardia m.
    mesocardia m.
    single ventricle m.
maltase deficiency
maltophilia
    Pseudallescheria m.
    Pseudomonas m.
    Xanthomonas m.
malum
    m. cordis
mammary
    m. artery
    m. artery graft
    m. souffle
    m. souffle murmur
    m. souffle sound
man
    radiation equivalent in m. (rem)
management
    data base m.
    postprocedural m.
    Trial of Antihypertensive Interventions and M. (TAIM)
    ventilator m.
mandatory minute volume (MMV)
Mandol
mandrel, mandril
    m. graft
mandrin

maneuver
    Addison m.
    cold pressor testing m.
    Ejrup m.
    Heimlich m.
    hemodynamic m.
    Hillis-Müller m.
    hyperventilation m.
    jaw thrust m.
    Jonnson m.
    Lecompte m.
    Mattox m.
    Mueller m.
    Müller m.
    Sellick m.
    Valsalva m.
maneuverability
manifest
    m. ischemia
    m. vector
manifold
    Morse m.
manipulation
    catheter m.
mannequin
manner
    m. of Creech
    m. of DeBakey-Creech
mannitol
Mannkopf sign
Mann-Whitney test
manofluorography (MFG)
manometer
    Dinamap ultrasound blood pressure m.
    Hürthle m.
manometer-tipped catheter
manometry
    esophageal m.
Manoplax
MANOVA
    multivariate analysis of variance
Mansfield
    M. Atri-Pace 1 catheter
    M. balloon
    M. bioptome

M

NOTES

Mansfield *(continued)*
M. orthogonal electrode
catheter
M. Polaris electrode
M. Scientific dilatation balloon
catheter
M. Valvuloplasty Registry
Mansfield-Webster catheter
Mantel-Haenszel
M.-H. statistic
M.-H. test
Mantoux test
manual edge detection
manubrium
MAO
monoamine oxidase
MAO inhibitor
MAOI
monoamine oxidase inhibitor
MAP
mean arterial pressure
monophasic action potential
map
polar coordinate m.
MAPD
monophasic action potential duration
maple bark disease
**Mapper hemostasis EP mapping
sheath**
mapping
activation-sequence m.
atrial activation m.
body surface Laplacian m.
(BSLM)
bull's-eye polar coordinate m.
cardiac m.
catheter m.
color-coded flow m.
color-flow m.
digital phase m. (DPM)
Doppler color flow m.
(DCFM)
electrophysiologic m.
endocardial m.
endocardial m. of ventricular
tachycardia
EP m.
flow m.
ice m.
intracardiac m.
intraoperative m.
Laplacian m.
pace-m.

pulsed-wave Doppler m.
retrograde atrial activation m.
spectral temporal m.
spectral turbulence m.
tachycardia pathway m.
ventricular m.
mapping/ablation catheter
maprotiline
MAPS
Multivessel Angioplasty Prognosis
Study
marantic
m. endocarditis
m. thrombosis
m. thrombus
marasmic
m. thrombosis
m. thrombus
marasmus
Marathon guiding catheter
Marax
M. bronchodilator
Marbach-Weil technique
Marburg virus
MARCATOR
Multicenter American Research
Trial with Cilazapril after
Angioplasty to Prevent
Transluminal Coronary Obstruction
and Restenosis
marcescens
Serratia m.
Marcillin
Marey law
Marfan syndrome
Margesic H
margin
costal m.
rib m.
marginal
m. arteries of Drummond
m. artery of colon
m. circumflex artery
obtuse m. (OM)
m. rales
marginatum
erythema m.
Marie-Bamberger syndrome
Marie syndrome
Marinol
marinum
Mycobacterium m.

Marion-Clatworthy side-to-end vena caval shunt
mark
- alignment m.
- M. VII cooling vest

marker
- m. catheter
- m. channel
- CYFRA 21-1 tumor m.
- gold m.
- lead-letter m.
- tumor m.
- vein graft ring m.

markings
- bronchial m.
- bronchovesicular m.
- interstitial m.
- lung m.
- perihilar m.
- pulmonary m.
- vascular m.

Marlex
Marmine Oral
Maroteaux-Lamy syndrome
Marpres
Marquest Respirgard II nebulizer
Marquette
- M. Case-12 electrocardiographic system
- M. Case-12 exercise system
- M. 3-channel laser holder
- M. 3-channel laser Holter
- M. electrocardiograph
- M. 8000 Holter monitor
- M. Holter recorder
- M. Responder 1500 multifunctional defibrillator
- M. Series 8000 Holter analyzer
- M. treadmill

Marriott method
Marshall
- M. fold
- M. ligament
- M. oblique vein

marsupialization
Marthritic

Martorell syndrome
Mary Allen Engle ventricle
mask
- AccurOx m.
- Aerochamber m.
- Bili m.
- BLB oxygen m.
- Boothby-Lovelace-Bulbulian oxygen m.
- ecchymotic m.
- Finney m.
- Inspiron AccurOx M.
- Kuhn m.
- meter m.
- nonrebreathing m.
- oxygen m.
- partial rebreathing m.
- PEP m.
- RBS face m.
- rebreathing m.
- reservoir face m.
- SCRAM face m.
- SealEasy resuscitation m.
- Venti m.
- ventilation m.
- Venturi m.
- Vickers Ventimask Mark 2 m.

masked hypertension
mask-mode
- m.-m. cardiac imaging
- m.-m. subtraction

Mason-Likar
- M.-L. 12-lead EKG system
- M.-L. limb lead modification
- M.-L. placement of EKG leads

mason's lung
mass
- cardiac m.
- echodense m.
- fungating m.
- intracardiac m.
- left ventricular m.
- myocardial m.
- pleural m.

massage
- cardiac m.
- carotid sinus m.

M

NOTES

massage *(continued)*
    closed chest cardiac m.
    direct cardiac m.
    external cardiac m.
    heart m.
    open chest cardiac m.
    vapor m.
Massier solution
massive
    m. collapse
    m. pneumonia
Masson
    M. bodies
    M. trichrome stain
MAST
    military anti-shock trousers
    MAST pants
    MAST suit
    MAST trousers
mast
    m. cell
    m. cell inhibitor
Master
    M. exercise stress test
    M. Flow Pumpette
    M. Flow Pumpette pump
    SpaceLabs Event M.
    M. two-step exercise test
mastocytosis syndrome
Masy angioscope
MAT
    multifocal atrial tachycardia
Matas
    M. aneurysmectomy
    M. test
match defect
matching
    afterload m.
material
    Biobrane/HF graft m.
    Biograft bovine heterograft m.
    Carbo-Seal graft m.
    Cellolite m.
    contrast m.
    embolized foreign m.
    fibrinohematic m.
    Haynes 25 m.
    Hexabrix contrast m.
    Kaltostat wound packing m.
    Kifa catheter m.
    low-osmolality contrast m.
    (LOCM)
    MycroMesh graft m.

    Myoview contrast m.
    nonionic contrast m.
    PermaMesh m.
    Soludrast contrast m.
    Stellite ring m.
    Zenotech graft m.
matrix
    extracellular m.
    m. mode
    myocardial collagen m.
Matson-Alexander rib stripper
Matson rib elevator
Matsuda titanium surgical instruments
Mattox maneuver
mattress
    apnea alarm m.
    Bedge antireflux m.
    eggcrate m.
    hypothermia m.
    Roho m.
maturation
    affinity m.
Maugeri syndrome
Mavik
max
    VO_2 m.
    maximum oxygen consumption
Maxair
Maxaquin Oral
Maxepa
MaxForce balloon dilatation catheter
Maxilith pacemaker pulse generator
maximal
    m. breathing capacity
    m. expiratory flow rate (MEFR)
    m. expiratory flow volume (MEFV)
    m. forced expiratory flow (FEFmax)
    m. inspiratory flow rate (MIFR)
    m. midexpiratory flow (MMEF)
    m. midexpiratory flow rate (MMEFR)
    m. sustainable ventilatory capacity (MSVC)
    m. velocity (V_{MAX})
    m. ventilation (MV)

m. ventilation rate (MVR)
m. vital capacity (MVC)
Maxima Plus plasma resistant fiber oxygenator
maximum
> m. breathing capacity (MBC)
> m. flow rate
> m. negative potential
> m. oxygen consumption (VO$_2$ max)
> m. oxygen uptake
> m. predicted heart rate (MPHR)
> m. ventricular elastance (Emax)
> m. voluntary ventilation (MVV)
> m. walking time

Maxi-Myst vaporizer
Maxivent
maxi-vessel loops
Maxzide
Mayaro virus
May-Grünwald-Giemsa stain
Mayo
> M. Asymptomatic Carotid Endarterectomy Study
> M. hemostat

Mayo-Gibbon heart-lung machine
maze procedure
Mazicon
mazindol
> hydrogen-3 m.

MB
> myocardial band
> myocardial bridging
> MB enzymes of CPK
> MB fraction

MBC
> maximum breathing capacity

MBF
> myocardial blood flow

MBq
> megabecquerel

MBV
> mitral balloon valvotomy

McArdle
> M. disease
> M. syndrome

McCort sign
McDowall reflex
MCE
> myocardial contrast echocardiography

MCG
> magnetocardiogram

McGinn-White sign
McGoon
> M. guidelines
> M. technique

McHenry protocol
mCi
> millicurie

MCL
> midclavicular line

MCM smart laser
McNaught keel
McNemar test
MCP-1
> monocyte chemotactic protein-1

McPheeters treatment
McQuigg-Mixter bronchial forceps
MCT Oil
MCV
> mean corpuscular volume

MDC
> metoprolol dilated cardiomyopathy

M/D 4 defibrillator system
MDF
> myocardial depressant factor

MDI
> metered-dose inhaler

MDP
> methylene diphosphonate

MDPIT
> Multicenter Diltiazem Post-Infarction Trial

MDR-TB
> multidrug-resistant tuberculosis

MDS
> myocardial depressant substance

Meadows syndrome

M

NOTES

Meadox
 M. graft
 M. graft sizer
 M. Teflon felt pledget
 M. woven velour prosthesis
Meadox-Cooley woven low-porosity prosthesis
mean
 arterial m.
 m. arterial blood pressure (MABP)
 m. arterial pressure (MAP)
 m. contrast enhancement
 m. corpuscular volume (MCV)
 m. diastolic left ventricular pressure
 m. electrical axis
 m. forced midexpiratory flow
 m. manifest vector
 m. midexpiratory flow rate ($FEF_{25-75\%}$)
 m. normalized systolic ejection rate
 m. pulmonary artery pressure (MPAP)
 m. pulmonary artery wedge pressure (MPAWP)
 m. QRS axis
 m. systolic left ventricular pressure
Means-Lernan mediastinal crunch
measles pneumonia
measure
 CD4+ m.
measurement
 blood flow m.
 cardiac output m.
 coronary blood flow m.
 Doppler m.
 gas clearance m.
 hemodynamic m.
 invasive pressure m.
 physiologic m.
 PR-AC m.
 pressure m.
 Reid index m.
 thermodilution m.
 transstenotic pressure gradient m.
 venous flow m.
Measurin
meat-wrapper's asthma
mebendazole

mecalil provocation
mecamylamine hydrochloride
mechanical
 m. alternation
 m. alternation of heart
 m. cough
 m. heart
 m. pleurodesis
 m. valve
 m. ventilation (MV)
mechanic bronchitis
mechanics
 fluid m.
 lung m.
mechanism
 m. of action
 compensatory m.
 coronary steal m.
 deglutition m.
 Frank-Starling m.
 gating m.
 peeling-back m.
 pinchcock m.
 reentrant m.
 sinus m.
 Starling m.
 steal m.
 wave-speed m.
mechanocardiography
mechanoelectrical feedback
mechanoreceptor
mechanoreflex
mechlorethamine hydrochloride
meclofenamate sodium
Meclomen Oral
meconium ileus
medazolam
MedGraphics
 M. Cardio O2 system
 M. CPX/D metabolic cart
media
 aortic tunica m.
 arterial m.
medial tear
median
 m. nerve injury
 m. sternotomy
 m. sternotomy incision
 m. survival time (MST)
medianus
 ramus m.
mediastinal
 m. amyloidosis

m. crunch
m. emphysema
m. flutter
m. lymph node biopsy
m. lymph nodes
m. pleurisy
m. shadow
m. shift
m. space
m. sump filter
m. wedge
mediastinitis
  descending necrotizing m.
  (DNM)
  fibrous m.
mediastinoscope
  Goldberg-MPC m.
mediastinoscopy
  Chamberlain m.
mediastinotomy
mediastinum
mediator
  vasoactive m.
medication
  prosyncopal m.
medicinalis
  Hirudo m.
Medicon rib spreader
Medicopaste
Medi-Facts system
Mediflex-Bookler device
Medigraphics 2000 analyzer
Medihaler-Epi
Medihaler Ergotamine
Medihaler-Iso
MEDILOG 4000 ambulatory ECG
  recorder
medionecrosis
  m. of aorta
  m. aortae idiopathica cystica
MediPort
Medipren
Medi-Quet tourniquet
Medi-Strumpf stockings
Meditape
Medi-Tech
  M.-T. balloon catheter

M.-T. catheter system
M.-T. guidewire
M.-T. multipurpose basket
M.-T. steerable catheter
Mediterranean anemia
Medi-Tuss AC
medium
  Adenoscan contrast m.
  m. chain triglycerides
  Conray contrast m.
  contrast m.
  Eagle m.
  iothalamate meglumine
    contrast m.
  ioxaglate meglumine
    contrast m.
  Isovue contrast m.
  Joklik m.
  metrizamide contrast m.
  nonionic contrast m.
  Optiray contrast m.
  polygelin colloid contrast m.
  SHU-454 contrast m.
Medi vascular stockings
Medivent
  M. self-expanding coronary
    stent
  M. vascular stent
Medlar bodies
Med-Neb respirator
Medrad Mark IV angiographic
  injector
Medralone injection
Medrol
  M. Dosepak
  M. Oral
medroxyprogesterone
  estrogen & m.
Medtel pacemaker
Medtronic
  M. Activitrax rate-responsive
    unipolar ventricular pacemaker
  M. cardiac cooling jacket
  M. connector
  M. defibrillator implant support
    device
  M. Elite DDDR pacemaker

M

NOTES

Medtronic *(continued)*
  M. Elite II pacemaker
  M. external cardioverter-
    defibrillator
  M. External Tachyarrhythmia
    Control Device
  M. Intact valve
  M. Interactive Tachycardia
    Terminating system
  M. interventional vascular stent
  M. Jewel 7219D and C
    device
  M. leads
  M. PCD implantable
    cardioverter-defibrillator
  M. prosthetic valve
  M. pulse generator
  M. Pulsor Intrasound pain
    reliever
  M. radiofrequency receiver
  M. RF 5998 pacemaker
  M. SPO pacemaker
  M. SP 502 pacemaker
  M. SynchroMed pump
  M. temporary pacemaker
  M. Thera "i-series" cardiac
    pacemaker
  M. tip
  M. Transvene
  M. Transvene electrode
  M. Transvene endocardial lead
    system
Medtronic-Hall
  M.-H. device
  M.-H. heart valve prosthesis
  M.-H. monocuspid tilting-disk
    valve
  M.-H. prosthetic heart valve
  M.-H. tilting-disk valve
    prosthesis
Medtronic-Hancock
  M.-H. device
medulla
  adrenal m.
  m. oblongata
medullary collecting duct
mefenamic acid
mefloquine hydrochloride
Mefoxin
MEFR
  maximal expiratory flow rate

MEFV
  maximal expiratory flow volume
megabecquerel (MBq)
megacardia
megaelectron volt (MeV)
megaesophagus
megahertz (MHz)
megaloblastic anemia
megalocardia
megaterium
  Bacillus m.
megaunit (MU)
meglumine
  m. diatrizoate enema study
    intracoronary sonicated m.
    ioxaglate m.
Meier-Magnum system
Meigs syndrome
meiosis
meizothrombin
melaninogenica
  Prevotella m.
melanoma
  Clark classification of
    malignant m.
melanotic carcinoma
melena
melenic stools
melioidosis
melitensis
  Brucella m.
Mellaril
mellitus
  diabetes m. (DM)
  insulin-dependent diabetes m.
    (IDDM)
  noninsulin-dependent
    diabetes m. (NIDDM)
melphalan
Melrose solution
Meltzer
  M. method
  M. sign
Melzack-Wall gate theory
membranacea
  angina m.
  pars m.
membranaceous
membrane
  alveolar-capillary m.,
    alveolocapillary m.
  antibasement m.
  basement m.

bronchial mucous m.
cell m.
m. channel
cuprophane m.
m. current
DeBove m.
Gore-Tex surgical m.
Henle elastic m.
Henle fenestrated m.
polyacrylonitrile m.
m. potential
Preclude pericardial m.
sarcolemmal m.
schneiderian respiratory m.
serous m.'s
syncytiovascular m. (SVM)
membrane-stabilizing activity
membranous
m. bronchitis
m. croup
m. laryngitis
m. pharyngitis
m. pulmonary atresia
m. septum
memory
cardiac m.
m. catheter
m. loop
MemoryTrace
M. AT
M. AT ambulatory cardiac
monitor
Menadol
mendelian disorder
Mendelson syndrome
Menghini needle
Mèniére syndrome
meningitic respiration
meningitidis
Neisseria m.
meningitis, pl. meningitides
meningococcal
m. pericarditis
m. vaccine
meningococcemia
meningococcus
meningoencephalitis

mental
m. clouding
m. status
m. stress
meperidine
m. hydrochloride
Mephyton Oral
mepivacaine hydrochloride
Mepron
mEq
milliequivalent
meralluride
mercaptomerin sodium
6-mercaptopurine
MERCATOR
Multicenter European Research Trial
with Cilazapril after Angioplasty to
Prevent Transluminal Coronary
Obstruction and Restenosis
Mercuhydrin
mercury (Hg)
millimeters of m. (mmHg)
m. poisoning
**mercury-in-rubber strain gauge
plethysmograph**
mercury-in-Silastic strain gauge
mercury-195m (^{195m}Hg)
Merendino technique
meridian
m. echocardiogram
m. echocardiography
meridional wall stress
merodiastolic
meromyosin
meropenem
merosystolic
**Mersilene braided nonabsorbable
suture**
mesangial
m. cell
m. immune injury
mesaortitis
mesarteritis
mesenchymal-derived tumor
mesenchymal intimal cell
mesenteric
m. angiography

M

NOTES

mesenteric *(continued)*
    m. arteritis
    m. artery
    m. artery occlusion
    m. bypass graft
    m. ischemia
    m. vascular occlusion
mesh stent
mesocardia
    m. malposition
mesocaval shunt
mesoderm
    precardiac m.
mesodermal tumor
mesodiastolic
mesophlebitis
mesosystolic
mesothelioma
    malignant m.
messenger
    m. ribonucleic acid (mRNA)
    second m.
Messerklinger endoscope
Mester test
Mestinon
mesylate
    bitolterol m.
    deferoxamine m.
    Desferal M.
    dihydroergotamine m.
    doxazosin m.
    phentolamine m.
    saquinavir m.
MET
    metabolic equivalents of task
Meta
    M. II pacemaker
    M. MV pacemaker
    M. rate-responsive pacemaker
metabolator
    Sanborn m.
metabolic
    m. acidosis
    m. alkalosis
    m. cart
    m. encephalopathy
    m. equivalents of task (MET, METs)
    m. parameter determination
    m. rate meter
    m. vasodilatory capacity
metabolism
    aerobic m.

    anaerobic m.
    arachidonate m.
    glucose m.
    myocardial m.
metabolite
    arachidonic acid m.'s
    prostacyclin m.
metaboreceptor
metacholin
metachronous lung cancer
Metahydrin
metaiodobenzylguanidine (MIBG)
    I-123 m.
    I-125 m. (I-125 MIBG)
metal
    heavy m.
    m. sewing ring
    trace m.
metallic
    m. breath sounds
    m. clicks
    m. echo
    m. rales
    m. tinkle
metamorphosing respiration
MetaPhor agarose
metaplasia
    goblet cell m.
metaplastic mucus-secreting cell
metapneumonic
    m. empyema
    m. pleurisy
Metaprel
metaproterenol
    Arm-a-Med M.
    Dey-Dose M.
    m. sulfate
metaraminol bitartrate
metarteriole
metastasectomy
    pulmonary m.
metastasis, pl. metastases
    cannonball metastases
    cardiac m.
    contact m.
    implantation m.
    tumor, nodes, m. (TNM)
metastatic
    m. carcinoid syndrome
    m. carcinoma
    m. disease
    m. phenotype

m. pneumonia
m. sarcoma
metazoal myocarditis
Metenix
metenkephalin
meter (*See also* flowmeter)
    Assess peak flow m.
    Astech peak flow m.
    ExacTech blood glucose m.
    kilopond m.'s (KPM)
    m. mask
    metabolic rate m.
    peak flow m.
    Periflux PF 1 D blood-
      flow m.
    m.'s per second (m/sec)
    m.'s per second squared
    Personal Best peak flow m.
    Pocketpeak peak flow m.
    TruZone peak flow m.
    Wright peak flow m.
    Youlten nasal inspiratory peak
      flow m.
metered-dose
    m.-d. inhaler (MDI)
    m.-d. spray
methacholine
    m. bronchoprovocation
      challenge
    m. chloride
    m. test
methamphetamine hydrochloride
methanesulfonate
    phentolamine m.
methemoglobinemia
methicillin
    m. sodium
methicillin-sensitive right-sided
  endocarditis
methimazole
methionine loading
method
    Allain m.
    Anderson-Keys m.
    Antyllus m.
    area-length m.
    Arvidsson dimension-length m.

atrial extrastimulus m.
Batch least-squares m.
Bland-Altman m.
Bohr isopleth m.
Brasdor m.
Brisbane m.
Brown-Dodge m.
Burow quantitative m.
catheter introduction m.
Celermajer m.
chromogenic m.
Cribier m.
CryoLife Single Step
  dilution m.
Cutler-Ederer m.
cyanogen bromide m.
Danielson m.
Defares rebreathing m.
Devereux-Reichek m.
Dodge area-length m.
Douglas bag collection m.
Dow m.
downstream sampling m.
dye-dilution m.
edge-detection m.
Eggleston m.
Eicken m.
estimated Fick m.
Eve m.
Fick oxygen m.
flow convergence m.
forward triangle m.
Galanti-Giusti colorimetric m.
Gärtner m.
gas clearance m.
Gräupner m.
half-time m.
Hanley-McNeil m.
Hatle m.
head-tilt m.
Heinecke m.
helium dilution m.
Hetzel forward triangle m.
Howard m.
Hugenholtz m.
immunometric sandwich m.
indocyanine green m.

M

NOTES

method *(continued)*
Kaplan-Meier m.
Kasser-Kennedy m.
Kennedy area-length m.
Kety-Schmidt m.
King biopsy m.
Kirstein m.
Konno biopsy m.
Laborde m.
Laurell m.
least-squares m.
Lee-White m.
Lown and Woolf m.
Marriott m.
Meltzer m.
Monte Carlo multiway sensitivity analysis m.
Murphy m.
Narula m.
Ogata m.
Oliver-Rosalki m.
Orsi-Grocco m.
oxygen step-up m.
Pachon m.
Penaz volume-clamp m.
Penn m.
polarographic m.
prick-test m.
prism m.
Purmann m.
pyramid m.
m. of Quinones
m. of Rackley, Rackley m.
Raff-Glantz derivative m.
Sandler-Dodge area-length m.
Satterthwaite m.
Scarpa m.
Schiller m.
Schüller m.
Shimazaki area-length m.
Sigma m.
Silvester m.
sliding scale m.
Stanford biopsy m.
Stegemann-Stalder m.
Strauss m.
Theden m.
thermodilution m.
Thom flap laryngeal reconstruction m.
Thompson-Hatina m.
Thrombo-Wellcotest m.
triphenyltetrazolium staining m.

von Claus chronometric m.
V-slope m.
Wardrop m.
Weiss logarithmic m.
Welcker m.
Westergren m.
Willett-Stampfer m.
Wilson-White m.
methohexital
methotrexate
methoxamine hydrochloride
methoxsalen
2-methoxyisobutyl isonitrile
technetium hexakis -m. i. (Tc-99 sestamibi)
methoxyisobutyl isonitrile (MIBI)
8-methoxypsoralen
methyclothiazide
m. and cryptenamine tannates
m. and deserpidine
m. and pargyline
methyl
m. isocyanate
m. prednisolone
methyldopa
chlorothiazide and m.
m. and hydrochlorothiazide
methylene
m. blue
m. diphosphonate (MDP)
methylphenidate
methylprednisolone
m. succinate
methylxanthine
methysergide
m. maleate
Meticorten Oral
metoclopramide hydrochloride
metocurine iodide
metolazone
metoprolol
m. dilated cardiomyopathy (MDC)
m. succinate
m. tartrate
Metras catheter
Metrix atrial defibrillation system
metrizamide
m. contrast medium
Metro I.V. injection
metronidazole
Metroxamine

METs
    metabolic equivalents of task
metyrosine
Metzenbaum scissors
MeV
    megaelectron volt
Mevacor
mevalonate acid
mevinolin
Mewissen infusion catheter
mexiletine
    m. hydrochloride
Mexitil
Mezlin
mezlocillin
    m. sodium
MFG
    manofluorography
MGA
    malposition of great arteries
Mgb
    myoglobulin
mg/kg
    milligrams per kilogram
MHA-TP
    microhemagglutination *Treponema pallidum*
        MHA-TP test
M-HEART
    Multi-Hospital Eastern Atlantic Restenosis Trial
MH valve
MHz
    megahertz
MI
    myocardial infarction
    myocardial ischemia
MIBG
    metaiodobenzylguanidine
        I-123 MIBG
        I-125 MIBG
           I-125 metaiodobenzylguanidine
MIBI
    methoxyisobutyl isonitrile
        MIBI stress test
        technetium-99m MIBI

MIC
    minimum inhibitory concentration
mica pneumoconiosis
micdadei
    Legionella m.
    Tatlockia m.
Michelson bronchoscope
miconazole
Micor catheter
MICRhoGAM
Micro
    M. Minix pacemaker
    M. Mist nebulizer
    M. Plus spirometer
    M. stent
    6 M. Stent PL
MicroAir Model NE U03
microalbuminuria
microanastomosis
    laser-assisted m. (LAMA)
microaneurysm
    Charcot-Bouchard m.
microangiopathic anemia
microangiopathy
    coronary m.
    thrombotic m.
microarousals
microatheroma
microballoon
    Rand m.
microbiologic
microbubbles
microbulldog clip
microcalcification
microcardia
microcatheter
    Terumo SP hydrophilic-polymer-coated m.
microcavitation
microcirculation
microcontaminant
microdensitophotometric quantification
MicroDigitrapper-HR
MicroDigitrapper-S apnea screening device
microembolism

NOTES

microembolization
microfibrillar collagen hemostat
microfilaria
MicroGard
Micro-Guide catheter
MicroHartzler ACS balloon catheter
  system
microhemagglutination *Treponema*
  pallidum (MHA-TP)
microinvasive
Microjet Quark portable pump
microjoule
Micro-K 10
Microknit
  M. patch graft
  M. vascular graft prosthesis
microlaryngoscope
  Dedo-Jako m.
microlaryngoscopy
  Thornell m.
Microlith
  M. pacemaker pulse generator
  M. P pacemaker
microlithiasis
  pulmonary alveolar m.
Micro-Loop II
micromanometer
  m. catheter
  m. catheter system
  catheter-tip m. system
micromanometry
Micronase
micronebulizer
  Bird m.
microNefrin
microneurography
micron needle
Micronor
microorganism
microparticle
microphages
  fat-laden m.
Micropolyspora faeni
Micropuncture Peel-Away introducer
microreentry
Microsampler device
microscope
  acoustic m.
  electron m.
  scanning electron m. (SEM)
microscopic polyangiitis
microscopy
  darkfield m.

electron m.
light m.
microsecond pulsed flashlamp
  pumped dye laser
Microsoftrac catheter
microsphere
  m. perfusion scintigraphy
  polystyrene latex m.'s
  radiolabeled m.
  Ultrasound Contrast M.
microsphygmy
microsphyxia
Micross
  M. dilatation catheter
  M. SL balloon
Microsulfon
MicroTach pneumotachometer
Microthin P2 pacemaker
microti
  Babesia m.
microtome
  Cryo-Cut m.
  Stadie-Riggs m.
Micro-Tracer
  M.-T. portable ECG
  M.-T. portable EKG
microvascular
  m. angina
  m. clamp
  m. free flap
Microvel double velour graft
MicroVent ventilator
Mictrin
micturition syncope
MIDA
  M. CoroNet instrumentation
  M. 1000 monitoring system
Midamor
MIDAS
  Myocardial Infarction Data
  Acquisition System
midazolam
midclavicular line (MCL)
mid-diastolic
  m.-d. murmur
  m.-d. rumble
middle
  m. lobe bronchus
  m. lobe syndrome
mid-infrared pulsed laser
midinspiratory
midline shift

midnodal
    m. extrasystole
    m. rhythm
midodrine
midsagittal plane
midsystolic
    m. buckling
    m. click syndrome
    m. dip
    m. murmur
    m. notching
mifarmonab
MIFR
    maximal inspiratory flow rate
migraine
    m. headache
    syncopal m.
    m. syncope
migrans
    erythema m.
    larva m.
    ocular larva m.
    thrombophlebitis m.
    visceral larva m.
migrated tumor
migrating
    m. pacemaker
    m. phlebitis
migration
    neural crest m.
migratory
    m. pneumonia
    m. pulmonary infiltrate
    m. thrombus
Mijnhard
    M. electrical cycloergometer
    M. Valugraph
Mikity-Wilson disease
Mikros pacemaker
Mikro-Tip
    M.-T. micromanometer-tipped
    catheter
    M.-T. transducer
Milano
    apolipoprotein A-I M., B. D.
    E

Miles vena cava clip
miliary
    m. embolism
    m. tuberculosis
milieu
MILIS
    Multicenter Investigation for the
    Limitation of Infarct Size
military anti-shock trousers (MAST)
milk
    m. scan
    m. spots
Millar
    M. asthma
    M. Doppler catheter
    M. Mikro-Tip catheter pressure
    transducer
    M. MPC-500 catheter
mille-feuilles effect
Miller
    M. elastic stain
    M. Fisher variant
    M. septostomy catheter
milleri
    Streptococcus m.
miller's asthma
mill-house murmur
milliamperage
milliampere (mA)
millicurie (mCi)
milliequivalent (mEq)
milligrams per kilogram (mg/kg)
millijoule (mJ)
Milliknit
    M. Dacron prosthesis
    M. vascular graft prosthesis
milliliter (mL)
    m. per kilogram (mL/kg)
millimeters of mercury (mmHg)
millimole (mmol)
millimoles per liter (mmol/L)
million
    m. international units (MIU)
    parts per m. (ppm)
milliosmole (mOsm)

M

NOTES

Millipore filter
millisecond (msec)
milliunit (mU)
millivolt (mV)
Mill-Rose
    M.-R. esophageal injector
    M.-R. Protected Specimen
      microbiology brush
mill-wheel murmur
milrinone
    m. lactate
Miltex rib spreader
Milton edema
mimetic
miner
    m.'s asthma
    m.'s phthisis
mineralocorticoid
    m. hormone
mineralocorticoid-induced
  hypertension
Mingograf
    M. 62 6-channel
      electrocardiograph
    M. 82 recorder
Mingograph
mini-arousals
miniballoon
Minibird II
Miniclinic
    A-V M.
minicoil
mini-defibrillator
    Liteguard m.-d.
Mini-Dose
    HypRho-D M.-D.
Mini-Gamulin Rh
Minilith pacemaker pulse generator
minimal
    m. leak technique
    m. luminal diameter (MLD)
Mini-Motionlogger Actigraph
minimum
    m. bactericidal concentration
    m. inhibitory concentration
      (MIC)
Mini-Neb nebulizer
MiniOX
    M. 1A oxygen analyzer
    M. 1000 oxygen analyzer
Minipress
Mini-Profile catheter
Miniscope MS-3

Mini Thin Asthma Relief
Minitran
    M. Patch
Minix pacemaker
Minizide
Minnesota
    M. classification of EKG
    M. code
    M. EKG classification
Minocin
    M. I.V. injection
    M. Oral
minocycline
    m. hydrochloride
Minodyl
minor
    pectoralis m.
minoxidil
Mintezol
Minuet DDD pacemaker
minute
    alveolar ventilation per m.
      (V_A)
    beats per m. (bpm)
    liters per m. (lpm)
    m. output
    oxygen consumption per m.
      (VO_2)
    physiological dead space
      ventilation per m. (V_D)
    10-m. supine/30-minute tilt test
    m. ventilation (V_E)
    6-M. Walk Test
minute-gun cough
miocardia
Miocardico
    L-Carnitine Ecocardiografia
    Digitalizzata Infarto M.
    (CEDIM)
Miochol
miosphygmia
Mipron digital computer-assisted
  calipers
mirabilis
    Proteus m.
Mirage over-the-wire balloon
  catheter
mirror-image
    m.-i. brachiocephalic branching
    m.-i. dextrocardia
    m.-i. laryngoscopy
    m.-i. lung syndrome

Mirsky
formula of M.
M. thick wall model
mismatch
ventilation/perfusion m.
V/Q m.
mismatching
afterload m.
missed beat
mist
Bronkaid m.
cool m.
Primatene m.
m. tent
Mistogen
M. nebulizer
M. passover humidifier
MITI
Myocardial Infarction Triage and
Intervention
MITI Classification of
Terminal Events in Patients
with Acute Myocardial
Infarction
mitis
Streptococcus m.
mitochondrial
m. calcium deposition
m. cardiomyopathy
m. enzymes
m. function
mitochondrion, pl. **mitochondria**
mitogen
mitomycin
mitoxantrone hydrochloride
mitral
m. annular calcification
m. annular calcium
m. atresia
m. balloon commissurotomy
m. balloon valvotomy (MBV)
m. buttonhole
m. click
m. E to F slope
m. facies
m. first sound (M_1)
m. funnel

m. incompetence
m. insufficiency
m. opening snap (MOS)
m. prolapse murmur
m. prosthesis
m. regurgitant jet
m. regurgitation (MR)
m. regurgitation murmur
m. restenosis
m. second sound (M_2)
m. stenosis (MS)
m. stenosis murmur
m. tap
m. valve (MV)
m. valve aneurysm
m. valve annulus
m. valve area (MVA)
m. valve closure index
m. valve echocardiography
m. valve endocarditis
m. valve gradient (MVG)
m. valve hypoplasia
m. valve leaflet
m. valve prolapse (MVP)
m. valve prolapse syndrome
m. valve regurgitation
m. valve replacement (MVR)
m. valve valvotomy
m. valvulitis
m. valvuloplasty
mitrale
P m.
mitralis
facies m.
mitralism
mitralization
mitral-septal apposition
Mitroflow
M. pericardial heart valve
M. pericardial prosthetic valve
MIU
million international units
mix
oncology m.
mixed
m. aneurysm
m. angina

M

NOTES

mixed *(continued)*
  m. asthma
  m. beat
  m. flora
  m. levocardia
  m. neurally-mediated syncope
  m. thrombus
  m. venous blood
  m. venous oxygen saturation
    (SvO_2)
MixOMask
  OEM Venturi M.
mixture
  helium-oxygen m. (heliox)
mizoribine
mJ
  millijoule
MK-383
MKIII
  Digitrapper M.
mL
  milliliter
MLD
  minimal luminal diameter
M-line protein
mL/kg
  milliliter per kilogram
MMEF
  maximal midexpiratory flow
MMEFR
  maximal midexpiratory flow rate
mmHg
  millimeters of mercury
M-mode
  motion mode
    M-mode echocardiogram
    M-mode echocardiography
    M-mode recording
    M-mode transducer
mmol
  millimole
mmol/L
  millimoles per liter
MMV
  mandatory minute volume
mobile
  carina sharp and m.
  cor m.
  m. coronary care unit
Mobin-Uddin
  M.-U. filter system
  M.-U. vena cava filter

Mobitz
  M. type I, II atrioventricular
    block
modafinil
modalities
  pacing m.
mode
  A-m.
  fixed-rate m.
  gated list m.
  histogram m.
  list m.
  matrix m.
  motion m. (M-mode)
  passive m.
  m. switching
model
  Cox proportional hazards m.
  Cox stepwise regression m.
  Hodgkin-Huxley m.
  Mirsky thick wall m.
  M. 40-400 Pruitt-Inahara shunt
  Torricelli m.
moderator band
modification
  A-V nodal m.
  Mason-Likar limb lead m.
  Mullins m.
modified
  m. brachial technique
  m. Bruce protocol
  m. Ellestad protocol
  m. Mark IV R-wave-triggered
    power injector
  m. multifactorial index of
    cardiac risk
  m. Seldinger technique
modulation
  autonomic m.
  brightness m.
module
  Capnostat Mainstream carbon
    dioxide m.
  Co-Oximeter m.
modulus
  impedance m.
Moduretic
Moersch bronchoscope
moexipril
  m. hydrochloride
mofetil
  mycophenolate m.
moiety-conserved cycle

moist
Nasal M.
m. rales
moisturizer
RoEzIt skin m.
mol
mole
mole (mol)
molecular-weight dextran
molecule
endothelium-leukocyte
adhesion m. (E-LAM)
molecule-1
intercellular adhesion m.
(ICAM-1)
vascular cell adhesion m.
(VCAM-1)
Molina needle catheter
Mol-Iron
Mollaret HSV
mollis
pulsus m.
molluscum contagiosum
Molnar disk
molsidomine
moment
magnetic m.
Monaghan
M. respirator
M. 300 ventilator
Monaldi drainage system
**Monarch Mini Mask nasal
interface**
Monark bicycle ergometer
Mönckeberg
M. arrhythmia
M. arteriosclerosis
M. degeneration
M. sclerosis
Monday
M. dyspnea
M. fever
**Mondini pulmonary arteriovenous
malformation**
Mondor
M. disease
M. syndrome

Monge disease
Monilia albicans
monilial esophagitis
moniliasis
chronic mucocutaneous m.
moniliformis
Streptobacillus m.
Monit
monitor
Accucap CO_2/O_2 m.
Accucom cardiac output m.
Accutorr A1, 3 blood
pressure m.
Accutracker II ambulatory
blood pressure m.
Acuson V5M transesophageal
echocardiographic m.
AID-Check m.
apnea m.
Arrhythmia Net arrhythmia m.
automatic oscillometric blood
pressure m.
Bedfont carbon monoxide m.
Biotrack coagulation m.
blood perfusion m. (BPM)
CA m.
Capintec nuclear VEST m.
cardiac m.
CardioDiary heart m.
Cardioguard 4000
electrocardiographic m.
Cardiovit AT-10 m.
3-channel Holter m.
Colin ambulatory BP m.
Commucor A+V Patient m.
Cricket pulse oximetry m.
Criticare $ETCO_2/SpO_2$ m.
DeltaTrac II metabolic m.
Digitrapper MkIII sleep m.
Dinamap blood pressure m.
Doplette m.
Doppler-Cavin m.
Doppler fetal heart m.
EcoCheck oxygen m.
electrocardiographic
transtelephonic m.
electronic fetal m.

M

NOTES

monitor *(continued)*
event m.
Finapres blood pressure m.
HeartCard m.
Heart Rate 1-2-3 m.
HemoTec activated clotting
time m.
Hewlett-Packard 78720 A
SDN m.
Holter m.
Homochron m.
Insta-Pulse heart rate m.
KinetiX ventilation m.
King of Hearts Holter m.
m. leads
Magellan m.
Marquette 8000 Holter m.
MemoryTrace AT ambulatory
cardiac m.
MRM-2 oxygen
consumption m.
Nellcor N1000 ETCO$_2$/SpO$_2$ m.
Nellcor Symphony N-3100
noninvasive blood
pressure m.
NoxBOX m.
Ohio Vortex respiration m.
Ohmeda 6200, 6300 CO$_2$ m.'s
Omega 5600 noninvasive blood
pressure m.
One Touch blood glucose m.
PAM2, PAM3 m.'s
Pick and Go m.
Polar Vantage XL heart
rate m.
Porta-Resp m.
Pressurometer blood
pressure m.
Puritan-Bennett 7250
metabolic m.
SpaceLabs Holter m.
TINA m.
transcutaneous oxygen m.
(TCOM)
Trans-Scan 2100 noninvasive
physiological m.
transtelephonic exercise m.
(TEM)
Tri-Met apnea m.
VenTrak respiratory
mechanics m.
VEST ambulatory ventricular
function m.

video m.
Vitalograph pulmonary m.
monitor/defibrillator
Lifepak 7 m.
monitoring
ambulatory
electrocardiographic m.
(AEM)
ambulatory Holter m. (AHM)
Doptone m.
Electrophysiology Study versus
Electrocardiographic M.
(ESVEM)
physiological m.
pulse oximetry m. (POM)
transtelephonic arrhythmia m.
(TTM)
Moniz carotid siphon
Monneret pulse
monoamine
m. oxidase (MAO)
m. oxidase inhibitor (MAO
inhibitor, MAOI)
monobactam
monoballoon
monocardiogram
Mono-Cedocard
Monocid
Monoclate-P
monoclonal
m. antibody 3G4
m. antimyosin antibody
m. hypothesis
m. theory of atherogenesis
MonoClone immunoenzymetric assay
monocrotaline
monocrotic
m. pulse
monocrotism
monocrotus
pulsus m.
monocyte
m. chemotactic protein-1
(MCP-1)
monocytogenes
Listeria m.
Monodox Oral
monofilament
m. absorbable suture
m. polypropylene suture
monofoil catheter
monoform tachycardia
Mono-Gesic

mononitrate
  isosorbide m.
mononuclear cell
mononucleosis
  infectious m.
monophasic
  m. action potential (MAP)
  m. action potential duration (MAPD)
  m. complex
monophonic wheeze
monophosphate
  adenosine m. (AMP)
  cyclic adenosine m. (cAMP)
  cyclic guanosine m. (cGMP)
  cyclic nucleotide adenosine m.
  guanosine m. (GMP)
monopolar temporary electrode
Monopril
Monorail
  M. imaging catheter
  M. Piccollino catheter
  M. Speedy balloon
Monostrut
  M. Bjdork-Shiley valve
  M. cardiac valve prosthesis
monosulfate
  guanethidine m.
monotest
  R-lactate enzyme m.
Monotest CK-MB NAC-act test
monotherapy
monotypic lesion
Mono-Vacc
monoxide
  carbon m. (CO)
  diffusing capacity of lung for carbon m. (DLCO)
monoxime
  butanedione m.
Monro
  foramen of M.
Monte Carlo multiway sensitivity analysis method
Montgomery
  M. Safe-T-Tube
  M. speaking valve
  M. tracheostomy

moon face
Moore
  M. procedure
  M. tracheostomy button
mopamidol
Moraxella
  M. catarrhalis
morbidity
morbid obesity
morcellation
Morch respirator
Moretz clip
Morgagni
  M. disease
  foramen of M.
  M. hernia
  M. nodules
Morgagni-Adams-Stokes syndrome
Morganella
moribund
moricizine
  m. hydrochloride
moriens
  ultimum m.
morphine
morphologic
morphology
  QRS m.
Morquio-Brailsford disease
Morquio syndrome
morrhuate sodium
Morsch-Retec respirator
Morse manifold
mortality rate
mortis
  myocardial rigor m.
Morton cough
MOS
  mitral opening snap
mosaic
  M. cardiac bioprosthesis
  m. jet
  m. perfusion
mosaic-jet signals
Moschcowitz
  M. disease
  M. test

M

mortality rate
mortis
    myocardial rigor m.
Morton cough
MOS
    mitral opening snap
mosaic
    M. cardiac bioprosthesis
    m. jet
    m. perfusion
mosaic-jet signals
Moschcowitz
    M. disease
    M. test
Mosher life-saving tracheal tube
mOsm
    milliosmole
mosquito
    m. clamp
    m. hemostat
moss-agate sputum
Mosso sphygmomanometer
motility
    esophageal m.
    receptor for hyaluronan-
       mediated m. (RHAMM)
motion
    atrioventricular junction m.
    cusp m.
    diastolic m.
    m. display echo
    interventricular septal m.
    m. mode (M-mode)
    paradoxic wall m.
    precordial m.
    regional wall m.
    segmental wall m.
    septal wall m.
    systolic anterior m. (SAM)
    ventricular wall m.
    wall m.
    whorl m.
motoricity
Motrin IB Sinus
mottling of extremities
Moulaert
    muscle of M.
moulin
    bruit de la roue de m.
Mounier-Kuhn syndrome
mountain sickness
Moure esophagoscope

mouse
    pleural m.
mousetail pulse
Mousseau-Barbin esophageal tube
mouth-to-mouth
    m.-t.-m. resuscitation
    m.-t.-m. ventilation
movable
    m. core straight safety wire
       guide
    m. heart
    m. pulse
Movat
    M. pentachrome
    M. stain
movement
    air m.
    ciliary m.
    m. disorder
    non-rapid eye m. (NREM)
    precordial m.
    rapid eye m. (REM)
moxalactam
Moxam
moyamoya disease
Moynahan syndrome
Moynihan respirator
MPA
    main pulmonary artery
MPAP
    mean pulmonary artery pressure
MPAWP
    mean pulmonary artery wedge
      pressure
MPHR
    maximum predicted heart rate
MPO
    myeloperoxidase
M-Prednisol injection
MPRG
    Multicenter Postinfarction Research
      Group
M-protein serotype
MPT
    multiple-parameter telemetry
MR
    mitral regurgitation
MRF
    magnetic resonance flowmetry
MRFIT
    Multiple Risk Factor Intervention
      Trial

MRI
magnetic resonance imaging
cine gradient-echo MRI
FLASH MRI
Gd-DTPA-enhanced MRI
GRASS MRI
spin-echo MRI
ThromboScan MRI
MRM-2
M. oxygen consumption
monitor
mRNA
messenger ribonucleic acid
skeletal alpha-actin mRNA
MRT Tidal Humidifier
MS
mitral stenosis
MS Classique balloon
dilatation catheter
MS-3
Miniscope MS-3
MS-857
m/sec
meters per second
msec
millisecond
MSI
magnetic source imaging
MSLT
Multiple Sleep Latency Test
MSNA
muscle sympathetic nerve activity
MSOF
multisystem organ failure
MST
median survival time
MST cryoprobe
MSVC
maximal sustainable ventilatory
capacity
MTC catheter
M-type alpha 1-antitrypsin
MU
megaunit
mU
milliunit
Much granules

mucicarmine stain
mucinous carcinoma
mucociliary
m. clearance
**mucocutaneous lymph node
syndrome**
mucoepidermoid carcinoma
mucogenicum
Mycobacterium m.
mucoid
m. exopolysaccharide
m. medial degeneration
mucolipidosis, pl. mucolipidoses
mucolytic
mucomembranous
Mucomyst
mucopolysaccharide
acid m. (AMP)
mucopolysaccharidosis,
pl. **mucopolysaccharidoses**
mucopurulent sputum
mucopus
Mucor
Mucoraceae
mucoretention cyst
mucormycosis
pulmonary m.
mucosal edema
mucoserous
Mucosol
mucous
m. desiccation
m. plugging
m. rales
m. sheets
m. threads
mucoviscidosis
mucus
m. hypersecretion
m. inhibitor
oyster mass of m.
m. plug
thick and sticky m.
viscid m.
Mueller
M. maneuver
M. sign

M

NOTES

Muerto Canyon virus
muffled heart sounds
MUGA
    multiple gated acquisition
    MUGA exercise stress test
    MUGA scan
Mui Scientific 6-channel esophageal
    pressure probe
Muller
    M. banding
    M. test
Müller
    M. experiment
    M. maneuver
    M. sign
    M. vena caval clamp
Mullins
    M. blade technique
    M. cardiac device
    M. dilator
    M. modification
    M. sheath/dilator
    M. sheath system
    M. transseptal catheter
    M. transseptal catheterization
      sheath
multi-access catheter (MAC)
Multicenter
    M. American Research Trial
      with Cilazapril after
      Angioplasty to Prevent
      Transluminal Coronary
      Obstruction and Restenosis
      (MARCATOR)
    M. Anti-Atheroma Study
      (MAAS)
    M. Diltiazem Post-Infarction
      Trial (MDPIT)
    M. European Research Trial
      with Cilazapril after
      Angioplasty to Prevent
      Transluminal Coronary
      Obstruction and Restenosis
      (MERCATOR)
    M. Investigation for the
      Limitation of Infarct Size
      (MILIS)
    M. Postinfarction Research
      Group (MPRG)
Multicor
    M. II cardiac pacemaker
multicrystal gamma camera

multidrug-resistance
multidrug-resistant tuberculosis
    (MDR-TB)
multi-element linear array
multifactorial
multiflanged Portnoy catheter
Multiflex catheter
multifocal atrial tachycardia (MAT)
multiform
    m. premature ventricular
      complex
    m. tachycardia
multiforme
    erythema m.
multigated angiography
Multi-Hospital Eastern Atlantic
    Restenosis Trial (M-HEART)
multi-infarct dementia
multilamellar body
multilayer design catheter
Multileaf collimator device
multilinear regression analysis
Multi Link stent
Multilith pacemaker
multilocular cyst
multimer assay
multinucleated giant cells
multiple
    m. embolism
    m. gated acquisition (MUGA)
    m. lentigines syndrome
    m. lipoprotein-type
      hyperlipidemia
    m. regression
    M. Risk Factor Intervention
      Trial (MRFIT)
    m. sclerosis
    m. shunt levels
    M. Sleep Latency Test
      (MSLT)
    m. system atrophy
multiple-balloon valvuloplasty
multiple-parameter telemetry (MPT)
multiplex
    m. catheter
    mononeuritis m.
    m. neuropathy
multipolar
    m. catheter
    m. catheter electrode
Multipurpose-SM catheter
multisensor catheter

Multistage Maximal Effort exercise stress test
multisystem organ failure (MSOF)
multivalve insufficiency
multivalvular
 m. disease
 m. disease murmur
multivariate analysis of variance (MANOVA)
Multi-Vent
 Hudson M.-V.
multivessel
 M. Angioplasty Prognosis Study (MAPS)
 m. coronary artery obstruction
 m. disease (MVD)
multiwire gamma camera
multocida
 Pasteurella m.
mupirocin
muqueux
 rales m.
mural
 m. aneurysm
 m. endocarditis
 m. thrombosis
 m. thrombus
Murat sign
Murgo pressure contours
mu rhythm
murine-derived monoclonal antibody 7E3 Fab
murine monoclonal antibody muromonab-CD3
murmur
 accidental m.
 amphoric m.
 anemic m.
 aneurysmal m.
 aortic-left ventricular tunnel m.
 aortic-mitral combined disease m.
 aortic regurgitation m.
 aortic stenosis m.
 apex m.
 apical mid-diastolic heart m.
 apical systolic heart m.

 arterial m.
 atriosystolic m.
 atrioventricular flow rumbling m.
 attrition m.
 Austin Flint m.
 basal diastolic m.'s
 bellows m.
 blood m.
 blowing m.
 blubbery diastolic m.
 brain m.
 Bright m.
 bronchial collateral artery m.
 Cabot-Locke m.
 carcinoid m.
 cardiac m.
 cardiopulmonary m.
 cardiorespiratory m.
 Carey Coombs short mid-diastolic m.
 carotid artery m.
 click m.
 coarse m.
 Cole-Cecil m.
 congenital m.
 continuous heart m.
 cooing m.
 Coombs m.
 crescendo m.
 crescendo-decrescendo m.
 Cruveilhier-Baumgarten m.
 decrescendo m.
 deglutition m.
 diamond ejection m.
 diamond-shaped m.
 diastolic m.
 direct m.
 Docke m.
 Duroziez m.
 dynamic m.
 early diastolic m.
 early-peaking systolic m.
 ejection m.
 end-diastolic m.
 endocardial m.
 end-systolic m.

M

NOTES

murmur *(continued)*
Eustace Smith m.
exit block m.
exocardial m.
expiratory m.
extracardiac m.
Fisher m.
Flint m.
Fräntzel m.
friction m.
functional m.
Gallavardin m.
Gibson m.
goose-honk m.
grade 1 through 6 m.
Graham Steell m.
groaning m.
Hamman m.
harsh m.
heart m.
hemic m.
high-frequency m.
high-pitched m.
Hodgkin-Key m.
holodiastolic m.
holosystolic m.
honking m.
hourglass m.
humming m.
humming-top m.
incidental m.
indirect m.
innocent m. of elderly
innocent heart m.
inorganic m.
lapping m.
late apical systolic m.
late diastolic m.
late-peaking systolic m.
left ventricular-right atrial
   communication m.
Levine gradation 1 through 6
   of cardiac m.'s
low-frequency m.
low-pitched m.
machinery m.
Makin m.
mammary souffle m.
mid-diastolic m.
midsystolic m.
mill-house m.
mill-wheel m.
mitral prolapse m.

mitral regurgitation m.
mitral stenosis m.
multivalvular disease m.
muscular m.
musical m.
noninvasive m.
nun's venous hum m.
obstructive m.
organic m.
outflow m.
pansystolic m.
Parrot m.
patent ductus arteriosus m.
pathologic m.
pericardial m.
physiologic m.
pleuropericardial m.
prediastolic m.
presystolic m.
primary pulmonary
   hypertension m.
protodiastolic m.
pulmonary m., pulmonic m.
rasping m.
reduplication m.
regurgitant m.
respiratory m.
Roger m.
rumbling diastolic m.
scratchy m.
seagull m.
seesaw m.
Steell m.
stenosal m.
Still m.
subclavian m.
subclavicular m.
systolic apical m.
systolic ejection m. (SEM)
systolic regurgitant m.
to-and-fro m.
transmitted m.
Traube m.
tricuspid m.
vascular m.
venous m.
ventricular septal defect m.
vesicular m.
water wheel m.
whooping m.
muromonab-CD3
murine monoclonal
   antibody m.-CD3

Murphy
   M. method
   M. percussion
muscarinic
   m. agonist
   m. receptor
muscle
   anterior papillary m. (APM)
   m. bridge
   bronchial smooth m.
   cardiac m.
   Chassaignac axillary m.
   m. immunocytochemical study
   latissimus dorsi m.
   m. of Moulaert
   papillary m.
   posterior papillary m. (PPM)
   rectus abdominis m.
   m. relaxant
   ribbon m.'s
   skeletal m.
   m. stiffness
   strap m.'s
   m. sympathetic nerve activity
    (MSNA)
   venous smooth m.
muscular
   m. dystrophy
   m. incompetence
   m. murmur
   m. subaortic stenosis
   m. venous pump
musculoskeletal pain
mush clamp
mushroom
   m. dust
   m. worker's lung
musical
   m. bruit
   m. murmur
   m. rales
Musset sign
mustard
   M. atrial baffle
   L-phenylalinine m.
   nitrogen m.

   M. operation
   M. procedure
Mustargen Hydrochloride
Mutamycin
mutant allele
mutation
mute
   m. reflexes
   m. toe signs
muzolimine
MV
   maximal ventilation
   mechanical ventilation
   mitral valve
mV
   millivolt
MVA
   malignant ventricular arrhythmia
   mitral valve area
MVC
   maximal vital capacity
MVD
   multivessel disease
MVE-50 implantable myocardial
   electrode
MVG
   mitral valve gradient
MVO$_2$
   myocardial oxygen consumption
MVP
   mitral valve prolapse
   MVP catheter
MVR
   maximal ventilation rate
   mitral valve replacement
MVV
   maximum voluntary ventilation
   MVV ventilator
myalgia gravis
Myambutol
myasthenia
   m. cordis
   m. gravis
   m. gravis pseudoparalytica
myasthenic crisis
mycetoma

M

NOTES

MycoAKT latex bead agglutination test
mycobacteria
mycobacterial
Mycobacterium
 M. *abscessus*
 M. *avium*
 M. *avium* complex (MAC)
 M. *avium* complex infection
 M. *avium-intracellulare* (MAI)
 M. *avium-intracellulare*
 infection
 M. *bovis*
 M. *chelonae*
 M. *fortuitum*
 M. *gordonae*
 M. *intracellulare*
 M. *kansasii*
 M. *leprae*
 M. *marinum*
 M. *mucogenicum*
 M. *peregrinum*
 M. *phlei*
 M. *smegmatis*
 M. *thermoresistable*
 M. *tuberculosis*
 M. *ulcerans*
 M. *vaccae*
Mycobutin
 M. Oral
mycophenolate mofetil
Mycoplasma
 M. *faucium*
 M. *hominis*
 M. *incognitus*
 M. *pneumoniae*
 M. *xenopi*
mycoplasmal pneumonia
mycoplasmosis
Mycoscint
mycosis
 m. fungoides
 Posadas m.
 pulmonary m.
Mycostatin Topical
mycotic
 m. aortic aneurysm
 m. aortography
 m. endocarditis
 m. infection
MycroMesh graft material
mydriatic

myectomy
 septal m.
myeloma
myelonecrosis
myeloperoxidase (MPO)
myelosuppression
Mykrox
Mylar catheter
Myleran
Myminic Expectorant
myocardial
 m. abscess
 m. anoxia
 m. band (MB)
 m. band enzymes of CPK
 (CPK-MB)
 m. bed
 m. blood flow (MBF)
 m. blush
 m. bridge
 m. bridging (MB)
 m. clamp
 m. cold-spot perfusion
 scintigraphy
 m. collagen matrix
 m. concussion
 m. contractility
 m. contrast echocardiography
 (MCE)
 m. contusion
 m. depolarization
 m. depressant factor (MDF)
 m. depressant substance (MDS)
 m. depression
 m. disease
 m. edema
 m. failure
 m. fiber shortening
 m. fibrosis
 m. function
 m. hamartoma
 m. hibernation
 m. hypertrophy
 m. infarction (MI)
 M. Infarction Data Acquisition
 System (MIDAS)
 m. infarction in dumbbell form
 m. infarction in H-form
 M. Infarction Triage and
 Intervention (MITI)
 M. Infarction Triage and
 Intervention project
 m. infundibular stenosis

m. injury
m. insufficiency
m. ischemia (MI)
m. ischemic syndrome
m. jeopardy index
m. lead
m. malnutrition
m. mass
m. metabolism
m. muscle creatine kinase isoenzyme (CK-MB)
m. necrosis
m. oxygen consumption (MVO$_2$)
m. oxygen demand
m. oxygen supply
m. oxygen uptake
m. perforation
m. perfusion
m. perfusion imaging
m. perfusion scintigraphy
m. perfusion study
m. protection
m. reserve
m. revascularization
m. rigor mortis
m. rupture
m. salvage
m. sparing
m. stiffness
m. stunning
m. tension
m. tissue
m. viability
m. viability scintigraphy
myocardiograph
myocardiopathy
alcoholic m.
chagasic m.
myocardiorrhaphy
myocarditic
myocarditis
acute isolated m.
bacterial m.
cardiac sarcoidosis m.
chronic m.
clostridial m.

coxsackievirus m.
cryptococcal m.
diphtheritic m.
echovirus m.
Fiedler m.
fragmentation m.
giant cell m.
helminthic m.
Histoplasma m.
hypersensitivity m.
idiopathic m.
indurative m.
metazoal m.
parenchymatous m.
peripartum m.
protozoal m.
rheumatic m.
rickettsial m.
spirochetal m.
syphilitic m.
toxic m.
tuberculoid m.
viral m.
myocardium
dysfunctional m.
fragmentation of m.
hibernating m.
ischemic m.
jeopardized m.
postischemic m.
senescent m.
stunned m.
underperfused m.
myocardosis
Reisman m.
myocyte
Anichkov m.
m. de-energization
m. hypertrophy
m. magnesium stores
m. metabolic activity
m. necrosis
myocytolysis
coagulative m.
m. of heart
myoendocarditis
myofascial

M

NOTES

myofibril
myofibrillar
  m. ATPase
    m. calcium level
myofibroblast
myofibrosis
  m. cordis
myofilament
    m. calcium responsiveness
    m. contractile activation
myogenic theory
myoglobin
  m. assay
myoglobulin (Mgb)
myoglobulinuria
myointimal plaque
myolysis
  cardiotoxic m.
myopathia cordis
myopathy
  centronuclear m.
  myotubular m.
  nemaline m.
myopericarditis
myoplasmic calcium
myoplasty
myopleuropericarditis
Myopore lead
Myoscint
myosin
  cardiac m.
  m. heavy chain
  m. light chain
myosin-specific antibody

myositis
myotomy
  septal m.
myotomy-myectomy-septal resection
myotonia
  m. congenita
myotonic muscular dystrophy
myotubular myopathy
Myoview contrast material
Myowire II cardiac electrode
Mytussin
myurous
myurus
  pulsus m.
myxedema
  m. heart
  pretibial m.
myxedematous
myxoma, pl. myxomata
  atrial m.
  cardiac m.
  infected m.
  left atrial m.
  left ventricular m.
  right atrial m.
  right ventricular m.
  m. tumor
  ventricular m.
myxomatous
  m. change
  m. degeneration
  m. proliferation
  m. pulmonary embolism

N
>N cell
>N region

N-13
>N-13 ammonia
>N-13 ammonia uptake

N₂
>nitrogen
>N_2 oximetry

n-3 fatty acid
n-6 fatty acid
N-acetylcysteine
N-acetylneuraminic acid
N-acetyl procainamide (NAPA)
Nachlas tube
NAD
>nicotinamide adenine dinucleotide

nadir
nadolol
nadroparin calcium
NAEP
>National Asthma Education Program

nafamostat
nafate
>cefamandole n.

nafazatrom
Nafcil
>N. injection

nafcillin
>n. sodium

Nagle exercise stress test
nail
>n. bed
>cyanosis of n. beds
>n. pulse
>n.-to-nail bed angle

NaK-ATPase
Nakayama anastomosis
nalbuphine hydrochloride
Naldecon
Nalfon
nalidixic acid
Nallpen injection
nalmefene hydrochloride
naloxone hydrochloride
naltrexone
NAME
>nevi, atrial myxoma, myxoid
>neurofibromas, and ephelides
>NAME syndrome

Namic
>N. angiographic syringe
>N. catheter

Nanos 01 pacemaker
NAPA
>N-acetyl procainamide

napkin-ring
>n.-r. calcification
>n.-r. defect
>n.-r. stenosis

Naprosyn
naproxen
Naqua
Narcan
>N. injection

Narco
>N. Biosystems recorder
>N. Physiograph-6B recorder

narcolepsy
Narcomatic flowmeter
narcosis
narcotic
narrow-complex tachycardia
narrowed pulse pressure
narrowing
>atherosclerotic n.
>eccentric n.
>luminal n.

Narula method
Nasabid
Nasacort
nasal
>n. airway
>n. asthma
>n. cannula
>Concentraid N.
>n. CPAP
>DDAVP N.
>n. flaring
>N. Moist
>n. polyposis
>n. prongs

Nasalcrom
>N. Nasal Solution

Nasalide
>N. Nasal Aerosol

Nasarel
NASCET
>North American Symptomatic
>Carotid Endarterectomy Trial

N

nasogastric tube
nasopharyngeal (NP)
  n. carcinoma
nasopharyngitis
nasopharynx
nasotracheal
  n. intubation
  n. suction
  n. tube
Nathan test
National
  N. Asthma Education Program
    (NAEP)
  N. Cholesterol Education
    Program (NCEP)
  N. Health and Nutrition
    Examination Survey
    (NHANES)
  N. Heart, Lung, and Blood
    Institute (NHLBI)
  N. Institutes of Health
  N. Registry of Myocardial
    Infarction (NRMI)
native
  n. coarctation
  n. coronary anatomy
  n. valve
  n. vessel
Natrecor
Natrilix
natriuresis
natriuretic
  n. hormone
  n. peptide
natural frequency
Naturetin
Naughton
  N. graded exercise stress test
  N. treadmill protocol
Nauheim
  N. bath
  N. treatment
Navelbine
Navidrex
Navier-Stokes equation
NBIH cardiac device
NBTE
  nonbacterial thrombotic endocarditis
NCEP
  National Cholesterol Education
  Program
Nd:YAG laser
near-fainting

near field
near-gain
near-infrared spectroscopy (NIS)
near-syncope
Nebcin
  N. injection
nebivolol
Nebules
  Ventolin N.
nebulization
  continuous albuterol n. (CAN)
nebulized
  n. bronchodilator
  n. tobramycin
nebulizer
  Acorn II n.
  aerosol n.
  AeroSonic personal
    ultrasonic n.
  AeroTech II n.
  air-powered n.
  Centimist n.
  Compu-Neb ultrasonic n.
  DeVilbiss n.
  hand-held n.
  Incenti-neb n.
  jet n.
  Marquest Respirgard II n.
  Micro Mist n.
  Mini-Neb n.
  Mistogen n.
  Pulmo-Aide n.
  Respirgard II n.
  Schuco n.
  Tote-A-Neb n.
  Twin Jet n.
  ultrasonic n.
NebuPent
  N. Inhalation
Necator americanus
necessitatis
  empyema n.
necrobiosis lipoidica diabeticorum
necrobiotic nodule
necrosis, pl. necroses
  avascular n.
  coagulation n.
  contraction band n.
  cystic medial n.
  digital n.
  dirty n.
  Erdheim cystic medial n.
  n. factor

fibrinoid n.
myocardial n.
myocyte n.
renal cortical n.
tissue n.
tubular n.
necrotic cyst
necrotisans
phlebitis nodularis n.
necrotizing
n. angiitis
n. arteriolitis
n. bronchopneumonia
n. pneumonia
n. vasculitis
nedocromil
n. sodium
needle
Abrams n.
Aldrete n.
argon n.
Arrow-Fischell EVAN n.
arterial n.
n. aspirate
aspirating n.
Atraloc n.
atraumatic n.
Becton-Dickinson Teflon-sheathed n.
Bengash n.
beveled thin-walled n.
Brockenbrough curved n.
Brughleman n.
butterfly n.
Cardiopoint cardiac surgery n.
Chiba n.
Cooley aortic vent n.
Cope pleural biopsy n.
Cope thoracentesis n.
Cournand n.
Cournand-Grino angiography n.
Cournand-Potts n.
Crown n.
Curry n.
DLP cardioplegic n.
Dos Santos n.

ergonomic vascular access n. (EVAN)
Ethalloy n.
eyeless n.
Fergie n.
Ferguson n.
Fischer pneumothoracic n.
Flynt n.
Frederick pneumothorax n.
front wall n.
n. holder
Hustead n.
Jamshidi n.
large-bore slotted aspirating n.
Lewy-Rubin n.
Lowell pleural n.
Luer-Lok n.
Menghini n.
micron n.
Nordenstrom Rotex II biopsy n.
O'Brien airway n.
olive-tipped n.
PercuCut biopsy n.
percutaneous cutting n.
pilot n.
Potts n.
Potts-Cournand n.
Quincke-point spinal n.
Ranfac n.
Rashkind septostomy n.
Riley n.
Ross n.
Rotex n.
Seldinger n.
slotted n.
standard n.
steel-winged butterfly n.
Stifcore aspiration n.
thin-walled n.
thoracentesis n.
Tru-Cut biopsy n.
UMI n.
Venflon n.
Vim-Silverman n.
Wang transbronchial n.

N

NOTES

needle *(continued)*
  Wasserman n.
  Zavala lung biopsy n.
needlepoint electrocautery
Needle-Pro needle protection device
NEEP
  negative end-expiratory pressure
NEET
  Nordic Enalapril Exercise Trial
NEFA
  nonesterified fatty acid
  NEFA scintigraphy
Neff percutaneous access set
negative
  n. chronotropism
  n. contrast
  n. end-expiratory pressure
    (NEEP)
  n. inotrope
  n. predictive value (NPV)
  n. pressure
  n. treppe
NegGram
Negri bodies
Negus bronchoscope
Negus-Broyles bronchoscope
Nehb D lead
Neisseria
  N. catarrhalis
  N. meningitidis
neisserial
Nellcor
  N. N2500 ETCO$_2$ multigas
    analyzer
  N. N1000 ETCO$_2$/SpO$_2$ monitor
  N. N200 pulse oximeter
  N. Symphony N-3100
    noninvasive blood pressure
    monitor
  N. Symphony N-3000 pulse
    oximeter
nemaline myopathy
Nembutal
neodymium:yttrium-aluminum-garnet
  laser (Nd:YAG laser)
Neofed
Neoflex bendable knife
neoformans
  Cryptococcus n.
neoglottis
neointima
neointimal
  n. hyperplastic response

  n. proliferation
  n. tear
NeoKnife electrosurgical instrument
neolumen
neomycin
  n. sulfate
neonatal
  Exosurf N.
  n. internal jugular puncture kit
  N. Y TrachCare
neonatorum
  apnea n.
  asphyxia n.
neoplasia
neoplasm
  extrathoracic n.
neoplastic
  n. disease
  n. pericarditis
neopterin
  serum n.
Neoral cyclosporine capsules
Neosar injection
Neo-Sert umbilical vessel catheter
  insertion set
Neos M pacemaker
Neo-Synephrine
Neo-Therm neonatal skin
  temperature probe
Neothylline
neovascularization
NeoVO-2-R volume control
  resuscitator
Nephril
nephritis, pl. **nephritides**
  familial n.
  immune-mediated
    membranous n.
Nephro-Fer
nephrogenic diabetes insipidus
nephrogram
nephron
nephropathic cardiomyopathy
nephropathy
  analgesic n.
  diabetic n.
  hypertensive n.
  hyperuricemic n.
nephrosclerosis
nephrotic syndrome
nephrotoxicity
Nernst equation

nerve
- cardiac sensory n.
- carotid sinus n.
- eleventh cranial n.
- n. of Hering
- hypoglossal n.
- n. of Kuntz
- laryngeal n.
- phrenic n.
- sensory n.
- thoracic n.
- vagus n.

Nervocaine
nervosa
- anorexia n.
- dysphagia n.

nervous
- n. asthma
- n. respiration
- n. system
- n. tachypnea

Nestor guiding catheter
Nestrex
nest of veins
net
- Arrhythmia N.
- Jahnke-Barron heart support n.

netilmicin sulfate
Netromycin injection
network
- Chiari n.
- fibrillar collagen n.
- interstitial and perivascular collagen n.
- local area n. (LAN)

Neubauer artery
neuf
- bruit de cuir n.

Neupogen
neural
- n. crest malformation
- n. crest migration

neuralgia
- glossopharyngeal n.

neurally-mediated syncope
neuritis
- optic n.

neuroblastoma
neurocardiac
neurocardiogenic syncope
neurocirculatory asthenia
neurodegenerative disease
neuroendocrine
- n. theory
- n. tumor

neurofibroma
neurofibromatosis
neurogenic
- n. abnormalities
- n. pulmonary edema
- n. theory
- n. tumor

neurohormonal function
neurohormone
neurohumoral
- n. factors
- n. stimulus

neuroleptic
neurologic
- n. examination
- n. status

neurological disorder
neuromediated syncope
neuromuscular
- n. disease
- n. disorder
- n. hypertension

neuromyopathic disorder
neuronal ceroid lipofuscinosis
neuropathy
- diabetic n.
- multiplex n.
- peripheral n.

neuropeptide Y
Neuroperfusion pump
neurosis, pl. neuroses
- anxiety n.
- cardiac n.

neurosyphilis
neuroticism
neurotoxic effect
Neuro-Trace instrument
neurotransmitter substance
neurovascular bundle

N

NOTES

neuroxanthoendothelioma
Neutrexin injection
neutropenia
neutropenic angina
neutrophil
  n. elastase
  segmented n.'s
neutrophilia
nevi (*pl. of* nevus)
Neville
  N. stent
  N. tracheal prosthesis
nevirapine
nevus, pl. nevi
  n. araneus
  nevi, atrial myxoma, myxoid
   neurofibromas, and ephelides
   (NAME)
New
  N. Orleans endarterectomy
   stripper
  N. Weavenit Dacron prosthesis
  N. York Heart Association
   (NYHA)
  N. York Heart Association
   classification (I-IV)
newborn
  persistent pulmonary
   hypertension of n. (PPHN)
  transient tachypnea of n.
   (TTNB)
NewLife oxygen concentrator
Newman-Keuls test
Newton
  N. guidewire
  N. law of motion and
   variables
NH
  NH region
  NH region of A-V node
NHANES
  National Health and Nutrition
   Examination Survey
NHLBI
  National Heart, Lung, and Blood
   Institute
Niacels
niacin
NiCad
  nickel-cadmium
nicardipine
  n. hydrochloride

nickel
  salt of n.
nickel-cadmium (NiCad)
  n.-c. battery
Nickerson-Kveim test
nicking
  arteriovenous n.
Nicks procedure
Nicobid
Nicoderm Patch
nicofuranose
Nicoladoni-Branham sign
Nicolar
nicorandil
Nicorette DS Gum
nicotinamide adenine dinucleotide
  (NAD)
2-nicotinamidoethyl nitrate
nicotine
Nicotinex
nicotinic acid
Nicotrol
  N. Patch
NIDDM
  noninsulin-dependent diabetes
   mellitus
nidulans
  Aspergillus n.
nidus
Niemann-Pick disease
nifedipine
  n. enzyme immunoassay
Niferex
NightBird nasal CPAP
nightsweats
night terrors
Niglycon
nigra
  cardiopathia n.
NIH
  N. cardiomarker catheter
  N. marking catheter
Nikaidoh-Bex technique
Nikaidoh translocation
Niko-Fix
Nilstat Topical
NIMBEX
Nimbus hemopump
nimodipine
Nimotop
NI-NR
  no infection-no rejection

nipple
aortic n.
Nipride
NIPS
noninvasive programmed stimulation
NIS
near-infrared spectroscopy
Nisocor
nisoldipine
Nissen 360-degree wrap
fundoplication
niter paper
nitinol
n. mesh stent
n. polymeric compound
n. thermal memory stent
nitrate
long-acting n.
2-nicotinamidoethyl n.
nitrendipine
nitric oxide (NO)
nitrite
amyl n.
sodium n.
Nitro-Bid
N.-B. I.V. injection
N.-B. Ointment
N.-B. Oral
nitroblue tetrazolium
Nitrocap
Nitrocels
Nitrocine
N. Oral
Nitro-Dial
Nitrodisc
N. Patch
Nitro-Dur Patch
Nitrodyl
nitrofurantoin
Nitrogard
N. Buccal
nitrogen (N_2)
blood urea n. (BUN)
n. curve
n. mustard
nitrogen-13 ammonia

nitroglycerin
n. transdermal patch
nitroglycerol
Nitroglyn
N. Oral
nitroimidazole
Nitrol
N. Ointment
Nitrolin
Nitrolingual
N. Translingual Spray
Nitromed
Nitronet
Nitrong
N. Oral Tablet
Nitropress
nitroprusside
n. infusion
sodium n.
n. sodium
nitrosothiol
Nitrospan
Nitrostat
N. Sublingual
Nitro TD
Nitrotym
nitrotyrosine
nitrous oxide
Nitrovas
nitrovasodilator
Nizoral
N. Oral
NK cells
NL3 guider
NMR
nuclear magnetic resonance
NMR relaxometry
NMR spectroscopy
NMRI
nuclear magnetic resonance imaging
NO
nitric oxide
no
n. infection-no rejection (NI-NR)
Nobis aortic occluder

N

NOTES

Nocardia
- *N. asteroides*
- *N. brasiliensis*
- *N. caviae*
- *N. israelii*
- *N. transvalensis*

nocardiosis
nociceptive threshold
nocturia
nocturnal
- n. angina
- n. asthma
- n. dyspnea

nod
- bishop's n.

nodal
- n. arrhythmia
- n. artery
- n. beat
- n. bigeminy
- n. bradycardia
- n. escape
- n. escape rhythm
- n. extrasystole
- n. paroxysmal tachycardia
- n. premature contraction
- n. reentrant tachycardia
- n. tissue

node
- Aschoff-Tawara n.
- atrioventricular n. (AVN)
- A-V n.
- axillary lymph n.'s
- Cruveilhier n.'s
- Delphian n.
- Flack n.
- Fraenkel n.'s
- Heberden n.'s
- His-Tawara n.
- Keith n.
- Keith-Flack n.
- Koch n.
- lymph n.
- mediastinal lymph n.'s
- NH region of A-V n.
- Osler n.
- paratracheal lymph n.'s
- perihilar lymph n.'s
- pretracheal lymph n.'s
- n. of Ranvier
- retropharyngeal lymph n.'s
- S-A n.
- sentinel n.
- shotty n.'s
- singer's n.
- sinus n., sinoatrial n. (SN)
- teacher's n.

nodo-Hisian bypass tract
nodosa
- arteritis n.
- periarteritis n.
- polyarteritis n.

nodose arteriosclerosis
nodosum
- erythema n.

nodoventricular
- n. fiber
- n. tract

nodular
- n. arteriosclerosis
- n. pulmonary amyloidosis
- n. sclerosis
- n. vasculitis

nodule
- acinar n.
- Albini n.'s
- Arantius n.
- Aschoff n.'s
- Bianchi n.'s
- calcified n.
- cold n.
- Morgagni n.'s
- necrobiotic n.
- solitary pulmonary n. (SPN)
- subcutaneous n.
- warm n.

nodus
- n. atrioventricularis
- n. sinuatrialis (NS)
- n. sinuatrialis echo

noisy chest
nolbufine
no-leak technique
Nolex LA
nomatopic stimulus
nomifensine maleate
nomogram
non
- conditio sine qua n.

nonacute total occlusion
nonbacteremic
nonbacterial
- n. thrombotic endocardial lesion

n. thrombotic endocarditis
(NBTE)
n. verrucous endocarditis
noncalcified valve
noncardiac
n. angiography
n. surgery
n. syncope
noncaseating
noncavitary
noncleaved cell lymphoma
noncollagenous pneumoconiosis
noncompensatory pause
noncoronary
n. cusp
n. sinus
nondisjunction
Non-Drowsy
Drixoral N.-D.
nonesterified fatty acid (NEFA)
nonexertional angina
nonexpansional dyspnea
nonflotation catheter
nonflow-directed catheter
nonglycoside inotropic agent
nonhemodynamic effect
non-Hodgkin lymphoma
nonimmunocompromised host
noninhalation
Nonin Onyx pulse oximeter
**noninsulin-dependent diabetes
mellitus (NIDDM)**
nonintegrated
n. transvenous defibrillation
lead
n. tripolar lead
noninvasive
n. assessment
n. evaluation
lower extremity n. (LENI)
n. murmur
n. programmed stimulation
(NIPS)
n. temporary pacemaker
n. test

nonionic
n. contrast material
n. contrast medium
nonischemic dilated cardiomyopathy
nonnecrotizing angiitis
nonocclusive mesenteric ischemia
nonoperative closure
**nonparoxysmal atrioventricular
junctional tachycardia**
nonpenetrating rupture
**nonpharmacologic measure of
treatment**
nonphasic sinus arrhythmia
nonpitting edema
nonpressor doses
**non-Q-wave myocardial infarction
(NQWMI)**
non-rapid eye movement (NREM)
nonrebreathing mask
nonreset nodus sinuatrialis
nonselective coronary angiography
non-sensing
atrial n.-s.
non-small
n.-s. cell carcinoma
n.-s. cell lung cancer
(NSCLC)
nonspecific climatic change
nonsteroidal anti-inflammatory agent
**nonsustained ventricular tachycardia
(NSVT)**
nonthoracotomy
n. defibrillation lead system
n. lead implantable
cardioverter-defibrillator
n. system antitachycardia
device (NTS-AICD)
nonthrombogenic
**nontransmural myocardial infarction
(NTMI)**
nontraumatizing catheter
nontuberculous
**nonuniform rotational defect
(NURD)**
Noonan syndrome
no-phase wrap
No Pour Pak suction catheter kit

NoProfile
N. balloon
N. balloon catheter
noradrenaline
Norcet
Norcuron
Nordach treatment
**Nordenstrom Rotex II biopsy
needle**
**Nordic Enalapril Exercise Trial
(NEET)**
Nordryl Oral
no-reflow phenomenon
norepinephrine
n. bitartrate
n. rometaraminol
n. uptake-1
norethindrone
norfloxacin
Norisodrine
Norlutate
Norlutin
normal
n. electrical axis
n. geometry
n. intravascular pressure
n. sinus rhythm (NSR)
n. vital capacity (NVC)
Normiflo
normocapnia
Normodyne
N. injection
N. Oral
normokinesia
normolipidemic
normomagnesemia
normonatremic
Normotensin
normotension
normotensive
normothermic cardioplegia
normovolemia
Normozide
Noroxin
N. Oral
Norpace
Norpramin
NOR-Q.D.
Norris test
Nor-tet Oral
North
N. American blastomycosis

N. American Symptomatic
Carotid Endarterectomy Trial
(NASCET)
Northwick Park Heart Study
**Norton flow-directed Swan-Ganz
thermodilution catheter**
nortriptyline
n. hydrochloride
Norvasc
norverapamil
Norwalk agent
Norwood
N. operation for hypoplastic
left-sided heart
N. univentricular heart
procedure
Nosema connori
nosocomial
n. endocarditis
n. infection
n. pneumonia
nosocomii
angina n.
nosology
Berlin n.
notch
anacrotic n.
aortic n.
atrial n.
cardiac n.
dicrotic n.
Sibson n.
sternal n.
thyroid n.
notching
midsystolic n.
rib n.
notha
angina n.
peripneumonia n.
Nottingham introducer
Nova
N. II pacemaker
N. MR pacemaker
Novacor
N. DIASYS cardiac device
N. left ventricular assist device
N. left ventricular assist
system
N. LVAD
Novafed

Novametrix
   N. ETCO$_2$ multigas analyzer
   N. pulse oximeter
Novantrone
Novastent stent
novo
   de n.
Novolin 70/30
NovoSeven
Novoste catheter
NoxBOX monitor
NP
   nasopharyngeal
NPH Iletin insulin
N-propanol
NPV
   negative predictive value
NQWMI
   non-Q-wave myocardial infarction
NREM
   non-rapid eye movement
     NREM sleep
NRMI
   National Registry of Myocardial
    Infarction
NS
   nodus sinuatrialis
     NS echo
NSCLC
   non-small cell lung cancer
NSR
   normal sinus rhythm
NSVT
   nonsustained ventricular tachycardia
N-terminal
   N.-t. proANF
   N.-t. proatrial natriuretic factor
NTMI
   nontransmural myocardial infarction
NTS-AICD
   nonthoracotomy system
    antitachycardia device
nuchal rigidity
nuclear
   n. magnetic resonance (NMR)
   n. magnetic resonance imaging
    (NMRI)

   n. pacemaker
   n. probe
   n. ventricular function study
    (NVFS)
nucleatum
   Fusobacterium n.
nucleotides
   total adenine n (TAN)
nucleus, pl. nuclei
   n. tractus solitarius
Nu-Iron
null
   n. hypothesis
   n. point
number
   Reynolds n.
   Strouhal n.
Numed intracoronary Doppler
  catheter
nummular
   n. aortitis
   n. sputum
nun's venous hum murmur
Nuprin
NURD
   nonuniform rotational defect
Nurolon suture
nutcracker esophagus
Nutracort
Nu-Trake Weiss emergency airway
  system
nutrient cardioplegia
Nu-Vois artificial larynx
NVC
   normal vital capacity
NVFS
   nuclear ventricular function study
Nyboer esophageal electrode
Nycore
   N. cardiac device
   N. pigtail catheter
Nydrazid injection
NYHA
   New York Heart Association
Nyomin
Nyquist limit
nystatin

N

NOTES

Nystat-Rx

Nystex Topical

O
O antigen
O point of cardiac apex pulse

O₂
oxygen
AVD O₂
arteriovenous oxygen
difference
hood O₂
O₂ radical
O₂ via nasal cannula

OAD
obstructive airway disease

oakridgensis
Legionella o.

OASIS
Organization to Assess Strategies for
Ischemic Syndromes

oat
o. cell
o. cell carcinoma

obesity
exogenous o.
morbid o.

obesity-hypoventilation syndrome

oblique
left anterior o. (LAO)
right anterior o. (RAO)
o. sinus

obliterans
arteriosclerosis o.
arteritis o.
bronchiolitis o.
bronchitis o.
endarteritis o.
pericarditis o.
phlebitis o.
thromboangiitis o.

obliterating
o. pericarditis
o. phlebitis

obliterative
o. bronchiolitis
o. cardiomyopathy
o. pleuritis

oblongata
medulla o.

O'Brien airway needle

obstruction
airflow o.

airway o.
aortic o.
chronic upper respiratory o.
coronary artery o.
dynamic intracavitary o.
fixed airflow o.
infundibular o.
irreversible airway o.
left ventricular inflow tract o.
left ventricular outflow tract o.
multivessel coronary artery o.
outflow tract o.
pulmonary vascular o.
right ventricular inflow o.
right ventricular outflow o.
stop-valve airway o.
subpulmonary o.
subvalvular o.
upper airway o.
vena cava o.
ventricular inflow tract o.
ventricular outflow tract o.

obstructive
o. airway disease (OAD)
o. atelectasis
o. emphysema
o. hypertrophic cardiomyopathy
o. lung disease
o. murmur
o. pneumonia
o. shock
o. sleep apnea (OSA)
o. thrombus
o. ventilatory defect

obturating embolism

obturator
Fitch o.
Hemaflex PTCA sheath
with o.
Hemaquet PTCA sheath
with o.

obtuse
o. marginal (OM)
o. marginal artery (OMA)
o. marginal branch (OMB)
o. marginal lymphatic

occluder
air clamp inflatable vessel o.
Bard Clamshell septal o.
Brockenbrough curved-tip o.

O

341

occluder *(continued)*
    catheter tip o.
    Clamshell septal o.
    Crile tip o.
    double-disk o.
    Flo-Rester vascular o.
    Hunter detachable balloon o.
    Nobis aortic o.
    tilting-disk o.
    tip o.
occluding thrombus
occlusion
    angioplasty-related vessel o.
    balloon o.
    branch retinal vein o. (BRVO)
    branch vessel o.
    coronary artery o.
    femoral artery o.
    femoral vein o.
    iliac artery o.
    inferior mesenteric vascular o.
    inferior vena cava o.
    intermittent coronary sinus o.
    mesenteric artery o.
    mesenteric vascular o.
    nonacute total o.
    recurrent mesenteric vascular o.
    side branch o.
    superior mesenteric vascular o.
    temporary unilateral pulmonary
      artery o.
    venous mesenteric vascular o.
occlusive
    o. disease
    o. thromboaortopathy
    o. thrombus
occult
    o. pericardial constriction
    o. pericarditis
occupational
    o. asthma
    o. lung disease
Ochrobacterium anthropi
ochrometer
ochronosis
Ochsner-Mahorner
    O.-M. echocardiogram
    O.-M. test
OCT
    optical coherence tomography
octapolar catheter
Octocaine
Octomyces etiennei

octreotide
ocular larva migrans
oculocardiac reflex
oculomucocutaneous syndrome
oculopharyngeal reflex
oculoplethysmography (OPG)
oculopneumoplethysmography
oculovagal reflex
Ocupress Ophthalmic
ODAM defibrillator
odorans
    Alcalgenes o.
odoratus
    Lathyrus o.
O'Dwyer intubation
odynophagia
Oehler symptoms
OEM
    O. 503 humidifier
    O. Venturi MixOMask
Oertel treatment
office
    o. angina
    o. hypertension
ofloxacin
Ogata method
Ohio
    O. Bubble humidifier
    O. critical care ventilator
    O. delux
    O. Hope resuscitator
    O. Vortex respiration monitor
ohm
    O. law
Ohmeda
    O. 6200, 6300 CO_2 monitors
    O. $ETCO_2$ multigas analyzer
    O. hand-held oximeter
    O. pulse oximeter
ohmic heating
ohmmeter
Ohnell
    X wave of O.
OHT
    orthotopic heart transplant
oil
    canola o.
    o. embolism
    fish o.
    MCT O.
    rapeseed o.
    trypsin, balsam peru, and
      castor o.

oil-aspiration pneumonia
ointment
    Nitro-Bid O.
    Nitrol O.
    Whitfield o.
OKT3
    O. antibody
    Orthoclone O.
OKT4A
Olbert
    O. balloon
    O. balloon catheter
Olean
oleate
    ethanolamine o.
olestra
Oligella
oligemia
oligemic
    o. shock
oligonucleotides
oliguria
Oliver-Rosalki method
Oliver sign
olive-tipped needle
olivopontocerebellar atrophy
Olympix II PTCA dilatation
  catheter
Olympus
    O. bioptome
    O. GIF-EUM2 echoendoscope
    O. One-Step Button tube
OM
  obtuse marginal
OM-1
  first obtuse marginal artery
OM-2
  second obtuse marginal artery
OMA
  obtuse marginal artery
OMB
  obtuse marginal branch
Omega 5600 noninvasive blood
  pressure monitor
Omega-NV balloon
omega-3 unsaturated fatty acids

Omni
    O. SST balloon
    O. tract retractor system
Omnicarbon
    O. heart valve prosthesis
    O. prosthetic heart valve
Omnicor
    O. pacemaker
    O. Programmer
Omniflex
    O. balloon
    O. balloon catheter
Omniflox
OmniHIB
Omni-Orthocor pacemaker
Omnipaque
Omnipen
OmniPlane TEE
Omniscience
    O. single leaflet cardiac valve
      prosthesis
    O. tilting-disk valve
    O. tilting-disk valve prosthesis
    O. valve device
Omni-Stanicor pacemaker
omphalitis
omphalocele
omphalomesenteric vein
Omsk hemorrhagic fever
Oncaspar
Oncet
oncology mix
Onconase
oncotic pressure
Oncovin injection
Ondine
    O. curse
    O. curse breathing
one-block claudication
one-flight exertional dyspnea
one-hole angiographic catheter
One Touch blood glucose monitor
one-ventricle heart
onion scale lesion
onychograph
Onyx

O

NOTES

oocytes
    Xenopus o.
opacification
    alveolar o.
    amorphous parenchymal o.
    ground-glass o.
opacify
opacity
    ground-glass o.
    vitreous o.
OPC-18790
open
    o. bronchus sign
    o. chest cardiac massage
    o. heart surgery
    o. lung biopsy
    o. pneumothorax
    o. tuberculosis
Open-Cath
    Abbokinase O.-C.
opening
    o. pressure
    o. snap
operation
    Abbe o.
    Anel o.
    arterial switch o.
    atrial baffle o.
    Babcock o.
    Barnard o.
    Beck I, II o.
    Berger o.
    Blalock-Hanlon o.
    Blalock-Taussig o.
    Brock o.
    Damus-Kaye-Stancel o.
    DKS o.
    Estlander o.
    fenestrated Fontan o.
    Fontan o.
    Freund o.
    Glenn o.
    Goldsmith o.
    Grondahl-Finney o.
    Heller-Belsey o.
    Heller-Nissen o.
    hemi-Fontan o.
    Hunter o.
    Konno o.
    Lindesmith o.
    Mustard o.
    Norwood o. for hypoplastic left-sided heart

    Palma o.
    Potts o.
    Ransohoff o.
    Rastan o.
    Rastelli o.
    Sawyer o.
    second-look o.
    Senning o.
    switch o.
    talc o.
    Tanner o.
    Trendelenburg o.
    Waterston o.
OPG
    oculoplethysmography
OPG-Gee instrument
Ophthalmic
    AK-Chlor O.
    Betimol O.
    Betoptic O.
    Chloroptic O.
    Ciloxan O.
    Gelfilm O.
    Ocupress O.
    Timoptic O.
ophthalmoplegia
ophthalmotonometry
opiate
opioid
Opitz syndrome
opportunistic
    o. infection
    o. pneumonia
opsonin
Opta 5 catheter
optic
    o. atrophy
    o. disk
    o. neuritis
optical
    o. coherence tomography (OCT)
    o. fiber catheter
Opticath oximeter catheter
Optichin disk test
Opti-Flex
OptiHaler drug delivery system
Optima
    O. MP pacemaker
    O. MPT Series III pacemaker
    O. SPT pacemaker
Optimine

Optiray
O. 320
O. contrast
O. contrast medium
Optiscope catheter
Opus
O. cardiac troponin I assay
O. pacemaker
Oracle
O. Focus PTCA catheter
O. Micro intravascular
ultrasound catheter
O. Micro Plus
O. Micro Plus PTCA catheter
oral
Achromycin V O.
Alazine O.
Aller-Chlor O.
AllerMax O.
Altace O.
o. anticoagulant therapy
Apresoline O.
Bactocill O.
Banophen O.
Beepen-VK O.
Belix O.
Benadryl O.
Betapace O.
Betapen-VK O.
Bio-Tab O.
Blocadren O.
Brethine O.
Bricanyl O.
Calm-X O.
o. candidiasis
Cardioquin O.
Cartrol O.
Catapres O.
CeeNU O.
Ceftin O.
Cerespan O.
Chlo-Amine O.
Chlorate O.
Chlor-Trimeton O.
Cipro O.
Compazine O.

o. contraceptive-induced
hypertension
Cortone Acetate O.
Curretab O.
Cycrin O.
Cyklokapron O.
Cytoxan O.
Delta-Cortef O.
Deltasone O.
Demadex O.
Diflucan O.
Dimetabs O.
Dormin O.
Doryx O.
Doxy O.
Doxychel O.
Dramamine O.
Dynacin O.
Edecrin O.
E.E.S. O.
E-Mycin O.
Eryc O.
EryPed O.
Ery-Tab O.
Erythrocin O.
Eryzole O.
Flagyl O.
Floxin O.
Flumadine O.
Gantrisin O.
Genabid O.
Genahist O.
Ilosone O.
Indocin O.
Kerlone O.
Laniazid O.
Lasix O.
Ledercillin VK O.
Lincocin O.
Liquid Pred O.
Marmine O.
Maxaquin O.
Meclomen O.
Medrol O.
Mephyton O.
Meticorten O.
Minocin O.

O

NOTES

oral *(continued)*
Monodox O.
Mycobutin O.
Nitro-Bid O.
Nitrocine O.
Nitroglyn O.
Nizoral O.
Nordryl O.
Normodyne O.
Noroxin O.
Nor-tet O.
Orasone O.
Orinase O.
Oxsoralen-Ultra O.
Panmycin O.
Pavabid O.
Pavased O.
Pavatine O.
Paverolan O.
PCE O.
PediaCare O.
Pediapred O.
Pediazole O.
Penetrex O.
Pen-Vee K O.
Phenameth O.
Phendry O.
Phenergan O.
Phenetron O.
poliovirus vaccine, live,
   trivalent, o.
Prednicen-M O.
Prelone O.
Proglycem O.
Prostaphlin O.
Prothazine O.
Protostat O.
Quinalan O.
Quinora O.
Retrovir O.
Rifadin O.
Rimactane O.
Robicillin VK O.
Robitet O.
Sporanox O.
Sterapred O.
Sumycin O.
Tega-Vert O.
Telachlor O.
Teldrin o.
Teline O.
Terramycin O.
Tetracap O.

Tetralan O.
Tetram O.
Trandate O.
o. tuberculosis
Unipen O.
Uri-Tet O.
Vancocin O.
Vasotec O.
V-Cillin K O.
Veetids O.
VePesid O.
Vibramycin O.
Videx O.
oralis
   Bacteroides o.
Orasone Oral
orciprenaline
order
   4th/5th/6th o. bronchi
Oregon tunneler
Oreopoulos-Zellerman catheter
Oretic
Oreticyl Forte
organic
   o. dust pneumoconiosis
   o. murmur
   o. phosphorus
organism
   Cox o.
   encapsulated o.
   gram-negative o.
   gram-positive o.
   pleuropneumonia-like o. (PPLO)
Organization
   O. to Assess Strategies for
      Ischemic Syndromes (OASIS)
   International Standards O.
      (ISO)
   World Health O. (WHO)
organized thrombus
organs
   Golgi tendon o.
oriental hemoptysis
orifice
   aortic o.
   atrioventricular o.
   cardiac o.
   effective regurgitant o.
   flow across o.
   valvular o.
orificial
   o. stenosis
   o. tuberculosis

origin
anomalous o.
Orimune
Orinase Oral
Orion balloon
Orlowski stent
Ormazine
Ornish
O. diet
O. theory
oroendotracheal tube
oropharyngeal tularemia
oropharynx
orphan
enterocytopathogenic human o. (ECHO)
respiratory and enteric o. (REO)
Orsi-Grocco method
ORT
orthodromic reciprocating tachycardia
orthoarteriotony
orthocardiac reflex
Orthoclone OKT3
Ortho Cytofluorograf 50-H flow cytometer
orthodeoxia
orthodox sleep
orthodromic
o. A-V reentrant tachycardia
o. circus movement tachycardia
o. reciprocating tachycardia (ORT)
orthogonal
o. electrocardiogram
o. lead system
o. plane
o. view
orthograde conduction
Orthomyxoviridae virus
orthopercussion
orthopnea
three-pillow o.
two-pillow o.
orthopneic

orthostatic
o. dyspnea
o. hypertension
o. hypopiesis
o. hypotension
o. syncope
o. tachycardia
orthotopic
o. biventricular artificial heart
o. cardiac transplant
o. heart transplant (OHT)
o. univentricular artificial heart
Orudis
Oruvail
oryzae
Aspergillus o.
Rhizopus o.
OSA
obstructive sleep apnea
Osborne wave
Osciflator balloon inflation syringe
oscillating saw
oscillation
high-frequency o. (HFO)
oscillator
Hayek o.
oscillatory afterpotential
oscillometer
oscilloscope
Oscor
O. atrial lead
O. pacing leads
OSD
Profilate OSD
OSF
outlet strut fracture
Osler
O. node
O. sign
O. triad
Osler-Weber-Rendu
O.-W.-R. disease
O.-W.-R. syndrome
Osmitrol
O. injection
osmolality
osmolarity

O

NOTES

347

osmometer
osmotic
    o. diuretic
    o. pressure
ossification
    pulmonary o.
ossifying pneumonitis
Ossoff-Karlan laryngoscope
osteoarthritis
osteoarthropathy
    hypertrophic pulmonary o.
    pulmonary hypertrophic o.
osteochondroma
osteogenesis imperfecta
osteoplastica
    tracheopathia o.
osteopontin
osteosarcoma
ostia
ostial lesion
ostium, pl. ostia
    coronary o.
    o. primum
    o. primum defect
    o. secundum
    o. secundum defect
    solitary coronary o.
Ostwald viscometer
Osypka
    O. atrial lead
    O. Cereblate electrode
    O. rotational angioplasty
Ototemp 3000
ototoxicity
OTW
    over-the-wire
    OTW perfusion catheter
ouabain
outflow
    o. murmur
    o. tract
    o. tract obstruction
outlet strut fracture (OSF)
output
    cardiac o. (CO)
    Fick cardiac o.
    left ventricular o.
    minute o.
    pacemaker o.
    stroke o.
    thermodilution cardiac o.

ovale
    foramen o.
    patent foramen o. (PFO)
oval foramen
ovalis
    annulus o.
    fossa o.
overdilation
overdrive
    o. pacing
    o. suppression
overflow wave
Overholt-Jackson bronchoscope
Overholt procedure
overinflation
    congenital lobar o.
overlay
    psychogenic o.
overload
    circulatory o.
    diastolic o.
    pressure o.
    volume o.
overreactivity
    physiological o.
override
    aortic o.
overriding aorta
oversampling
oversensing
    afterpotential o.
    o. pacemaker
oversewing
over-the-wire (OTW)
    o.-t.-w. balloon dilatation
        system
    Buchbinder Thruflex o.-t.-w.
    o.-t.-w. probe
    o.-t.-w. PTCA balloon catheter
overventilation
Owens
    O. balloon
    O. balloon catheter
    O. Lo-Profile dilatation
        catheter
Owren
    O. disease
    O. factor V deficiency
oxacillin
    o. sodium
oxalate
    calcium o.
oxalosis

oxalotransaminase
  glutamic o.
oxamniquine
oxandralone
oxazepam
Oxford
  O. Medilog frequency-
    modulated recorder
  O. technique
ox heart
oxidase
  cytochrome c o.
  monoamine o. (MAO)
  xanthine o.
oxidative phosphorylation
oxide
  endothelium-derived nitric o.
  magnesium o.
  nitric o. (NO)
  nitrous o.
oxidized
  o. cellulose
OxiFlow
OxiLink oximeter probe cover
oximeter
  American Optical o.
  BI-OX III ear o.
  Cricket recording pulse o.
  Criticare pulse o.
  ear o.
  Hewlett-Packard ear o.
  Nellcor N200 pulse o.
  Nellcor Symphony N-3000
    pulse o.
  Nonin Onyx pulse o.
  Novametrix pulse o.
  Ohmeda hand-held o.
  Ohmeda pulse o.
  Oxypleth pulse o.
  OxyTemp hand-held pulse o.
  Oxytrak pulse o.
  pulse o.
  SpaceLabs pulse o.
  SpotCheck+ hand-held pulse o.
oximetric catheter
Oximetrix 3 System

oximetry
  CO o.
  CO_2 o.
  finger o.
  Hb o.
  $HbCO_2$ o.
  HbO_2 o.
  N_2 o.
  oxygen saturation as measured
    using pulse o. (SpO_2)
  PCO_2 o.
  PO_2 o.
  reflectance o.
  spectrophotometric o.
oxotremorine
oxprenolol
Oxsoralen Topical
Oxsoralen-Ultra Oral
oxtriphylline
Oxycel
Oxycure topical oxygen system
Oxyfill oxygen refilling system
oxygen (O_2)
  blood o.
  blow-by o.
  o. consumption (VO_2)
  o. consumption index
  o. consumption per minute
    (VO_2)
  o. content
  o. cost
  o. debt
  o. delivery
  o. dissociation curve
  fraction of inspired o. (FIO_2)
  humidified o.
  hyperbaric o.
  o. inhalation
  o. mask
  o. paradox
  partial pressure of o. (PO_2)
  o. radical
  o. radical scavenger
  o. saturation
  o. saturation as measured
    using pulse oximetry (SpO_2)

O

NOTES

oxygen *(continued)*
  o. saturation of the
    hemoglobin of arterial blood
  o. step-up method
  o. tension
  o. tent
  o. therapy
  T-piece o.
  o. transport
  o. uptake
oxygen-15
oxygenation
  bubble o.
  disk o.
  extracorporeal membrane o.
    (ECMO)
  film o.
  hyperbaric o.
  pump o.
  rotating disk o.
  screen o.
oxygenator
  Bentley o.
  bubble o.
  Capiox-E bypass system o.
  Cobe Optima hollow-fiber
    membrane o.
  DeBakey heart pump o.
  disk o.
  extracorporeal membrane o.
  extracorporeal pump o.
  Gambro o.
  intravascular o. (IVOX)
  Lilliput o.

  Maxima Plus plasma resistant
    fiber o.
  Monolyth o.
  plasma-resistant fiber o. (PRF)
  pump o.
  Sarns membrane o. (SMO)
oxygen-binding capacity
oxygen-carrying
  o.-c. capacity
  o.-c. perfluorochemical liquid
oxygen-diffusing capacity
oxyhemoglobin (HbO$_2$)
  o. dissociation curve
Oxy-Hood pressurizer
OxyLead interconnect cable
Oxylite
Oxymax
Oxymizer
  O. device
Oxypleth pulse oximeter
oxypurinol
oxysterol inhibitor
OxyTemp hand-held pulse oximeter
oxytetracycline
  o. hydrochloride
OxyTip
  O. sensor
oxytoca
  Klebsiella o.
Oxytrak pulse oximeter
**Oxy-Ultra-Lite ambulatory oxygen
system**
oyster mass of mucus

P

P cell
P congenitale
P loop
P mitrale
P terminal force
P vector
P wave
P wave amplitude
P wave axis
P wave triggered ventricular pacemaker

p24

p. antigen
p. antigen test

P-A

P-A conduction time
P-A interval

PA

pulmonary artery
PA banding
PA filling pressure
PA 120 Osypka radiofrequency probe
PA Watch position-monitoring catheter

P&A

percussion and auscultation

pAAT

plasma alpha 1-antitrypsin

PAC

premature atrial contraction

Paceart complete pacemaker patient testing system

paced

p. cycle length
p. rhythm
p. ventricular evoked response

Pacejector

pacemaker

AAI p.
AAT p.
Accufix p.
Acculith p.
Activitrax II p.
activity-sensing p.
p. adaptive rate
AEC p.
Aequitron p.
AFP II p.

p. afterpotential
AICD-B p.
AICD-BR p.
Alcatel p.
American Optical Cardiocare p.
American Optical R-inhibited p.
p. amplifier refractory period
Amtech-Killeen p.
antitachycardia p. (ATP)
AOO p.
Arco atomic p.
Arco lithium p.
p. artifact
artificial p.
Arzco p.
Astra T4, T6 p.
atrial asynchronous p.
atrial demand-inhibited p.
atrial demand-triggered p.
atrial synchronous ventricular inhibited p.
atrial tracking p.
atrial triggered ventricular-inhibited p.
atrial VOO p.
Atricor Cordis p.
atrioventricular sequential p.
Aurora dual-chamber p.
Autima II dual-chamber p.
automatic p.
p. automaticity
Avius sequential p.
A-V sequential p.
A-V synchronous p.
Axios 04 p.
Basix p.
Betacel-Biotronik p.
bifocal demand DVI p.
Biorate p.
Biotronik p.
bipolar p.
breathing p.
p. burst pacing
Byrel SX p.
Byrel-SX/Versatrax p.
p. capture
cardiac p.
Cardio-Pace Medical Durapulse p.

P

pacemaker *(continued)*
p. catheter
Chardack-Greatbatch p.
Chardack Medtronic p.
Chorus DDD p.
Chorus RM rate-responsive
  dual-chamber p.
Chronocor IV external p.
Chronos 04 p.
Circadia dual-chamber rate-
  adaptive p.
Classix p.
p. code system
Command PS p.
committed mode p.
Cook p.
Coratomic R wave inhibited p.
Cordis Atricor p.
Cordis Chronocor IV p.
Cordis Ectocor p.
Cordis fixed-rate p.
Cordis Gemini cardiac p.
Cordis Multicor p.
Cordis Omni Stanicor Theta
  transvenous p.
Cordis Sequicor cardiac p.
Cordis Stanicor unipolar
  ventricular p.
Cordis Synchrocor p.
Cordis Ventricor p.
Cosmos 283 DDD p.
Cosmos II DDD p.
Cosmos pulse-generator p.
CPI Astra p.
CPI DDD p.
CPI Maxilith p.
CPI Microthin DI, DII
  lithium-powered
  programmable p.
CPI Minilith p.
CPI Ultra II p.
CPI Vista-T p.
cross-talk p.
Cyberlith p.
Cybertach automatic-burst
  atrial p.
Cybertach 60 bipolar p.
Daig ESI-II or DSI-III screw-
  in lead p.
Dart p.
Dash single-chamber rate-
  adaptic p.
Delta TRS p.

demand p.
Devices, Ltd. p.
Dialog p.
Diplos M 05 p.
Dromos p.
dual-chamber p.
dual-demand p.
Durapulse p.
ECT p.
Ectocor p.
ectopic p.
Ela Chorus DDD p.
Elecath p.
electric cardiac p.
p. electrodes
electronic p.
Elema p.
Elema-Schonander p.
Elevath p.
Elite p.
Encor p.
end-of-life p.
Enertrax 7100 p.
Ergos O_2 dual-chamber rate-
  responsive p.
escape p.
p. escape interval
external p.
p. failure
fixed-rate p.
fully automatic p.
Galaxy p.
Gemini DDD p.
Gen2 p.
Genisis p.
Guardian p.
Hancock bipolar balloon p.
p. hysteresis
p. impedance
Intermedics Stride p.
Intertach p.
Kalos p.
Kantrowitz p.
Kelvin Sensor p.
p. lead fracture
p. leads
Legend p.
Leukos p.
lithium p.
Maestro implantable cardiac p.
p. malfunction
Mallory RM-1 cell p.
Medtel p.

Medtronic Activitrax rate-
responsive unipolar
ventricular p.
Medtronic Elite DDDR p.
Medtronic Elite II p.
Medtronic RF 5998 p.
Medtronic SP 502 p.
Medtronic SPO p.
Medtronic temporary p.
Medtronic Thera "i-series"
cardiac p.
Meta II p.
Meta MV p.
Meta rate-responsive p.
Microlith P p.
Micro Minix p.
Microthin P2 p.
migrating p.
Mikros p.
Minix p.
Minuet DDD p.
Multicor II cardiac p.
Multilith p.
Nanos 01 p.
Neos M p.
noninvasive temporary p.
Nova II p.
Nova MR p.
nuclear p.
Omnicor p.
Omni-Orthocor p.
Omni-Stanicor p.
Optima MP p.
Optima MPT Series III p.
Optima SPT p.
Opus p.
p. output
oversensing p.
Paragon II p.
PASAR tachycardia
reversion p.
PDx pacing and diagnostic p.
pervenous p.
phantom p.
Phoenix 2 p.
Phymos 3D p.
Pinnacle p.

p. pocket
PolyFlex p.
p. potential
Precept DR p.
Prima p.
Prism-CL p.
Programalith III p.
programmable p.
Programmer III p.
Prolog p.
Pulsar NI implantable p.
P wave triggered ventricular p.
Q-T interval sensing p.
Quantum p.
rate-modulated p.
rate-responsive p.
p. reedswitch
Reflex 8220 p.
refractory period of
electronic p.
Relay cardiac p.
Seecor p.
p. sensitivity
Sensolog II, III p.
Sensor p.
Sequicor III p.
shifting p.
Siemens-Elema p.
Solus p.
p. sound
Spectrax SX, SX-HT, SXT,
VL, VM, VS p.
p. spike
Stanicor p.
Stride cardiac p.
subsidiary atrial p.
Swing DR1 DDDR p.
Symbios 7006 p.
Synchrony I, II p.
p. syndrome
Synergyst DDD p.
Synergyst II p.
Tachylog p.
temperature-sensing p.
Thermos p.
p. threshold
transthoracic p.

NOTES

P

pacemaker *(continued)*
  Trios M p.
  Triumph VR p.
  p. undersensing
  Unilith p.
  Unity-C cardiac p.
  Unity VDDR p.
  universal p.
  VAT p.
  Ventak AICD p.
  ventricular asynchronous p.
  ventricular demand-inhibited p.
  ventricular demand-triggered p.
  Versatrax II 7000A p.
  Vicor p.
  Vista 4, T, TRS p.
  Vitatron Diamond p.
  VOO p.
  VVD mode p.
  VVI p.
  VVIR p.
  wandering p.
  Zoll NTP noninvasive p.
pacemaker-mediated tachycardia (PMT)
Paceport catheter
pacer
  Intertach II p.
Pacer-Tracer
pace-terminable
pace-terminate
Pacewedge dual-pressure bipolar pacing catheter
Pachon
  P. method
  P. test
pacing
  AAI p.
  AAI-RR p.
  AAT p.
  antitachycardia p.
  AOO p.
  asynchronous p.
  atrial overdrive p.
  atrial train p.
  autodecremental p.
  burst atrial p.
  p. catheter
  p. code
  p. cycle length
  DDD p.
  DDDR p.
  DDI p.

DDIR p.
decremental atrial p.
diaphragmatic p.
dual-chamber p.
DVI p.
p. hysteresis
implantable cardioverter-defibrillator/atrial tachycardia p. (ICD-ATP)
incremental atrial p.
incremental ventricular p.
inhibited p.
intracardiac p.
p. modalities
overdrive p.
pacemaker burst p.
permanent p.
ramp p.
rapid atrial p.
rapid-burst p.
rate-responsive p.
p. stimulus
p. system analyzer
temporary p.
p. threshold
threshold p.
trains of ventricular p.
transatrial p.
transesophageal atrial p. (TAP, TEAP)
transesophageal echocardiography with p. (TEEP)
triggered p.
underdrive p.
VAT p.
VDD p.
ventricular p.
VOO p.
VVI p.
VVIR p.
VVI-RR p.
VVI/VVIR p.
VVT p.
pacing-induced angina
pack-year smoking history
pack-years of smoking
PaCO$_2$
  arterial partial pressure of CO$_2$
PAD
  peripheral arterial disease
  pulsatile assist device

pad
electrode p.
Littman defibrillation p.
pericardial fat p.
p. sign
Signa P.
SomaSensor p.
paddles
anteroposterior p.
cardioversion p.
defibrillation p.
defibrillator p.
electrode p.
Paecilomyces
P. variotii
PAF
paroxysmal atrial fibrillation
platelet activating factor
Page episodic hypertension
Paget
P. disease
P. disease of bone
Paget-Schroetter venous thrombosis
Paget-von Schrötter syndrome
PAI
plasminogen activator inhibitor
PAI-1
plasminogen activator inhibitor-1
pain
atypical chest p.
chest p.
crushing chest p.
dream p.
functional p.
musculoskeletal p.
phantom p.
pleuritic chest p.
psychogenic p.
pulmonary p.
rest p.
staccato p.
pain-free walking time (PFWT)
pain, pallor, paraesthesia, pulselessness, paralysis, prostration (PPPPPP)
paired
p. beats

p. electrical stimulation
p. *t* test
PAK
percutaneous access kit
Denver PAK
palatopharyngeal sphincter
pale
p. hypertension
p. thrombus
paleopneumoniae
Peptostreptococcus p.
palestinensis
Acanthamoeba p.
palisading
palisading histiocyte
palliation
palliative
p. surgery
pallida
asphyxia p.
pallidum
microhemagglutination
Treponema p. (MHA-TP)
Treponema p.
pallor
palm
liver p.
tripe p.
Palma operation
palmar
p. arch
p. erythema
p. xanthoma
palmare
xanthoma striatum p.
Palmaz
P. balloon-expandable iliac stent
P. vascular stent
Palmaz-Schatz (PS)
P.-S. balloon-expandable stent
P.-S. coronary stent
palmi (*pl. of* palmus)
palmic
palmitate
C-11 p.

NOTES

palmitate *(continued)*
  clofazimine p.
  colfosceril p.
palmitic acid
palmitoylcarnitine
palmodic
palmoscopy
palmus, pl. palmi
palpation
  bimanual precordial p.
palpitatio cordis
palpitation
  paroxysmal p.
  premonitory p.
PAM2, PAM3 monitors
Pamelor
PAMI
  Primary Angioplasty in Myocardial
  Infarction
pamoate
  pyrantel p.
Panacet 5/500
panacinar emphysema
pancarditis
panchamber enlargement
Pancoast syndrome
panconduction defect
pancreas
pancreatic
  p. extract
  p. polypeptide (PP)
pancreatitis
pancuronium
  p. bromide
pandiastolic
panel
  Cholestech LDX system with
  TC and Glucose P.
  lipid p.
  South Florida RAST p.
  thyroid p.
pang
  breast p.
Panhematin
panic disorder
paninspiratory
Panje voice button
panlobular emphysema
Panmycin Oral
panniculitis
panning
panophthalmitis

pansystolic
  p. flow
  p. murmur
pantaloon
  p. embolism
  p. patch
pantothenate synthetase
pants
  MAST p.
pantyhose
  Glattelast compression p.
Panwarfin
panzerherz
PAO$_2$
  alveolar oxygen partial pressure
PaO$_2$
  arterial oxygen partial pressure
PAOP
  pulmonary artery occlusion pressure
PAP
  positive airway pressure
  pulmonary artery pressure
papain
Papanicolaou solution
papaverine
  p. hydrochloride
paper
  asthma p.
  niter p.
Papercuff
papilla
  Bergmeister p.
papillary
  p. adenocarcinoma
  p. carcinoma
  p. fibroelastoma
  p. muscle
  p. muscle abscess
  p. muscle dysfunction
  p. muscle syndrome
  p. muscle tip
  p. tumor
papilledema
papillitis
papillomatosis
  recurrent respiratory p.
papillomavirus
  human p. (HPV)
papillotome
  Wilson-Cook p.
papulonecrotic tuberculosis
papulosis
  atrophic p.

PAPVD
partial anomalous pulmonary venous drainage
PAPVR
partial anomalous pulmonary venous return
paraaminobenzoic acid
paraaminosalicylate sodium
paraaminosalicylic acid (PAS, PASA)
para-aortic bodies
paracentesis
p. pericardii
p. thoracis
paracetamol sensitivity
parachute
p. deformity
p. mitral valve
paracicatricial emphysema
Paracoccidioides brasiliensis
paracoccidioidin skin test
paracoccidioidomycosis
paracorporeal heart
paracrine
paradox
calcium p.
French p.
p. image
oxygen p.
thoracoabdominal p.
paradoxic
p. rocking impulse
p. split of S_2
p. wall motion
paradoxical
p. cerebral embolism
p. embolization
p. embolus
p. pulse
p. respiration
paradoxically split S_2 sound
paradoxus
p. parvus et tardus
pulsus p.
paraesophageal hernia
paraffin block
paraffinoma

paraganglioma
p. tumor
Paragon II pacemaker
paragonimiasis
Paragonimus westermani
parahaemolyticus
Haemophilus p.
Vibrio p.
parainfluenza
p. virus
parainfluenzae
Haemophilus p.
parallel shunt
paralysis
diphtheric p., diphtheritic p.
ischemic p.
periodic p.
phrenic nerve p.
respiratory p.
tick p.
vasomotor p.
Volkmann ischemic p.
paralytica
dysphagia p.
paralytic chest
paralyticus
laryngismus p.
thorax p.
paramagnetic substance
paramedian
paramedic
parameters
systemic hemodynamic p.
paramethasone acetate
parametric
p. image
p. imaging
Paramyxoviridae virus
paraplane echocardiography
Paraplatin
parapneumonic effusion
parapsilosis
Candida p.
paraquat
pararrhythmia
parasagittal plane
paraseptal emphysema

NOTES

P

parasitic
    p. cardiomyopathy
    p. infestation
parasternal
    p. examination
    p. heave
    p. long-axis view
    p. long-axis view
      echocardiogram
    p. short-axis view
    p. short-axis view
      echocardiogram
    p. systolic lift
    p. systolic thrill
    p. view
parasympathetic
    p. function
    p. nerve fibers
    p. nervous system
parasympathomimetic
parasystole
    pure p.
parasystolic
    p. beat
    p. ventricular tachycardia
parathyroid hormone
paratracheal
    p. chain
    p. lymph nodes
    p. region
paravalvular
parchemin
    bruit de p.
parchment heart
parenchyma
parenchymal
    p. amyloidosis
    p. fibrosis
parenchymatous
    p. myocarditis
    p. pneumonia
Parenteral
    Coly-Mycin M P.
pargyline
    methyclothiazide and p.
Parham bands
parietal
    p. endocarditis
    p. pericardiectomy
    p. pericardium
    p. pleura
    p. thrombus
parieto-occipital artery

Park
    P. aneurysm
    P. blade septostomy catheter
Parlodel
parnaparin
paromomycin sulfate
paroxysm
    p. of coughing
paroxysmal
    p. atrial fibrillation (PAF)
    p. atrial tachycardia (PAT)
    p. burst
    p. cough
    p. junctional tachycardia
    p. nocturnal dyspnea (PND)
    p. nocturnal hemoglobinuria
      (PNH)
    p. nodal tachycardia
    p. palpitation
    p. pulmonary edema
    p. reentrant supraventricular
      tachycardia
    p. sinus tachycardia
    p. sleep
    p. supraventricular arrhythmia
    p. supraventricular tachycardia
      (PSVT)
    p. ventricular tachycardia
parrot
    p. fever
    P. murmur
pars membranacea
Parsonnet
    P. coronary probe
    P. pulse generator pouch
partial
    p. anomalous pulmonary
      venous drainage (PAPVD)
    p. anomalous pulmonary
      venous return (PAPVR)
    p. atrioventricular canal
    p. encircling endocardial
      ventriculotomy
    p. heart block
    p. intermixed fibrosis
    p. liquid ventilation
    p. occlusion inferior vena cava
      clip
    p. pressure of carbon dioxide
      (PCO_2)
    p. pressure of CO gas (PCO)
    p. pressure of CO_2 gas
    p. pressure of oxygen (PO_2)

p. rebreathing mask
p. thromboplastin time (PTT)
particle
Amberlite p.'s
Dane p.'s
partitioning
left atrial p.
parts per million (ppm)
Partuss LA
parvus
p. alternans
p. et tardus pulse
pulsus p.
Parzen window
PAS
paraaminosalicylic acid
peripheral access system
PAS port
PASA
paraaminosalicylic acid
PASAR tachycardia reversion pacemaker
PASG
pneumatic antishock garment
P.A.S. Port
P. P. catheter
P. P. Fluoro-Free
passage
adiabatic fast p.
passive
p. clot
p. congestion
p. edema
p. hyperemia
p. interval
p. mode
p. smoking
passover humidifier
Passy-Muir tracheostomy speaking valve
paste
electrode p.
Pasteurella
P. aerogenes
P. multocida
pasteurellosis

PAT
paroxysmal atrial tachycardia
patch
autologous pericardial p.
cardiac p.
Carrel p.
Dacron intracardiac p.
defibrillation p.
Deponit P.
electrodispersive skin p.
epicardial defibrillator p.
Gore-Tex cardiovascular p.
Habitrol P.
Ionescu-Shiley pericardial p.
MacCallum p.
Minitran P.
Nicoderm P.
Nicotrol P.
Nitrodisc P.
Nitro-Dur P.
nitroglycerin transdermal p.
pantaloon p.
pericardial p.
Peyer p.
polypropylene intracardiac p.
ProStep P.
sandwich p.
soldier's p.'s
Teflon intracardiac p.
Transdermal-NTG P.
Transderm-Nitro P.
patch-graft
p.-g. angioplasty
Dacron onlay p.-g.
patchplasty
patchy
p. atelectasis
p. infiltrate
p. infiltration
Patella disease
patency
catheter p.
epicardial vessel p.
probe p.
PATENT
Prourokinase and t-PA Enhancement of Thrombolysis

NOTES

P

359

patent
>p. bronchus sign
>p. ductus arteriosus (PDA)
>p. ductus arteriosus murmur
>p. ductus arteriosus umbrella
>p. foramen ovale (PFO)

Pathfinder catheter
Pathocil
pathogenesis
pathogenicity
pathologic murmur
pathology
>coexistent p.

pathophysiology
pathostimulation
pathway
>accessory p.
>antegrade internodal p.
>anterior internodal p.
>atrio-His p.
>atrioventricular node p.'s
>Bachmann p.
>conduction p.
>diacylglycerate p.
>fast p.
>final common p.
>internodal p.'s
>Kent p.
>reentrant p.
>retrograde fast p.
>scavenger cell p.
>selective past p.
>septal p.
>shunt p.
>slow A-V node p.
>Thorel p.

patient compliance
patient-controlled analgesic (PCA)
Patil stereotactic system
pattern
>ballerina-foot p.
>cephalization of pulmonary
>>flow p.
>circadian p.
>contraction p.
>crochetage p.
>deer-antler vascular p.
>dip-and-plateau p.
>eggshell p.
>fishnet p.
>ground-glass p.
>hourglass p.
>intraventricular conduction p.

>juvenile p.
>Poincar plot p.
>QR p.
>QS p.
>respiratory p.
>reticular p.
>sawtooth p.
>scintillating speckle p.
>sine-wave p.
>torpedo-shaped p.
>uptake-mismatch p.
>vascular p.
>W p.

patty
>cottonoid p.

pause
>compensatory p.
>noncompensatory p.
>postextrasystolic p.
>preautomatic p.
>sinus exit p.

pause-dependent arrhythmia
PAV
>proportional assist ventilation

Pavabid Oral
Pavased Oral
Pavatine Oral
pavementing
Paverolan Oral
Pavlov reflex
PAVM
>pulmonary arteriovenous
>>malformation

Pavulon
PAW
>pulmonary artery wedge

PAWP
>pulmonary artery wedge pressure

Paykel scale
PBC
>perfusion balloon catheter

PBP
>percutaneous balloon pericardiotomy

PBV
>pulmonary blood volume

PBZ
>Pyribenzamine

PC
>posterior circumflex artery

PCA
>patient-controlled analgesic
>PCA system

PCBS
    percutaneous cardiopulmonary
      bypass support
PCD
    programmable cardioverter-
      defibrillator
      Jewel PCD
      PCD Transvene implantable
        cardioverter-defibrillator system
PCE Oral
PCIRV
    pressure-controlled inverse ratio
      ventilation
PCNA
    proliferating cell nuclear antigen
PCO
    partial pressure of CO gas
PCO$_2$
    partial pressure of carbon dioxide
      PCO$_2$ oximetry
P congenitale
PCP
    Pneumocystis carinii pneumonia
PCPB
    percutaneous cardiopulmonary
      bypass
PCPS
    percutaneous cardiopulmonary
      support
PCR
    polymerase chain reaction
      PCR assay
PCRA
    percutaneous coronary rotational
      atherectomy
PCS
    proximal coronary sinus
PCWP
    pulmonary capillary wedge pressure
PD
    postural drainage
PDA
    patent ductus arteriosus
    posterior descending artery
      PDA umbrella
PDB preperitoneal distention
balloon system

PDE
    phosphodiesterase inhibitor
      PDE isoenzyme inhibitor
P-dextrocardiale
PDF
    probability density function
PDGF
    platelet-derived growth factor
PD&P
    postural drainage and percussion
PDT
    percutaneous dilational tracheostomy
      PDT guidewire
PDx pacing and diagnostic
pacemaker
PE
      PE Plus II peripheral balloon
      catheter
PE-60-I-2 implantable pronged
unipolar electrode
PE-60-K-10 implantable unipolar
endocardial electrode
PE-60-KB implantable unipolar
endocardial electrode
PE-85-I-2 implantable pronged
unipolar electrode
PE-85-K-10 implantable unipolar
endocardial electrode
PE-85-KB implantable unipolar
endocardial electrode
PE-85-KS-10 implantable unipolar
endocardial electrode
PEA
    pulseless electrical activity
peak
      p. A velocity
      p. diastolic filling rate
      p. emptying rate
      p. E velocity
      p. exercise
      p. exercise oxygen
        consumption (VO$_2$)
      p. expiratory flow (PEF)
      p. expiratory flow rate (PEFR)
      p. filling rate (PFR)
      p. flow meter
      p. flowmeter

NOTES

P

peak *(continued)*
    h p.
    p. incidence
    p. inspiratory flow (PIF)
    p. inspiratory flow rate (PIFR)
    p. instantaneous gradient
    p. jet flow rate
    p. magnitude
    p. systolic aortic pressure
     (PSAP)
    p. systolic gradient (PSG)
    p. systolic gradient pressure
    p. systolic velocity
    p. tidal inspiratory flow (PTIF)
    p. transaortic valve gradient
    p. and trough
    p. twitch force
    p. work load
peaked P wave
peak and trough levels
PEAP
    positive end-airway pressure
pearls
    Laennec p.
pear-shaped heart
Pearson-Clopper value
Pearson correlation coefficient
peau d'orange
pectoral
    p. fremitus
    p. heart
    p. tea
pectoralgia
pectoralis
    p. major
    p. minor
pectoriloquous bronchophony
pectoriloquy
    aphonic p.
    whispering p.
pectoris
    angina p.
    angor p.
    variant angina p.
pectorophony
pectus
    p. carinatum
    p. excavatum
    p. gallinatum
    p. recurvatum
pedal
    p. edema
    p. pulse

pedal-mode ergometer
PediaCare Oral
Pediapred Oral
pediatric
    p. cardiomyopathy
    Cleocin P.
    Exosurf P.
    Fedahist Expectorant P.
    p. hypertension
    p. pigtail catheter
    Robitussin P.
Pediazole Oral
pedicle graft
Pedi-Dri
Pedoff continuous wave transducer
pedunculated thrombus
PedvaxHIB
peel
    pericardial p.
    pleural p.
    visceral p.
Peel-Away
    P.-A. catheter
    P.-A. introducer set
peeling-back mechanism
PEEP
    positive end-expiratory pressure
    PEEP valve
Peep-Keep II adapter
PEF
    peak expiratory flow
pefloxacin
PEFR
    peak expiratory flow rate
PEG-ADA
    pegademase bovine
pegademase bovine (PEG-ADA)
pegaspargase
PEG interleukin-2
Pelger-Huet cells
pellagra
Pelorus stereotactic system
Pemco prosthetic valve
PE-MT balloon dilatation catheter
pen
    light p.
Penaz volume-clamp method
penbutolol
    p. sulfate
penciclovir
pencil percussion
Penderluft syndrome
pendulous heart

pendulum
    cor p.
    p. rhythm
penetrating
    p. injury
    p. rupture
penetration
Penetrex Oral
penicillin
    benzathine benzyl p.
    p. g
    p. g benzathine
    p. g benzathine and procaine
      combined
    p. g, parenteral, aqueous
    p. g procaine
    p. phenoxymethyl
    semisynthetic p.
    p. VK
    p. v potassium
Penicillium
penile-brachial pressure index
Penlon infant resuscitator
Penn
    P. Convention criteria
    P. method
    P. State TAH
    P. State total artificial heart
    P. State ventricular assist
      device
Pentacarinat injection
PentaCath catheter
Pentacef
pentachrome
    Movat p.
pentaerythritol tetranitrate
pentalogy
    Cantrell p.
    p. of Fallot, Fallot p.
Pentalumen catheter
Pentam-300 injection
pentamidine
    p. in aerosol form
    aerosolized p.
    p. isethionate
PentaPace QRS catheter
Pentatrichomonas hominis

Pentax bronchoscope
pentazocine
pentetate
    imciromab p.
pentobarbital
Pentothal
    P. Sodium
pentoxifylline
Pen.Vee K Oral
PEP
    positive expiratory pressure
    preejection period
    PEP mask
peppermint test
peptic
    p. aspiration pneumonitis
    p. esophagitis
    p. ulcer
peptide
    adrenomedullin p.
    atrial natriuretic p.
    brain natriuretic p. (BNP)
    calcitonin gene-related p.
    C-type natriuretic p. (CNP)
    human atrial natriuretic p.
      (hANP)
    natriuretic p.
    procollagen type III
      aminoterminal p. (PIIIP)
    tick anticoagulant p.
    vasoactive intestinal p.'s (VIP)
    vasoconstrictor p.
peptidoglycan
peptidomimetic
Peptococcus
    P. constellatus
Peptostreptococcus
    P. anaerobius
    P. asaccharolyticus
    P. evolutus
    P. paleopneumoniae
    P. prevotii
    P. productus
    P. saccharolyticus
per
    p. primam healing
    p. primam intentionem

NOTES

P

per *(continued)*
  p. secondam healing
  p. secondam intentionem
Per-C-Cath
perceived exertion
perchloric acid
Percor-Stat-DL catheter
PercuCut biopsy needle
PercuGuide
percussion
  p. and auscultation (P&A)
  chest p.
  coin p.
  p. dullness
  fist p.
  Goldscheider p.
  Murphy p.
  pencil p.
  piano p.
  Plesch p.
  p. and postural drainage
  (P&PD)
  postural drainage and p.
  (PD&P)
  slapping p.
  p. sound
  strip p.
  tangential p.
  threshold p.
  p. wave
percussor
  G5 Neocussor p.
percutaneous
  p. access kit (PAK)
  p. approach
  p. balloon angioplasty
  p. balloon aortic valvuloplasty
  p. balloon mitral valvuloplasty
  p. balloon pericardiotomy
  (PBP)
  p. balloon pulmonic
  valvuloplasty
  p. brachial sheath
  p. cardiopulmonary bypass
  (PCPB)
  p. cardiopulmonary bypass
  support (PCBS)
  p. cardiopulmonary support
  (PCPS)
  p. catheter insertion
  p. catheter introducer kit
  p. coronary rotational
  atherectomy (PCRA)

  p. cutting needle
  p. dilational tracheostomy
  (PDT)
  p. intra-aortic balloon
  counterpulsation
  p. intra-aortic balloon
  counterpulsation catheter
  p. left heart bypass (PLHB)
  p. mitral balloon
  commissurotomy (PMBC)
  p. mitral balloon valvotomy
  (PMBV)
  p. mitral balloon valvuloplasty
  (PMBV)
  p. mitral commissurotomy
  (PMC)
  p. mitral valvuloplasty (PMV)
  p. needle biopsy
  p. patent ductus arteriosus
  closure
  p. radiofrequency catheter
  ablation
  p. rotational thrombectomy
  (PRT)
  p. rotational thrombectomy
  catheter
  p. technique
  p. transatrial mitral
  commissurotomy
  p. transhepatic cardiac
  catheterization
  p. transluminal angioscopy
  (PTAS)
  p. transluminal balloon
  valvuloplasty
  p. transluminal coronary
  angioplasty (PTCA)
  p. transluminal coronary
  revascularization (PTCR)
  p. transtracheal bronchography
  p. transvenous mitral
  commissurotomy (PTMC)
  p. tunnel
peregrinum
  Mycobacterium p.
perennial allergic rhinitis
Perez sign
**Per-fit percutaneous tracheostomy
  kit**
perflubron
**perfluorocarbon-exposed sonicated
  dextrose albumin (PESDA)**
perforating arteries

perforation
    cardiac p.
    guidewire p.
    myocardial p.
    septal p.
    ventricular p.
perforator
    gaiter p.'s
    septal p.
performance
    cardiac p.
    left ventricular systolic p.
    ventricular p.
perfringens
    Clostridium p.
perfusion
    p. balloon catheter (PBC)
    p. bed
    blood p.
    cardiac p.
    cerebral p.
    p. defect
    isolated heat p.
    mosaic p.
    myocardial p.
    p. pressure
    root p.
    p. scintigraphy
    splanchnic bed p.
    stuttering of p.
perfusion/ventilation
periaccretio pericardii
Periactin
periaortic abscess
periapical
periarteritis nodosa
peribronchial
    p. cuffing
    p. desquamation
    p. fibrosis
    p. pneumonia
pericarbon bioprosthesis
pericardectomy
pericardia (*pl. of* pericardium)
pericardiac tumor
pericardial
    p. baffle

    p. basket
    p. biopsy
    p. calcification
    p. cyst
    p. disease
    p. ccho
    p. effusion
    p. fat pad
    p. flap
    p. fluid
    p. fremitus
    p. friction rub
    p. friction sound
    p. knock
    p. lavage
    p. murmur
    p. patch
    p. peel
    p. poudrage
    p. pressure
    p. reflex
    p. sac
    p. sling
    p. tamponade
    p. tap
    p. teratoma
    p. well
    p. window
pericardicentesis
pericardiectomy
    parietal p.
    visceral p.
pericardii
    accretio p.
    concretio p.
    hydrops p.
    paracentesis p.
    periaccretio p.
    synechia p.
pericardiocentesis
pericardiophrenic artery
pericardioplasty in pectus
    excavatum repair
pericardiorrhaphy
pericardioscopy
pericardiosternal ligament
pericardiostomy

NOTES

P

365

pericardiotomy
   percutaneous balloon p. (PBP)
   p. scissors
   subxiphoid limited p.
pericarditic
pericarditis
   acute fibrinous p.
   adhesive p.
   amebic p.
   bacterial p.
   calcific p.
   p. calculosa
   p. callosa
   carcinomatous p.
   cholesterol p.
   chronic constrictive p.
   constrictive p.
   drug-associated p.
   drug-induced p.
   dry p.
   effusive-constrictive p.
   p. epistenocardica
   fibrinous p.
   fibrous p.
   gram-negative p.
   hemorrhagic p.
   histoplasmic p.
   idiopathic p.
   infective p.
   inflammatory p.
   internal adhesive p.
   ischemic p.
   localized p.
   meningococcal p.
   neoplastic p.
   p. obliterans
   obliterating p.
   occult p.
   postinfarction p.
   postoperative p.
   purulent p.
   radiation-induced p.
   rheumatic p.
   serofibrinous p.
   p. sicca
   Sternberg p.
   subacute p.
   suppurative p.
   transient p.
   traumatic p.
   tuberculous p.
   uremic p.

   p. villosa
   viral p.
pericarditis-myocarditis syndrome
pericardium, pl. pericardia
   absent p.
   adherent p.
   bread-and-butter p.
   calcified p.
   congenitally absent p.
   diaphragmatic p.
   dropsy of p.
   empyema of p.
   p. externum
   p. fibrosum
   fibrous p.
   p. internum
   parietal p.
   p. serosum
   shaggy p.
   thickened p.
   visceral p.
pericardotomy
perielectrode fibrosis
**Periflow peripheral balloon
   angioplasty-infusion catheter**
Periflux PF 1 D blood-flow meter
perihilar
   p. lymph nodes
   p. markings
peri-infarction block
**perimembranous ventricular septal
   defect**
**Perimount RSR pericardial
   bioprosthesis**
perimuscular plexus
perimyocarditis
perimyoendocarditis
perimysial plexus
perimysium
perindopril
   p. erbumine
perindoprilat
perineal artery
perinodal tissue
period
   absolute refractory p. (ARP)
   accessory pathway effective
     refractory p. (APERP)
   antegrade refractory p.
   atrial effective refractory p.
   atrioventricular refractory p.
   diastolic filling p.
   effective refractory p. (ERP)

ejection p.
functional refractory p. (FRP)
intersystolic p.
isoelectric p.
isometric p. of cardiac cycle
isometric contraction p.
isometric relaxation p.
isovolumetric relaxation p.
   (IVRP)
isovolumic relaxation p.
pacemaker amplifier
   refractory p.
postinfarction p.
postsphygmic p.
preejection p. (PEP)
presphygmic p.
pulse p.
refractory p.
relative refractory p. (RRP)
systolic ejection p. (SEP)
ventricular effective
   refractory p. (VERP)
vulnerable p.
Wenckebach p.
periodic
   p. breathing
   p. edema
   p. paralysis
   p. respiration
periodicity
   A-V node Wenckebach p.
periorbital edema
periosteotome
   Alexander-Farabeuf p.
periosteum
peripartum
   p. cardiomyopathy
   p. myocarditis
peripheral
   p. access system (PAS)
   p. airspaces
   P. AngioJet system
   p. arterial disease (PAD)
   p. arteriosclerosis
   p. atherectomy system
   p. atherosclerotic disease
   p. blood eosinophilia

p. circulation
p. cyanosis
p. edema
p. laser angioplasty (PLA)
p. neuropathy
p. pulmonic stenosis
p. resistance unit (PRU)
p. stigmata
p. vascular disease (PVD)
p. vascular resistance
peripherally inserted catheter (PIC)
peripneumonia notha
peristaltic wave
peristasis
peristatic hyperemia
Peri-Strips
perisystole
perisystolic
peritoneal dialysis
Peritrate
perivalvular leak
perivascular
   p. canal
   p. edema
   p. eosinophilic infiltrates
   p. fibrosis
   p. spaces
Perles
   Tessalon P.
Perma-Flow coronary graft
PermaMesh material
permanent
   p. cardiac pacing lead
   p. junctional reciprocating
      tachycardia (PJRT)
   p. pacemaker placement
   p. pacing
Permapen injection
Permathane lead
permeability
permissive hypercapnia
pernio
   lupus p.
peroneal
   p. artery
   p. muscular atrophy

NOTES

P

367

peroxidase
 avidin-biotin p.
peroxide
 hydrogen p.
peroxynitrite
perpetual arrhythmia
perpetuus
 pulsus irregularis p.
Per-Q-Cath percutaneously inserted central venous catheter
Persantine
 I.V. P.
Persantine-isonitrile stress test
persistent
 p. common atrioventricular canal
 p. ductus arteriosus
 p. fetal circulation
 p. ostium primum
 p. pulmonary hypertension of newborn (PPHN)
 p. truncus arteriosus
Personal Best peak flow meter
Perspex button
persulfate
 p. salt
pertechnate
 sodium p.
pertechnetate sodium
Perthes test
Pertofrane
pertubation
perturbed
 p. autonomic nervous system function
 p. carotid baroreceptor
Pertussin CS
pertussis
 Bordetella p.
 Haemophilus p.
 p. toxin
peruana
 verruga p.
pervenous
 p. catheter
 p. pacemaker
PES
 programmed electrical stimulation
PESDA
 perfluorocarbon-exposed sonicated dextrose albumin
PET
 polyethylene terephthalate

positron emission tomography
 PET balloon
 PET balloon atherectomy device
petal-fugal flow
petechia, pl. **petechiae**
pethidine
petiolous epiglottiditis
Petit sinuses
Peto-Prentice log-rank test
Petrillium
Peyer patch
Peyrot thorax
PF
 pulmonary function
Pfizerpen-AS injection
PFO
 patent foramen ovale
PFR
 peak filling rate
PFT
 pulmonary function test
Pfuhl-Jaffé sign
PFWT
 pain-free walking time
P-H
 P-H conduction time
 P-H interval
pH
 hydrogen ion concentration
 scalp pH
phacoma
phagocyte
phagocytic function
phagocytosis
Phalen stress test
Phanatuss
Phantom
 P. cardiac guidewire
 P. V Plus catheter
phantom
 p. aneurysm
 p. pacemaker
 p. pain
 p. sponge
 p. tumor
pharmacodynamics
pharmacokinetics
pharmacologic
 p. stress
 p. stress echocardiography
 p. stress perfusion imaging
pharmacological cardioversion

Pharmacopeia
  United States P. (USP)
pharmacotherapy
pharyngalgia
pharyngeal
  p. arch
  p. artery
  p. crisis
  p. pouch
  p. pouch syndrome
  p. reflex
pharyngis
  globus p.
pharyngitis
  acute p.
  arcanobacterial p.
  atrophic p.
  catarrhal p.
  chronic p.
  croupous p.
  diphtheric p., diphtheritic p.
  follicular p.
  gangrenous p.
  glandular p.
  granular p.
  herpangina p.
  membranous p.
  phlegmonous p.
  plague p.
  p. sicca
  p. ulcerosa
pharyngoconjunctival fever
pharyngoesophageal sphincter
pharyngoparalysis
pharyngoplasty
  Hynes p.
pharyngoscopy
pharyngospasm
pharynx
  constrictor muscle of p.
  raphe of p.
phase
  p. angle
  ejection p.
  p. image
  p. image analysis
  p. imaging

  Korotkoff p.
  plateau p.
  supernormal recovery p.
  venous p.
  vulnerable p.
  washout p.
phased
  p. array sector scanner
  p. array sector transducer
  p. array study
  p. array system
  p. array technology
  p. array ultrasonographic
  device
phase-encoded velocity image
phasic sinus arrhythmia
Phemister elevator
Phenameth
  P. DM
  P. Oral
Phenazine injection
phenazopyridine
  sulfisoxazole and p.
Phendry Oral
Phenergan
  P. injection
  P. Oral
  P. VC with Codeine
  P. with Dextromethorphan
Phenetron Oral
phenindamine tartrate
phenindione
  p. sensitivity
phenobarbital
  theophylline, ephedrine, and p.
phenolformaldehyde
phenomenon, pl. phenomena
  AFORMED p.
  Anrep p.
  Aschner p.
  Ashley p.
  Ashman p.
  Austin Flint p.
  blush p.
  Bowditch p.
  cascade p.
  coronary steal p.

NOTES

P

phenomenon *(continued)*
diaphragm p.
diaphragmatic p.
dip p.
Duckworth p.
Ehret p.
embolic p.
Gallavardin p.
gap conduction p.
Gärtner vein p.
Goldblatt p.
Gregg p.
Hering p.
Hill p.
Katz-Wachtel p.
Kienbock p.
Koch p.
Litten p.
no-reflow p.
Raynaud p.
reentry p.
R on T p.
Schellong-Strisower p.
Splendore-Hoeppli p.
staircase p.
steal p.
treppe p.
warm-up p.
washout p.
Wenckebach p.
Williams p.
Woodworth p.
phenothiazine
phenotype
high-risk p.
metastatic p.
phenoxybenzamine
p. hydrochloride
phenoxymethyl
penicillin p.
phenprocoumon
phentolamine
p. hydrochloride
p. mesylate
p. methanesulfonate
phenylbutazone
p. sensitivity
phenylephrine
guaifenesin,
phenylpropanolamine, and p.
(ULR)
p. hydrochloride
isoproterenol and p.

Phenylfenesin L.A.
phenylpropanolamine
guaifenesin and p.
p. hydrochloride
p. toxicity
phenytoin
pheochromocytoma
Phe-Pro-boro-Arg
Pherazine w/DM
Pherazine with Codeine
Phialophora
P. verrucosa
phlebarteriectasia
phlebectasia
p. laryngis
phlebemphraxis
phlebitis
adhesive p.
blue p.
chlorotic p.
gouty p.
migrating p.
p. nodularis necrotisans
p. obliterans
obliterating p.
plastic p.
puerperal p.
sclerosing p.
superficial p.
phlebodynamics
phlebogram
phlebograph
phlebography
phlebolithiasis
phlebomanometer
phleborrheogram
Cranley-Grass p.
phlebostasis
phlebotomize
phlebotomy
bloodless p.
phlegmasia
p. alba dolens
p. cerulea dolens
phlegmonosa
angina p.
phlegmonous
p. laryngitis
p. pharyngitis
phlei
Mycobacterium p.

Phoenix
   P. 2 pacemaker
   P. total artificial heart
phonarteriogram
phonarteriography
Phonate
phonoangiography
   carotid p.
phonocardiogram
phonocardiograph
   linear p.
   logarithmic p.
   spectral p.
   stethoscopic p.
phonocardiographic transducer
phonocardiography
phonocatheter
phonoscope
phonoscopy
phosducin
phosgene
phosphatase
   acid p.
   alkaline p.
phosphate
   Aralen P.
   azapetine p.
   chloroquine p.
   Cleocin P.
   codeine p.
   Decadron P.
   dexamethasone sodium p.
    (DSP)
   disopyramide p.
   Hexadrol P.
   Hydrocortone P.
phosphatidylcholine (PtdCho)
   dipalmitoyl p. (DPPC)
phosphinic acid
phosphocreatine
phosphodiesterase
   p. enzyme
   p. inhibitor (PDE)
   p. isoenzyme inhibitors
phosphofructokinase
Phosphoinositol

phosphokinase
   creatine p. (CPK)
phospholamban
phospholipase B, C
phospholipid
phosphomonoesterase
phosphorus
   organic p.
phosphorylase
   glycogen p.
   p. kinase
phosphorylation
   oxidative p.
photoablation
photocoagulation
PhotoDerm VL device
photodisruption
photodynamic therapy
PhotoFix alpha pericardial
   bioprosthesis
photometer
   HemoCue p.
photomicrography
photomultiplier
photon
   annihilation p.
photopeak
photoplethysmography (PPG)
photoresection
photostethoscope
phrenic
   p. artery
   p. nerve
   p. nerve paralysis
phrenocardia
phthinoid
   p. bronchitis
   p. chest
phthisis
   aneurysmal p.
   bacillary p.
   black p.
   collier's p.
   diabetic p.
   fibroid p.
   grinders' p.
   miner's p.

NOTES

P

phthisis *(continued)*
  potter's p.
  pulmonary p.
  stone-cutter's p.
phycomycosis
phylaxis
Phyllocontin Tablet
Phymos 3D pacemaker
physical
  p. inactivity
  p. stimulus
Physical Work Capacity exercise
  stress test
Physio-Control Lifestat
  sphygmomanometer
physiodensitometry
physiologic
  p. congestion
  p. measurement
  p. murmur
  p. pattern release (PPR)
  p. third heart sound
physiological
  p. dead space
  p. dead space ventilation per
    minute (V_D)
  p. monitoring
  p. overreactivity
  p. split of S_2
  p. stress
physiologically split S_2 sound
physiology
  constrictive p.
  Damus-Kaye-Stancel procedure
    for single ventricle p.
phytanic acid accumulation
phytohemagglutinin
phytonadione
piano percussion
piaulement
  bruit de p.
PIC
  peripherally inserted catheter
PICA
  posterior inferior communicating
    artery
Piccolino
  P. balloon
  P. Monorail catheter
pi cell
Pick
  P. and Go monitor
  P. syndrome

Picker
  P. Dyna Mo collimator
  P. Magnascanner
pickwickian syndrome
Picornaviridae
  P. virus
PIE
  pulmonary infiltration with
    eosinophilia
  pulmonary interstitial emphysema
  PIE syndrome
piechaudii
  Alcaligenes p.
Pielograf
Pierce-Donachy Thoratec ventricular
  assist device
Pierre Robin syndrome
piesimeter
  Hales p.
piesis
piezoelectric
PIF
  peak inspiratory flow
PIFR
  peak inspiratory flow rate
pig bronchus
pigeon-breast deformity
pigeon-breeder's
  p.-b. disease
  p.-b. lung
pigeon chest
piggyback
pigskin
pigtail catheter
PIH
  pregnancy-induced hypertension
PIIIP
  procollagen type III aminoterminal
    peptide
pillar
  tonsillar p.
Pilling
  P. bronchoscope
  P. microanastomosis clamp
pillow-shaped balloon
pilocarpine iontophoresis test
pilot
  p. needle
Pilotip
  P. catheter
  P. catheter guide
pilsicainide
Pima

pimobendan
PIMS
   programmable implantable
   medication system
pinacidil
pinchcock mechanism
pincushion distortion
pindolol
pinc resin-colophony
pinhole VSD
pink
   p. puffer
   p. sputum
   p. tetralogy of Fallot
pinked up
Pinkerton .018 balloon catheter
Pinnacle
   P. introducer sheath
   P. pacemaker
Pins
   P. sign
   P. syndrome
PIP
   positive inspiratory pressure
pipecuronium bromide
piperacillin sodium and tazobactam
   sodium
Piperanometozine
piperazine
   p. citrate
pipobroman
Pipracil
pirbuterol
   p. acetate
pirenzepine
piretanide
piriform sinus
pirmenol
Pirogoff angle
pirolazamide
piroximone
PISA
   proximal isovelocity surface area
pistol-shot femoral sound
piston pulse
Pitressin injection
pitting edema

Pittsburgh pneumonia
Pitt talking tracheostomy tube
pixel
Pizzolatto stain
P-J interval
PJRT
   permanent junctional reciprocating
   tachycardia
PLA
   peripheral laser angioplasty
PLAC
   Pravastatin Limitation of
   Atherosclerosis in Coronary
   Arteries
   Pravastatin, Lipids, and
   Atherosclerosis in the Carotids
placebo
placement
   lead p.
   permanent pacemaker p.
   temporary pacemaker p.
   Thoracoport p.
placental
   p. barrier
   p. circulation
   p. respiration
plague
   bubonic p.
   p. pharyngitis
   p. pneumonia
   pneumonic p.
PLA-I platelet antigen
planar
   p. myocardial imaging
   p. thallium scintigraphy
   p. thallium test
   p. xanthoma
plane
   Addison p.
   axial p.
   coronal p.
   cove p.
   midsagittal p.
   orthogonal p.
   parasagittal p.
   sagittal p.
   short-axis p.

NOTES

P

plane *(continued)*
  sternal p.
  sternoxiphoid p.
  transaxial p.
planimeter
planimetry
plantar ischemia test
plant toxicity
plaque
  atheromatous p.
  atherosclerotic p.
  calcified p.
  carcinoid p.
  carotid p.
  p. disruption
  echogenic p.
  echolucent p.
  fibrofatty p.
  fibrous p.
  p. fissuring
  p. fracture
  Hollenhorst p.'s
  intraluminal p.
  lipid-rich p.
  myointimal p.
  pleural p.
  p. rupture
  shelf of p.
  p. strutting
  submucosal p.
  unstable p.
plaque-cracker
  LeVeen p.-c.
Plaquenil
plaquing
plasma
  p. alpha 1-antitrypsin (pAAT)
  p. beta-thromboglobulin
  p. catecholamine
  p. cell pneumonia
  p. coagulation system
  p. colloid osmotic pressure
  p. endothelin
  p. endothelin concentration
  p. erythropoietin
  p. exchange column
  p. fibrinogen
  fresh frozen p. (FFP)
  p. glycocalicin
  platelet-poor p. (PPP)
  platelet-rich p. (PRP)
  p. renin
  p. renin activity (PRA)

  p. skimming
  p. thromboplastin antecedent
  p. thromboplastin component
  p. volume
  p. volume expander
  zoster immune p. (ZIP)
plasmalemma
Plasma-Lyte A
Plasmanate
plasmapheresis
Plasma-Plex
**plasma-resistant fiber oxygenator
(PRF)**
Plasmatein
plasmatic vascular destruction
plasmin
α_2-**plasmin inhibitor**
plasminogen
  p. activator
  p. activator inhibitor (PAI)
  p. activator inhibitor-1 (PAI-1)
plasminogen-streptokinase complex
Plasmodium
  P. embolism
plastic
  p. bronchitis
  p. endocarditis
  p. phlebitis
  p. pleurisy
  p. polymer
  p. sewing ring
plasticity
  skeletal muscle p.
plasty
  endoventricular circular
    patch p.
  sliding p.
plate
  p. thrombosis
  p. thrombus
plateau
  h p.
  p. phase
  p. pulse
  p. response
  ventricular p.
platelet
  p. activating factor (PAF)
  p. aggregation
  p. antibody
  p. factor 4
  p. imaging
  p. receptor glycoprotein

p. thrombosis
p. thrombus
platelet-aggregating factor
platelet-derived growth factor
(PDGF)
plateletpheresis
platelet-poor plasma (PPP)
platelet-rich plasma (PRP)
platelike atelectasis
platform
TomTec echo p.
Platinol
platinum
P. PLUS guidewire
salt of p.
platypnea
platysma
pledget
Dacron p.
Meadox Teflon felt p.
polypropylene p.
Teflon p.
pledgeted mattress suture
PlegiaGuard
Plendil
pleomorphic
p. premature ventricular
complex
p. tachycardia
Plesch
P. percussion
P. test
plethora
plethoric
plethysmograph
body p.
jerkin p.
mercury-in-rubber strain
gauge p.
Respitrace inductive p.
plethysmography
cuff p.
impedance p. (IPG)
strain-gauge p.
thermistor p.
pleura
black p.

cervical p.
costodiaphragmatic recess of p.
costomediastinal recess of p.
cupula of p.
discission of p.
fibrin bodies of p.
parietal p.
visceral p.
pleuracentesis
pleuracotomy
pleural
p. abrasion
p. adhesion
p. amyloidosis
p. biopsy
p. bleb
p. cap
p. crackles
p. cupula
p. effusion
p. empyema
p. fibrin balls
p. fluid
p. fremitus
p. friction rub
p. lavage
p. mass
p. meniscus sign
p. mouse
p. peel
p. plaque
p. poudrage
p. rales
p. rings
p. sac
p. scarring
p. shock
p. space
p. tag
p. tap
p. tents
p. thickening
p. tube
pleuralgia
pleurectomy
thoracoscopic apical p.
Pleur-evac

NOTES

P

Pleur-evac
P.-e. autotransfusion system
P.-e. device
P.-e. suction
pleurisy
acute p.
adhesive p.
blocked p.
cholesterol p.
chronic p.
chyliform p.
chylous p.
circumscribed p.
costal p.
diaphragmatic p.
diffuse p.
double p.
dry p.
encysted p.
exudative p.
fibrinous p.
hemorrhagic p.
ichorous p.
indurative p.
interlobar p.
interlobular p.
latent p.
mediastinal p.
metapneumonic p.
plastic p.
primary p.
proliferating p.
pulmonary p.
pulsating p.
purulent p.
sacculated p.
secondary p.
serofibrinous p.
serous p.
single p.
suppurative p.
tuberculous p.
typhoid p.
visceral p.
wet p.
pleuritic
p. chest pain
p. pneumonia
p. rub
pleuritis
fibrinous acute p.
lupus p.
obliterative p.

pleurocentesis
pleurodesis
chemical p.
doxycycline p.
mechanical p.
talc p.
thoracoscopic talc p.
pleurodynia
pleuroesophageal fistula
pleurogenic pneumonia
pleurolith
pleuroparietopexy
pleuropericardial
p. murmur
p. rub
p. window
pleuropneumonectomy
pleuropneumonia-like organism (PPLO)
pleuropulmonary
pleuroscopy
plexectomy
plexiform lesion
PlexiPulse
P. device
plexogenic pulmonary arteriopathy
plexus
Batson p.
brachial p.
perimuscular p.
perimysial p.
PLHB
percutaneous left heart bypass
pliability
plication
plombage
plop
cardiac tumor p.
tumor p.
plot
bull's-eye p.
plug
Alcock catheter p.
collagen p.
Dittrich p.'s
Ivalon p.
mucus p.
plugging
mucous p.
plumb-line sign
Plummer
P. disease

P. water-filled pneumatic
esophageal dilator
Plummer-Vinson syndrome
plunging goiter
plurilocular
plus
Lorcet P.
Oracle Micro P.
PMBC
percutaneous mitral balloon
commissurotomy
PMBV
percutaneous mitral balloon
valvotomy
percutaneous mitral balloon
valvuloplasty
PMC
percutaneous mitral
commissurotomy
PMI
point of maximum impulse
P mitrate
PML
progressive multifocal
leukoencephalopathy
PMT
pacemaker-mediated tachycardia
PMT AccuSpan tissue
expander
PMV
percutaneous mitral valvuloplasty
PND
paroxysmal nocturnal dyspnea
pneocardiac reflex
pneumatic
p. antishock garment (PASG)
p. compression stockings
p. cuff
p. tourniquet
p. trousers
pneumatocardia
pneumatocele
pneumatohemia
pneumatonometer
Digibind p.
pneumectomy

pneumobacillus
Friedländer p.
pneumocentesis
pneumococcal
p. empyema
p. pneumonia
p. vaccine
pneumococci
pneumococcosis
pneumococcus, pl. **pneumococci**
pneumoconiosis
asbestos p.
bauxite p.
coal workers' p.
collagenous p.
hard metal p.
kaolin p.
mica p.
noncollagenous p.
organic dust p.
rheumatoid p.
p. siderotica
silicotic p.
talc p.
pneumocystic
Pneumocystis
P. carinii
P. carinii pneumonia (PCP)
P. pneumonitis
pneumocystis
p. pneumonia
pneumocystosis
pneumocytes
type II p.
pneumohemia
pneumohemothorax
pneumohydropericardium
pneumohydrothorax
pneumomediastinography
pneumomediastinum
pneumonectomy
Pneumo-Needle reusable instrument
pneumonia
abortive p.
acute interstitial p.
adenoviral p.
p. alba

NOTES

P

pneumonia *(continued)*
alcoholic p.
amebic p.
anthrax p.
apex p.
apical p.
p. aposthematosa
aspiration p.
atypical p.
bacillary p.
bacterial pneumococcal p.
bilious p.
bronchial p.
bronchiolitis obliterans
    organizing p. (BOOP)
Buhl desquamative p.
Carrington p.
caseous p.
catarrhal p.
central p.
cerebral p.
cheesy p.
Chlamydia p.
chronic eosinophilic p. (CEP)
chronic fibrous p.
cold agglutinin p.
community-acquired p. (CAP)
congenital aspiration p.
contusion p.
core p.
Corrigan p.
croupous p.
deglutition p.
Desnos p.
desquamative interstitial p.
    (DIP)
p. dissecans
double p.
Eaton agent p.
embolic p.
eosinophilic p.
ephemeral p.
ether p.
fibrinous acute lobar p.
fibrous p.
Friedländer bacillus p.
gangrenous p.
gelatinous acute p.
giant cell p.
Hecht p.
herpes p.
hypersensitivity p.
hypostatic p.

idiopathic acute eosinophilic p.
idiopathic interstitial p.
indurative p.
influenzal p.
influenza virus p.
inhalation p.
p. interlobularis purulenta
interstitial plasma cell p.
intrauterine p.
Kaufman p.
Klebsiella p.
Legionella p.
Legionnaire p.
lingular p.
lipid p.
lipoid p.
lobar p.
lobular p.
Löffler p.
Louisiana p.
lymphoid interstitial p.
massive p.
measles p.
metastatic p.
migratory p.
mycoplasmal p.
necrotizing p.
nosocomial p.
obstructive p.
oil-aspiration p.
opportunistic p.
parenchymatous p.
peribronchial p.
Pittsburgh p.
plague p.
plasma cell p.
pleuritic p.
pleurogenic p.
pneumococcal p.
pneumocystis p.
Pneumocystis carinii p. (PCP)
polymicrobial p.
primary atypical p.
primary eosinophilic p.
progressive p.
Proteus p.
purulent p.
Reisman p.
rheumatic p.
rickettsial p.
secondary p.
septic p.
Serratia p.

staphylococcal p.
Stoll p.
streptococcal p.
superficial p.
suppurative p.
terminal p.
toxemic p.
transplant p.
traumatic p.
tuberculous p.
tularemic p.
TWAR p.
typhoid p.
vagus p.
varicella p.
ventilator-associated p.
viral p.
walking p.
wandering p.
white p.
woolsorter's p.
pneumoniae
   Bacillus p.
   Chlamydia p.
   Diplococcus p.
   Klebsiella p.
   Mycoplasma p.
   Streptococcus p.
pneumonic
   p. fever
   p. plague
pneumonitis
   acute interstitial p.
   acute radiation p.
   aspiration p.
   chemical p.
   cholesterol p.
   CMV p.
   cytomegalovirus p.
   desquamative interstitial p.
    (DIP)
   eosinophilic p.
   granulomatous p.
   herpes simplex p.
   hypersensitivity p. (HP)
   interstitial p.
   kerosene p.

lymphocytic interstitial p. (LIP)
malarial p.
ossifying p.
peptic aspiration p.
Pneumocystis p.
radiation p.
uremic p.
pneumonoconiosis
   bauxite p.
   rheumatoid p.
pneumonopathy
   eosinophilic p.
pneumonoresection
pneumonotherapy
pneumopathy
   seropositive nonsyphilitic p.
Pneumopent
pneumopericardium
   tension p.
   ventilator-induced p.
pneumoperitoneum
pneumopexy
pneumophila
   Legionella p.
pneumoplethysmography
pneumopleuritis
pneumopleuroparietopexy
pneumoresection
Pneumoscope
pneumosilicosis
pneumotachograph
   Fleisch p.
pneumotachometer
   hot-wire p.
   MicroTach p.
pneumotaxic center
pneumotherapy
pneumothorax, pl. **pneumothoraces**
   artificial p.
   clicking p.
   closed chest p.
   extrapleural p.
   iatrogenic p.
   induced p.
   open p.
   pressure p.
   spontaneous p.

NOTES

P

pneumothorax *(continued)*
  tension p.
  therapeutic p.
  valvular p.
  ventilator-induced p.
pneumotomy
Pneumotron ventilator
Pneumovax 23
pneumovirus
pneuPAC
  p. resuscitator
  p. ventilator
PNH
  paroxysmal nocturnal
    hemoglobinuria
PNS Unna boot
Pnu-Imune 23
PO₂
  partial pressure of oxygen
    PO₂ oximetry
POC
  polyolefin copolymer
    POC balloon
pocket
  abdominal p.
  pacemaker p.
  regurgitant p.'s
  retropectoral p.
  P. SPO₂T
  p.'s of Zahn
Pocket-Dop II
Pockethaler
  Vancenase P.
Pocketpeak peak flow meter
pod
  rigid p.
podagra
POET
  pulse oximeter/end tidal CO₂
poikilocytosis
Poincar plot pattern
point
  p. of Arrhigi
  Boyd p.
  Castellani p.
  p. of critical stenosis
  cut p.
  D p.
  de Mussy p.
  E p.
  Erb p.
  exit p.
  Guéneau de Mussy p.

  isoelectric p.
  J p.
  p. of maximum impulse (PMI)
  null p.
  Z p.
pointes
  torsade de p.
Poiseuille
  P. law
  P. resistance formula
poisoning
  arsenic p.
  arsine gas p.
  fluorocarbon p.
  lead p.
  mercury p.
polacrilex chewing gum
Poladex
polar
  p. coordinate map
  P. Vantage XL heart rate
    monitor
Polaramine
polarcardiography
Polaris
  P. electrode
  P. Mansfield/Webster
    deflectable tip
  P. steerable diagnostic catheter
polarity
polarization
  electrochemical p.
  fluorescence p.
polarographic method
Polhemus-Schafer-Ivemark syndrome
polichinelle
  voix de p.
poliomyelitis
poliovirus
  p. vaccine, live, trivalent, oral
Polisar-Lyons tracheal tube
polixus
  Rhodnius p.
pollen asthma
poloxamer 188
polyacrylamide gel electrophoresis
polyacrylonitrile membrane
polyangiitis
  microscopic p.
polyarteritis
  disseminated p.
  p. nodosa
polyarthritis

polycardia
polychondritis
  relapsing p.
Polycillin
polyclonal gammopathy
polycrotic
polycrotism
polycystic
  p. kidney
  p. kidney disease
  p. lung
  p. tumor
polycythemia
  p. hypertonica
  p. vera
polydactyly
polyene
polyethylene
  p. terephthalate (PET)
  p. terephthalate balloon
PolyFlex pacemaker
Polygam S/D
polygelin colloid contrast medium
polygenic
  p. hypercholesterolemia
  p. hyperlipidemia
polygonal
polygraph
  Mackenzie p.
polyhedral surface reconstruction
PolyHeme
polymer
  plastic p.
polymerase
  p. chain reaction (PCR)
  Taq DNA p.
polymeric endoluminal paving stent
polymicrobial pneumonia
polymorphic
  p. premature ventricular
    complex
  p. slow wave
polymorphism
  restriction fragment length p.
    (RFLP)
polymorphonuclear leukocyte

polymorphous ventricular
  tachycardia
Polymox
polymyalgia rheumatica syndrome
polymyositis
polymyxa
  Bacillus p.
polymyxin
polyneuritiformis
  heredopathia atactica p.
polyneuropathy
  ascending p.
  Roussy-Lévy p.
polyolefin copolymer (POC)
  p. c. balloon
polyostotic fibrous dysplasia
polyp
  cardiac p.
polypeptide
  atrial natriuretic p. (ANP)
  pancreatic p. (PP)
polyphaga
  Acanthamoeba p.
polyphosphoinositide
polyploidy
Poly-Plus Dacron vascular graft
polypoidal lesion
polypoid bronchitis
polyposis
  nasal p.
polypous endocarditis
polypropylene
  p. intracardiac patch
  p. pledget
polysaccharide-iron complex
polysaccharide storage disease
polysome
polysomnogram (PSG)
polysomnographic study
polysomnography
polysplenia
Polystan cardiotomy reservoir
polystyrene latex microspheres
polytef
polytetrafluoroethylene (PTFE)
  expanded p. (EPTFE, ePTFE)

NOTES

P

polythiazide
  prazosin and p.
polyurethane
  p. foam
  p. foam embolus
polyuria
polyvinyl
  p. chloride (PVC)
  p. chloride balloon
  p. chloride tube
  p. prosthesis
POM
  pulse oximetry monitoring
Pompe disease
POMS 20/50 oxygen conservation device
ponderal index
ponderance
  ventricular p.
ponopalmosis
Ponstel
Pontiac fever
pool
  blood p.
poorly-differentiated carcinoma
poorly reversible asthma
poor R wave progression
popliteal
  p. aneurysm
  p. artery
  p. pulse
poppet
  ball p.
  barium-impregnated p.
  prosthetic p.
popping sensation
porcelain aorta
porcine
  p. bioprosthesis
  p. heterograft
  p. prosthesis
  p. prosthetic valve
pores
  Kohn p.
pork
  p. insulin
  P. NPH Iletin II
  P. Regular Iletin II
porphyria
  acute intermittent p. (AIP)
porphyrin
Porstmann technique

port
  chest p.
  Luer-Lok p.
  PAS p.
  Q P.
  SEA p.
  side p.
porta, pl. **portae**
  p. hepatis
  p. lienis
  p. pulmonaris
portable
  Pulsair .5 liquid oxygen p.
Port-A-Cath
  P.-A.-C. device
  P.-A.-C. implantable catheter system
portacaval
  p. anastomosis
  p. H graft
  p. shunt
port-access
  p.-a. coronary artery bypass grafting
  St. Jude Medical P.-a.
portae (*pl. of* porta)
portal
  p. circulation
  p. hypertension
  p. vein
  p. vein thrombosis
Porta-Resp monitor
Porter sign
Portex
  P. Neo-Vac meconium suction device
  P. Per-Fit tracheostomy kit
  P. Per-Fit tracheostomy tube
  P. Soft-Seal cuff system
  P. ThermoVent heat and moisture exchanger
portion
  infradiaphragmatic p.
Portmanteau test
portogram
portography
  computed tomography angiographic p. (CTAP)
  splenic p.
portoportal anastomosis
portopulmonary shunt
portosystemic anastomosis
portovenography

Posadas mycosis
Posadas-Wernicke disease
POSCH
Program on the Surgical Control of
Hyperlipidemias
position
body p.
electrical heart p.
heart p.
LAO p.
left anterior oblique p.
levo-transposed p.
RAO p.
right anterior oblique p.
shock p.
Trendelenburg p.
tricuspid p.
positioner
CAS-8000V general
angiography p.
positive
p. afterpotential
p. airway pressure (PAP)
p. chronotropism
p. end-airway pressure (PEAP)
p. end-expiratory pressure
(PEEP)
p. expiratory pressure (PEP)
p. inspiratory pressure (PIP)
p. treppe
Positrol
P. cardiac device
P. II catheter
positron emission tomography
(PET)
postabsorptive state
postanesthesia pulmonary edema
postangioplasty
post-balloon angioplasty restenosis
postcardiotomy syndrome
postcardioversion pulmonary edema
postcatheterization
postcommissurotomy syndrome
postdiastolic
postdicrotic
postdiphtheritic stenosis
postdrive depression

postductal
posterior
p. approach
p. circumflex artery (PC)
p. descending artery (PDA)
p. inferior communicating
artery (PICA)
p. leaflet
p. myocardial infarction
p. papillary muscle (PPM)
posteroinferior dyskinesis
posteroseptal wall
postextrasystolic
p. aberrancy
p. beat
p. pause
p. potentiation
p. T wave
posthyperventilation apnea
postictal state
postinfarction
p. angina
p. pericarditis
p. period
p. syndrome
postinfectious bradycardia
postinfective bradycardia
postinflammatory
postintervention
postischemic
p. heart
p. myocardium
postmicturition syncope
postmortem
p. clot
p. thrombus
postmyocardial
p. infarction
p. infarction syndrome
postnasal catarrh
postobstructive atelectasis
Post-Op
Emerson P.-O.
postoperative pericarditis
postpartum
p. cardiomyopathy
p. hypertension

NOTES

P

383

postperfusion
p. arrhythmia
p. lung
p. psychosis
p. syndrome
postpericardiotomy syndrome (PPS)
postphlebitic syndrome
postpneumonectomy tuberculous
empyema
postpneumonic
postprandial
p. angina
p. blood sugar
postprimary tuberculosis
postprocedural management
postpump syndrome
postrenal azotemia
postsphygmic
p. interval
p. period
poststenotic dilation
posttest
Tukey-Kramer p.
posttransfusion syndrome
posttussive
p. emesis
p. syncope
postural
p. drainage (PD)
p. drainage and percussion (PD&P)
p. hypotension
p. syncope
posture
Stern p.
posturing
decerebrate p.
Potain sign
potassium (K)
canrenoate p.
p. chloride (KCl)
p. gluconate
glucose, insulin, and p. (GIK)
p. hydroxide (KOH)
p. inhibition
p. iodide
P. Iodide Enseals
p. ion
losartan p.
penicillin v p.
p. wasting
potassium/HCTZ
losartan p.

potassium/hydrochlorothiazide
losartan p.
potassium-sparing diuretic
potassium-wasting diuretic
potential
action p.
bioelectric p.
cardiac action p.
electrical p.
fibrillation p.
Kent p.
maximum negative p.
membrane p.
monophasic action p. (MAP)
pacemaker p.
putative slow pathway p.
resting membrane p.
transmembrane p.
potentiation
postextrasystolic p.
Pott aneurysm
Pottenger sign
potter's
p. asthma
p. phthisis
Potts
P. anastomosis
P. bronchial forceps
P. needle
P. operation
P. procedure
P. shunt
Potts-Cournand needle
Potts-Smith anastomosis
pouch
Cardio-Cool myocardial protection p.
laryngeal p.
Parsonnet pulse generator p.
pharyngeal p.
poudrage
Beck epicardial p.
pericardial p.
pleural p.
talc p.
pounds
p. per square inch (psi)
p. per square inch gauge (psig)
Pourcelot index
povidone-iodine
powder
Evans blue p.
lyophilized p.

powdered tantalum
power
  p. Doppler ultrasound
  p. injector
  left ventricular p.
  resolving p.
  spectral p.
  ventricular p.
PP
  pancreatic polypeptide
PPACK
  D-Phe-L-Pro-L-Arg-chloromethyl
  ketone
PPD
  purified protein derivative
  PPD skin test
P&PD
  percussion and postural drainage
PPG
  photoplethysmography
PPHN
  persistent pulmonary hypertension of
  newborn
P-P interval
PPLO
  pleuropneumonia-like organism
PPL skin test
PPM
  posterior papillary muscle
ppm
  parts per million
PPP
  platelet-poor plasma
PPPPPP
  pain, pallor, paraesthesia,
  pulselessness, paralysis, prostration
PPR
  physiologic pattern release
  PPR verapamil
PPS
  postpericardiotomy syndrome
P pulmonale
P-Q
  P-Q interval
  P-Q segment depression

P-R
  P-R interval
  P-R segment
PRA
  plasma renin activity
PR-AC measurement
practolol
praecox
  ascites p.
  lymphedema p.
Pravachol
pravastatin
  P. Limitation of
    Atherosclerosis in Coronary
    Arteries (PLAC)
  P., Lipids, and Atherosclerosis
    in the Carotids (PLAC)
  p. sodium
praziquantel
prazosin
  p. hydrochloride
  p. and polythiazide
prearterioles
preautomatic pause
pre-beta lipoprotein
precapillary
  p. arterioles
  p. sphincter
precardiac mesoderm
precatheterization
Preceder interventional guidewire
Precept
  P. DR pacemaker
  P. lead
precipitation
  heparin-induced extracorporeal
    low-density lipoprotein p.
    (HELP)
precipitin
Preclude pericardial membrane
preconditioning
precordial
  p. A wave
  p. bulge
  p. catch syndrome
  p. electrocardiography
  p. heave

NOTES

P

precordial *(continued)*
 p. honk
 p. leads
 p. motion
 p. movement
 p. pulse
 p. thrill
 p. thump
precordialgia
precordium
 quiet p.
Precose
Predaject injection
Predalone injection
Predator balloon catheter
Predcor injection
prediastole
prediastolic
 p. murmur
Predicort-50 injection
predicrotic
predictive value
predictor
 Corazonix P.
 univariate p.
Prednicen-M Oral
prednisolone
 methyl p.
Prednisol TBA injection
prednisone
predominant emphysema
predose level
preductal
preeclampsia
preejection period (PEP)
preexcitation
 p. syndrome
 ventricular p.
preexisting condition
pregnancy-induced hypertension
 (PIH)
preinfarction
 p. angina
 p. syndrome
prekallikrein
preload
 p. reduction
 p. reserve
 ventricular p.
Prelone Oral
Premarin
premature
 p. atherosclerosis

 p. atrial beat
 p. atrial complex
 p. atrial contraction (PAC)
 p. atrioventricular junctional
 complex
 p. excitation
 p. junctional beat
 p. systole
 p. ventricular beat (PVB)
 p. ventricular complex
 p. ventricular complex-trigger
 hypothesis
 p. ventricular contraction
 (PVC)
prematurity
 chronic pulmonary insufficiency
 of p.
premedication
Premo guidewire
premonitory
 p. palpitation
 p. syndrome
prenalterol hydrochloride
prenylamine
preparation
 insulin p.
 Langendorff heart p.
preprandial
prerenal azotemia
presacral edema
presbycardia
presbyesophagus
presbylaryngia
prescription
 exercise p.
presentation
 roentgenographic p.
preservation
 tissue p.
preshaped catheter
presphygmic
 p. interval
 p. period
pressor drug
pressoreceptive
pressoreceptor
 p. reflex
pressosensitive
pressosensitivity
 reflexogenic p.
pressure
 Alladin InfantFlow nasal
 continuous positive air p.

alveolar carbon dioxide p.
alveolar oxygen partial p.
(PAO$_2$)
aortic blood p. (AoBP)
aortic dicrotic notch p.
aortic pullback p.
arterial blood p. (ABP)
arterial carbon dioxide p.
arterial dicrotic notch p.
arterial oxygen partial p.
(PaO$_2$)
ascending aortic p.
atmospheres of p.
atrial filling p.
average mean p. (AMP)
barometric p.
bi-level positive airway p.
(BiPAP)
BiPAP nasal continuous
positive airway p.
blood p. (BP)
capillary wedge p.
carbon dioxide p.
cardiovascular p.
central venous p. (CVP)
cerebral perfusion p. (CPP)
coaxial p.
colloid osmotic p.
compliance, rate, oxygenation,
and p. (CROP)
continuous positive air p.
continuous positive airway p.
(CPAP)
p. conversion
coronary perfusion p.
coronary venous p.
p. decay
diastolic blood p. (DBP)
diastolic filling p. (DFP)
differential blood p.
Donders p.
downstream venous p.
dynamic p.
elastic recoil p.
end-diastolic p. (EDP)
end-diastolic left ventricular p.
end-systolic left ventricular p.

expiratory positive airway p.
(EPAP)
p. gradient
P. guide guidewire
p. half-time
p. half time technique
high blood p.
hyperbaric p.
p. injector
inspiratory positive airway p.
(IPAP)
intermittent positive p. (IPP)
intracardiac p.
intramyocardial p.
intrapericardial p.
intrathoracic p.
intravascular p.
jugular venous p. (JVP)
juxtacardiac pleural p.
labile blood p.
left atrial p.
left ventricular diastolic p.
left ventricular end-diastolic p.
(LVEDP)
left ventricular filling p.
left ventricular systolic p.
lower body negative p.
(LBNP)
mean arterial p. (MAP)
mean arterial blood p.
(MABP)
mean diastolic left
ventricular p.
mean pulmonary artery p.
(MPAP)
mean pulmonary artery
wedge p. (MPAWP)
mean systolic left
ventricular p.
p. measurement
narrowed pulse p.
negative p.
negative end-expiratory p.
(NEEP)
normal intravascular p.
oncotic p.
opening p.

NOTES

P

pressure *(continued)*
    osmotic p.
    p. overload
    PA filling p.
    peak systolic aortic p. (PSAP)
    peak systolic gradient p.
    perfusion p.
    pericardial p.
    plasma colloid osmotic p.
    p. pneumothorax
    positive airway p. (PAP)
    positive end-airway p. (PEAP)
    positive end-expiratory p. (PEEP)
    positive expiratory p. (PEP)
    positive inspiratory p. (PIP)
    PSG p.
    pullback p.
    pulmonary artery p. (PAP)
    pulmonary artery occlusion p. (PAOP)
    pulmonary artery occlusive wedge p.
    pulmonary artery wedge p. (PAWP)
    pulmonary capillary wedge p. (PCWP)
    pulmonary hypertension p.
    pulmonary vascular p.
    pulmonary wedge p. (PWP)
    pulse p.
    p. recovery
    resting p.
    right atrial p. (RAP)
    right ventricular diastolic p.
    right ventricular end-diastolic p. (RVEDP)
    right ventricular systolic p.
    p. sling
    p. stasis
    stump p.
    p. support ventilation
    systemic mean arterial p. (SMAP)
    systolic blood p. (SBP)
    systolic left ventricular p.
    torr p.
    p. tracing
    p. transducer
    transmural p.
    transmyocardial perfusion p.
    p. urticaria
    variable positive airway p. (VPAP)
    venous p.
    p. ventilator
    ventricular diastolic p.
    ventricular filling p.
    p. wave
    p. waveform
    wedge p.
    zero end-expiratory p. (ZEEP)
    zero end-inspiratory p.
    z point p.
pressure-controlled inverse ratio ventilation (PCIRV)
pressure-cycled ventilator
pressure-flow relationship
pressure-natriuresis curve
pressure-regulated volume control ventilation (PRVC)
pressure-volume
    p.-v. analysis
    p.-v. curve
    p.-v. diagram
    p.-v. relation
pressurizer
    Oxy-Hood p.
Pressurometer blood pressure monitor
PresTab
    Glynase P.
Presto
    P. cardiac device
    P. spirometry system
Presto-Flash spirometry system
presyncopal
    p. episode
    p. spell
presyncope
presystole
presystolic
    p. gallop
    p. murmur
    p. pressure and volume
    p. thrill
pretibial
    p. edema
    p. myxedema
pretracheal lymph nodes
prevalence
Prevel sign
prevention
    Bezafibrate Infarction P. (BIP)
    secondary p.

Trials of Hypertension P.
(TOHP)
preventricular stenosis
prevertebral space
Prevotella
　　P. melaninogenica
prevotii
　　Peptostreptococcus p.
Prevue system
PRF
　　plasma-resistant fiber oxygenator
　　pulse repetition frequency
Price-Thomas bronchial forceps
prickle cell carcinoma
prick-test method
Prima
　　P. pacemaker
　　P. Total Occlusion Device
Primacor
primaquine phosphate antimalarial
primary
　　P. Angioplasty in Myocardial
　　Infarction (PAMI)
　　p. atelectasis
　　p. atypical pneumonia
　　p. cardiomyopathy
　　p. closure
　　p. coccidioidomycosis
　　p. eosinophilic pneumonia
　　p. pleurisy
　　p. pulmonary histiocytosis X
　　p. pulmonary hypertension
　　murmur
　　p. pulmonary parenchymal
　　disease
　　p. systemic amyloidosis
　　p. thrombus
　　p. tuberculosis
　　p. ventricular tachycardia
　　(PVT)
Primatene mist
Primaxin
prime
　　P. balloon
　　crystalloid p.
　　R-R p.
　　RSR p. (RSR')

primed lymphocyte test
PRIMI
　　Prourokinase in Myocardial
　　Infarction
priming dose
primitive aorta
primordial catheter tube
primum
　　p. atrial septal defect
　　ostium p.
　　persistent ostium p.
　　septum p.
Principen
principle
　　Beer-Lambert p.
　　Castaneda p.
　　Fick p.
　　Frank-Straub-Wiggers-Starling p.
　　hemodynamic p.
　　Huygens p.
Prinivil
Prinzide
Prinzmetal
　　P. effect
　　P. variant angina
Priscoline
　　P. injection
Prism-CL pacemaker
prism method
privet cough
proaccelerin
Pro-Air
Pro-Amatine
proANF
　　proatrial natriuretic factor
　　N-terminal proANF
proarrhythmia
proarrhythmic effect
proatrial natriuretic factor
　　(proANF)
probability
　　p. analysis
　　Cooperman event p.
　　p. density function (PDF)
proband

NOTES

probe
acradinium-ester-labeled nucleic
acid p.
AngeLase combined mapping-
laser p.
p. balloon catheter
Bard p.
blood-flow p.
cardiac p.
P. cardiac device
Chandler V-pacing p.
coronary artery p.
digoxigenin-labeled DNA p.
DNA p.
Doppler velocity p.
Dymer excimer delivery p.
esophageal temperature p.
four-beam laser Doppler p.
Gallagher bipolar mapping p.
Hagar p.
Hoffrel transesophageal p.
hot-tipped laser p.
Mui Scientific 6-channel
esophageal pressure p.
Neo-Therm neonatal skin
temperature p.
nuclear p.
over-the-wire p.
PA 120 Osypka
radiofrequency p.
Parsonnet coronary p.
p. patency
Radiometer p.
Robicsek vascular p.
scintillation p.
p. shield
Silverstein stimulator p.
transcranial Doppler p.
transesophageal p.
transesophageal echo p.
Typ Vasocope III Doppler p.
Probeta
Probing sheath exchange catheter
probucol
procainamide
N-acetyl p. (NAPA)
p. hydrochloride
procaine
p. hydrochloride
penicillin g p.
PRO-CAM
Prospective Cardiovascular Munster
study

Procanbid
Procan SR
Procardia
procaterol
Procath electrophysiology catheter
procedure
Alliston p.
Anderson p.
arterial switch p.
Bentall p.
Bing-Taussig heart p.
Björk method of Fontan p.
Blalock-Taussig p.
Brock p.
Charles p.
cherry-picking p.
Cockett p.
compartment p.
corridor p.
Damian graft p.
Damus-Kaye-Stancel p.
Damus-Stancel-Kaye p.
de-airing p.
debubbling p.
debulking p.
domino p.
Effler-Groves mode of
Allison p.
esophageal sling p.
Fontan-Baudet p.
Fontan-Kreutzer p.
Fontan modification of
Norwood p.
Gill-Jonas modification of
Norwood p.
Glenn p.
hemi-Fontan p.
His-Hass p.
Jacobaeus p.
Jatene arterial switch p.
Jonas modification of
Norwood p.
Junod p.
Karhunen-Loeve p.
Ko-Airan bleeding control p.
Kolmogorov-Smirnov p.
Kondoleon-Sistrunk
elephantiasis p.
Konno p.
Lam p.
Langevin updating p.
latissimus dorsi p.
left atrial isolation p.

Lewis-Tanner p.
Luke p.
Lyon-Horgan p.
maze p.
Moore p.
Mustard p.
Nicks p.
Norwood univentricular
  heart p.
Overholt p.
Potts p. *Heart rate - blood pressure*
Quaegebeur p.
Rashkind p.
Rastan-Konno p.
Rastelli p.
Ross p.
Sade modification of
  Norwood p.
salting-out p.
Schenk-Eichelter vena cava
  plastic filter p.
Schonander p.
Senning transposition p.
septation p.
Simplate p.
Sondergaard p.
Stancel p.
Sugiura p.
switch p.
Thal p.
Vineberg p.
Waterston-Cooley p.
Womack p.
process
consolidative p.
xiphisternal p.
xiphoid p.
processing
film p.
signal p.
Processor
Cobe 2991 cell P.
prochlorperazine
procollagen
type III p.
p. type III aminoterminal
  peptide (PIIIP)

**proconvertin prothrombin
  conversion accelerator**
Procort
Pro-Depo injection
prodromal symptom
prodrome
Prodrox injection
product
Autoplex Factor VIII inhibitor
  bypass p.
calcium p.
double p.
fibrinogen degradation p.
fibrinogen-fibrin degradation p.
fibrin split p.
lipid peroxidation p.
rate pressure p.
production
carbon dioxide p.
energy p.
sputum p.
venous carbon dioxide p.
  (VCO_2)
productive
p. bronchitis
p. cough
p. sputum
p. tuberculosis
productus
Peptostreptococcus p.
Profen LA
Profilate OSD
profile
aortic valve velocity p.
Astra p.
deflated p.
P. Plus balloon dilatation
  catheter
serum lipid p.
The Sickness Impact P.
ultra-low p. (ULP)
Profilnine Heat-Treated
Proflex 5 catheter
Pro-Flo XT catheter
profunda
p. femoris artery
p. femoris vein

NOTES

P

profundaplasty
progeria
progesterone
progestin
Proglycem Oral
prognosis
Prograf
program
   CAPRI p.
   Expedited Recovery P.
   Hypertension Detection and
      Follow-Up P. (HDFP)
   Linde Walker Oxygen P.
   National Asthma Education P.
      (NAEP)
   National Cholesterol
      Education P. (NCEP)
   P. on the Surgical Control of
      Hyperlipidemias (POSCH)
   Systolic Hypertension in the
      Elderly P. (SHEP)
   WALK p.
Programalith
   P. III pacemaker
   P. III pulse generator
programmability
programmable
   p. cardioverter-defibrillator
      (PCD)
   p. implantable medication
      system (PIMS)
   p. pacemaker
programmed electrical stimulation
   (PES)
Programmer
   P. III pacemaker
   Omnicor P.
progression
   poor R wave p.
   R wave p.
progressive
   p. interstitial pulmonary
      fibrosis
   p. multifocal
      leukoencephalopathy (PML)
   p. multiple hyaloserositis
   p. parenchymal restriction
   p. pneumonia
   p. scanning
   p. systemic sclerosis (PSS)
   p. thrombus
ProHIBiT
pro-inflammatory substance

proiosystole, proiosystolia
Project
   European Myocardial
      Infarction P. (EMIP)
   Harvard Atherosclerosis
      Reversibility P. (HARP)
   Myocardial Infarction Triage
      and Intervention P.
   Stanford Coronary Risk
      Intervention P. (SCRIP)
projection
   anterior oblique p.
   anteroposterior p.
   left anterior oblique p.
   left lateral p.
   right anterior oblique p.
   spider p.
projector
   Tagarno 3SD
      cineangiography p.
prolapse
   mitral valve p. (MVP)
   tricuspid valve p.
   valvular p.
prolapsed mitral valve syndrome
Prolastin
prolate ellipse
proliferans
   endarteritis p.
proliferating
   p. cell nuclear antigen (PCNA)
   p. pleurisy
proliferation
   myxomatous p.
   neointimal p.
Prolog pacemaker
prolongation of expiration
prolonged Q-T interval syndrome
Proloprim
Prometa
promethazine
   p. hydrochloride
   p., phenylephrine, and codeine
   p. with dextromethorphan
Prometh injection
Promine
PROMISE
   Prospective Randomized Milrinone
      Survival Evaluation
Promit
Pronestyl
prongs
   nasal p.

propafenone hydrochloride
propagated thrombus
propagating thrombosis
propagation
    impulse p.
    p. of R wave
propantheline
Pro/Pel
    P. coating
    P. coating cardiac device
    Hi-Torque Floppy with P.
propellant
    halogenated hydrocarbon p.
propeptide
    aminoterminal p.
property
    p.'s of lipophilicity
    vagolytic p.
prophylactic
    p. antibiotic
    p. therapy
prophylaxis
    SBE p.
propionate
    fluticasone p.
Propionibacterium acnes
propionyl L carnitine
propionyl-L-carnitine
Proplex T
propofol
proportional assist ventilation (PAV)
propranolol
    p. hydrochloride
    p. and hydrochlorothiazide
Propulsid
propylthiouracil (PTU)
Prorex injection
ProSom
Prospective
    P. Cardiovascular Munster
    study (PRO-CAM)
    P. Randomized Milrinone
    Survival Evaluation
    (PROMISE)
    P. Randomized Study of
    Ventricular Failure and

    Efficacy of Digoxin
    (PROVED)
prostacyclin
    p. metabolite
prostaglandin
    p. E, E1
Prostaphlin
    P. injection
    P. Oral
ProStep
    P. Patch
prosthesis, pl. prostheses
    Alvarez p.
    Angelchik antireflux p.
    antireflux p.
    aortic p.
    ball-and-cage p.
    ball-cage p.
    ball valve p.
    Barnard mitral valve p.
    Baxter mechanical valve p.
    Beall disk valve p.
    Beall mitral valve p.
    Bentall cardiovascular p.
    Bionit vascular p.
    Bivona-Colorado voice p.
    Björk-Shiley aortic valve p.
    Björk-Shiley convexoconcave
    60-degree valve p.
    Björk-Shiley floating disk p.
    Blom-Singer indwelling low-
    pressure voice p.
    Braunwald-Cutter ball valve p.
    caged ball valve p.
    Capetown aortic valve p.
    CarboMedics cardiac valve p.
    cardiac valve p.
    Carpentier annuloplasty ring p.
    Carpentier-Edwards aortic
    valve p.
    Carpentier-Edwards
    glutaraldehyde-preserved
    porcine xenograft p.
    Carpentier-Rhone-Poulenc mitral
    ring p.
    Cartwright heart p.
    Cartwright valve p.

NOTES

P

prosthesis *(continued)*
collar p.
Cooley-Bloodwell mitral
valve p.
Cooley Dacron p.
Cross-Jones disk valve p.
Cutter aortic valve p.
Cutter-Smeloff aortic valve p.
DeBakey ball valve p.
DeBakey Vasculour-II
vascular p.
Delrin frame of valve p.
De Vega p.
duckbill voice p.
Duromedics valve p.
Edwards Teflon intracardiac
patch p.
esophageal p.
Golaski-UMI vascular p.
Gott-Daggett heart valve p.
Groningen voice p.
Hammersmith mitral p.
Hancock mitral valve p.
heart valve p.
Ionescu-Shiley valve p.
Kaster mitral valve p.
knitted vascular p.
Lillehei-Cruz-Kaster p.
Lillehei-Kaster cardiac valve p.
Lillehei-Kaster mitral valve p.
Meadox-Cooley woven low-
porosity p.
Meadox woven velour p.
Medtronic-Hall heart valve p.
Medtronic-Hall tilting-disk
valve p.
Microknit vascular graft p.
Milliknit Dacron p.
Milliknit vascular graft p.
mitral p.
Monostrut cardiac valve p.
Neville tracheal p.
New Weavenit Dacron p.
Omnicarbon heart valve p.
Omniscience single leaflet
cardiac valve p.
Omniscience tilting-disk
valve p.
polyvinyl p.
porcine p.
Rashkind double-disk
occluder p.
Sauvage filamentous p.

Sorin mitral valve p.
Starr-Edwards aortic valve p.
Starr-Edwards ball valve p.
Starr-Edwards cardiac valve p.
Starr-Edwards disk valve p.
Starr-Edwards heart valve p.
Starr-Edwards mitral p.
stentless porcine aortic
valve p.
St. Jude heart valve p.
supra-annular p.
tilting-disk aortic valve p.
Ultra Low resistance voice p.
USCI Sauvage EXS side-
limb p.
vascular graft p.
Weavenit p.
Wesolowski vascular p.
woven Teflon p.
prosthetic
p. aortic valve
p. cardiac valve
p. poppet
p. ring annuloplasty
p. valve endocarditis
p. valve sewing ring
p. valve thrombosis
p. valve vegetation
Prostin VR Pediatric injection
prostration
pain, pallor, paraesthesia,
pulselessness, paralysis, p.
(PPPPP)
prosyncopal medication
protamine
p. sulfate
Protara
protease
p. inhibitor
protease-antiprotease imbalance
protected brush
protection
automated boundary p. (ABP)
myocardial p.
protective
p. block
p. zone
Protegra
protein
amyloid A p.
bone morphogenetic p. type 2
(BMP-2)
BvgS p.

p. C
cardiac gap junction p.
coagulation p.
contractile p.
cytosolic p.
p. electrophoresis
eosinophil cationic p.
ESAT-6 p.
G p.'s
Gc p.
glycosylation of
  intracellular p.'s
heat shock p. (HSP)
45-kilodalton p.
p. kinase
p. kinase A, C
M p.
M-line p.
rat urine p.
recognition p.
rhoGDI p.
p. S
p. S deficiency
secretory leukoprotease
  inhibitor p.
Tamm-Horsfall p.
thrombus precursor p. (TpT)
ToxR p.
protein-1
monocyte chemotactic p.
  (MCP-1)
proteinase
α₁-proteinase inhibitor (α₁-AT)
protein-calorie
p.-c. deficiency
p.-c. malnutrition
proteinosis
alveolar p.
pulmonary alveolar p.
proteinuria
proteoglycan
proteolysis
proteolytic enzyme
Proteus
P. *mirabilis*
P. pneumonia
P. *vulgaris*

Protex swivel adapter
Prothazine
P. injection
P. Oral
prothrombin
p. time (PT)
p. time/partial thromboplastin
  time (PT/PTT)
prothrombinase complex
protocol
ABC p.
Astrand-Rhyming p.
Balke treadmill p.
Balke-Ware treadmill p.
Bruce treadmill p.
continuous ramp p.
Cornell exercise p.
Ellestad p.
exsanguination p.
Global Utilization of
  Streptokinase and t-PA for
  Occluded Coronary
  Arteries p.
GUSTO p.
Hixson-Vernier p.
James exercise p.
Kattus treadmill p.
McHenry p.
modified Bruce p.
modified Ellestad p.
Naughton treadmill p.
RAMP antitachycardia
  pacing p.
Reeves treadmill p.
reinjection p.
rest metabolism/stress
  perfusion p.
SCAN antitachycardia
  pacing p.
Sheffield treadmill p.
standard Bruce p.
TAMI p.
USAFSAM treadmill p.
Weber-Janicki cardiopulmonary
  exercise p.
Westminster drug-free p.

NOTES

P

protodiastolic
  p. gallop
  p. murmur
  p. rumble
proton
  p. density
  p. spectroscopy
proto-oncogene
proto-oncogenic effect
Protostat Oral
protoveratrine A and B
protozoal myocarditis
protozoan
protriptyline
  p. hydrochloride
prourokinase
  P. in Myocardial Infarction
  (PRIMI)
  P. and t-PA Enhancement of
  Thrombolysis (PATENT)
PROVED
  Prospective Randomized Study of
  Ventricular Failure and Efficacy of
  Digoxin
Pro-Vent
  P.-V. arterial blood gas kit
  P.-V. arterial blood sampling
  kit
Proventil
Providencia
Provigil
provocation
  bronchial p.
  mecalil p.
  p. test
Provocholine
Provox speaking valve
prowazekii
  Rickettsia p.
proxetil
  cefpodoxime p.
proximal
  p. convoluted tubule
  p. coronary sinus (PCS)
  p. isovelocity surface area
  (PISA)
PRP
  platelet-rich plasma
PRP-D vaccine
PRP-OMPC vaccine
PRT
  percutaneous rotational
  thrombectomy

PRU
  peripheral resistance unit
prudent diet
Pruitt-Inahara
  P.-I. balloon-tipped perfusion
  catheter
  P.-I. carotid shunt
Pruitt vascular shunt
prune juice sputum
pruning
  branch vessel p.
Prussian helmet sign
PRVC
  pressure-regulated volume control
  ventilation
PRx Endotak-Sub-Q array
PS
  Palmaz-Schatz
psammoma bodies
psammosarcoma
PSAP
  peak systolic aortic pressure
Pseudallescheria
  P. boydii
  P. maltophilia
  P. stutzeri
pseudallescheriasis
pseudangina, pseudoangina
pseudoalternating current
pseudoaneurysm
pseudoangina (*var. of* pseudangina)
pseudoapoplexy
pseudoasthma
pseudo-AV block
pseudobronchiectasis
pseudocavitation
pseudocirrhosis
pseudocoarctation
  p. of aorta
pseudocomplications
pseudocroup
pseudocylindrical bronchiectasis
pseudodextrocardia
pseudodiastolic
pseudodiphtheriticum
  Bacillus p.
pseudodisappearance criterion
pseudoephedrine
  carbinoxamine and p.
  p. and dextromethorphan
  guaifenesin and p.
  p. HCl
  p. and ibuprofen

pseudofusion beat
pseudohypoparathyroidism
pseudohypotension
pseudoinfarction
pseudo-Kaposi sarcoma
pseudolupus
pseudo-Mahaim fiber
pseudomallei
 p. group
 Pseudomonas p.
pseudomembranous
 p. angina
 p. bronchitis
 p. croup
pseudomonads
Pseudomonas
 P. aeruginosa
 P. cepacia
 P. elastase
 P. exotoxin
 P. maltophilia
 P. pseudomallei
 P. stutzeri
pseudomucinous
pseudonormalization of T wave
pseudoparalytica
 myasthenia gravis p.
pseudopericarditis
pseudopneumonia
pseudothrombocytopenia
pseudotruncus arteriosus
pseudotuberculosis
 Yersinia p.
pseudotumor
pseudotumoral mediastinal amyloidosis
pseudoxanthoma
 p. elasticum
 p. elasticum syndrome
PSG
 peak systolic gradient
 polysomnogram
  PSG pressure
psi
 pounds per square inch
psig
 pounds per square inch gauge

P-sinistrocardiale
psittaci
 Chlamydia p.
psittacosis
psoriasis
PSS
 progressive systemic sclerosis
PSVT
 paroxysmal supraventricular tachycardia
psychocardiac reflex
psychogenic
 p. dyspnea
 p. overlay
 p. pain
psychological
 p. factor
 p. stimulus
psychosis
 postperfusion p.
psychosocial
 P. Adjustment to Illness Scale
 p. factor
psychostimulant
psychotherapy
psychotropic agent
psyllium
PT
 prothrombin time
PTAS
 percutaneous transluminal angioscopy
PTCA
 percutaneous transluminal coronary angioplasty
PTCR
 percutaneous transluminal coronary revascularization
PtdCho
 phosphatidylcholine
pterygoid chest
PTFE
 polytetrafluoroethylene
PTIF
 peak tidal inspiratory flow

NOTES

P

PTMC
 percutaneous transvenous mitral
  commissurotomy
PTP-gamma
PT/PTT
 prothrombin time/partial
  thromboplastin time
PTT
 partial thromboplastin time
PTU
 propylthiouracil
puerile respiration
puerperal
 p. phlebitis
 p. thrombosis
puff
 p. of smoke
 veiled p.
puffer
 pink p.
puffing sound
Puig
 P. Massana annuloplasty ring
 P. Massana-Shiley annuloplasty
  ring
 P. Massana-Shiley annuloplasty
  valve
pullback
 aortic p.
 p. pressure
pull-through
 station p.-t.
Pulmanex
Pulmo-Aide
 P.-A. nebulizer
 P.-A. Traveler
pulmoaortic canal
Pulmocare
Pulmo-Graph
pulmonale
 atrium p.
 cor p.
 P pulmonale
 pseudo-P pulmonale
pulmonaris
 porta p.
pulmonary
 p. acid aspiration syndrome
 p. agenesis
 p. alveolar hemorrhage
 p. alveolar microlithiasis
 p. alveolar proteinosis
 p. amebiasis

p. amyloidosis
p. anthrax
p. aplasia
p. arch
p. arterial web
p. arteriolar resistance
p. arteriovenous fistula
p. arteriovenous malformation
 (PAVM)
p. artery (PA)
p. artery band
p. artery banding (PA banding)
p. artery catheterization
p. artery occlusion pressure
 (PAOP)
p. artery occlusive wedge
 pressure
p. artery pressure (PAP)
p. artery sling
p. artery steal
p. artery stenosis
p. artery wedge (PAW)
p. artery wedge pressure
 (PAWP)
p. aspergillosis
p. atresia
p. autograft valve
p. barotrauma
p. bed
p. blastoma
p. blood flow
p. blood volume (PBV)
p. botryomycosis
p. branch stenosis
p. capillary wedge pressure
 (PCWP)
p. cavitation
p. circulation
p. coccidioidomycosis
p. cyanosis
p. disease anemia syndrome
p. dysmaturity syndrome
p. effusion
p. embolectomy
p. embolism
p. embolization
p. embolus
p. failure
p. fever
p. fibrosis
p. flotation catheter
p. function (PF)
p. function test (PFT)

p. gas exchange
p. hamartoma
p. heart
p. hemosiderosis
p. hypertension
p. hypertension pressure
p. hypertrophic osteoarthropathy
p. incompetence
p. infarct
p. infarction
p. infarction syndrome
p. infiltration with eosinophilia (PIE)
p. insufficiency
p. interstitial edema
p. interstitial emphysema (PIE)
p. lymphoma
p. markings
p. meniscus sign
p. metastasectomy
p. mucormycosis
p. murmur
p. mycosis
p. notch sign
p. ossification
p. pain
p. parenchymal window
p. phthisis
p. pleurisy
p. pulse
p. rales
p. scintigraphy
p. sequestration
p. sling syndrome
p. surfactant
p. systemic blood flow ratio
p. target sign
p. thromboembolism
p. toilet
p. tuberculosis
p. valve anomaly
p. valve area
p. valve disease
p. valve echocardiography
p. valve gradient
p. valve restenosis
p. valve stenosis

p. valve vegetation
p. valvular regurgitation
p. valvular stenosis
p. valvuloplasty
p. vascular obstruction
p. vascular obstructive disease
p. vascular pressure
p. vascular reactivity
p. vascular redistribution
p. vascular resistance (PVR)
p. vascular resistance index (PVRI)
p. vasculature
p. vasculitis
p. vasoconstriction
p. vein
p. veno-occlusive disease (PVOD)
p. venous connection
p. venous connection anomaly
p. venous drainage
p. venous return
p. venous return anomaly
p. wedge angiography
p. wedge pressure (PWP)
pulmonic
    p. area
    p. closure sound
    p. endocarditis
    p. incompetence
    p. insufficiency
    p. murmur
    p. regurgitation
    p. second sound
    p. valve
    p. valve closure sound
    p. valve stenosis
pulmonis
    alveoli p.
    basis p.
pulmonocoronary reflex
Pulmopak pump
PulmoSonic
pulmowrap
Pulmozyme
Pulsair .5 liquid oxygen portable
Pulsar NI implantable pacemaker

NOTES

P

pulsate
pulsatile
   p. assist device (PAD)
   p. flow
pulsating
   p. empyema
   p. pleurisy
pulsation
   suprasternal p.
Pulsator
   P. dry heparin arterial blood
     gas kit
   P. syringe
pulse
   alternating p.
   p. amplitude
   anacrotic p., anadicrotic p.
   arterial p.
   atrial liver p.
   atrial venous p.
   Bamberger bulbar p.
   biferious p.
   bigeminal p.
   bigeminal bisferious p.
   bisferious p.
   bounding p.
   brachial p.
   bulbar p.
   cannonball p.
   capillary p.
   carotid p.
   catacrotic p.
   catadicrotic p.
   catatricrotic p.
   centripetal venous p.
   collapsing p.
   cordy p.
   Corrigan p.
   coupled p.
   p. curve
   CV wave of jugular venous p.
   p. deficit
   dicrotic p.
   digitalate p.
   dorsalis pedis p.
   p. duration
   elastic p.
   entoptic p.
   filiform p.
   formicant p.
   F point of cardiac apex p.
   funic p.
   f wave of jugular venous p.

   gaseous p.
   p. generator
   guttural p.
   hard p.
   hyperkinetic p.
   hypokinetic p.
   incisura p.
   intermittent p.
   irregularly irregular p.
   jerky p.
   jugular venous p.
   Kussmaul paradoxical p.
   labile p.
   long p.
   Monneret p.
   monocrotic p.
   mousetail p.
   movable p.
   nail p.
   O point of cardiac apex p.
   p. oximeter
   p. oximeter/end tidal CO_2
     (POET)
   p. oximetry device
   p. oximetry monitoring (POM)
   paradoxical p.
   parvus et tardus p.
   pedal p.
   p. period
   piston p.
   plateau p.
   popliteal p.
   precordial p.
   p. pressure
   pulmonary p.
   quadrigeminal p.
   Quincke p.
   radial p.
   p. rate
   p. repetition
   p. repetition frequency (PRF)
   respiratory p.
   reversed paradoxical p.
   Riegel p.
   SF wave of cardiac apex p.
   soft p.
   spike-and-dome p.
   tense p.
   thready p.
   tibial p.
   tidal wave p.
   p. tracing
   trigeminal p.

trip-hammer p.
triple-humped pressure p.
p. trisection
undulating p.
unequal p.
vagus p.
venous p.
vermicular p.
water-hammer p.
p. wave
p. wave velocity (PWV)
p. width
wiry p.
y depression of jugular
    venous p.
y descent of jugular venous p.
pulsed
p. Doppler echocardiography
p. Doppler flowmetry
p. dye laser
p. laser ablation
PulseDose
P. oxygen delivery technology
P. portable compressed oxygen
    systems
pulsed-wave Doppler mapping
pulse-height analyzer
pulseless
p. bradycardia
p. disease
p. electrical activity (PEA)
p. idioventricular rhythm
PulseSpray
P. infusion system
pulsimeter, pulsometer
pulsus
p. alternans
p. anadicrotus
p. bigeminus
p. bisferiens
p. caprisans
p. catacrotus
p. catadicrotus
p. celer
p. celerrimus
p. cordis
p. debilis

p. differens
p. duplex
p. durus
p. filiformis
p. fluens
p. formicans
p. fortis
p. frequens
p. heterochronicus
p. inaequalis
p. incongruens
p. infrequens
p. intercidens
p. intercurrens
p. irregularis perpetuus
p. magnus
p. mollis
p. monocrotus
p. myurus
p. paradoxus
p. parvus
p. parvus et tardus
p. quadrigeminus
p. rarus
p. respiratione intermittens
p. tardus
p. tremulus
p. trigeminus
p. vacuus
p. venosus
pultaceous debris
Pulvules
Cinobac P.
Seromycin P.
pumilus
Bacillus p.
pump
Abbott infusion p.
abdominothoracic p.
Accupressure infusion p.
angle port p.
aortic balloon p.
AVCO balloon p.
Axiom double sump p.
balloon p.
Bard cardiopulmonary
    support p.

NOTES

pump *(continued)*
Bard TransAct intra-aortic
balloon p.
Barron p.
Baxter Flo-Gard 8200
volumetric infusion p.
Bio-Medicus p.
blood p.
BVS p.
CADD-Plus intravenous
infusion p.
cardiac balloon p.
Cobe double blood p.
Cordis Hakim p.
Cormed ambulatory infusion p.
p. current
Datascope intra-aortic
balloon p.
Datascope system 90 intra-
aortic balloon p.
ECMO p.
p. failure
Flowtron DVT p.
p. function
Gomco thoracic drainage p.
Hakim-Cordis p.
Harvard p.
heart p.
HeartMate p.
IMED infusion p.
Infusaid infusion p.
Infuse-A-Port p.
ion p.
IVAC volumetric infusion p.
Jobst extremity p.
KAAT II Plus intra-aortic
balloon p.
Kangaroo p.
Kontron intra-aortic balloon p.
left ventricular bypass p.
Life Care P.
Lindbergh p.
p. lung
Master Flow Pumpette p.
Medtronic SynchroMed p.
Microjet Quark portable p.
muscular venous p.
Neuroperfusion p.
p. oxygenation
p. oxygenator
Pulmopak p.
roller p.
sump p.

SynchroMed programmable p.
Thoratec p.
Travenol infusion p.
volumetric infusion p.
Pumpette
Master Flow P.
Stat 2 P.
pumpkin-seeding
pump-oxygenator
punch
Abrams pleural biopsy p.
p. biopsy
Goosen vascular p.
puncture
apical left ventricular p.
direct cardiac p.
left ventricular p.
tracheoesophageal p.
transseptal p.
venous p.
pup cell
pupils
Argyll Robertson p.
pure
p. flutter
p. parasystole
purified protein derivative (PPD)
**purine nucleotides adenosine
triphosphate**
Puritan
P. All Purpose
P. Bennett ETCO$_2$ multigas
analyzer
P. Bubble-Jet
Puritan-Bennett
P.-B. 7250 metabolic monitor
P.-B. ventilator
Purkinje
P. cells
P. conduction
P. fibers
P. system
P. tumor
Purmann method
puromucous
Purpose
Puritan All P.
purpura
anaphylactoid p.
p. fulminans
Henoch-Schönlein p.
idiopathic thrombocytopenic p.
(ITP)

thrombotic thrombocytopenic p. (TTP)

purpurea
  Digitalis p.

purr

purring thrill

pursed-lip breathing

pursestring suture

pursing
  lip p.

purulent
  p. pericarditis
  p. pleurisy
  p. pneumonia
  p. sputum

purulenta
  pneumonia interlobularis p.

pushability

putative slow pathway potential

putrid
  p. bronchitis
  p. empyema

PVB
  premature ventricular beat

PVC
  polyvinyl chloride
  premature ventricular contraction

PVD
  peripheral vascular disease

PVOD
  pulmonary veno-occlusive disease

PVR
  pulmonary vascular resistance

PVRI
  pulmonary vascular resistance index

PVT
  primary ventricular tachycardia

PWP
  pulmonary wedge pressure

PWV
  pulse wave velocity

pyemic embolism

pyknosis

pyloric incompetence

pyocyanines

pyogenes
  Streptococcus p.

Pyopen

pyopneumopericardium

pyopneumothorax

pyothorax

PYP
  pyrophosphate
  PYP imaging
  PYP scan

pyramid method

pyrantel pamoate

pyrazinamide (PZA)
  rifampin, isoniazid, and p.

Pyribenzamine (PBZ)

pyridazinone dinitrile

pyridoxilated stroma-free
  hemoglobin (SFHb)

pyridoxine hydrochloride

pyriform thorax

pyrimethamine
  sulfadoxine and p.

pyrogen reaction

pyroglycolic acid suture

pyrolytic carbon

pyrophosphate (PYP)
  p. imaging
  p. scintigram
  p. scintigraphy
  technetium-99m p.

pyruvate
  p. dehydrogenase

pyruvic acid

PZA
  pyrazinamide

NOTES

P

403

Q

Q fever
Q Port
Q wave
Q wave myocardial infarction
Q wave regression

QCA

quantitative coronary angiography

Q-cath

Q-c. catheter
Q-c. catheterization recording
system

QCT

quantitative computed tomography

Q-H interval
Q-M interval
Qp/Qs

flow ratio

Q-RB interval
Q-R interval
QR pattern
QRS

QRS alternans
QRS axis
QRS complex
QRS interval
QRS loop
QRS morphology
slurring of QRS
QRS synchronous atrial
defibrillation shocks
QRS vector

QRS-ST junction
QRS-T

QRS-T angle
QRS-T complex
QRS-T interval
QRS-T value

QS

QS complex
QS deflection
QS pattern
QS wave

Q-S₂ interval

Q-S$_2$ interval
Q-Stress

Q-S. treadmill
Q-S. treadmill stress test

Q-switched Nd:YAG laser
Q-T

Q-T interval

Q-T interval sensing pacemaker
Q-T syndrome

QT

QT corrected for heart rate
(QTc)
QT dispersion

QTc

QT corrected for heart rate
QTc interval

QTp/QTe

ratio of QTp/QTe

QT/QTc dispersion
Q-TU interval syndrome
quad

q. coughing
q. screen format

QuadPolar

Q. electrode

quadpolar w/Damato curve catheter
quadrangulation of Frouin
quadricuspid
quadrigeminal

q. pulse
q. rhythm

quadrigeminus

pulsus q.

quadrigeminy
quadriparesis
quadriplegia
quadripolar

q. Itrel 2 pulse generator
q. Quad electrode
q. steerable electrode catheter

quadruple rhythm
quadruplet
Quaegebeur procedure
Quain

Q. fatty degeneration
Q. fatty heart

quality

q. control

Quality of Well-Being Index
Quanticor catheter
quantification

acoustic q. (AQ)
microdensitophotometric q.
shunt q.

quantify
quanti-Pirquet reaction

quantitative
- q. arteriography
- q. computed tomography (QCT)
- q. coronary angiographic analysis
- q. coronary angiography (QCA)
- q. Doppler
- q. left ventriculography
- q. two-dimensional echocardiography

Quantum
- Q. pacemaker
- Q. PSV

QuantX color quantification tool
quartile range
quartisternal
quartz transducer
quasi-sinusoidal biphasic waveform
quaternary
Queckenstedt sign
Queensland
- Q. fever
- Q. tick typhus

quellung reaction
Queltuss
Quénu-Muret sign
quenuthoracoplasty
query fever
Quest
- Tranquility Q.

questionnaire
- Coping Strategies q.
- Kellner q.
- Rose q.
- Seattle angina q. (SAQ)

Questran
- Q. Light

Quetelet index
Quibron
quick
- q. prothrombin time
- Q. test

QuickFlash arterial catheter
QuickFurl
- Q. DL
- Q. SL balloon

quiet
- q. breath sounds
- q. chest
- q. heart sounds
- q. precordium

Quik-Chek external pacer tester
Quik-Prep
quinacrine
Quinaglute
- Q. Dura-Tabs

Quinalan
- Q. Oral

quinaprilat
quinapril hydrochloride
Quinatime
Quincke
- Q. disease
- Q. edema
- Q. pulse
- Q. sign

Quincke-point spinal needle
quinestrol
quinethazone
Quinidex
- Q. Extentabs

quinidine
- q. gluconate
- q. sulfate

quinine
- q. sulfate

quinolones
Quinones
- method of Q.

Quinora
- Q. Oral

quinsy
- lingual q.

Q-U interval
Quinton
- Q. PermCath catheter
- Q. tube

Quinton-Scribner shunt
quotient
- respiratory q. (RQ)
- V/Q q.

R
    gas constant
    roentgen
        R on T phenomenon
        R unit
        R wave
        R wave amplitude
        R wave gating
        R wave progression
RA
    rheumatoid arthritis
    right atrium
        RA cell
RAA
    right atrial appendage
RAAS
    renin-angiotensin-aldosterone system
rAAT
    recombinant alpha$_1$ antitrypsin
rabbit antithymocyte globulin
rabbit-ear sign
rabies
RACAT
    rapid acquisition computed axial
        tomography
racemic epinephrine
racemose aneurysm
Rackley
    method of R., R. method
racquet incision
RAD
    reactive airways disease
    right axis deviation
rad
    radiation absorbed dose
radarkymography
radial
    r. artery
    r. pulse
RADIANCE
    Randomized Assessment of Digoxin
        on Inhibitors of Angiotensin
        Converting Enzyme
radiant heat device (RHD)
radiation
    r. absorbed dose (rad)
    r. equivalent in man (rem)
    ionizing r. (IR)
    r. lung disease
    r. pneumonitis

    r. safety
    secondary r.
    r. therapy
radiation-induced pericarditis
radical
    hydroxyl r.
    O_2 r.
    oxygen r.
radicle
radiculitis
    cervical r.
Radifocus catheter guidewire
**RadiMedical fiberoptic pressure-
    monitoring wire**
**radioactive iodinated serum albumin
    (RISA)**
radioallergosorbent test (RAST)
radiocardiogram
radiocardiography
radiocontrast dye
radiodense
radiodermatitis
radiofrequency (RF)
    r. ablater
    r. ablation (RFA)
    r. catheter ablation
    r. current (RFC)
    r. electrophrenic respiration
    r. hot balloon
radiographic
    r. technique
radiography
radioimmunoassay
    Coat-a-Count r.
    Mallinckrodt r.
radioisotope
radioisotopic study
radiolabeled
    r. fibrinogen
    r. iodine
    r. microsphere
radioligand
    r. binding assay
radiologic scimitar syndrome
Radiometer probe
radiometry
    BACTEC r.
Radionics RFG-35
radionuclide
    r. angiocardiography

R

radionuclide *(continued)*
r. angiography
r. cineangiocardiography
gold-195m r.
r. imaging
r. scanning
r. study
r. technique
r. ventriculography (RNV)
radiopacity
radiopaque
r. calibrated catheter
r. tantalum stent
radiopharmaceutical
radiotracer
radius
thrombocytopenia-absent r.
(TAR)
radon
RADS
reactive airways disease syndrome
RAE
right atrial enlargement
RAE endotracheal tube
Raeder-Harbitz syndrome
Raff-Glantz derivative method
ragpicker's disease
ragsorter's disease
railroad track sign
rain of collaterals
rake retractor
rale
amphoric r.
atelectatic r.
basilar r.
bibasilar r.
border r.
bronchial r.
bronchiectatic r.
bubbling r.
cavernous r.
cellophane r.
clicking r.
coarse r.
collapse r.
consonating r.
crackling r.
crepitant r.
r. de retour
dry r.
extrathoracic r.
gurgling r.
guttural r.

Hirtz r.
r. indux
inspiratory r.
laryngeal r.
marginal r.
metallic r.
moist r.
mucous r.
r. muqueux
musical r.
pleural r.
pulmonary r.
r. redux
r. and rhonchi
sibilant r.
Skoda r.
snoring r.
sonorous r.
subcrepitant r.
tracheal r.
Velcro r.
vesicular r.
wet r.
whistling r.
Raman
R. spectography
R. spectroscopy
rami (*pl. of* ramus)
ramipril
Ramirez shunt
Ramond sign
RAMP
R. antitachycardia pacing
protocol
ramp pacing
ramus, pl. **rami**
r. intermedius
r. intermedius artery
r. medianus
Randall-Baker Soucek (RBS)
Rand microballoon
randomized
R. Assessment of Digoxin on
Inhibitors of Angiotensin
Converting Enzyme
(RADIANCE)
R. Evaluation of Salvage
Angioplasty with Combined
Utilization of Endpoints
(RESCUE)
R. Intervention in the
Treatment of Angina (RITA)
r. trials

R

random-zero sphygmomanometer
Ranfac needle
range
>   dynamic r.
>   interquartile r.
>   logarithmic dynamic r.
>   quartile r.
range-alternating current
ranging
>   echo r.
Ranke complex
ranolazine
Ransohoff operation
Ranvier
>   node of R.
RAO
>   right anterior oblique
>   RAO angulation
>   RAO position
>   RAO view
RAP
>   right atrial pressure
rapamycin
rape
>   bruit de scie ou de r.
rapeseed oil
raphe of pharynx
rapid
>   r. acquisition computed axial
>   tomography (RACAT)
>   r. atrial pacing
>   r. depolarization
>   r. eye movement (REM)
>   r. filling wave
>   r. nonsustained ventricular
>   tachycardia
>   r. sequence induction (RSI)
>   r. y descent
rapid-burst pacing
rappel
>   bruit de r.
rarus
>   pulsus r.
RAS
>   rotational atherectomy system

rash
>   erythematous, maculopapular r.
>   maculopapular r.
Rashkind
>   R. balloon technique
>   R. cardiac device
>   R. double-disk occluder
>   prosthesis
>   R. double umbrella
>   R. double umbrella device
>   R. procedure
>   R. septostomy balloon catheter
>   R. septostomy needle
Rasmussen aneurysm
Rasor Blood Pumping system
raspatory
>   Coryllos rib r.
>   rib r.
rasping murmur
RAST
>   radioallergosorbent test
Rastan-Konno procedure
Rastan operation
Rastelli
>   R. conduit
>   R. operation
>   R. procedure
rate
>   baseline variability of fetal
>   heart r.
>   beat-to-beat variability of fetal
>   heart r.
>   complication r.
>   count r.
>   critical r.
>   disintegration r.
>   ejection r.
>   erythrocyte sedimentation r.
>   (ESR)
>   expiratory flow r.
>   fetal heart r.
>   flow r.
>   heart r. (HR)
>   r. hysteresis
>   r. immunonephelometry
>   inspiratory flow r.
>   low flow r.

NOTES

rate *(continued)*
magnet r.
maximal expiratory flow r.
(MEFR)
maximal inspiratory flow r.
(MIFR)
maximal midexpiratory flow r.
(MMEFR)
maximal ventilation r. (MVR)
maximum flow r.
maximum predicted heart r.
(MPHR)
mean midexpiratory flow r.
(FEF$_{25-75\%}$)
mean normalized systolic
ejection r.
mortality r.
pacemaker adaptive r.
peak diastolic filling r.
peak emptying r.
peak expiratory flow r.
(PEFR)
peak filling r. (PFR)
peak inspiratory flow r. (PIFR)
peak jet flow r.
r. pressure product
pulse r.
QT corrected for heart r.
(QTc)
repetition r.
respiratory r.
sedimentation r.
slew r.
stroke ejection r.
systolic ejection r. (SER)
target heart r. (THR)
Westergren erythrocyte
sedimentation r.
Wintrobe sedimentation r.
rate-adaptive device
rate-dependent angina
rate-modulated pacemaker
rate-responsive
dual-chamber r.-r. (DR)
r.-r. pacemaker
r.-r. pacing
single-chamber, r.-r.
Rathke pouch tumor
ratings of perceived exertion (RPE)
ratio
AH:HA r.
ankle-brachial blood pressure r.

aorta-left atrium r.
aortic root r.
cardiothoracic r. (CT, CTR)
0 to 10 category r. (CR-10)
conduction r.
contrast r.
dead space:tidal volume r.
E:A wave r.
E:I r.
flow r. (Qp/Qs)
forced expiratory volume timed
to forced capacity r.
forced expiratory volume timed
to forced vital capacity r.
(FEV/FVC)
I:E r.
inspiratory to expiratory r.
(I:E)
international normalized r.
(INR)
La:A r.
L/S r.
pulmonary systemic blood
flow r.
r. of QTp/QTe
renal vein renin r.
residual volume to total lung
capacity r. (RV/TLC)
resistance r.
RV/TLC r.
sex r.
shunt r.
signal-to-noise r.
systolic velocity r.
transmitral Doppler E:A r.
transmitral E:A r.
V/C r.
ventilation/perfusion r.
rationalization
Ratliff criteria for myocarditis
rattle of return
rat urine protein
Rauchfuss triangle
Raudilan PB
Raudixin
Raudolfin
Raulerson syringe
Rautaharju ECG criteria
Rauwolfia
R. alkaloid
R. extract
R. serpentina

RAVES
   Reduced Anticoagulation in Vein
   Graft Stent
ray
   beta r.
   gamma r.
   r. sum
   x-r.
Raynaud
   R. disease
   R. phenomenon
   R. syndrome
RayTec sponge
Razi cannula introducer
RBBB
   right bundle-branch block
RBS
   Randall-Baker Soucek
   RBS face mask
RCA
   right coronary artery
   rotational coronary atherectomy
RDI
   respiratory disturbance index
RDS
   respiratory distress syndrome
reabsorbable suture
reaction
   allergic r.
   anaphylactoid r.
   Arthus-type r.
   cholera vaccine r.
   egg-yellow r.
   Eisenmenger r.
   Fernandez r.
   fibrinolytic r.
   fight-or-flight r.
   Haber-Weiss r.
   hexokinase r.
   inflammatory r.
   Kveim r.
   polymerase chain r. (PCR)
   pyrogen r.
   quanti-Pirquet r.
   quellung r.
   reverse transcriptase polymerase
      chain r. (RT-PCR)

   smallpox vaccine r.
   vagal r.
   vasovagal r.
   Weil-Felix r.
   xanthine oxidase r.
reactivation tuberculosis
reactive
   r. airways disease (RAD)
   r. airways disease syndrome
      (RADS)
   r. dilation
   r. hyperemia
reactivity
   pulmonary vascular r.
reagin
real-time three-dimensional
   echocardiography
rebound angina
rebreathing
   r. bag
   r. mask
recainam
recalcitrant hypertension
recanalization
   balloon occlusive intravascular
      lysis enhanced r. (BOILER)
   excimer vascular r.
   r. vs. recannulization
recannulization
   recanalization vs. r.
receiver
   Medtronic radiofrequency r.
receptive aphasia
receptor
   adrenergic r.
   A-II r.
   alpha r.
   beta r.
   beta-adrenergic r. (BAR)
   cholinergic r.
   chylomicron remnant r.
   endothelin A, B r.'s
   epithelial 5'-nucleotide r.
   Fc r.'s
   glycoprotein IIb/IIIa r.
   H1 r.

R

NOTES

receptor *(continued)*
    r. for hyaluronan-mediated
      motility (RHAMM)
    irritant r.
    juxtacapillary r.
    muscarinic r.
    ryanodine r.
    stretch r.
receptor-operated calcium channel
recessed balloon septostomy catheter
recipient heart
reciprocal
    r. beat
    r. bigeminy
    r. rhythm
    r. ST depression
reciprocating
    r. macroreentry orthodromic
      tachycardia
    r. rhythm
reciprocity
reclosure
recoarctation of aorta
recognition protein
recoil
    elastic r.
    r. wave
recombinant
    r. alpha$_1$ antitrypsin (rAAT)
    r. alteplase
    r. desulfatohirudin
    r. hirudin (r-hirudin)
    r. lys-plasminogen
    r. tissue plasminogen activator
      (rt-PA)
    r. tissue-type plasminogen
      activator
Recombinate
reconstitution
    homocollateral r.
reconstruction
    bifurcated vein graft for
      vascular r.
    Cabral coronary r.
    polyhedral surface r.
    Sheen airway r.
recorder
    circadian event r.
    Del Mar Avionics three-
      channel r.
    Eigon CardioLoop r.
    event r.

    24-hour ambulatory
      electrocardiographic r.
    King of Hearts event r.
    Marquette Holter r.
    MEDILOG 4000 ambulatory
      ECG r.
    Mingograf 82 r.
    Narco Biosystems r.
    Narco Physiograph-6B r.
    Oxford Medilog frequency-
      modulated r.
    Scole Alta II 3-channel
      precalibrated Holter AM r.
    SNAP sleep r.
    Vas r.
    videotape r.
recording
    bipolar esophageal r.
    cineloop r.
    Doppler r.
    M-mode r.
    X, Y, Z r.'s
recovery
    pressure r.
recrudescence
recruitable collateral vessel
recruitment
    host-generated neutrophils r.
rectification
    anomalous r.
    inward-going r.
rectocardiac reflex
rectus abdominis muscle
recurrence risk
recurrent
    r. mesenteric ischemia
    r. mesenteric vascular
      occlusion
    r. myocardial infarction
    r. respiratory papillomatosis
recursion
    Levinson-Durbin r.
recurvatum
    pectus r.
red
    r. atrophy
    r. hypertension
    r. infarct
    r. thrombus
Redifocus guidewire
RediFurl
    R. DL, SL
    R. TaperSeal IAB catheter

redilation
redistribution
    r. imaging
    pulmonary vascular r.
    vascular r.
Reduced Anticoagulation in Vein Graft Stent (RAVES)
reductase
    3-hydroxy-3-methylglutaryl
        coenzyme A r.
reduction
    afterload r.
    gradient r.
    preload r.
    stapled lung r.
redundant cusp syndrome
reduplication murmur
redux
    rale r.
reedswitch
    pacemaker r.
reendothelialization
reentrant
    r. arrhythmia
    r. atrial tachycardia
    r. circuit
    r. loop
    r. mechanism
    r. pathway
    r. supraventricular tachycardia
reentry
    atrioventricular nodal r.
    A-V nodal r.
    bundle-branch r.
    r. phenomenon
    Schmitt-Erlanger model of r.
    sinus nodal r.
    r. theory
    ventricular r.
Reeves treadmill protocol
reference
    r. electrode
    r. value
refill
    transcapillary r.
reflectance oximetry
reflecting level

reflection
    guidewire r.
reflex
    abdominocardiac r.
    Abrams heart r.
    r. angina
    aortic r.
    Aschner r.
    Aschner-Dagnini r.
    r. asthma
    atriopressor r.
    auriculopressor r.
    Babinski r.
    Bainbridge r.
    baroreceptor r.
    Bezold-Jarisch r.
    bregmocardiac r.
    Breuer-Hering inflation r.
    cardiac depressor r.
    carotid sinus r.
    chemoreceptor r.
    Churchill-Cope r.
    coronary r.
    cough r.
    r. cough
    craniocardiac r.
    Cushing r.
    depressor r.
    diving r.
    Erben r.
    esophagosalivary r.
    eyeball compression r.
    eyeball-heart r.
    gag r.
    gasp r.
    Head paradoxical r.
    heart r.
    hepatojugular r.
    Hering-Breuer r.
    Hoffman r.
    hypochondrial r.
    inflation r.
    Kisch r.
    Kocher-Cushing r.
    laryngeal r.
    Livierato r.
    Loven r.

NOTES

413

reflex *(continued)*
McDowall r.
mute r.'s
oculocardiac r.
oculopharyngeal r.
oculovagal r.
orthocardiac r.
R. 8220 pacemaker
Pavlov r.
pericardial r.
pharyngeal r.
pneocardiac r.
pressoreceptor r.
psychocardiac r.
pulmonocoronary r.
rectocardiac r.
respiratory r.'s
sinus r.
sneeze r.
R. SuperSoft steerable
guidewire
r. sympathetic dystrophy
r. sympathoexcitation
r. tachycardia
vagal r.
vascular r.
r. vasodilation
vasopressor r.
venorespiratory r.
viscerocardiac r.
Re/Flex filter
reflexogenic pressosensitivity
Reflotron bedside theophylline test
reflux
abdominojugular r.
cardioesophageal r.
erosive r.
esophageal r.
r. esophagitis
extraesophageal r.
gastroesophageal r. (GER)
hepatojugular r. (HJR)
refractoriness
refractory
r. period
r. period of electronic
pacemaker
r. tachycardia
Refsum disease
regimen
dosage r.
exercise r.
stepped-care antihypertensive r.

region
AN r.
N r.
NH r.
paratracheal r.
watershed r.
regional
r. myocardial blood flow
(RMBF)
r. wall motion
**Regionally Organized Cardiac Key
European Trial (ROCKET)**
Registry
Balloon Valvuloplasty R.
Mansfield Valvuloplasty R.
Regitine
regression
r. analysis
arteriographic r.
r. equation
least-squares r.
linear r.
multiple r.
Q wave r.
regular
R. (Concentrated) Iletin II U-
500
R. Iletin I
r. purified pork insulin
r. rate and rhythm (RRR)
r. sinus rhythm (RSR)
regularly irregular rhythm
regulator
cystic fibrosis
transmembrane r. (CFTR)
regulon
BvgAS r.
regurgitant
r. fraction
r. jet
r. jet area (RJA)
r. murmur
r. pockets
r. wave
regurgitation
aortic r. (AR)
aortic valve r.
ischemic mitral r.
mitral r. (MR)
mitral valve r.
pulmonary valvular r.
pulmonic r.
semilunar valve r.

tricuspid r. (TR)
valvular r.
rehabilitation
cardiac r.
vocational r.
work r.
rehalation
Rehbein rib spreader
Reid
R. index
R. index measurement
reinfarction
reinfection tuberculosis
reinfusion
reinjection protocol
Reisman
R. myocardosis
R. pneumonia
Reiter
R. disease
R. syndrome
reject control
rejection
acute allograft r.
acute lung r.
r. cardiomyopathy
r. cardiomyopathy transplant
graft r.
no infection-no r. (NI-NR)
rejection-associated pulmonary
fibrosis
relapsing
r. fever
r. polychondritis
relation
concentration-effect r.
diastolic pressure-volume r.
end-systolic pressure-volume r.
end-systolic stress-dimension r.
force-frequency r.
force-length r.
force-velocity r.
force-velocity-length r.
force-velocity-volume r.
interval-strength r.
length-resting tension r.
length-tension r.

pressure-volume r.
resting length-tension r.
tension-length r.
ventilation/perfusion r.
ventricular end-systolic
pressure-volume r.
relationship
Laplace r.
pressure-flow r.
stress-shortening r.
relative
r. cardiac volume
r. incompetence
r. refractory period (RRP)
r. risk
r. wall thickness (RWT)
relaxant
muscle r.
relaxation
r. atelectasis
diastolic r.
dynamic r.
endothelium-mediated r.
isovolumetric r.
isovolumic r.
left ventricular diastolic r.
r. loading
smooth muscle r.
stress r.
r. technique
r. time
r. time index
ventricular r.
relaxometry
NMR r.
Relay cardiac pacemaker
release
Acutrim Precision R.
allergen-induced mediator r.
physiologic pattern r. (PPR)
sustained r.
Relia-Vac drain
Relief
Mini Thin Asthma R.
Vicks DayQuil Sinus Pressure
& Congestion R.

R

NOTES

Relief *(continued)*
Vicks 44D Cough & Head Congestion R.
Relief
reliever
Arthritis Foundation Pain R.
Medtronic Pulsor Intrasound pain r.
REM
rapid eye movement
REM sleep
REM sleep-related hypoxemia
rem
radiation equivalent in man
Remac system
remission
Legroux r.
remnant
chylomicron r.
remodeling
arterial r.
concentric r.
ventricular r.
Renaissance spirometry system
renal
r. angiography
r. arteriography
r. artery
r. artery bypass graft
r. artery disease
r. artery-reverse saphenous vein bypass
r. azotemia
r. blood vessel
r. cortical necrosis
r. cyst
r. dialysis
r. diet
r. dyspnea
r. failure
r. fistula
r. function
r. hypertension
r. insufficiency
r. parenchymal disease
r. transplant
r. tuberculosis
r. vein
r. vein renin ratio
renal-splanchnic steal
Rendu-Osler-Weber
R.-O.-W. disease
R.-O.-W. syndrome

Renese
renin
r. angiotensin
r. inhibitor
plasma r.
renin-angiotensin-aldosterone
r.-a.-a. cascade
r.-a.-a. system (RAAS)
renin-angiotensin blocker
Renografin-76
sonicated R.
renography
renomedullary lipid
renoprival hypertension
Renormax
renovascular
r. angiography
r. hypertension
Renovist
Rentrop
R. catheter
R. classification
REO
respiratory and enteric orphan
REO virus
reocclusion
ReoPro
Reovirus
repair
Allison hiatal hernia r.
Boerema hernia r.
Brom r.
DeBakey-Creech aneurysm r.
Effler hiatal hernia r.
Fontan r.
Hatafuku fundus onlay patch esophageal r.
pericardioplasty in pectus excavatum r.
reparative cardiac surgery
repeat
r. balloon mitral valvotomy
r. revascularization
reperfusion
r. arrhythmia
r. catheter
emergency r.
r. injury
late r.
reperfusion-induced hemorrhage
repetition
pulse r.

r. rate
r. time (TR)
repetitive
r. monomorphic ventricular
tachycardia
r. paroxysmal ventricular
tachycardia
replacement
aortic valve r. (AVR)
Cosgrove mitral valve r.
mitral valve r. (MVR)
supra-annular mitral valve r.
(SMVR)
valve r.
repletion
replication
repolarization
benign early r. (BER)
early rapid r.
final rapid r.
repression
reptilase
RES-701-1
RESCUE
Randomized Evaluation of Salvage
Angioplasty with Combined
Utilization of Endpoints
rescue
r. angioplasty
citrovorum r.
ResCue Key
**Research Medical straight multiple-
holed aortic cannula**
resection
activation map-guided
surgical r.
bronchial sleeve r.
endocardial r.
infundibular wedge r.
lesser r.
myotomy-myectomy-septal r.
segmental lung r.
septal r.
Torek r. of thoracic esophagus
reserpine
chlorothiazide and r.

hydralazine, hydrochlorothiazide,
and r.
hydrochlorothiazide and r.
hydroflumethiazide and r.
reserve
breathing r. (BR)
cardiac r.
cardiopulmonary r.
r. cell carcinoma
coronary arterial r.
coronary flow r. (CFR)
coronary vascular r.
coronary vasodilator r.
diastolic r.
extraction r.
Frank-Starling r.
heart rate r. (HRR)
myocardial r.
preload r.
respiratory r.
systolic r.
vasodilator r.
reservoir
Cardiometrics cardiotomy r.
cardiotomy r.
Cobe cardiotomy r.
double bubble flushing r.
r. face mask
Intersept cardiotomy r.
Jostra cardiotomy r.
Polystan cardiotomy r.
Scimed extracorporeal silicone
rubber r.
Shiley cardiotomy r.
William Harvey cardiotomy r.
reset nodus sinuatrialis
residual
r. gradient
r. jet
r. lung capacity
r. stenosis
r. volume (RV)
r. volume/total lung capacity
(RV/TLC)
r. volume to total lung
capacity ratio (RV/TLC)

R

NOTES

417

resin
anion exchange r.
bile acid binding r.
cholestyramine r.
thermosetting r.
resin-colophony
pine r.-c.
resistance
afterload r.
airway r.
aortic valve r.
cerebrovascular r. (CVR)
coronary vascular r.
elastic r.
hydraulic r.
peripheral vascular r.
pulmonary arteriolar r.
pulmonary vascular r. (PVR)
r. ratio
systemic vascular r. (SVR)
total peripheral r. (TPR)
total pulmonary r.
vascular peripheral r.
r. vessel
resistant hypertension
Resistex expiratory resistance exerciser
resistive heating
resolution
energy r.
spatial r.
temporal r.
resolving power
resonance
bandbox r.
bell-metal r.
cough r.
cracked-pot r.
nuclear magnetic r. (NMR)
shoulder-strap r.
skodaic r.
whispering r.
wooden r.
resonant frequency
resorption atelectasis
Respa-DM
Respaire-120 SR
Respaire-60 SR
Respa-1st
Respbid
RespiGam
Respinol-G
Respiradyne

respiration
abdominal r.
absent r.
accelerated r.
accessory muscles of r.
aerobic r.
agonal r.
amphoric r.
anaerobic r.
apneustic r.
artificial r.
asthmoid r.
Austin Flint r.
Biot r.
Bouchut r.
bronchial r.
bronchocavernous r.
r. bronchoscope
bronchovesicular r.
cavernous r.
central r.
cerebral r.
Cheyne-Stokes r.
cogwheel r.
collateral r.
controlled diaphragmatic r.
Corrigan r.
costal r.
cyclic r.
decreased r.
diaphragmatic r.
direct r.
divided r.
electrophrenic r.
external r.
forced r.
granular r.
harsh r.
internal r.
interrupted r.
intrauterine r.
jerky r.
Kussmaul r.
Kussmaul-Kien r.
labored r.
meningitic r.
metamorphosing r.
nervous r.
paradoxical r.
periodic r.
placental r.
puerile r.
radiofrequency electrophrenic r.

R

rude r.
Schafer method of artificial r.
Seitz metamorphosing r.
shallow r.
sighing r.
slow r.
sonorous r.
stertorous r.
stridulous r.
supplementary r.
suppressed r.
temperature, pulse, and r.
   (TPR)
thoracic r.
transitional r.
tubular r.
vesiculocavernous r.
vicarious r.
wavy r.
respiratometer
Collins r.
respirator
Ambu r.
BABYbird r.
Bear 5 r.
Bourns infant r.
Bragg-Paul r.
cabinet r.
cuirass r.
Drinker r.
Emerson cuirass r.
Engstrom r.
Gill I r.
r. lung
Med-Neb r.
Monaghan r.
Morch r.
Morsch-Retec r.
Moynihan r.
Sanders jet ventilation
   device r.
respiratory
r. acidosis
r. alkalosis
r. arrest
r. arrhythmia
r. burst

r. capacity
r. center
r. collapse
r. distress
r. distress syndrome (RDS)
r. disturbance index (RDI)
r. drive
r. embarrassment
r. and enteric orphan (REO)
r. exchange
r. excursion
r. failure
r. feedback (RFb)
r. flora
r. function
r. infection
r. insufficiency
r. murmur
r. ordered phase encoding
   (ROPE)
r. paralysis
r. pattern
r. pulse
r. quotient (RQ)
r. rate
r. reflexes
r. reserve
r. sound
r. standstill
r. stridor
r. support
r. swing
r. syncytial virus (RSV)
r. syncytial virus conduit
r. syncytial virus IV immune
   globulin
Taiwan acute r. (TWAR)
r. toilet
r. tract
Respirgard II nebulizer
respirometer
Fraser Harlake r.
Haloscale r.
Wright r.
Respiromonitor RM-300
Respironics CPAP machine

NOTES

Respitrace
R. inductive plethysmograph
R. machine
Respivir
response
acute r.
cholinergic r.
chronotropic r.
controlled ventricular r.
Cushing pressure r.
dynamic frequency r.
endothelium-dependent dilator r.
to substance P
fight-or-flight r.
frequency r.
giving-up/given-up r.
Henry-Gauer r.
implantation r.
incrementing r.
neointimal hyperplastic r.
paced ventricular evoked r.
plateau r.
slow r.
square wave r.
thyrotropin-releasing hormone r.
vagal r.
ventricular r.
vigilance r.
response-to-injury
r.-t.-i. hypothesis
r.-t.-i. hypothesis of
atherogenesis
r.-t.-i. theory
responsiveness
myofilament calcium r.
Res-Q
R.-Q ACD
R.-Q ACD implantable
cardioverter-defibrillator
R.-Q AICD
R.-Q arrhythmia control device
rest
r. angina
r. dyspnea
r. ejection fraction
r. and exercise gated nuclear
angiography
r. hypoxemia
r. metabolism/stress perfusion
protocol
r. pain
r. radionuclide angiography

restenosis
aortic valve r.
intrastent r.
r. lesion
mitral r.
Multicenter American Research
Trial with Cilazapril after
Angioplasty to Prevent
Transluminal Coronary
Obstruction and R.
(MARCATOR)
Multicenter European Research
Trial with Cilazapril after
Angioplasty to Prevent
Transluminal Coronary
Obstruction and R.
(MERCATOR)
post-balloon angioplasty r.
pulmonary valve r.
tricuspid r.
rest-exercise- equilibrium
radionuclide ventriculography
resting
r. length-tension relation
r. membrane potential
r. pressure
r. tachycardia
r. value
Reston subtype
restored cycle
Restoril
rest-redistribution thallium-201
imaging
restriction
r. endonuclease
r. fragment length
polymorphism (RFLP)
progressive parenchymal r.
restrictive
r. airways defect
r. airways disease
r. cardiomyopathy
r. functional impairment
r. heart disease
r. lung disease
r. ventilatory defect
restrictus
Aspergillus r.
result
true-negative test r.
true-positive test r.
resuscitate
do not r. (DNR)

resuscitation
    cardiac r.
    cardiopulmonary r. (CPR)
    r. cart
    heart-lung r.
    mouth-to-mouth r.
resuscitator
    ACD r.
    BagEasy disposable manual r.
    First Response manual r.
    High Oxygen PRM r.
    Hope r.
    Hudson Lifesaver r.
    infant Ambu r.
    Laerdal infant r.
    NeoVO-2-R volume control r.
    Ohio Hope r.
    Penlon infant r.
    pneuPAC r.
    Robertshaw bag r.
    Safe Response manual r.
    SureGrip manual r.
retained lung fluid (RLF)
retard
    expiratory r.
retention
    sodium r.
    water r.
reticularis
    livedo r.
reticular pattern
reticuloendothelial system
reticulonodular
reticulum
    sarcoplasmic r.
retina
retinae
    cyanosis r.
retinal
    r. artery
    r. vessel
retinopathy
    diabetic r.
    hypertensive r.
retour
    rale de r.

retractor
    Allison lung r.
    Andrews r.
    Bahnson sternal r.
    Benedict r.
    Bookwalter r.
    Burford rib r.
    Carten mitral valve r.
    Carter r.
    Cooley r.
    Cooley-Merz sternum r.
    Cosgrove r.
    DeBakey chest r.
    Finochietto r.
    Finochietto-Geissendorfer rib r.
    Frater intracardiac r.
    Gelpi r.
    Gerbode sternal r.
    Gross-Pomeranz-Watkins r.
    Haight-Finochietto rib r.
    Hartzler rib r.
    Lukens thymus r.
    rake r.
    Sellor rib r.
    Semb lung r.
    Theis rib r.
    Zalkind lung r.
    Zimberg esophageal hiatal r.
Retract-O-Tape
retraining
    computerized diaphragmatic
    breathing r. (CDBR)
retrieval
    intravascular foreign body r.
retrocardiac space
retroconduction
retroesophageal aorta
retrograde
    r. aortography
    r. atrial activation mapping
    r. beat
    r. block
    r. catheter insertion
    r. catheterization
    r. conduction
    r. embolism
    r. fast pathway

NOTES

retrograde *(continued)*
  r. femoral approach
  r. P wave
retropectoral pocket
retroperfusion
  coronary sinus r.
retropharyngeal
  r. abscess
  r. lymph nodes
  r. space
retropharyngitis
Retroscan
retrosternal thyroid
retrotracheal space
Retrovir
  R. injection
  R. Oral
retrovirus
return
  anomalous pulmonary
    venous r.
  r. extrasystole
  partial anomalous pulmonary
    venous r. (PAPVR)
  pulmonary venous r.
  rattle of r.
  systemic venous r.
  total anomalous pulmonary
    venous r. (TAPVR)
  venous r.
returning cycle
Retzius veins
revascularization
  coronary r.
  heart laser r.
  myocardial r.
  percutaneous transluminal
    coronary r. (PTCR)
  repeat r.
  transmyocardial r. (TMR)
  transmyocardial laser r.
Revase
reverberation
  r. artifact
  echo r.
reversal
  lead r.
reverse
  r. saphenous vein
  r. transcriptase polymerase
    chain reaction (RT-PCR)
  r. transcriptase polymerase
    chain reaction test

reversed
  r. arm leads
  r. bypass
  r. coarctation
  r. ductus arteriosus
  r. paradoxical pulse
  r. reciprocal rhythm
  r. saphenous vein graft
  r. shunt
  r. three sign
reversible
  r. bronchospasm
  r. ischemic neurologic defect
    (RIND)
  r. obstructive airways disease
    (ROAD)
reversion
Reversol injection
Revex
Revitalizer Soft-Start nasal CPAP
Reye syndrome
Reynolds number
Reynold-Southwick H-graft
  portacaval shunt
RF
  radiofrequency
  rheumatic fever
    RF ablation
    RF Ablatr ablation catheter
    RF wave
RFA
  radiofrequency ablation
RFb
  respiratory feedback
    RFb system
RFB System-I for CDBR
RFC
  radiofrequency current
RFG-35
  Radionics R.
RF-generated thermal balloon
  catheter
RFLP
  restriction fragment length
    polymorphism
RG-201
Rh
  Rhesus
    Rh antibody
    Rh factor
    Mini-Gamulin Rh
rhabdomyolysis
rhabdomyoma

rhabdomyosarcoma
RHAMM
    receptor for hyaluronan-mediated
    motility
RHD
    radiant heat device
    rheumatic heart disease
rheocardiography
rheologic
    r. change
    r. therapy
rheology
Rheomacrodex
RheothRx
Rhesus (Rh)
rheumatic
    r. aortitis
    r. arteritis
    r. carditis
    r. endocarditis
    r. fever (RF)
    r. heart disease (RHD)
    r. mitral insufficiency
    r. mitral valve stenosis
    r. myocarditis
    r. pericarditis
    r. pneumonia
    r. valvulitis
rheumatica
    angina r.
rheumatism of heart
rheumatoid
    r. arteritis
    r. arthritis (RA)
    r. factor
    r. lung
    r. pneumoconiosis
    r. pneumonoconiosis
Rheumatrex
rhinitis
    allergic r.
    perennial allergic r.
    seasonal allergic r.
rhinocerebral infection
Rhinocort
Rhinosyn-DMX
rhinovirus

r-hirudin
    recombinant hirudin
Rhizopus
    R. oryzae
rhodesiense
    Trypanosoma r.
Rho(D) immune globulin
Rhodnius polixus
Rhodococcus
    R. equi
RhoGAM
rhoGDI protein
rhonchal fremitus
rhonchi, sing. **rhonchus**
    expiratory r.
    rales and r.
    sibilant r.
    sonorous r.
rhonchorous cough
rhysodes
    Acanthamoeba r.
rhythm
    accelerated idioventricular r.
    (AIVR)
    accelerated junctional r.
    agonal r.
    atrial r.
    atrioventricular junctional r.
    atrioventricular nodal r., A-V
    nodal r.
    A-V junctional r.
    baseline r.
    bigeminal r.
    cantering r.
    cardiac r.
    circadian r.
    concealed r.
    coronary nodal r.
    coronary sinus r.
    coupled r.
    r. disturbance
    diurnal r.
    ectopic r.
    embryocardia r.
    escape r.
    fibrillation r.
    gallop r.

R

NOTES

rhythm *(continued)*
  irregularly irregular r.
  junctional escape r.
  lower nodal r.
  midnodal r.
  mu r.
  nodal escape r.
  normal sinus r. (NSR)
  paced r.
  pendulum r.
  pulseless idioventricular r.
  quadrigeminal r.
  quadruple r.
  reciprocal r.
  reciprocating r.
  regularly irregular r.
  regular rate and r. (RRR)
  regular sinus r. (RSR)
  reversed reciprocal r.
  sinus r.
  slow escape r.
  r. strip
  systolic gallop r.
  tic-tac r.
  trainwheel r.
  trigeminal r.
  triple r.
  ventricular r.
  wide complex r.
rhythmicity
Rhythmin
Rhythmonorm
rhythmophone
RhythmScan
rib
  r. approximator
  r. cage
  r. margin
  r. notching
  r. raspatory
  r. shears
  r. spreader
ribavirin
Ribbert thrombosis
ribbon
  r. muscles
  safety r.
ribonucleic acid (RNA)
riboprobe
  CMV IE-2 r.
  HIV-1 r.
  IE-2 r.

riboside
  AICA r.
ribosome
Richet aneurysm
Ricketts-Abrams technique
Rickettsia
  R. australis
  R. prowazekii
rickettsial
  r. endocarditis
  r. myocarditis
  r. pneumonia
riding
  r. embolism
  r. embolus
Riecker respiration bronchoscope
Riedel
  R. struma
  R. thyroiditis
Riegel pulse
Riesman
  R. myocardosis
  R. pneumonia
rifabutin
Rifadin
  R. injection
  R. Oral
Rifamate
rifampin
  r. and isoniazid
  r., isoniazid, and pyrazinamide
rifamycin
rifapentine
Rifater
Rift Valley fever virus
right
  r. anterior oblique (RAO)
  r. anterior oblique equivalent
  r. anterior oblique position
  r. anterior oblique projection
  r. aortic arch
  r. atrial appendage (RAA)
  r. atrial enlargement (RAE)
  r. atrial myxoma
  r. atrial pressure (RAP)
  r. atrial thrombus
  r. atrium (RA)
  r. axis deviation (RAD)
  r. bundle branch block (RBBB)
  r. common carotid artery
  r. coronary artery (RCA)
  r. coronary catheter

R

r. heart
r. heart bypass
r. heart catheter
r. heart catheterization
r. heart failure
r. internal mammary artery (RIMA)
r. Judkins catheter
r. parasternal impulse
r. pulmonary artery (RPA)
r. ventricle (RV)
r. ventricular apex (RVA)
r. ventricular assist device (RVAD)
r. ventricular cardiomyopathy
r. ventricular diastolic collapse
r. ventricular diastolic pressure
r. ventricular dimension
r. ventricular dysplasia
r. ventricular ejection fraction (RVEF)
r. ventricular end-diastolic pressure (RVEDP)
r. ventricular failure
r. ventricular function
r. ventricular heave
r. ventricular hypertrophy (RVH)
r. ventricular hypoplasia
r. ventricular infarction
r. ventricular inflow obstruction
r. ventricular myxoma
r. ventricular outflow obstruction
r. ventricular outflow tract (RVOT)
r. ventricular outflow tract tachycardia
r. ventricular systolic pressure
r. ventricular systolic time interval
right-angle chest tube
right-sided heart failure
right-to-left shunt
rightward axis
rigid
r. bronchoscopy

r. pod
r. thoracoscope
rigidity
nuchal r.
Rigiflex TTS balloon catheter
rigor
calcium r.
Riley-Cournand equation
Riley-Day syndrome
Riley needle
RIMA
right internal mammary artery
Rimactane Oral
rimantadine
r. hydrochloride
RIND
reversible ischemic neurologic defect
ring
r. abscess
aortic r.
atrial r.
atrioventricular r.
Bickel r.
Carpentier r.
coronary r.
Crawford suture r.
double-flanged valve sewing r.
Duran annuloplasty r.
r. electrode
esophageal contraction r.
knitted sewing r.
Lower r.'s
metal sewing r.
plastic sewing r.
pleural r.'s
prosthetic valve sewing r.
Puig Massana annuloplasty r.
Puig Massana-Shiley annuloplasty r.
Schatzki esophageal r.
Sculptor annuloplasty r.
sewing r.
r. shadow
r. sign
St. Jude annuloplasty r.
tracheal r.'s

NOTES

425

ring *(continued)*
    vascular r.
    Waldeyer tonsillar r.
Ringer
    R. lactate
    R. solution
Riolan
    anastomosis of R.
RISA
    radioactive iodinated serum albumin
rise time
risk
    r. factor
    r. index
    modified multifactorial index
      of cardiac r.
    recurrence r.
    relative r.
    stochastic r.
    r. stratification
    surgical r.
RITA
    Randomized Intervention in the
    Treatment of Angina
Ritchie catheter
ritodrine
Riva-Rocci sphygmomanometer
Rivero-Carvallo
    R.-C. effect
    R.-C. sign
Riviere sign
RJA
    regurgitant jet area
R-lactate enzyme monotest
RLF
    retained lung fluid
RM-300
    Respiromonitor R.
RMBF
    regional myocardial blood flow
RNA
    ribonucleic acid
    RNA glycosidase toxin
RNV
    radionuclide ventriculography
Ro-13-6438
Ro 4483
ROAD
    reversible obstructive airways
    disease
roadmapping
    coronary r.
Roadrunner PC guidewire

Robertshaw bag resuscitator
Robertson sign
Robicillin VK Oral
Robicsek vascular probe
Robinson index
Robinul
    R. Forte
Robitet Oral
Robitussin
    R. Cough Calmers
    R. Pediatric
    R. Severe Congestion Liqui-
      Gels
Robodoc robot
robot
    Robodoc r.
Rocephin
Rochalimaea
Rocha-Lima inclusion
Rochester-Kocher clamp
Rochester-Péan clamp
rocker
    hematology r.
ROCKET
    Regionally Organized Cardiac Key
    European Trial
Rockey mediastinal cannula
Rocky Mountain spotted fever
rodhaini
    Babesia r.
Rodrigo equation
Rodriguez
    R. aneurysm
    R. catheter
Rodriguez-Alvarez catheter
roentgen (R)
    r. knife
roentgenogram
    apical lordotic r.
    chest r.
roentgenographic presentation
roentgenography
Roesler-Bressler infarction
RoEzIt skin moisturizer
Roferon-A
Rogaine
Roger
    R. bruit
    bruit de R.
    R. disease
    maladie de R.
    R. murmur
Rogers sphygmomanometer

Roho mattress
Rokitansky disease
roller pump
Rolleston rule
rolling hernia
Romaña sign
Romano-Ward syndrome
rometaraminol
    norepinephrine r.
Romhilt-Estes
    R.-E. point score criteria
    R.-E. point scoring system
    R.-E. score
ROMI
    rule out myocardial infarction
Ronase
Rondec
    R. Drops
    R. Filmtab
    R. Syrup
R-on-T premature ventricular
  complex
Roos test
root
    aortic r.
    r. injection
    r. perfusion
root-mean-square voltage
ROPE
    respiratory ordered phase encoding
Rosai-Dorfman disease
Rosalki technique
rose
    R. questionnaire
    r. spot
    R. tamponade
Rosenbach syndrome
Rosenblum rotating adapter
rosette
Ross
    R. needle
    R. procedure
    R. River virus
Rossetti modification of Nissen
  fundoplication
Rostan asthma

rotablator
    R. atherectomy device
    R. catheter
    Heart Technology R.
    r. wire
Rotacamera
Rotacaps
    Ventolin R.
Rotacs
    R. guidewire
    R. motorized catheter
    R. rotational atherectomy
      device
    R. system
Rotahaler
rotary atherectomy device
rotating disk oxygenation
rotation
    clockwise r.
    counterclockwise r.
    shoulder r.
rotational
    r. ablation
    r. ablation laser
    r. atherectomy device
    r. atherectomy system (RAS)
    r. coronary atherectomy (RCA)
    r. dynamic angioplasty catheter
Rotch sign
Rotex needle
Rothia dentocariosa
Rothschild sign
Roth spot
rotoslide
Roubin-Gianturco flexible coil stent
Rougnon-Heberden disease
rouleaux formation
rounded atelectasis
round heart
round-robin classification
roundworm
Roussy-Lévy
    R.-L. disease
    R.-L. polyneuropathy
    R.-L. syndrome
route of insertion
rove magnetic catheter

R

NOTES

427

roxithromycin
Royal Flush catheter
RPA
   right pulmonary artery
RPE
   ratings of perceived exertion
R-P interval
R-Port implantable vascular access
   system
RQ
   respiratory quotient
R-R
      R-R interval
      R-R prime
      R-R prime interval
RR cycle
RRP
   relative refractory period
RRR
   regular rate and rhythm
RS complex
RSI
   rapid sequence induction
      RSI orotracheal intubation
RSR
   regular sinus rhythm
      RSR prime (RSR')
RSR'
   RSR prime
RS-T
      RS-T interval
      RS-T segment
RSV
   respiratory syncytial virus
rt-PA
   recombinant tissue plasminogen
   activator
      catabolism of rt-PA
      double-chain rt-PA
RT-PCR
   reverse transcriptase polymerase
   chain reaction
RTV total artificial heart
rub
      friction r.
      pericardial friction r.
      pleural friction r.
      pleuritic r.
      pleuropericardial r.
      saddle leather friction r.
rubella syndrome
rubeola
Rubex

rubidium-81
rubidium-82
   r. imaging
Rubinol
Rubinstein-Taybi syndrome
rubor
   dependent r.
ruby laser
rude respiration
Ruel forceps
Ruiz-Cohen round expander
rule
   r. of bigeminy
   Gibson r.
   Liebermeister r.
   r. out myocardial infarction
      (ROMI)
   Rolleston r.
   Simpson r.
rumble
   Austin Flint r.
   booming r.
   diastolic r.
   filling r.
   mid-diastolic r.
   protodiastolic r.
rumbling diastolic murmur
Rumel
   R. clamp
   R. thoracic forceps
   R. tourniquet
Rumpel-Leede test
runoff
   aortofemoral arterial r.
   aortogram with distal r.
   arterial r.
   r. arteriogram
   digital r.
   distal r.
   venous r.
rupture
   aortic r.
   balloon r.
   cardiac r.
   chamber r.
   chordae tendineae r.
   chordal r.
   esophageal r.
   interventricular septal r.
   intraperitoneal r.
   intrapleural r.
   myocardial r.
   nonpenetrating r.

penetrating r.
plaque r.
traumatic r.
valve r.
ventricular septal r.
ruptured
  r. aortic aneurysm
  r. sinus of Valsalva
Ruschelit polyvinyl chloride endotracheal tube
Russian influenza
rusty sputum
Ru-Tuss DE
RV
  residual volume
  right ventricle
RVA
  right ventricular apex
RVAD
  right ventricular assist device
RVEDP
  right ventricular end-diastolic pressure
RVEF
  right ventricular ejection fraction

RVH
  right ventricular hypertrophy
RVOT
  right ventricular outflow tract
RV/TLC
  residual volume/total lung capacity
  residual volume to total lung capacity ratio
    RV/TLC ratio
RWT
  relative wall thickness
RX
  RX stent delivery system
Rx
  Rx perfusion catheter
  Rx Streak balloon catheter
Rx5000 cardiac pacing system
ryanodine receptor
Rymed
Rynatan
Rythmodan
Rythmol

R

NOTES

S

septum
S wave

S₁

first heart sound

S₂

second heart sound

S₃

third heart sound
S_3 gallop

S₄

fourth heart sound
S_4 gallop

S₇

summation gallop
S_7 gallop

S-A, SA

sinoatrial
S-A nodal reentrant tachycardia
S-A node

Sabin-Feldman dye test
sabot

coeur en s.
s. heart

sac

aortic s. (AS)
Hilton s.
Lap S.
lateral s.
pericardial s.
pleural s.
truncoaortic s.

saccharolyticus

Peptostreptococcus s.

Saccharomyces

S. anginae

Saccomanno fixative
saccular

s. aneurysm
s. bronchiectasis

sacculated

s. empyema
s. pleurisy

sacculation

localized s.

sacral edema
sacrococcygeal aorta
SACT

sinoatrial conduction time

saddle

s. embolism
s. embolus
s. leather friction rub
s. thrombus

Sade modification of Norwood procedure
Sadowsky hook wire
Safar bronchoscope
Safar-S airway
Safe Response manual resuscitator
Safe-T-Coat heparin-coated thermodilution catheter
Safe-T-Tube

Montgomery S.-T.-T.

safety

s. guidewire
radiation s.
s. ribbon

SafTouch catheter
sag

ST s.

sagittal

s. cuts
s. plane
s. view

sail sound
Sala cells
salbutamol
Saleto-200
Salflex
Salgesic
salicylate
saline

Broncho S.
heparinized s.
iced s.
s. loading
s. slush

salivarius

Streptococcus s.

Salkowski test
salmeterol

s. xinafoate

Salmonella

S. choleraesuis

salmon skin
salsalate
Salsitab

S

salt
dietary s.
ethylenediaminetetraacetic acid disodium s.
gold s.
s. of nickel
persulfate s.
s. of platinum
s. wasting
salt-and-pepper appearance
salt-and-water dependent hypertension
saltans
thrombophlebitis s.
salt-depletion syndrome
salt-free diet
salting-out procedure
saluresis
saluretic agent
Saluron
salute
allergic s.
Salutensin-Demi
saluting
salvage
s. balloon angioplasty
limb s.
myocardial s.
Salvatore-Maloney tracheotome
salves
tachycardia en s.
salvo
s. of beats
s. of ventricular tachycardia
SAM
systolic anterior motion
SAM system
Sam
S. Levine sign
S. Roberts bronchial biopsy forceps
sampling
bioptic s.
blood s.
chorionic villus s.
San
S. Joaquin Valley disease
S. Joaquin Valley fever
Sanborn metabolator
Sanchez-Cascos cardioauditory syndrome
Sanders
S. bed

S. intubation laryngoscope
S. jet ventilation device respirator
Sandhoff disease
Sandifer syndrome
Sandler-Dodge area-length method
Sandman system
Sandoglobulin
Sandostatin
Sandoz suction/feeding tube
Sandrock test
sandwich
s. enzyme-linked immunosorbent assay
s. patch
sanguinis
ictus s.
Sansert
Sansom sign
SaO$_2$
arterial oxygen saturation
saphenofemoral
s. junction
s. system
saphenous
s. vein
s. vein bypass graft angiography
s. vein cannula
s. vein graft
s. vein varicosity
SAQ
Seattle angina questionnaire
saquinavir mesylate
saralasin
sarcoid
Boeck s.
s. granuloma
sarcoidosis
fibrocystic s.
sarcolemmal
s. calcium channel
s. level
s. membrane
sarcolemma lipid
sarcoma
cardiac s.
Kaposi s. (KS)
metastatic s.
pseudo-Kaposi s.
soft tissue s.
sarcomatous tumor
sarcomere

Sarcophaga
sarcoplasmic
    s. reticulum
    s. reticulum-associated
      glycolytic enzymes
sarcosporidiosis
sarcotubular system
Sarnoff aortic clamp
Sarns
    S. electric saw
    S. intracardiac suction tube
    S. membrane oxygenator
      (SMO)
    S. soft-flow aortic cannula
    S. ventricular assist device
    S. wire-reinforced catheter
Sarot bronchus clamp
SART
    sinoatrial recovery time
saruplase
    Liquaemin in Myocardial
    Infarction during
    Thrombolysis with S.
    (LIMITS)
SAS
    sleep apnea syndrome
satellite lesion
Satinsky clamp
Satterthwaite method
saturated solution of potassium
  iodide (SSKI)
saturation
    arterial s.
    arterial oxygen s. (SaO_2)
    s. index
    mixed venous oxygen s.
    (SvO_2)
    oxygen s.
    step-up in oxygen s.
    s. time
    venous s.
saucerize
Sauerbruch-Herrmannsdorfer-Gerson
  diet
Sauerbruch rib guillotine
sausaging of vein
Sauvage filamentous prosthesis

Savary-Gilliard esophageal dilator
SAVE
    Survival and Ventricular Ectopy
      SAVE trial
Saventrine Intravenous
Saver
    Cell S.
    Haemonetics Cell S.
saw
    oscillating s.
    Sarns electric s.
    sternum s.
    Stryker s.
sawtooth
    s. pattern
    s. wave
Sawyer operation
SAX
    short axis
SBE
    subacute bacterial endocarditis
      SBE prophylaxis
SBF
    systemic blood flow
SBP
    systolic blood pressure
SBSE
    supine bicycle stress
    echocardiography
SBT
    serum bactericidal titer
scabbard trachea
SCAD
    spontaneous coronary artery
    dissection
SCA-EX
    S.-E. 7F graft
    S.-E. ShortCutter catheter
    S.-E. ShortCutter catheter with
      rotating blades
scalar
    s. electrocardiogram
    s. leads
scale
    activity s.
    Borg numerical s.
    Borg treadmill exertion s.

S

NOTES

scale *(continued)*
  cardiac adjustment s.
  dyspnea s.
  French s.
  Glasgow Coma S.
  gray s.
  Grossman s.
  Health Locus of Control S.
  Holmes-Rahe s.
  Karnovsky rating s.
  Paykel s.
  Psychosocial Adjustment to
    Illness S.
  Tennant distress s.
  Toronto Alexithymia S.
  visual analogue s. (VAS)
  voxel gray s.
  Wigle s.
scalene
  s. fat pad biopsy
  s. lymph node biopsy
scalenectomy
scalenotomy
  Adson-Coffey s.
scalenus
  s. anterior syndrome
  s. anticus syndrome
scalloping
scalp
  s. electrode
  s. pH
SCAN
  S. antitachycardia pacing
    protocol
scan
  CardioTec s.
  carotid duplex s.
  s. converter
  CT s.
  gallium s.
  gated cardiac s.
  HRCT s.
  lung s.
  milk s.
  MUGA s.
  PYP s.
  scintillation s.
  sector s.
  sestamibi s.
  tebo s.
  teboroxime s.
  technetium-99m hexamibi s.
  thin-slice CT s.

  ventilation/perfusion s.
  ventilation/perfusion lung s.
    (V/Q lung scan)
  V/Q lung s.
  ventilation/perfusion lung scan
**Scandinavian Simvastatin Survival
  Study (SSSS)**
Scanlan vessel dilator
scanner
  Biosound wide-angle monoplane
    ultrasound s.
  CardioData MK-3 Holter s.
  computed tomography s.
  Corometrics Doppler s.
  Del Mar Avionics S.
  Diasonics Cardiovue SectOR s.
  Imatron C-100 tomographic s.
  Imatron Ultrafast CT s.
  phased array sector s.
  ultrafast computed
    tomographic s.
  Ultrafast CT s.
scanning
  duplex s.
  electronic s.
  s. electron microscope (SEM)
  fluorodopamine positron
    emission tomographic s.
  s. format
  gated blood-pool s.
  interlaced s.
  lung s.
  progressive s.
  radionuclide s.
Scanning-Beam Digital x-ray
scar
  s. emphysema
  infarct s.
  zipper s.
scarlatinosa
  angina s.
scarlet fever
Scarpa
  S. fascia
  S. method
scarring
  apical s.
  pleural s.
SCAT
  Simvastatin/Enalapril Coronary
    Atherosclerosis Regression Trial
Scatchard plot analysis

scatter
  Compton s.
scattered echo
scattergram
scatterplot smoothing technique
scavenger
  s. cell pathway
  lysophosphatidylcholine s.
  oxygen radical s.
scavenging tube
SCD
  sudden cardiac death
Schafer method of artificial
  respiration
Schapiro sign
Schapiro-Wilks test
Schatzki esophageal ring
Schatz-Palmaz
  S.-P. intravascular stent
  S.-P. tubular mesh stent
Schaumann disease
Schede-thoracoplasty
Scheffé test
Scheie syndrome
Scheinmann laryngeal forceps
Schellong-Strisower phenomenon
Schellong test
Schenk-Eichelter vena cava plastic
  filter procedure
Schepelmann sign
Schick sign
Schiff test
Schiller method
Schindler esophagoscope
Schistosoma
schistosomiasis
schistothorax
Schlesinger solution
Schlichter test
Schmidt-Lanterman clefts
Schmitt-Erlanger model of reentry
Schmorl furrow
Schneider
  S. catheter
  S. index
  S. stent
  S. Wallstent

schneiderian respiratory membrane
Schneider-Meier-Magnum system
Schneider-Shiley balloon
Scholten
  S. endomyocardial bioptome
  S. endomyocardial bioptome
    and biopsy forceps
Schonander
  S. procedure
  S. technique
Schoonmaker catheter
Schoonmaker-King single catheter
  technique
Schott treatment
Schuco nebulizer
Schüller method
Schultz angina
Schultze test
Schumacher aorta clamp
Schwarten
  S. LP balloon catheter
  S. LP guidewire
Schwartz test
scie
  bruit de s.
Scimed
  S. angioplasty catheter
  S. extracorporeal silicone
    rubber reservoir
scimitar syndrome
scintigram
  pyrophosphate s.
scintigraphic perfusion defect
scintigraphy
  AMA-Fab s.
  antimyosin infarct-avid s.
  dipyridamole thallium-201 s.
  exercise thallium-201 s.
  FFA-labeled s.
  gallium 67 s.
  gated blood-pool s.
  indium-111 s.
  infarct-avid hot-spot s.
  infarct-avid myocardial s.
  iodine-131 MIBG s.
  labeled FFA s.
  microsphere perfusion s.

S

NOTES

scintigraphy *(continued)*
    myocardial cold-spot
      perfusion s.
    myocardial perfusion s.
    myocardial viability s.
    NEFA s.
    perfusion s.
    planar thallium s.
    pulmonary s.
    pyrophosphate s.
    single-photon gamma s.
    SPECT s.
    stress thallium s.
    Tc-99 sestamibi s.
    thallium-201 perfusion s.
    thallium-201 planar s.
    thallium-201 SPECT s.
    ventilation s.
scintillating speckle pattern
scintillation
    s. camera
    s. cocktail
    s. probe
    s. scan
scintiphotography
scintiscan
    technetium-99m stannous
      pyrophosphate s.
scintiscanner
scintiview
scirrhous carcinoma
scissors
    Beall s.
    Blum arterial s.
    Crafoord lobectomy s.
    De Martel s.
    Duffield cardiovascular s.
    Dumont thoracic s.
    Haimovici arteriotomy s.
    Jabaley-Stille Super Cut S.
    Jorgenson thoracic s.
    Karmody venous s.
    Metzenbaum s.
    pericardiotomy s.
sclera
    blue s.
scleredema
    s. adultorum
    s. of Buschke
sclerodactyly
scleroderma
    s. lung
ScleroLaser

Scleromate
sclerosant
sclerosing
    s. agent
    s. cholangitis
    s. hemangioma
    s. phlebitis
    variceal s.
sclerosis, pl. **scleroses**
    aortic s.
    arterial s.
    arteriocapillary s.
    arteriolar s.
    endocardial s.
    Mönckeberg s.
    multiple s.
    nodular s.
    progressive systemic s. (PSS)
    tuberous s.
    valvular s.
    vascular s.
sclerotherapy
    variceal s.
Scole Alta II 3-channel
    precalibrated Holter AM
    recorder
Scoop 1, 2 catheter
scooping
score
    Aldrich s.
    APACHE II, III s.
    Berning and Steensgaard-
      Hansen s.
    Brasfield chest radiograph s.
    Brush electrocardiographic s.
    calcium s.
    Califf s.
    Detsky s.
    Dripps-American Surgical
      Association s.
    Duke treadmill prognostic s.
    echo s.
    Estes s.
    Gensini s.
    Goldman cardiac risk index s.
    Hollenberg treadmill s.
    jeopardy s.
    lung injury s. (LIS)
    Romhilt-Estes s.
    Selvester QRS s.
    VAMC prognostic s.
    wall motion s.

scorpion venom
scotoma, pl. **scotomata**
Scot-Tussin DM Cough Chasers
scout
    s. film
    s. view
SCRAM face mask
scratch
    Lerman-Means s.
scratchy murmur
screening
    spirometric s.
screen oxygenation
screw-in
    s.-i. epicardial electrode
    s.-i. lead
screw-on lead
SCRIP
    Stanford Coronary Risk Intervention
    Project
scrub typhus
Sculptor annuloplasty ring
scurvy
SCV-CPR
    simultaneous compression-
    ventilation CPR
SDS-PAGE
SE
    spin-echo
        SE image
SEA
    side-entry access
        SEA port
sea
    s. fronds
seagull
    s. bruit
    s. murmur
seal
    Asherman chest s.
    watertight s.
seal-bark cough
SealEasy resuscitation mask
Sealy-Laragh technique
searcher
    Allport-Babcock s.
Searle volume ventilator

seasonal
    s. allergic rhinitis
    s. allergies
Seattle angina questionnaire (SAQ)
Sebastiani syndrome
SEC
    spontaneous echo contrast
Sechrist IV-100 infant ventilator
second
    dyne s.'s
    forced expiratory volume in
        1 s. (FEV$_1$)
    s. heart sound (S$_2$)
    S. International Study of
        Infarct Survival (ISIS-2)
    s. messenger
    meters per s. (m/sec)
    s. mitral sound
    s. obtuse marginal artery (OM-
        2)
    s. through fifth shock count
secondary
    s. aortic area
    s. asphyxia
    s. atelectasis
    s. bronchitis
    s. bronchus
    s. cardiomyopathy
    s. chemoprophylaxis
    s. dextrocardia
    s. hypertension
    s. infection
    s. pleurisy
    s. pneumonia
    s. prevention
    S. Prevention Reinfarction
        Israeli Nifedipine Trial
        (SPRINT)
    s. radiation
    s. thrombus
second-degree
    s.-d. A-V block
    s.-d. heart block
second-hand smoke
second-look operation
secretor
    gene s.

NOTES

secretory
   s. leukoprotease inhibitor
     protein
   s. leukoproteinase inhibitor
sector
   s. scan
   s. scan echocardiography
Sectral
secundum
   s. atrial septal defect
   foramen s.
   ostium s.
   septum s.
Securon SR
sedentary lifestyle
sedimentation
   s. rate
Seecor pacemaker
seeding
   pumpkin-s.
Seeker guidewire
seesaw murmur
segment
   apicoposterior s.
   bronchopulmonary s.
   coving of ST s.'s
   dyssynergic myocardial s.
   flail s.'s
   P-R s.
   RS-T s.
   ST s.
   Ta s.
   TP s.
   T-P-Q s.
   TQ s.
segmental
   s. arterial disorganization
   s. atelectasis
   s. bronchus
   s. lung resection
   s. pressure index
   s. stenosis
   s. wall motion
segmentation
   k-space s.
   time-resolved imaging by
     automatic data s. (TRIADS)
segmentectomy
segmented
   s. hyalinizing vasculitis
   s. neutrophils
   s. ring tripolar lead
seismic wave

seismocardiogram
seismocardiography
Seitz
   S. metamorphosing respiration
   S. sign
seizure
Seldane
Seldinger
   S. needle
   S. percutaneous technique
Selecon coronary angiography
   catheter
Selecor
Selectan
selective
   s. angiography
   s. aortography
   s. arteriography
   s. intracoronary thrombolysis
     (SICT)
   s. past pathway
selenium
   s. deficiency
   s. sulfide
Selestoject
self-expanding stent
self-guiding catheter
self-positioning balloon catheter
self-powered treadmill
self-terminating tachycardia
Sellick maneuver
Sellor rib retractor
Seloken ZOC
Selvester QRS score
SEM
   scanning electron microscope
   systolic ejection murmur
sematilide hydrochloride
Semb
   S. apicolysis
   S. lung retractor
semidirect leads
semihorizontal heart
semilunar
   s. valve
   s. valve regurgitation
semisynthetic penicillin
semivertical heart
Semliki Forest virus
Semon sign
Sendai virus
senescent
   s. aortic stenosis

s. heart
s. myocardium

senile

s. amyloidosis
s. arrhythmia
s. arteriosclerosis
s. emphysema

senilis

arcus s.
circus s.

senility
Senning

S. intra-atrial baffle
S. operation
S. transposition procedure

sensation

elephant-on-the-chest s.
S. intra-aortic balloon catheter
popping s.

sensing

integrated bipolar s.
s. spike

sensitivity

s. analysis
atrial s.
aureomycin s.
chlortetracycline s.
digitalis s.
pacemaker s.
paracetamol s.
phenindione s.
phenylbutazone s.
sulfonamide s.
ventricular s.

sensitization

baroreceptor s.

sensitized cell
Sensiv endotracheal tube
Sensolog II, III pacemaker
sensor

ClipTip reusable s.
Cross Top replacement
oxygen s.
OxyTip s.
S. pacemaker
SpiroSense flow s.

sensorium

clouded s.

sensory nerve
sentinel node
**Sentron pigtail angiographic
micromanometer catheter**
SEP

systolic ejection period

separation

aortic cusp s.
E point to septal s. (EPSS)

Sepracoat coating solution
sepsis

alcoholism, leukopenia,
pneumococcal s. (ALPS)

septa (*pl. of* septum)

interlobular s.

septal

s. arcade
s. defect
s. dip
s. dropout
s. hypertrophy
s. myectomy
s. myotomy
s. pathway
s. perforating arteries
s. perforation
s. perforator
s. resection
s. wall motion

septation

s. of heart
s. procedure

septectomy

atrial s.
Blalock-Hanlon atrial s.
Edwards s.

septic

s. embolization
s. endocarditis
s. fever
s. pneumonia
s. shock

septicemia sputum
septicum

Clostridium s.

NOTES

S

septomarginalis
    trabecula s.
septostomy
    atrial s.
    atrial balloon s.
    balloon atrial s.
    blade atrial s.
Septra
septum, pl. **septa (S)**
    atrial s.
    conal s.
    interarterial s.
    interatrial s.
    interventricular s.
    membranous s.
    s. primum
    s. secundum
    sigmoid s.
    s. spurium
    Swiss cheese interventricular s.
    ventricular s.
SEQOL
    Study of Economics and Quality of Life
sequela, pl. **sequelae**
Sequel compression system
sequence
    anaplerotic s.
    direct mapping s.
    FLASH s.'s
    intra-atrial activation s.
    intracardiac atrial activation s.
    spin-echo imaging s.
sequencing
    DNA s.
Sequential Compression Device
sequestrant
    bile acid s.
Sequestra 1000 system
sequestration
    s. bronchopneumonia
    pulmonary s.
sequestrectomy
Sequicor III pacemaker
SER
    systolic ejection rate
sera (pl. of serum)
Serafini hernia
Ser-A-Gen
Ser-Ap-Es
Serathide
Serevent

serial
    s. cut films
    s. dilation
serialographic filming
series elastic element
seroconversion
seroeffusive
serofibrinous
    s. pericarditis
    s. pleurisy
serological test
Seroma-Cath catheter
Seromycin Pulvules
seronegative spondyloarthropathy
seropneumothorax
seropositive nonsyphilitic pneumopathy
serosanguineous
serosum
    pericardium s.
serothorax
serotonin
serotype
    M-protein s.
serotyping
serous
    s. membranes
    s. pleurisy
Serpalan
Serpasil
serpentina
    Rauwolfia s.
serpentine aneurysm
serpiginous
serrated catheter
Serratia
    S. liquefaciens
    S. marcescens
    S. pneumonia
serraticus
    stridor s.
sertraline hydrochloride
serum, pl. **sera**
    s. amylase
    antilymphocyte s.
    s. bactericidal titer (SBT)
    s. creatine kinase
    s. enzyme study
    ERIG s.
    s. glutamic-oxaloacetic transaminase (SGOT)
    s. glutamic-pyruvic transaminase (SGPT)

s. IgE
s. iron
s. lipid profile
s. Mgb assay
s. neopterin
s. prothrombin conversion accelerator (SPCA)
s. renin level
s. shock
s. sickness
s. triglycerides

service
HeartLine s.
Servo ventilator 300
sestamibi
s. imaging
s. scan
s. stress test
Tc-99 s.
technetium hexakis 2-methoxyisobutyl isonitrile

set
Acland-Banis arteriotomy s.
ACS percutaneous introducer s.
Arrow Hi-flow infusion s.
Borst side-arm introducer s.
Diethrich coronary artery s.
Dotter Intravascular Retrieval S.
Neff percutaneous access s.
Neo-Sert umbilical vessel catheter insertion s.
Peel-Away introducer s.
Sobel-Kaplitt-Sawyer gas endarterectomy s.
U-Mid-O_2 Jet S.

seven
health level s. (HL7)
seven-pinhole tomography
sevoflurane
Sewall technique
sewing
s. ring
s. ring loop
sex
s. ratio
s. steroid

sexual
s. angina
s. asthma
s. syncope
SFHb
pyridoxilated stroma-free hemoglobin
SF wave of cardiac apex pulse
SGOT
serum glutamic-oxaloacetic transaminase
SGPT
serum glutamic-pyruvic transaminase
shadow
acoustic s.
S. balloon
bat wing s.
butterfly s.
cardiac s.
mediastinal s.
S. over-the-wire balloon catheter
ring s.
snowstorm s.
summation s.
shadow-free laryngoscope
shadowing
acoustic s.
shaggy pericardium
Shaher-Puddu classification
shake test
shaking sound
shallow
s. respiration
s. water blackout
shape
echo-signal s.
Shapshay-Healy laryngoscope
Sharing
United Network for Organ S. (UNOS)
shaver
s. catheter
S. disease
shear
atrial s.

NOTES

S

441

shear *(continued)*
    s. force
    s. rate of blood
    s. stress
    s. thinning
shears
    Bethune rib s.
    Brunner rib s.
    Coryllos-Bethune rib s.
    Coryllos-Moure rib s.
    Coryllos-Shoemaker rib s.
    Duval-Coryllos rib s.
    Eccentric locked rib s.
    Frey-Sauerbruch rib s.
    Giertz-Shoemaker rib s.
    Gluck rib s.
    rib s.
    Shoemaker rib s.
sheath
    Arrow s.
    ArrowFlex s.
    arterial s.
    carotid s.
    check-valve s.
    Cordis s.
    Desilets-Hoffman s.
    s. and dilator system
    French s.
    Hemaflex s.
    Hemaquet s.
    introducer s.
    888 introducer s.
    IVT percutaneous catheter
      introducer s.
    Klein transseptal introducer s.
    Mapper hemostasis EP
      mapping s.
    Mullins transseptal
      catheterization s.
    percutaneous brachial s.
    Pinnacle introducer s.
    Super ArrowFlex
      catheterization s.
    Terumo Radiofocus s.
    vascular s.
    venous s.
sheath/dilator
    Mullins s.
sheathing
    halo s.
Sheehan and Dodge technique
Sheen airway reconstruction
sheep antidigoxin Fab antibody

sheepskin boot
sheet
    mucous s.'s
    s. sign
Sheffield
    S. exercise stress test
    S. treadmill protocol
Shekelton aneurysm
shelf of plaque
Shenstone tourniquet
SHEP
    Systolic Hypertension in the Elderly
      Program
shepherd's crook deformity
Sherpa guiding catheter
Shibley sign
shield
    bronchoscopic face s.
    chest s.
    face s.
    probe s.
shift
    axis s.
    Doppler s.
    mediastinal s.
    midline s.
shifter
    frequency s.
shifting pacemaker
Shigella
shiitake mushroom extract
Shiley
    S. cardiotomy reservoir
    S. catheter
    S. convexoconcave heart valve
    S. Phonate speaking valve
    S. Tetraflex vascular graft
    S. tracheostomy tube
Shimadzu cardiac ultrasound
Shimazaki area-length method
shiners
    allergic s.
SHJR4
    side-hole Judkins right, curve 4
      SHJR4 catheter
SHJR4s
    side-hole Judkins right, curve 4,
      short
shock
    biphasic s.
    s. blocks
    burst s.
    cardiac s.

cardiogenic s.
chronic s.
compensated s.
s. count
DC electric s.
declamping s.
decompensated s.
defibrillation s.
diastolic s.
distributive s.
high-energy transthoracic s.
hypovolemic s.
s. index
insulin s.
irreversible s.
s. lung
obstructive s.
oligemic s.
pleural s.
s. position
QRS synchronous atrial
    defibrillation s.'s
septic s.
serum s.
systolic s.
s. therapy
toxic s.
vasogenic s.
shocky
shoddy fever
Shoemaker rib shears
Shone
    S. anomaly
    S. complex
short
    s. axis (SAX)
    side-hole Judkins right, curve
        4, s. (SHJR4s)
short-axis
    s.-a. parasternal view
    s.-a. plane
ShortCutter catheter
shortening
    circumferential fiber s.
    fiber s.
    s. fraction
    fractional myocardial s.

myocardial fiber s.
s. velocity
velocity of circumferential
    fiber s. (VCF)
ventricular wall s.
short-long-short cycle
shortness of breath (SOB)
Short Speedy balloon
short-term
    flow-assisted, s.-t. (FAST)
short-winded
Shoshin disease
shot
    fast low-angle s. (FLASH)
    sinus s.
shotty nodes
shoulder
    s. horizontal flexion
    s. rotation
shoulder-hand syndrome
shoulder-strap resonance
Should We Intervene Following
    Thrombolysis (SWIFT)
shower
    embolic s.
Shprintzen syndrome
shrinker
    Juzo s.
SHU-454 contrast medium
SHU-508A contrast agent
shudder
    carotid s.
shunt
    Allen-Brown s.
    aortofemoral artery s.
    aortopulmonary s.
    arteriovenous s.
    ascending aorta-to-pulmonary
        artery s.
    atrial ventricular s.
    atriopulmonary s.
    balloon s.
    bidirectional s.
    Blalock-Taussig s.
    Brenner carotid bypass s.
    cardiac s.
    carotid artery s.

S

NOTES

shunt *(continued)*
   cavocaval s.
   Cimino arteriovenous s.
   Cordis-Hakim s.
   s. cyanosis
   Denver pleuroperitoneal s.
   s. detection
   distal splenorenal s.
   Drapanas mesocaval s.
   extracardiac s.
   Glenn s.
   Gott s.
   interarterial s.
   intracardiac s.
   Javid s.
   left-to-right s.
   LeVeen peritoneovenous s.
   Marion-Clatworthy side-to-end
     vena caval s.
   mesocaval s.
   Model 40-400 Pruitt-Inahara s.
   parallel s.
   s. pathway
   portacaval s.
   portopulmonary s.
   Potts s.
   Pruitt-Inahara carotid s.
   Pruitt vascular s.
   s. quantification
   Quinton-Scribner s.
   Ramirez s.
   s. ratio
   reversed s.
   Reynold-Southwick H-graft
     portacaval s.
   right-to-left s.
   Simeone-Erlik side-to-end
     portorenal s.
   splenorenal s.
   Sundt carotid endarterectomy s.
   systemic to pulmonary s.
   Thomas s.
   transjugular intrahepatic
     portosystemic s. (TIPS)
   USCI s.
   Vascu-Flo carotid s.
   Vitagraft arteriovenous s.
   Waterston s.
shunted blood
shunting
   venoarterial s.
shuttlemaker's disease
Shy-Drager syndrome

SIADH
   syndrome of inappropriate
     antidiuretic hormone
sialic acid
sibilance
sibilant
   s. rales
   s. rhonchi
Sibson
   S. notch
   S. vestibule
Sicar sign
sicca
   bronchitis s.
   laryngitis s.
   pericarditis s.
   pharyngitis s.
   s. syndrome
sickle
   s. cell anemia
   s. cell crisis
   s. cell disease
   s. cell-thalassemia
   s. cell trait
Sickledex
sicklemia
sickling
sickness
   African sleeping s.
   cave s.
   compressed-air s.
   decompression s.
   mountain s.
   serum s.
   sleeping s.
sick sinus syndrome (SSS)
**SICOR cardiac catheterization
   recording system**
SICT
   selective intracoronary thrombolysis
side
   s. branch compromise
   s. branch occlusion
   s. lobe
   s. lobe artifact
   s. port
   s. stretching
side-entry access (SEA)
side-hole
   s.-h. Judkins right, curve 4
     (SHJR4)
   s.-h. Judkins right, curve 4
     catheter

s.-h. Judkins right, curve 4,
short (SHJR4s)
sideport
sideropenic dysphagia
siderophage
siderosis
siderotica
pneumoconiosis s.
sidewinder percutaneous intra-aortic
balloon catheter
SIDS
sudden infant death syndrome
Siemens
S. BICOR cardioscope
S. HICOR cardioscope
S. open heart table
S. Orbiter gamma camera
S. Siecure implantable
cardioverter-defibrillator
S. ventilator
Siemens-Albis bicycle ergometer
Siemens-Elema
S.-E. AG bicycle ergometer
S.-E. pacemaker
SIESTA
snooze-induced excitation of
sympathetic triggered activity
sigh function
sighing
s. dyspnea
s. respiration
Sigma
S. method
unipolar Pisces S.
sigmoid septum
sign
Abrahams s.
ace of spades s.
air bronchogram s.
antler s.
applesauce s.
Aschner s.
atrioseptal s.
Auenbrugger s.
Aufrecht s.
auscultatory s.
Baccelli s.

bagpipe s.
Bamberger s.
Bard s.
B6 bronchus s.
Béhier-Hardy s.
bent bronchus s.
Bethea s.
Biermer s.
Biot s.
Bird s.
black pleura s.
Bouillaud s.
Boyce s.
Bozzolo s.
Branham s.
Braunwald s.
bread-and-butter textbook s.
Broadbent inverted s.
Brockenbrough s.
Brockenbrough-Braunwald s.
bronchial meniscus s.
calcium s.
Carabello s.
Cardarelli s.
Carvallo s.
Castellino s.
Cegka s.
Charcot s.
Cheyne-Stokes s.
clenched fist s.
cooing s.
Corrigan s.
Cruveilhier s.
Cruveilhier-Baumgarten s.
cuff s.
D'Amato s.
Davis s.
de la Camp s.
Delbet s.
Delmege s.
Demarquay s.
de Musset s. (aortic aneurysm)
de Mussy s. (pleurisy)
d'Espine s.
Dew s.
Dieuaide s.
Dorendorf s.

S

NOTES

sign *(continued)*
doughnut s.
Drummond s.
Duchenne s.
Duroziez s.
E s.
Ebstein s.
Ellis s.
Erni s.
Ewart s.
Ewing s.
Faget s.
failing lung s.
Federici s.
Fischer s.
flying W s.
Friedreich s.
Glasgow s.
Gowers s.
Grancher s.
Greene s.
Griesinger s.
Grocco s.
Grossman s.
Gunn crossing s.
Hall s.
Hamman s.
Heim-Kreysig s.
Heimlich s.
Hill s.
hilum convergence s.
hilum overlay s.
Homans s.
Hoover s.
Hope s.
Huchard s.
intravascular fetal air s.
Jaccoud s.
Jackson s.
Jürgensen s.
Karplus s.
Kellock s.
knuckle s.
Korányi s.
Kreysig s.
Kussmaul s.
Laennec s.
Lancisi s.
Landolfi s.
Levine s.
Litten diaphragm s.
Livierato s.
Lombardi s.

Löwenberg cuff s.
Macewen s.
Mahler s.
Mannkopf s.
McCort s.
McGinn-White s.
s. mechanism for ventilator
  breathing
Meltzer s.
Mueller s.
Müller s.
Murat s.
Musset s.
mute toe s.'s
Nicoladoni-Branham s.
Oliver s.
open bronchus s.
Osler s.
pad s.
patent bronchus s.
Perez s.
Pfuhl-Jaffé s.
Pins s.
pleural meniscus s.
plumb-line s.
Porter s.
Potain s.
Pottenger s.
Prevel s.
Prussian helmet s.
pulmonary meniscus s.
pulmonary notch s.
pulmonary target s.
Queckenstedt s.
Quénu-Muret s.
Quincke s.
rabbit-ear s.
railroad track s.
Ramond s.
reversed three s.
ring s.
Rivero-Carvallo s.
Riviere s.
Robertson s.
Romaña s.
Rotch s.
Rothschild s.
Sam Levine s.
Sansom s.
Schapiro s.
Schepelmann s.
Schick s.
Seitz s.

Semon s.
S s. of Golden
sheet s.
Shibley s.
Sicar s.
silhouette s.
Skoda s.
Smith s.
snake-tongue s.
square root s.
steeple s.
Steinberg thumb s.
Sterles s.
Sternberg s.
stretched bronchus s.
string s.
T s.
tail s.
tenting s.
thumbprint bronchus s.
trapezius ridge s.
Traube s.
Trimadeau s.
Troisier s.
Trunecek s.
Unschuld s.
Walker-Murdoch wrist s.
Weill s.
Wenckebach s.
Westermark s.
Williams s.
Williamson s.
windsock s.
Wintrich s.
3-sign
signal
s. averaging
Doppler s.
gating s.
magnetic resonance s.
mosaic-jet s.'s
s. processing
signal-averaged
s.-a. echocardiogram
s.-a. echocardiography
s.-a. electrocardiogram
s.-a. electrocardiography

signaling
transmembrane s.
signal-to-noise ratio
Signa Pad
signet-ring cell carcinoma
Sigvaris
S. compression stockings
S. medical stockings
Silaminic Expectorant
Silastic
S. bead embolization
S. catheter
S. strain gauge
Sildicon-E
silence
EKG s.
silent
s. angina
s. electrode
s. gap
s. mitral stenosis
s. myocardial infarction (SMI)
s. myocardial ischemia
s. pericardial effusion
Silfedrine
Children's S.
silhouette
cardiac s.
cardiomediastinal s.
s. sign
silica
silicoanthracosis
silicone
Silicore catheter
silicosis
silicotic pneumoconiosis
silicotuberculosis
silk
s. guidewire
silo-filler's lung
Silon tent
Silphen DM
Siltussin DM
silver (Ag)
s. bead electrode
Grocott methenamine s.

S

NOTES

silver *(continued)*
s. bead electrode
Grocott methenamine s.
s. sulfadiazine
S. syndrome
silver-methenamine stain
silver-silver chloride electrode
Silverstein stimulator probe
silver-wire effect
silver-wiring of retinal arteries
Silvester method
Simeone-Erlik side-to-end portorenal shunt
Simmons II, III catheter
Simmons-type sidewinder catheter
Simon
S. foci
S. nitinol inferior vena cava filter
Simon-nitinol IVC filter
Simplate procedure
simplex
angina s.
carcinoma s.
herpes s.
Simplus PE/t dilatation catheter
Simpson
S. atherectomy catheter
S. Coronary AtheroCath catheter
S. Coronary AtheroCath system
S. peripheral AtheroCath
S. rule
S. Ultra Lo-Profile II catheter
Simpson-Robert
S.-R. catheter
S.-R. vascular dilation system
Simron
simultaneous compression-ventilation CPR (SCV-CPR)
SIMV
synchronized intermittent mandatory ventilation
simvastatin
Simvastatin/Enalapril Coronary Atherosclerosis Regression Trial (SCAT)
Sindbis virus
Sine-Aid IB
Sinequan
Sine-U-View nasal endoscope
sine wave
sine-wave pattern

Singer-Blom valve
singer's node
Singh-Vaughan Williams
S.-V. W. antiarrhythmic drug classification
S.-V. W. classification of arrhythmias
single
s. atrium
s. lumen
s. papillary muscle syndrome
s. pleurisy
s. premature extrastimulation
s. ventricle
s. ventricle malposition
single-balloon
s.-b. valvotomy
s.-b. valvuloplasty
single-breath
s.-b. diffusion
s.-b. nitrogen curve
s.-b. nitrogen washout test
single-chamber, rate-responsive
single-crystal gamma camera
single-gene disorder
single-lung transplant (SLT)
single-pass lead
single-photon
s.-p. detection
s.-p. emission
s.-p. emission computed tomography (SPECT)
s.-p. emission tomography (SPET)
s.-p. emission tomography imaging (SPET imaging)
s.-p. gamma scintigraphy
single-plane aortography
single-stage exercise stress test
single-vessel
s.-v. coronary stenosis
s.-v. disease
sinister
bronchus principalis s.
sinistrocardia
sinistrum
atrium s.
cor s.
sinoaortic baroreflex activity
sinoatrial (S-A, SA)
s. arrest
s. block
s. bradycardia
s. conduction time (SACT)
s. exit block
s. nodal artery

sinoauricular
  s. block
sinobronchial
  s. syndrome
sinobronchitis
sinopulmonary
sino-tubular junction
sinoventricular conduction
sinuatrialis
  nodus s. (NS)
  nonreset nodus s.
  reset nodus s.
Sinufed Timecelles
sinus
  aortic s.
  s. arrest
  s. arrhythmia
  s. bradycardia
  carotid s.
  s. catarrh
  coronary s.
  s. cycle length
  s. exit block
  s. exit pause
  s. mechanism
  s. nodal automaticity
  s. nodal reentrant tachycardia
  s. nodal reentry
  s. node (SN)
  s. node artery
  s. node/AV conduction
   abnormality
  s. node disease
  s. node dysfunction
  s. node function
  s. node recovery time (SNRT)
  noncoronary s.
  oblique s.
  Petit s.'s
  piriform s.
  proximal coronary s. (PCS)
  s. reflex
  s. rhythm
  s. shot
  s. standstill
  s. thrombosis
  Valsalva s., s. of Valsalva

  s. of Valsalva aneurysm
  s. of Valsalva aortography
  s. venosus
  s. venosus atrial septal defect
  s. x-ray
SinuScope system
sinusitis
siphon
  carotid s.
  Duguet s.
  Moniz carotid s.
Sippy esophageal dilator
Sirius red stain
SIRS
  systemic inflammatory response
   syndrome
site
  arterial entry s.
  entry s.
  extrapulmonary s.
  target s.
sitting-up view
in situ
  carcinoma i. s.
situational syncope
situs
  s. ambiguus
  s. inversus
  s. solitus
  s. transversus
  visceroatrial s.
size
  French s.
  Multicenter Investigation for
   the Limitation of Infarct S.
   (MILIS)
sizer
  Björk-Shiley heart valve s.
  Meadox graft s.
sizing
  s. balloon
  French s. of catheter
SJM X-Cell cardiac bioprosthesis
Sjögren syndrome
SK
  streptokinase

S

NOTES

skeletal
>s. alpha-actin mRNA
>s. muscle
>s. muscle plasticity

skeleton
>fibrous s.

skeletonization

skewer technique

skimming
>plasma s.

skin
>s. button
>s. gun
>s. heart
>salmon s.
>tenting of s.
>s. turgor

Skinny
>S. dilatation catheter
>S. over-the-wire balloon catheter

skip graft

skipped beat

Skoda
>S. rales
>S. sign

skodaic resonance

SK-Pramine

SKY epidural pain control system

Skylark surface electrode

Slalom balloon

slant-hole tomography

slapping percussion

slaved programmed electrical stimulation

SLE
>systemic lupus erythematosus

Sleek catheter

sleep
>s. apnea
>s. apnea/hypopnea syndrome
>s. apnea syndrome (SAS)
>crescendo s.
>D s.
>deep s.
>s. deprivation
>desynchronized s.
>dreaming s.
>fast wave s.
>s. hypoxia
>NREM s.
>orthodox s.
>paroxysmal s.

>REM s.
>s. spindles
>s. study
>synchronized s. (S-sleep)

sleep-disordered breathing

sleeping
>s. sickness
>s. tachycardia

sleeve
>s. lobectomy
>LocalMed catheter infusion s.

Sleuth
>CO S.
>ETO S.
>HBT S.

slew rate

slice
>coronal s.
>transaxial s.

Slick stylette endotracheal tube guide

Slider
>S. balloon
>S. catheter

Slidewire extension guide

sliding
>s. filament theory
>s. hiatal hernia
>s. plasty
>s. rail catheter
>s. scale method

slim disease

sling
>cardiac s.
>pericardial s.
>pressure s.
>pulmonary artery s.
>s. ring complex
>vascular s.

Slinky
>S. balloon
>S. balloon catheter
>S. PTCA catheter

slipping rib syndrome

Slip/Stream
>Bennett S.

slit ventricle syndrome

Slo-bid

Slo-Niacin

slope
>D to E s.
>E to F s.
>mitral E to F s.

Slo-Phyllin
slotted needle
slough
sloughed bronchial epithelium
slow
    s. A-V node pathway
    s. channel
    s. channel blocker
    s. escape rhythm
    S. FE
    s. respiration
    s. response
    s. vital capacity (SVC)
    s. zone
slow-fast tachycardia
slowing
    diffuse paroxysmal s.
slow-pathway ablation
slow-reacting substance of
  anaphylaxis (SRS-A)
SLT
    single-lung transplant
sludged blood
sludging
slurred speech
slurring
    s. of ST
    s. of QRS
slurry
    gelatin sponge s.
    talc s.
slush
    ice s.
    saline s.
slushed ice
Sly disease
SM
    sonomicrometry
small
    s. airways disease
    s. cell carcinoma
small-lunged emphysema
smallpox vaccine reaction
SMAP
    systemic mean arterial pressure
smart
    s. defibrillator

    S. position-sensing catheter
    S. Trigger
    S. Trigger Bear 1000
      ventilator
SmartNeedle
SMC
    smooth muscle cell
smear
    buffy coat s.
    sputum s.
Smec balloon catheter
smegmatis
    Mycobacterium s.
Smeloff-Cutter ball-cage prosthetic
  valve
Smeloff heart valve
SMI
    silent myocardial infarction
SMILE
    Survival of Myocardial Infarction
    Long-Term Evaluation
Smith-Lemli-Opitz syndrome
Smith sign
SMO
    Sarns membrane oxygenator
smoke
    puff of s.
    second-hand s.
smokelike echoes
smoker's
    s. bronchitis
    s. cough
    s. tongue
smoking
    s. cessation
    cigarette s.
    s. history
    pack-years of s.
    passive s.
smoking-induced angina
smooth
    s. muscle cell (SMC)
    s. muscle relaxation
smoothing
    digital s.

S

NOTES

SMVR
    supra-annular mitral valve
      replacement
SMVT
    sustained monomorphic ventricular
      tachycardia
SN
    sinoatrial node
    sinus node
snake
    s. graft
    s. venom
snake-tongue sign
snap
    closing s.
    mitral opening s. (MOS)
    opening s.
    tricuspid opening s.
Snaplets-EX
SNAP sleep recorder
snare
    s. catheter
    s. device
    s. technique
sneeze
    s. reflex
    s. syncope
Snider match test
sniffling bronchophony
sniff test
S-nitrosothiols
snooze-induced excitation of
    sympathetic triggered activity
    (SIESTA)
snoring rales
snowman
    s. abnormality
    s. heart
snowplow effect
snowstorm shadow
SNRT
    sinus node recovery time
Snuggle Warm convective warming
    system
Snyder Surgivac drainage
SO$_2$
    sulfur dioxide
^{82}So
    strontium-82
SOB
    shortness of breath
Sobel-Kaplitt-Sawyer gas
    endarterectomy set

sobria
    Aeromonas s.
Society
    American Cancer S.
    American Thoracic S. (ATS)
    Canadian Cardiovascular S.
      (CCS)
sock array
sodium
    aminosalicylate s.
    s. bicarbonate
    brequinar s.
    cefazolin s.
    cefmetazole s.
    cefonicid s.
    cefoperazone s.
    cefotaxime s.
    cefoxitin s.
    ceftizoxime s.
    ceftriaxone s.
    cephalothin s.
    cephapirin s.
    s. channel
    cloxacillin s.
    colistimethate s.
    cromolyn s.
    dalteparin s.
    dantrolene s.
    dextrothyroxine s.
    s. dichloroacetate
    dicloxacillin s.
    dietary s.
    s. dodecylsulfate polyacrylamide
      gel electrophoresis
    enoxaparin s.
    epoprostenol s.
    fluvastatin s.
    s. ion
    ioxaglate s.
    meclofenamate s.
    s. meglumine diatrizoate
    s. meglumine ioxaglate
    mercaptomerin s.
    methicillin s.
    mezlocillin s.
    morrhuate s.
    nafcillin s.
    nedocromil s.
    s. nitrite
    s. nitroprusside
    nitroprusside s.
    oxacillin s.
    paraaminosalicylate s.

S. P.A.S.
Pentothal S.
s. pertechnate
pertechnetate s.
piperacillin sodium and
tazobactam s.
s. polystyrene sulfonate
s. polystyrene sulfonate enema
pravastatin s.
s. retention
stibogluconate s.
s. tetradecyl sulfate
thiamylal s.
thiopental s.
thiopentone s.
warfarin s.
sodium-potassium exchange
Soemmerring
arterial vein of S.
**Sofamor spinal instrumentation
device**
Sofarin
soft
s. event
s. pulse
s. tissue sarcoma
Softech endotracheal tube
Soft-EZ reusable electrode
SOF-T guidewire
Softip catheter
**Softouch UHF cardiac pigtail
catheter**
Softrac-PTA catheter
Soft-Vu Omni flush catheter
software
Image-Measure morphometry s.
Sokolow electrocardiographic index
Sokolow-Lyon
S.-L. voltage
S.-L. voltage criteria
Solcotrans autotransfusion unit
soldered bond
soldering
s. flux
s. fumes

soldier
s. heart
s. patches
Sole Primeur 33D analyzer
solid angle concept
solitarius
nucleus tractus s.
solitary
s. coronary ostium
s. pulmonary arteriovenous
fistula
s. pulmonary nodule (SPN)
solitus
situs s.
ventricular situs s.
visceroatrial situs s.
Solo
S. balloon
S. catheter
solubility
lipid s.
Solu-Cortef
Soludrast contrast material
Solu-Medrol
S.-M. injection
Solurex
Solus pacemaker
Soluspan
Celestone S.
solution
Anti-Sept bactericidal scrub s.
Atrovent Inhalation S.
Belzer s.
Betadine Helafoam s.
Bretschneider-HTK
cardioplegic s.
Brompton s.
Burow s.
cardioplegic s.
Collins s.
Crolom Ophthalmic S.
crystalloid cardioplegic s.
Dakin s.
Denhardt s.
ECS cardioplegic s.
extracellular-like, calcium-
free s. (ECS)

S

NOTES

solution *(continued)*
  Gey s.
  Hank balanced salt s.
  Hartmann s.
  ICS cardioplegic s.
  Intal Nebulizer S.
  intracellular-like, calcium-
    bearing crystalloid s. (ICS)
  Krebs s.
  Krebs-Henseleit s.
  Lugol s.
  Massier s.
  Melrose s.
  Nasalcrom Nasal S.
  Papanicolaou s.
  Ringer s.
  Schlesinger s.
  Sepracoat coating s.
  stroma-free hemoglobin s.
  St. Thomas s.
  Tyrode s.
  University of Wisconsin s.
SOLVD
  Studies of Left Ventricular
  Dysfunction
SomaSensor
  S. device
  S. pad
somatic
somatomedin
somatostatin
somnambulism
somniloquism
somniloquy
SomnoStar apnea testing device
Sondergaard procedure
Sones
  S. Cardio-Marker catheter
  S. coronary catheter
  S. guidewire
  S. hemostatic bag
  S. Hi-Flow catheter
  S. Positrol catheter
  S. selective coronary
    arteriography
  S. technique
  S. woven Dacron catheter
sonicated
  s. contrast agent
  s. dextrose albumin
  s. Renografin-76
Sonicath imaging catheter
sonication technique

sonicator
sonogram
sonography
  Acuson computed s.
  transcranial contrast Doppler s.
sonolucency
sonomicrometer piezoelectric crystals
sonomicrometry (SM)
sonorous
  s. rales
  s. respiration
  s. rhonchi
Sonos
  S. 500 imaging system
  S. 2000 ultrasound imager
Sopha Medical gamma camera
Sophy high-resolution collimator
Sorbitrate
Sorenson thermodilution catheter
Sorin
  S. mitral valve prosthesis
  S. prosthetic valve
Sorivudine
soroche
sorter
  cell s.
Sos guidewire
Sotacor
sotalol
  s. hydrochloride
Sotradecol injection
Soucek
  Randall-Baker S. (RBS)
souffle
  cardiac s.
  fetal s.
  funic s.
  mammary s.
soufflet
  bruit de s.
sound
  absent breath s.'s
  adventitious breath s.'s
  aortic closure s.
  aortic second s. (A_2)
  atrial s.
  auscultatory s.
  bandbox s.
  Beatty-Bright friction s.
  bell s.
  bellows s.
  bottle s.
  bronchial breath s.'s

bronchovesicular breath s.'s
cannon s.
cardiac s.
coarse breath s.'s
coin s.
cracked-pot s.
crowing breath s.'s
crunching s.
decreased breath s.'s
distant breath s.'s
distant heart s.'s
double-shock s.
eddy s.'s
ejection s.'s (ES)
esophageal s.
first heart s. (S$_1$)
flapping s.
fourth heart s. (S$_4$)
friction s.
gallop s.
heart s.'s S$_1$, S$_2$, S$_3$, S$_4$
hippocratic s.
Korotkoff s.
mammary souffle s.
metallic breath s.'s
mitral first s. (M$_1$)
mitral second s. (M$_2$)
muffled heart s.'s
pacemaker s.
paradoxically split S$_2$ s.
percussion s.
pericardial friction s.
physiologically split S$_2$ s.
physiologic third heart s.
pistol-shot femoral s.
puffing s.
pulmonic closure s.
pulmonic second s.
pulmonic valve closure s.
quiet breath s.'s
quiet heart s.'s
respiratory s.
sail s.
second heart s. (S$_2$)
second mitral s.
shaking s.
splitting of heart s.'s

squeaky-leather s.
succussion s.'s
tambour s.
third heart s. (S$_3$)
tic-tac s.'s
to-and-fro s.
tracheal s.
tricuspid valve closure s.
tubular breath s.'s
tumor plop s.
tympanitic s.
vesicular breath s.'s
waterwheel s.
s. wave cycle
xiphisternal crunching s.

South Florida RAST panel
Souttar tube
SP1005
    Cardiomyostimulator SP1005
SP-10 spirometer
space
    air s.
    alveolar dead s.
    anatomical dead s.
    antecubital s.
    s. of Burns
    echo-free s.
    extrapleural s.
    H s.
    His perivascular s.
    Holzknecht s.
    intercostal s.
    interstitial s.
    Larrey s.'s
    mediastinal s.
    perivascular s.'s
    physiological dead s.
    pleural s.
    prevertebral s.
    retrocardiac s.
    retropharyngeal s.
    retrotracheal s.
    subphrenic s.
    Traube semilunar s.
    Westberg s.
    Zang s.

S

NOTES

SpaceLabs
> S. Event Master
> S. Holter monitor
> S. pulse oximeter

Spacemaker balloon dissector
space-occupying lesion
spacer
> Ellipse compact s.

spacing
spadelike configuration
SPAF
> Stroke Prevention in Atrial Fibrillation

Span-FF
spannungs-P
sparfloxacin
sparing
> myocardial s.

spark erosion
Sparks mandrel technique
spasm
> arterial s.
> bronchial s.
> bronchopulmonary s.
> carpopedal s.
> catheter-related peripheral vessel s.
> catheter-tip s.
> coronary artery s.
> diffuse esophageal s.
> ergonovine-induced s.
> esophageal s.
> vascular s.
> venous s.

spasmodic
> s. asthma
> s. croup

spastica
> dysphagia s.

spasticity
spatial
> s. intensity
> s. resolution
> s. tracking
> s. vector
> s. vectorcardiography

SPCA
> serum prothrombin conversion accelerator

Spearman
> S. nonparametric univariate correlation
> S. rho test

Spears laser balloon
specificity
speckling
SPECT
> single-photon emission computed tomography
> adenosine ^{99m}Tc sestamibi SPECT
> SPECT scintigraphy
> stress perfusion and rest function by sestamibi-gated SPECT

spectography
> magnetic resonance s.
> Raman s.

spectra (*pl. of* spectrum)
Spectra-Cath
> S.-C. STP catheter

spectral
> s. analysis
> S. Cardiac STATus Test
> s. envelope
> s. leakage
> s. phonocardiograph
> s. power
> s. temporal mapping
> s. turbulence mapping
> s. waveform

Spectranetic P23 Statham transducer
Spectranetics laser
Spectraprobe
Spectrax SX, SX-HT, SXT, VL, VM, VS pacemaker
Spectrobid
spectrometer
> Amis 2000 respiratory mass s.

spectrophotometer
> Hitachi U-2000 s.
> liquid scintillation s.

spectrophotometric oximetry
spectroscopy
> electron paramagnetic resonance s.
> flame emission s. (FES)
> fluorescence s.
> magnetic resonance s.
> near-infrared s. (NIS)
> NMR s.
> proton s.
> Raman s.

spectroscopy-directed laser
spectrum, pl. **spectra**

SpectRx test
specular echo
speculum
　　Yankauer pharyngeal s.
speech
　　alaryngeal s.
　　esophageal s.
　　slurred s.
Speedy balloon catheter
spell
　　blackout s.
　　greyout s.
　　hypercyanotic s.
　　hypoxic s.
　　presyncopal s.
　　syncopal s.
　　tet s.
　　tetrad s.
Spembly cryoprobe
Spencer plication of vena cava
Spens syndrome
SPET
　　single-photon emission tomography
　　SPET imaging
Spexil
sphaericus
　　Bacillus s.
sphericity index
sphincter
　　cardioesophageal s.
　　esophageal s.
　　gastroesophageal s.
　　hepatic s.
　　palatopharyngeal s.
　　pharyngoesophageal s.
　　precapillary s.
Sphingobacterium
sphingolipidosis
sphygmic
　　s. interval
sphygmocardiograph
sphygmocardioscope
sphygmochronograph
sphygmogram
sphygmograph
sphygmography
sphygmoid

sphygmomanometer
　　Ayers s.
　　Erlanger s.
　　Faught s.
　　Hawksley random zero
　　　　mercury s.
　　Mosso s.
　　Physio-Control Lifestat s.
　　random-zero s.
　　Riva-Rocci s.
　　Rogers s.
sphygmomanometry
sphygmometer
sphygmometroscope
sphygmo-oscillometer
sphygmopalpation
sphygmophone
sphygmoscope
　　Bishop s.
sphygmoscopy
sphygmosystole
sphygmotonograph
sphygmotonometer
sphygmoviscosimetry
spider
　　s. angioma
　　arterial s.
　　s. burst
　　s. projection
　　vascular s.
　　s. venom
spike
　　s. activity
　　H s.
　　pacemaker s.
　　sensing s.
spike-and-dome
　　s.-a.-d. configuration
　　s.-a.-d. pulse
spillover
　　jugular venous catechol s.
spinal muscular atrophy
spin density
spindle
　　aortic s.

S

NOTES

spindle *(continued)*
s. cell carcinoma
His s.
sleep s.'s
spin-echo (SE)
s.-e. imaging
s.-e. imaging sequence
s.-e. MRI
Spinhaler
spin-lattice time
spinocerebellar
s. ataxia
s. degeneration
spin-spin time
spiral
Curschmann s.'s
s. dissection
S. Mark V portable ultrasonic
drug inhaler
spiramycin
spirapril
s. hydrochloride
spirochetal
s. disease
s. infection
s. myocarditis
spirochete
spirogram
forced expiratory s. (FES)
spirography
spiro-index
Spirolite 201 spirometer
spirometer
Benedict-Roth s.
Bennett monitoring s.
Calculair s.
Coach incentive s.
Collins Dry s.
Collins Survey s.
Douglas bag s.
Eagle s.
Flash portable s.
incentive s.
Inspirx incentive s.
Krogh apparatus s.
Micro Plus s.
SP-10 s.
Spirolite 201 s.
Spirovit SP-1 portable s.
Tissot s.
Venturi s.
Vitalograph s.

Vitalor incentive s.
Wright s.
spirometric screening
spirometry
incentive s.
Tri-flow incentive s.
Spironazide
spironolactone
hydrochlorothiazide and s.
SpiroSense
S. flow sensor
S. system
Spirovit
S. SP-1 portable spirometer
Spirozide
Spitzer theory
splanchnic
s. bed perfusion
s. blood flow
s. vessel
splanchnicotomy
splayed
carina not s.
Splendore-Hoeppli phenomenon
splenic
s. anemia
s. flexure syndrome
s. portography
splenomegaly
splenopneumonia
splenoportal hypertension
splenoportography
splenorenal shunt
splice
breakaway s.
splinter hemorrhages
splinting
split
paradoxic s. of S$_2$
physiological s. of S$_2$
split-function lung test
split-lung ventilation
split-sheath introducer
splitter
beam s.
splitting
commissural s.
s. of heart sounds
SPN
solitary pulmonary nodule
SpO$_2$
oxygen saturation as measured using
pulse oximetry

spondylitis
    ankylosing s. (AS)
spondyloarthropathy
    seronegative s.
sponge
    Collostat s.
    Ivalon s.
    phantom s.
    RayTec s.
spontaneous
    s. coronary artery dissection
    (SCAD)
    s. echo contrast (SEC)
    s. pneumothorax
    s. reentrant sustained
    ventricular tachycardia
Sporanox
    S. Oral
SPO₂T
    Pocket SPO$_2$T
spot
    Brushfield s.
    café-au-lait s.
    Campbell de Morgan s.'s
    cotton-wool s.
    De Morgan s.'s
    Horder s.'s
    hot s.
    milk s.'s
    rose s.
    Roth s.
    tendinous s.
    ventricular milk s.'s
    white s.
SpotCheck+ hand-held pulse oximeter
spot-film fluorography
spray
    Astelin nasal s.
    Hurricaine s.
    metered-dose s.
    Nitrolingual Translingual S.
spread
    lymphangitic s.
    venous s.
spreader
    Bailey rib s.

    Burford-Finochietto rib s.
    Davis rib s.
    DeBakey rib s.
    Favaloro-Morse rib s.
    Harken rib s.
    Mcdicon rib s.
    Miltex rib s.
    Rehbein rib s.
    rib s.
spring
    S. catheter
    disk s.
spring-loaded stent
springwater cyst
SPRINT
    Secondary Prevention Reinfarction
    Israeli Nifedipine Trial
Sprint catheter
SPTI
    systolic pressure time index
spuria
    angina s.
spurious aneurysm
spurium
    septum s.
sputum, pl. sputa
    s. aerogenosum
    albuminoid s.
    s. analysis
    blood-tinged s.
    bloody s.
    brown s.
    s. coctum
    copious s.
    s. crudum
    s. cruentum
    currant jelly s.
    s. cytology
    egg-yolk s.
    elastic fibers in s.
    frothy s.
    globular s.
    green s.
    hemorrhagic s.
    icteric s.
    s. induction
    moss-agate s.

S

NOTES

sputum *(continued)*
  mucopurulent s.
  nummular s.
  pink s.
  s. production
  productive s.
  prune juice s.
  purulent s.
  rusty s.
  septicemia s.
  s. smear
  tenacious s.
  s. viscosity and elasticity
  white s.
  yellow s.
S-QRS interval
squamous
  s. cell
  s. cell carcinoma
square
  s. root sign
  s. wave response
  s. wave stimulus
squared
  kilogram per meter s. (kg/m2)
  liters per minute per meter s.
  meters per second s.
squatting
squeak
squeaky-leather sound
squeeze
  s. effect
  thoracic s.
  tussive s.
squeezer
  lemon s.
Sramek formula
SR calcium ATPase
SRS-A
  slow-reacting substance of
  anaphylaxis
SSKI
  saturated solution of potassium
  iodide
S-sleep
  synchronized sleep
SSS
  sick sinus syndrome
SSSS
  Scandinavian Simvastatin Survival
  Study
S-sulfate

ST
  ST alterations
  ST interval
  ST junction
  ST sag
  ST segment
  ST segment alternans
  ST segment changes
  ST segment depression
  ST segment elevation
  slurring of ST
  ST vector
  ST wave
St.
  St. Joseph Adult Chewable
  Aspirin
  St. Joseph Cough Suppressant
  St. Jude annuloplasty ring
  St. Jude bileaflet prosthetic
  valve
  St. Jude cardiac device
  St. Jude heart valve prosthesis
  St. Jude Medical bileaflet
  tilting-disk aortic valve
  St. Jude Medical Port-Access
  St. Jude mitral valve
  St. Jude prosthetic aortic valve
  St. Thomas Hospital
  cardioplegia
  St. Thomas solution
  St. Vitus dance
stab
  s. incision
  s. wound
stability
stab-in epicardial electrode
stable angina
staccato pain
Stachrom PAI chromogenic assay
Stack
  S. autoperfusion balloon
  S. perfusion catheter
Stadie-Riggs microtome
Stagesic
staging
  TNM s.
stagnant
  s. anoxia
  s. hypoxia
stagnation
stain, staining
  calcofluor s.
  Dieterle s.

Diff-Quik s.
endocardial s.
Gomori methenamine silver s.
Gram s.
H&E s.
hematoxylin-cosin s.
immunoperoxidase s.
Kinyoun s.
Mallory s.
Masson trichrome s.
May-Grünwald-Giemsa s.
Miller elastic s.
Movat s.
mucicarmine s.
Pizzolatto s.
silver-methenamine s.
Sirius red s.
TTC s.
van Gieson s.
Wright s.
Ziehl-Neelsen s.
stainless
s. steel guidewire
s. steel mesh stent
staircase phenomenon
Stamey test
Stancel procedure
stand-alone laser treatment
standard
Boehringer Mannheim s.
s. Bruce protocol
s. deviations
s. Lehman catheter
s. limb lead
s. needle
standby pulse generator
standstill
atrial s.
auricular s.
cardiac s.
respiratory s.
sinus s.
ventricular s.
Stanford
S. biopsy method
S. bioptome

S. Coronary Risk Intervention
Project (SCRIP)
Stanford-Caves bioptome
Stanford-type aortic dissection
Stanicor pacemaker
Stannius ligature
Staphcillin
staphyledema
staphylococcal
s. bronchitis
s. endocarditis
s. infection
s. pneumonia
Staphylococcus
S. aureus
S. epidermidis
staphylopharyngorrhaphy
stapled lung reduction
stapler
Androsov vascular s.
Inokucki vascular s.
stapling
bleb s.
starch
hydroxyethyl s.
Starling
S. curve
S. equation
S. force
S. law
S. mechanism
Starr-Edwards
S.-E. aortic valve prosthesis
S.-E. ball-and-cage valve
S.-E. ball valve prosthesis
S.-E. cardiac valve prosthesis
S.-E. disk valve prosthesis
S.-E. heart valve prosthesis
S.-E. mitral prosthesis
S.-E. mitral valve
S.-E. prosthetic valve
S.-E. Silastic valve
Star Sync
stasis, pl. **stases**
s. cirrhosis
s. dermatitis
s. edema

NOTES

stasis *(continued)*
    pressure s.
    s. ulcer
    venous s.
state
    cardiovascular steady s.
    gradient-recalled acquisition in
      the steady s. (GRASS)
    hypercoagulable s.
    hyperdynamic s.
    hyperkinetic s.
    postabsorptive s.
    postictal s.
    S. Trait Anxiety Inventory
static dilation technique
statins
station pull-through
statistic
    Gehan s.
    Lee-Desu s.
    Mantel-Haenszel s.
    Wei-Lachin s.
Stat 2 Pumpette
status
    s. anginosus
    s. asthmaticus
    cardiac s.
    s. epilepticus
    mental s.
    neurologic s.
    work s.
staurosporine
stavudine
Stay Trim Diet Gum
steal
    coronary s.
    endoperoxide s.
    iliac s.
    s. mechanism
    s. phenomenon
    pulmonary artery s.
    renal-splanchnic s.
    subclavian s.
    transmural s.
steam-fitter's asthma
steam tent
stearothermophilus
    Bacillus s.
steatorrhea
steatosis
    s. cardiaca
    s. cordis
Steele bronchial dilator

Steell murmur
steel-winged butterfly needle
steeple sign
steepling
    s. of trachea
    tracheal s.
steerable
    s. angioplastic guidewire
    s. electrode catheter
    s. guidewire catheter
Steerocath catheter
Stegemann-Stalder method
Steidele complex
Steinberg thumb sign
Steinert disease
Stela electrode lead
stellate
    s. ganglion
    s. ganglion blockade
Stellite
    S. ring material
    S. ring material of prosthetic
      valve
stem bronchus
Stemphyllium
stems
    transposition of arterial s.
stenocardia
stenosal murmur
stenosis, pl. stenoses
    airway s.
    aortic s. (AS)
    bottle-neck s.
    branch pulmonary artery s.
    bronchial s.
    buttonhole mitral s.
    calcific mitral s.
    calcific nodular aortic s.
    caroticovertebral s.
    carotid s.
    chronic aortic s.
    cicatricial s.
    congenital aortic s.
    congenital mitral s.
    coronary artery s.
    coronary ostial s.
    discrete subvalvular aortic s.
    distal s.
    Dittrich s.
    double aortic s.
    eccentric s.
    enucleation of subaortic s.
    fibrous subaortic s.

fish-mouth mitral s.
flow-limiting s.
focal eccentric s.
geometry of s.
granulation s.
hemodynamically significant s.
high-grade s.
hourglass s.
hypertrophic subaortic s. (HSS)
idiopathic hypertrophic
  subaortic s. (IHSS)
left main coronary s.
mitral s. (MS)
muscular subaortic s.
myocardial infundibular s.
napkin-ring s.
orificial s.
peripheral pulmonic s.
point of critical s.
postdiphtheritic s.
preventricular s.
pulmonary artery s.
pulmonary branch s.
pulmonary valve s.
pulmonary valvular s.
pulmonic valve s.
residual s.
rheumatic mitral valve s.
segmental s.
senescent aortic s.
silent mitral s.
single-vessel coronary s.
subaortic s.
subpulmonary s.
subpulmonic s.
subvalvar s.
subvalvular aortic s.
subvalvular mitral s.
supravalvar s.
supravalvular aortic s. (SVAS)
tight s.
tricuspid s.
valvular aortic s.
valvular pulmonic s.
vascular s.
stenothorax
stenotic lesion

stent
ACS Multi-Link coronary s.
activated balloon expandable
  intravascular s.
s. apposition
Atkinson tube s.
AVE Micro s.
bailout s.
balloon-expandable flexible
  coil s.
balloon-expandable
  intravascular s.
biodegradable s.
CardioCoil coronary s.
carotid s.
Carpentier s.
coil s.
Cook intracoronary s.
Cordis radiopaque tantalum s.
s. deployment
double-J s.
Dumon tracheobronchial s.
Dynamic Y s.
eluting s.
emergency bailout s.
Endocoil s.
EsophaCoil self-expanding
  esophageal s.
s. expansion
Flex s.
Freitag s.
Gianturco-Roubin s.
Gianturco Z s.
heat-activated recoverable
  temporary s. (HARTS)
heat-expandable s.
helical coil s.
Hood stoma s.
Hood-Westaby T-Y s.
s. implantation
InStent CarotidCoil s.
interdigitating coil s.
intravascular s.
Medivent self-expanding
  coronary s.
Medivent vascular s.

S

NOTES

stent *(continued)*
Medtronic interventional vascular s.
mesh s.
Micro s.
6 Micro S. PL
Multi Link s.
Neville s.
nitinol mesh s.
nitinol thermal memory s.
Novastent s.
Orlowski s.
Palmaz balloon-expandable iliac s.
Palmaz-Schatz balloon-expandable s.
Palmaz-Schatz coronary s.
Palmaz vascular s.
polymeric endoluminal paving s.
radiopaque tantalum s.
Reduced Anticoagulation in Vein Graft S. (RAVES)
Roubin-Gianturco flexible coil s.
Schatz-Palmaz intravascular s.
Schatz-Palmaz tubular mesh s.
Schneider s.
self-expanding s.
spring-loaded s.
stainless steel mesh s.
Strecker balloon-expandable s.
Strecker coronary s.
Strecker tantalum s.
s. strut
tantalum s.
thermal memory s.
Tower s.
T-Y s.
Ultraflex self-expanding s.
VascuCoil peripheral vascular s.
Wallstent flexible, self-expanding wire-mesh s.
Wallstent spring-loaded s.
Wiktor coronary s.
wire mesh self-expandable s.
Y s.
Z s.
zig-zag s.
stenting
bailout s.

coronary s.
endoluminal s.
stentless
s. porcine aortic valve
s. porcine aortic valve prosthesis
s. porcine xenograft
stent-mounted
s.-m. allograft valve
s.-m. heterograft valve
step-down therapy
Step-One Diet
stepped-care antihypertensive regimen
steps
Krönig s.
step-up in oxygen saturation
stepwise
Sterapred Oral
stereoauscultation
stereolithography
stereoscopic interrogation
Sterges carditis
Steri-Cath catheter
Sterles sign
Sterna-Band self-locking suture
sternad
sternal
s. border
s. dehiscence
s. notch
s. plane
s. synchondrosis
s. wiring
sternalgia
sternal-splitting incision
Sternberg
S. myocardial insufficiency
S. pericarditis
S. sign
Sterneedle tuberculin test
sternochondral junction
sternoclavicular angle
sternocleidomastoid
s. artery
sternocostal triangle
sternodynia
sternomastoid
sternotome
sternotomy
median s.
sternotracheal
sternoxiphoid plane

Stern posture
sternum
  s. saw
  wiring of s.
steroid
  s. aerosol
  anabolic s.
  high-dose s.
  sex s.
steroid-dependent
  s.-d. asthma
  s.-d. asthmatic
steroid-eluting pacemaker lead
steroid-sparing agent
Ster-O₂-Mist ultrasonic cup
stertor
  hen-cluck s.
stertorous respiration
Stertzer
  S. brachial catheter
  S. guiding catheter
Stertzer-Myler extension wire
stethoscope
  Acoustascope esophageal s.
  Doppler fetal s.
stethoscopic phonocardiograph
Stevens-Johnson syndrome
Stewart-Hamilton cardiac output
  technique
sthenic fever
STI
  systolic time interval
stibogluconate sodium
stick
  arterial s.
Stifcore
  S. aspiration needle
stiff
  s. heart
  s. heart syndrome
  s. lung
stiffness
  active dynamic s.
  chamber s.
  diastolic s.
  elastic s.
  s. index

  muscle s.
  myocardial s.
  vascular s.
  volume s.
stigma, pl. stigmata
  peripheral stigmata
Stilith implantable cardiac pulse
  generator
Still
  S. disease
  S. murmur
stimulant
  adrenergic s.
stimulation
  β-adrenergic s.
  alpha-adrenergic s.
  beta-adrenergic s.
  beta adrenoceptor s.
  noninvasive programmed s.
   (NIPS)
  paired electrical s.
  programmed electrical s. (PES)
  slaved programmed electrical s.
  subthreshold s.
  supramaximal tetanic s.
  s. threshold
  transcutaneous electrical s.
   (TES)
  transesophageal atrial s.
   (TRAS)
  ultrarapid subthreshold s.
  vagal s.
  ventricular-programmed s.
stimulator
  Arzco model 7 cardiac s.
  Atrostim phrenic nerve s.
  Bloom programmable s.
  Grass S88 muscle s.
stimulus, pl. stimuli
  chemical s.
  heterotopic s.
  neurohumoral s.
  nomatopic s.
  pacing s.
  physical s.
  psychological s.

S

NOTES

stimulus *(continued)*
    square wave s.
    triple s.
stippling
stochastic risk
Stockert cardiac pacing electrode
Stockholm
    Angina Prognosis Study in S.
      (APSIS)
stocking-glove distribution
stockings
    antiembolism s.
    A-T antiembolism s.
    Bellavar medical support s.
    Camp-Sigvaris s.
    Carolon life support
      antiembolism s.
    compression s.
    Comtesse medical support s.
    elastic s.
    Fast-Fit vascular s.
    Florex medical compression s.
    graduated compression s.
      (GCS)
    Jobst-Stride support s.
    Jobst-Stridette support s.
    Jobst VPGS s.
    Juzo s.
    Kendall compression s.
    Linton elastic s.
    Medi-Strumpf s.
    Medi vascular s.
    pneumatic compression s.
    Sigvaris compression s.
    Sigvaris medical s.
    Stride support s.
    TED antiembolism s.
    thigh-high antiembolic s.
    True Form support s.
    Twee alternating cut-off
      compressor s.
    Vairox high compression
      vascular s.
    VenES II Medical s.
    Venofit medical compression s.
    Venoflex medical
      compression s.
    venous pressure gradient
      support s.
    Zimmer antiembolism
      support s.
stocking-seam incision
stoichiometric fashion

Stokes
    collar of S.
    S. expectorant
Stokes-Adams
    S.-A. disease
    S.-A. syndrome
Stokvis-Talma syndrome
Stoll pneumonia
stoma
    tracheostomy s.
stomach cough
Stomatococcus
stone
    s. asthma
    s. heart
    lung s.
stone-cutter's phthisis
stone-stripper's asthma
stools
    melenic s.
stopcock
    three-way s.
stop-valve airway obstruction
stores
    myocyte magnesium s.
storm
    thyroid s.
Storz
    S. bronchoscope
    S. bronchoscopic telescope
    S. tracheoscope
Storz-Hopkins laryngoscope
Storz-Shapshay tracheoscope
straddling
    s. aorta
    s. atrioventricular valve
    s. embolism
    s. thrombus
    s. tricuspid valve
straight
    s. back syndrome
    s. flush percutaneous catheter
    s. hemostat
straight-line EKG
strain
    s. gauge
    0157-H7 s.
    Lagrangian s.
strain-gauge plethysmography
strand
    iridium s.
stranding
strandy infiltrate

strap muscles
stratification
    risk s.
stratified thrombus
Strauss method
streak
    fatty s.
streaky infiltrate
Strecker
    S. balloon-expandable stent
    S. coronary stent
    S. tantalum stent
Strength
    Bayer Low Adult S.
strenuous exercise
Streptase
streptavidin
Streptobacillus moniliformis
streptococcal
    s. antibody
    s. bronchitis
    s. carditis
    s. empyema
    s. endocarditis
    s. infection
    s. pneumonia
Streptococcus
    S. *agalactiae*
    S. *anginosus*
    S. *faecalis*
    S. *milleri*
    S. *mitis*
    S. *pneumoniae*
    S. *pyogenes*
    S. *salivarius*
    S. *viridans*
streptokinase (SK)
    s. antibody
streptokinase-plasminogen complex
streptokinase-streptodornase
streptolysin-O
streptomycin
    s. sulfate
stress
    circumferential wall s. (CWS)
    S. Echo bed
    s. echocardiography

emotional s.
left ventricular end-systolic s.
left ventricular wall s.
mental s.
meridional wall s.
s. MUGA electrocardiogram
s. perfusion and rest function
    by sestamibi-gated SPECT
pharmacologic s.
physiological s.
s. relaxation
shear s.
tensile s.
s. test
s. thallium-201 myocardial
    perfusion imaging
s. thallium scintigraphy
s. thallium study
ventricular wall s.
wall s.
s. washout myocardial
    perfusion image
stress-injected sestamibi-gated
  SPECT with echocardiography
stress-redistribution-reinjection
  thallium-201 imaging
stress-related
    s.-r. arrhythmia
    s.-r. hypertension
stress-shortening relationship
stretch
    S. balloon
    S. cardiac device
    s. receptor
stretched
    s. bronchus sign
    s. diameter
stretching
    side s.
    s. syncope
stria, pl. striae
Striadyne
striation
    tabby cat s.
stricture
    esophageal s.
    Wickwitz esophageal s.

NOTES

S

Stride
    S. cardiac pacemaker
    S. support stockings
strident
stridor
    biphasic s.
    congenital laryngeal s.
    inspiratory s.
    laryngeal s.
    respiratory s.
    s. serraticus
stridulosa
    laryngitis s.
stridulous respiration
stridulus
    laryngismus s.
string of pearls fashion
string sign
strip
    bovine pericardium s.'s
    Breathe Right nasal s.
    Cover-Strip wound closure s.'s
    EKG monitor s.
    Flu-Glow s.
    s. percussion
    rhythm s.
stripe
    subepicardial fat s.
stripper
    Alexander rib s.
    Cole polyethylene vein s.
    Dorian rib s.
    Doyle vein s.
    Dunlop thrombus s.
    hydraulic vein s.
    Kurten vein s.
    Matson-Alexander rib s.
    New Orleans endarterectomy s.
    thrombus s.
    Trace vein s.
    Zollinger-Gilmore intraluminal
      vein s.
stroke
    cardioembolic s.
    s. ejection rate
    embolic s.
    heart s.
    heat s.
    lacunar s.
    s. output
    S. Prevention in Atrial
      Fibrillation (SPAF)

    s. volume (SV)
    s. volume index (SVI)
    s. work
    s. work index (SWI)
stroma-free hemoglobin solution
Strong unbridling of celiac artery axis
Strongyloides
strontium-82 (^{82}So)
Stroop color word conflict test
Strophanthus gratus
Strouhal number
structure
    echo-dense s.
    wall s.
struma
    Riedel s.
strut
    George Washington s.
    stent s.
strutting
    plaque s.
Stryker saw
ST-T
    ST-T deviation
    ST-T wave
    ST-T wave changes
Stuart-Prower factor
Student-Newman-Keuls test
Student *t* test
study
    altitude simulation s.
    amyl nitrite s.
    Asymptomatic Carotid
      Atherosclerosis S. (ACAS)
    Asymptomatic Carotid
      Atherosclerosis Plaque S.
      (ACAPS)
    atrial pacing s.
    Captopril and Thrombolysis S.
      (CATS)
    Cardiac Arrhythmia Pilot S.
      (CAPS)
    Cardiolite cardiac perfusion s.
    Carotid Artery Stenosis with
      Asymptomatic Narrowing:
      Operation Versus Aspirin S.
      (CASANOVA)
    case-control s.
    Cholesterol Lowering
      Atherosclerosis S. (CLAS)
    cohort s.

Cooperative North Scandinavian
Enalapril Survival S.
(CONSENSUS)
Coronary Artery Surgery S.
(CASS)
dipyridamole thallium-201
cardiac perfusion s.
Doppler s.
Duke University Clinical
Cardiology S. (DUCCS)
S. of Economics and Quality
of Life (SEQOL)
electrophysiologic s. (EPS)
equilibrium-gated blood pool s.
European Coronary Surgery S.
exercise s.
Expanded Clinical Evaluation
of Lovastatin S. (EXCEL)
Familial Atherosclerosis
Treatment S. (FATS)
floating wall motion s.
Framingham Heart s.
gated blood-pool s. (GBPS)
Helsinki Heart S.
hemodynamic-angiographic s.
HOT s.
hypertension optimal
treatment s.
hypoxic response s.
imaging s.
interventional s.
intracardiac
electrophysiologic s.
Intravenous Streptokinase in
Acute Myocardial
Infarction S. (ISAM)
LATE s.
Late Potential Italian S.
(LAPIS)
S.'s of Left Ventricular
Dysfunction (SOLVD)
Mayo Asymptomatic Carotid
Endarterectomy S.
meglumine diatrizoate enema s.
Multicenter Anti-Atheroma S.
(MAAS)

Multivessel Angioplasty
Prognosis S. (MAPS)
muscle immunocytochemical s.
myocardial perfusion s.
Northwick Park Heart S.
nuclear ventricular function s.
(NVFS)
phased array s.
polysomnographic s.
Prospective Cardiovascular
Munster s. (PRO-CAM)
radioisotopic s.
radionuclide s.
Scandinavian Simvastatin
Survival S. (SSSS)
Second International S. of
Infarct Survival (ISIS-2)
serum enzyme s.
sleep s.
stress thallium s.
Total Ischemic Burden
Bisoprolol S. (TIBBS)
VeHF s.
Veterans Administration
Cooperative s.
wall motion s.
West of Scotland Coronary
Prevention S. (WOSCOPS)
Zutphen s.

stump
bronchial s.
cardiac s.
s. pressure
stunned
s. atrium
s. myocardium
stunning
myocardial s.
Sturge-Weber syndrome
stuttering
s. myocardial infarction
s. of perfusion
stutzeri
Pseudallescheria s.
Pseudomonas s.
stylet
Bing s.

NOTES

S

stylet *(continued)*
  cardiovascular s.
  transmyocardial pacing s.
  transthoracic pacing s.
Stylus cardiovascular suture
Sub-4
  S. Platinum Plus wire kit
  S. small vessel balloon
    dilatation catheter
subacute
  s. bacterial endocarditis (SBE)
  s. bronchopneumonia
  s. infective endocarditis
  s. myocardial infarction
  s. pericarditis
  s. tamponade
subannular mattress suture
subaortic stenosis
subclavian
  s. arteriovenous fistula
  s. artery
  s. artery bypass graft
  s. lymphatic
  s. murmur
  s. steal
  s. steal syndrome
  s. triangle
  s. vein
subclavian-carotid bypass
subclavian-subclavian bypass
subclavicular murmur
subclinical asthma
subcostal
  s. view
  s. zone
subcrepitant rales
subcutaneous
  s. emphysema
  s. nodule
  s. suture
  s. tunneling device
subcuticular suture
subendocardial
  s. ischemia
  s. layer
  s. myocardial infarction
  s. zone
subendocardium
subepicardial fat stripe
suberosis
subglottic
  s. laryngitis
subjective fremitus

subjunctional heart block
Sublimaze
Sublingual
  Nitrostat S.
submassive pulmonary embolism
submucosa
submucosal
  s. gland hypertrophy
  s. plaque
submucous
subpectoral implantation of
  cardioverter-defibrillator
subphrenic space
subpleural edema
subpulmonary
  s. obstruction
  s. stenosis
subpulmonic stenosis
Sub-Q-Set subcutaneous continuous
  infusion device
Subramanian clamp
subsalicylate
  bismuth s.
subsarcolemma cisterna
subsartorial tunnel
subsegmental bronchus
subsidiary atrial pacemaker
substance
  myocardial depressant s.
    (MDS)
  neurotransmitter s.
  s. P
  paramagnetic s.
  pro-inflammatory s.
  thiobarbituric acid reactive s.
    (TBARS)
  vasodepressor s.
substernal thyroid
substitutional cardiac surgery
substrate
  arrhythmogenic s.
  tachyarrhythmic s.
subthreshold stimulation
subtilis
  Bacillus s.
subtraction
  s. angiography
  digital s.
  functional s.
  intraoperative digital s. (IDIS)
  mask-mode s.
subtype
  Reston s.

Sudan s.
Zaire s.
subvalvar stenosis
subvalvular
    s. aortic stenosis
    s. mitral stenosis
    s. obstruction
subxiphoid
    s. area
    s. limited pericardiotomy
succinate
    cifenline s.
    hydrocortisone sodium s.
    methylprednisolone s.
    metoprolol s.
succinylcholine
    s. chloride
succussion
    hippocratic s.
    s. sounds
sucker
    Churchill s.
    intracardiac s.
sucking wound
Sucquet-Hoyer anastomosis
Sucrets Cough Calmers
suction
    diastolic s.
    nasotracheal s.
    Pleur-evac s.
Sudafed
Sudan subtype
sudden
    s. cardiac death (SCD)
    s. infant death syndrome
      (SIDS)
Sudex
Sufedrin
sufentanil
    s. citrate
suffocative
    s. bronchitis
    s. catarrh
    s. goiter
sugar
    capillary blood s. (CBS)

postprandial blood s.
    s. tumor
Sugiura procedure
suicide ventricle
suis
    Actinobacillus s.
suit
    anti-G s.
    Life S.
    MAST s.
Sular
sulbactam
    ampicillin and s.
sulcus, pl. sulci
    atrioventricular s.
    bulboventricular s.
    coronary s.
    costophrenic sulci
    interventricular s.
    s. terminalis
sulfadiazine
    silver s.
    s., sulfamethazine, and
      sulfamerazine
sulfadoxine and pyrimethamine
sulfamerazine
    sulfadiazine, sulfamethazine,
      and s.
Sulfamethoprim
sulfamethoxazole
sulfasalazine
sulfate
    amikacin s.
    amphetamine s.
    atropine s.
    bleomycin s.
    Capastat S.
    capreomycin s.
    chondroitin s.
    debrisoquine s.
    dermatan s.
    dextroamphetamine s.
    ephedrine s.
    ferrous s.
    gentamicin s.
    guanadrel s.
    guanethidine s.

S

NOTES

sulfate *(continued)*
    hydroxychloroquine s.
    magnesium s.
    metaproterenol s.
    neomycin s.
    netilmicin s.
    paromomycin s.
    penbutolol s.
    protamine s.
    quinidine s.
    quinine s.
    sodium tetradecyl s.
    streptomycin s.
    terbutaline s.
    trimethoprim s.
    trospectomycin s.
    vinblastine s.
    vincristine s.
Sulfatrim
sulfhydryl depletion hypothesis
sulfide
    hydrogen s.
    selenium s.
sulfinpyrazone
sulfisoxazole
    erythromycin and s.
    s. and phenazopyridine
sulfonamides
sulfonamide sensitivity
sulfonate
    sodium polystyrene s.
sulfonylurea
sulfoxide
    albendazole s.
    dimethyl s.
sulfur dioxide (SO$_2$)
sulindac
Sullivan
    S. III nasal continuous positive air pressure device
    S. nasal variable positive airway pressure unit
    S. VPAP II
sulmazole
Sulphan Blue
sulphur hexafluoride
SULP II balloon catheter
sum
    ray s.
sumatriptan
Summagraphics digitizing tablet
summation
    s. beat

    s. gallop (S$_7$)
    impulse s.
    s. shadow
sump pump
Sumycin Oral
sundowning
Sundt carotid endarterectomy shunt
Super-9
    S. guiding cardiac device
    S. guiding catheter
Super ArrowFlex catheterization sheath
superdicrotic
superficial
    s. femoral artery
    s. phlebitis
    s. pneumonia
superficialis
    esophagitis dissecans s.
Superflow guiding catheter
superimposed echodensity
superimposition
superior
    s. carotid artery
    s. mesenteric artery bypass
    s. mesenteric artery syndrome
    s. mesenteric vascular occlusion
    s. QRS axis
    s. thyroid artery
    s. vena cava (SVC)
    s. vena cava syndrome
supernatant
supernormal recovery phase
superoinferior heart
superoxide
    s. anion
    s. dismutase
Superselector Y-K guidewire
supertension
supine
    s. bicycle stress echocardiography (SBSE)
    s. exercise
    s. rest gated equilibrium image
supplement
    Vivonex Plus nutritional s.
supplementary respiration
supply
    Air S.
    energy s.
    myocardial oxygen s.

support
Abee s.
advanced cardiac life s. (ACLS)
advanced life s. (ALS)
advanced trauma life s. (ATLS)
basic cardiac life s. (BCLS)
basic life s. (BLS)
biventricular s. (BVS)
cardiopulmonary s. (CPS)
Dr. Gibaud thermal health s.
extracorporeal life s. (ECLS)
IMP-Capello arm s.
inotropic s.
percutaneous cardiopulmonary s. (PCPS)
percutaneous cardiopulmonary bypass s. (PCBS)
respiratory s.
ventilatory s.
volume-assured pressure s. (VAPS)
Suppository
Truphylline S.
Suppress
suppressant
cough s.
St. Joseph Cough S.
suppressed respiration
suppression
overdrive s.
suppurative
s. pericarditis
s. pleurisy
s. pneumonia
supra-annular
s.-a. mitral valve replacement (SMVR)
s.-a. prosthesis
supraclavicular
s. examination
s. fossa
s. lymph node biopsy
supraglottoplasty
supra-Hisian block
supramaximal tetanic stimulation

supranormal
s. conduction
s. excitability
s. excitation
suprasellar aneurysm
suprasternal
s. examination
s. pulsation
s. view
supravalvar
s. aortic stenosis-infantile hypercalcemia syndrome
s. aortic stenosis syndrome
s. stenosis
supravalvular
s. aortic stenosis (SVAS)
s. aortic stenosis-infantile hypercalcemia syndrome
s. aortic stenosis syndrome
supraventricular
s. arrhythmia
s. crest
s. ectopy
s. extrasystole
s. premature contraction
s. tachyarrhythmia
s. tachycardia (SVT)
supraventricularis
crista s.
Suprax
surcingle
Von Lackum s.
surdocardiac syndrome
SureGrip
S. breathing bag
S. manual resuscitator
surf
Human S.
Surface
Carmeda BioActive S.
surfactant
bovine lavage extract s. (BLES)
s. deficiency
hydrolysis of s.
pulmonary s.
surf test

S

NOTES

surgery
> ablative cardiac s.
> bypass s.
> cardiac s.
> cardiothoracic s. (CTS)
> coronary artery bypass grafting s.
> excisional cardiac s.
> keyhole s.
> lung volume reduction s. (LVRS)
> noncardiac s.
> open heart s.
> palliative s.
> reparative cardiac s.
> substitutional cardiac s.
> video-assisted thoracic s. (VATS)

Surgica K6 laser
surgical
> s. s.
> s. emphysema
> s. risk
> s. tuberculosis

Surgicel
Surgiclip
> Auto Suture S.

Surgicraft
> S. pacemaker electrode
> S. suture

Surgilase 150 laser
Surgilon suture
Surgitool prosthetic valve
Surgitron unit
Surital
Surmontil
Survanta
surveillance angiography
survey
> environmental s.
> Jenkins Activity S.
> National Health and Nutrition Examination S. (NHANES)

Survival
> First American Study of Infarct S. (ASIS-1)
> S. of Myocardial Infarction Long-Term Evaluation (SMILE)
> S. and Ventricular Ectopy (SAVE)
> S. with Oral d-sotalol (SWORD)

susceptibility
suspended
> s. heart
> s. heart syndrome

Suspension
> Aristocort Intralesional S.
> Children's Motrin S.

suspension laryngoscopy
Sus-Phrine
sustained
> s. monomorphic ventricular tachycardia (SMVT)
> s. release

Sustaire
susurrus
Sutton law
suture
> Cardioflon s.
> cardiovascular silk s.
> chromic catgut s.
> Cooley U s.'s
> Endoknot s.
> end-to-side s.
> EPTFE vascular s.'s
> Ethibond s.
> everting mattress s.
> figure-of-eight s.
> Frater s.
> interrupted pledgeted s.
> Mersilene braided nonabsorbable s.
> monofilament absorbable s.
> monofilament polypropylene s.
> Nurolon s.
> pledgeted mattress s.
> pursestring s.
> pyroglycolic acid s.
> reabsorbable s.
> Sterna-Band self-locking s.
> Stylus cardiovascular s.
> subannular mattress s.
> subcutaneous s.
> subcuticular s.
> Surgicraft s.
> Surgilon s.
> through-the-wall mattress s.
> Ti-Cron s.
> U s.'s

suturing
> coupled s.

SV
> stroke volume

SVAS
supravalvular aortic stenosis
SVC
slow vital capacity
superior vena cava
SVI
stroke volume index
SVM
syncytiovascular membrane
SvO₂
mixed venous oxygen saturation
SVR
systemic vascular resistance
SVRI
systemic vascular resistance index
SVT
supraventricular tachycardia
swallow
barium s.
s. syncope
wet s.
swallowing
Swan-Ganz
S.-G. balloon flotation catheter
S.-G. bipolar pacing catheter
S.-G. flow-directed catheter
S.-G. Pacing TD catheter
S.-G. syndrome
Swank high-flow arterial blood filter
sweat
s. chloride
s. chloride test
sweating
sweep
Sweet Tip lead
SWI
stroke work index
SWIFT
Should We Intervene Following Thrombolysis
swimmer's view
swimming
hypoxic lap s.
swing
S. DR1 DDDR pacemaker
respiratory s.

swinging heart
Swiss
S. cheese defect
S. cheese interventricular septum
S. Kiss intrastent balloon inflation device
switch
DNA s.
isoactin s.
isomyosin s.
s. operation
s. procedure
switching
automatic mode s. (AMS)
mode s.
SWORD
Survival with Oral d-sotalol
Swyer-James syndrome
Sydenham
S. chorea
S. cough
sydowi
Aspergillus s.
Sylvest disease
Sylvius
valve of S.
Symadine
Symbion
S. cardiac device
S. Jarvik-7 artificial heart
S. J-7 70-mL ventricle total artificial heart
Symbion/CardioWest 100 mL total artificial heart
Symbios 7006 pacemaker
Symcor
Symmetrel
symmetric
s. asphyxia
s. vitiligo
symmetrical phased array
sympathectomy, sympathetectomy
cervicothoracic s.
lumbar s.

S

NOTES

sympathetic
    s. activity
    s. nervous system
sympathoadrenal system
sympathoexcitation
    reflex s.
sympathoexcitatory
sympathoinhibition
sympatholytic
sympathomimetic
    s. amine
    s. drug
sympathovagal
    s. balance
    s. imbalance
    s. transition
Symphony patient monitoring system
symphysis, gen. **symphyses**
    cardiac s.
symptom
    Baumès s.
    Burghart s.
    Duroziez s.
    Fischer s.
    gastrointestinal s.
    Kussmaul s.
    Oehler s.'s
    prodromal s.
    Trunecek s.
symptomatic asthma
symptom-free interval
symptom-limited
    s.-l. treadmill exercise test
Synapse electrocardiographic cream
Sync
    Star S.
synchondrosis
    sternal s.
SynchroMed programmable pump
synchronization
synchronized
    s. intermittent mandatory ventilation (SIMV)
    s. sleep (S-sleep)
synchronizer
    CardioSync cardiac s.
synchronous
    s. airway lesions
synchrony
    atrial s.
    atrioventricular s.

    A-V s.
    S. I, II pacemaker
synchrotron-based transvenous angiography
syncopal
    s. migraine
    s. migraine headache
    s. spell
syncope
    Adams-Stokes s.
    s. anginosa
    cardiac s.
    cardiogenic s.
    cardioinhibitory s.
    carotid sinus s.
    cerebrovascular s.
    cough s.
    defecation s.
    deglutition s.
    diver's s.
    exertional s.
    hypoglycemic s.
    hypoxic s.
    hysterical s.
    laryngeal s.
    local s.
    micturition s.
    migraine s.
    mixed neurally-mediated s.
    near-s.
    neurally-mediated s.
    neurocardiogenic s.
    neuromediated s.
    noncardiac s.
    orthostatic s.
    postmicturition s.
    posttussive s.
    postural s.
    sexual s.
    situational s.
    sneeze s.
    stretching s.
    swallow s.
    toilet-seat s.
    transient s.
    tussive s.
    vasodepressor-cardioinhibitory s.
    vasovagal s.
syncytial virus
syncytiovascular membrane (SVM)
syndactyly

syndrome
acquired immunodeficiency s. (AIDS)
acute chest s.
acute respiratory distress s.
acute retroviral s.
Adams-Stokes s.
adrenogenital s.
adult respiratory distress s. (ARDS)
Albright s.
Alport s.
ALPS s.
amniotic fluid s.
Andersen s.
anomalous first rib thoracic s.
antiphospholipid s.
aortic arch s.
aortic arteritis s.
apallic s.
Apert s.
arteriohepatic dysplasia s.
Asherson s.
Ask-Upmark s.
Austrian s.
Ayerza s.
Babinski s.
ballooning mitral cusp s.
bangungot s.
Bannwarth s.
Barlow s.
Barsony-Polgar s.
Barth s.
Bartter s.
Bauer s.
beer and cobalt s.
Behçet s.
Bernheim s.
Beuren s.
billowing mitral valve s.
Blackfan-Diamond s.
Bland-Garland-White s.
Bloom s.
blue finger s.
blue toe s.
blue velvet s.
Boerhaave s.

brachial s.
Bradbury-Eggleston s.
bradycardia-tachycardia s.
brady-tachy s.
bradytachycardia s.
Brett s.
Brock s.
bubbly lung s.
Budd-Chiari s.
Bürger-Grütz s.
busulfan lung s.
capillary leak s.
Caplan s.
carcinoid s.
cardioauditory s.
cardiofacial s.
carotid sinus s.
carotid steal s.
Carpenter s.
CATCH 22 s.
cauda equina s.
cervical rib s.
Charcot s.
Charcot-Weiss-Baker s.
CHARGE s.
Chiari s.
Chiari-Budd s.
Chinese restaurant s.
chronic hyperventilation s.
Churg-Strauss s. (CSS)
click s.
click-murmur s.
Cockayne s.
Cogan s.
compartment s.
congenital central hypoventilation s.
Conn s.
Conradi-Hünermann s.
Cornelia de Lange s.
costochondral s.
costoclavicular rib s.
costosternal s.
cricopharyngeal achalasia s.
cri-du-chat s.
cryptophthalmos s.
Curracino-Silverman s.

S

NOTES

syndrome *(continued)*
Cushing s.
cutis laxa s.
Cyriax s.
DaCosta s.
declamping shock s.
DeGimard s.
de Lange s.
Determann s.
DiGeorge s.
distal intestinal obstruction s.
(DIOS)
Down s.
Dressler s.
drowned newborn s.
drug-induced lupus s.
Duncan s.
Dysshwannian s.
Eaton-Lambert s.
effort s.
Ehlers-Danlos s.
Eisenmenger s.
elfin facies s.
Ellis-van Creveld s.
eosinophilia-myalgia s. (EMS)
eosinophilic pulmonary s.
epibronchial right pulmonary
artery s.
euthyroid sick s.
familial cholestasis s.
fat embolism s. (FES)
fetal alcohol s. (FAS)
fibrinogen-fibrin conversion s.
flapping valve s.
Fleischner s.
floppy valve s.
Forney s.
Forrester s.
four-day s.
Gailliard s.
Gaisböck s.
gastrocardiac s.
Gerhardt s.
Goldenhar s.
Goodpasture s.
Gorlin s.
Gowers s.
Grönblad-Strandberg s.
Guillain-Barré s.
Gulf War s.
Halbrecht s.
Hamman-Rich s.
Hantavirus pulmonary s. (HPS)

Hare s.
heart and hand s.
heart-hand s.
Hegglin s.
Heiner s.
hemangioma-
thrombocytopenia s.
Henoch-Schönlein s.
Hermansky-Pudlak s.
Herner s.
heterotaxy s.
holiday heart s.
Holt-Oram s.
homocystinuria s.
Horner s.
Howel-Evans s.
Hughes-Stovin s.
Hunter s.
Hunter-Hurler s.
Hurler s.
hyperabduction s.
hyperapolipoprotein B s.
hypereosinophilia s.
hypereosinophilic s.
hyperkinetic heart s.
hyperlucent lung s.
hypersensitive carotid sinus s.
hyperventilation s.
hyperviscosity s.
hypoplastic left heart s.
(HLHS)
idiopathic hypereosinophilic s.
(IHES)
idiopathic long Q-T interval s.
immotile cilia s.
s. of inappropriate antidiuretic
hormone (SIADH)
incontinentia pigmenti s.
infant respiratory distress s.
(IRDS)
intermediate coronary s.
Ivemark s.
Jackson s.
Janus s.
Jervell and Lange-Nielsen s.
Jeune s.
Job s.
Kallmann s.
Kartagener s.
Kasabach-Merritt s.
Kawasaki s.
Kearns s.
Kearns-Sayre s.

Kimmelstiel-Wilson s.
Klein-Waardenburg s.
Klinefelter s.
Klippel-Feil s.
Klippel-Trenaunay-Weber s.
Kostmann s.
Kugelberg-Welander s.
LAMB s.
Landouzy-Déjérine s.
Landry-Guillain-Barre s.
Laubry-Soulle s.
Laurence-Moon-Bardet-Biedl s.
Laurence-Moon-Biedl s.
Leitner s.
Lenègre s.
Lenz s.
LEOPARD s.
Leredde s.
Leriche s.
Lev s.
Libman-Sacks s.
Löffler s.
long Q-T s. (LQTS)
long Q-TU s.
Lown-Ganong-Levine s.
low-salt s., low-sodium s.
Lutembacher s.
Macleod s.
malignant carcinoid s.
Mallory-Weiss s.
Marfan s.
Marie s.
Marie-Bamberger s.
Maroteaux-Lamy s.
Martorell s.
mastocytosis s.
Maugeri s.
McArdle s.
Meadows s.
Meigs s.
Mendelson s.
Mèniére s.
metastatic carcinoid s.
middle lobe s.
midsystolic click s.
mirror-image lung s.
mitral valve prolapse s.

Mondor s.
Morgagni-Adams-Stokes s.
Morquio s.
Mounier-Kuhn s.
Moynahan s.
mucocutaneous lymph node s.
multiple lentigines s.
myocardial ischemic s.
NAME s.
nephrotic s.
Noonan s.
obesity-hypoventilation s.
oculomucocutaneous s.
Opitz s.
Organization to Assess
 Strategies for Ischemic S.'s
 (OASIS)
Osler-Weber-Rendu s.
pacemaker s.
Paget-von Schrötter s.
Pancoast s.
papillary muscle s.
Penderluft s.
pericarditis-myocarditis s.
pharyngeal pouch s.
Pick s.
pickwickian s.
PIE s.
Pierre Robin s.
Pins s.
Plummer-Vinson s.
Polhemus-Schafer-Ivemark s.
polymyalgia rheumatica s.
postcardiotomy s.
postcommissurotomy s.
postinfarction s.
postmyocardial infarction s.
postperfusion s.
postpericardiotomy s. (PPS)
postphlebitic s.
postpump s.
posttransfusion s.
precordial catch s.
preexcitation s.
preinfarction s.
premonitory s.
prolapsed mitral valve s.

S

NOTES

syndrome *(continued)*
   prolonged Q-T interval s.
   pseudoxanthoma elasticum s.
   pulmonary acid aspiration s.
   pulmonary disease anemia s.
   pulmonary dysmaturity s.
   pulmonary infarction s.
   pulmonary sling s.
   Q-T s.
   Q-TU interval s.
   radiologic scimitar s.
   Raeder-Harbitz s.
   Raynaud s.
   reactive airways disease s.
    (RADS)
   redundant cusp s.
   Reiter s.
   Rendu-Osler-Weber s.
   respiratory distress s. (RDS)
   Reye s.
   Riley-Day s.
   Romano-Ward s.
   Rosenbach s.
   Roussy-Lévy s.
   rubella s.
   Rubinstein-Taybi s.
   salt-depletion s.
   Sanchez-Cascos
    cardioauditory s.
   Sandifer s.
   scalenus anterior s.
   scalenus anticus s.
   Scheie s.
   scimitar s.
   Sebastiani s.
   shoulder-hand s.
   Shprintzen s.
   Shy-Drager s.
   sicca s.
   sick sinus s. (SSS)
   Silver s.
   single papillary muscle s.
   sinobronchial s.
   Sjögren s.
   sleep apnea s. (SAS)
   sleep apnea/hypopnea s.
   slipping rib s.
   slit ventricle s.
   Smith-Lemli-Opitz s.
   Spens s.
   splenic flexure s.
   Stevens-Johnson s.
   stiff heart s.
   Stokes-Adams s.
   Stokvis-Talma s.
   straight back s.
   Sturge-Weber s.
   subclavian steal s.
   sudden infant death s. (SIDS)
   superior mesenteric artery s.
   superior vena cava s.
   supravalvar aortic stenosis s.
   supravalvar aortic stenosis-
    infantile hypercalcemia s.
   supravalvular aortic stenosis s.
   supravalvular aortic stenosis-
    infantile hypercalcemia s.
   surdocardiac s.
   suspended heart s.
   Swan-Ganz s.
   Swyer-James s.
   systemic inflammatory
    response s. (SIRS)
   systolic click-murmur s.
   tachybradycardia s.
   tachycardia-bradycardia s.
   tachycardia-polyuria s.
   Takayasu s.
   TAR s.
   Taussig-Bing s.
   Taybi s.
   thoracic endometriosis s.
   thoracic outlet s.
   thrombocytopenia-absent
    radius s.
   Tietze s.
   toxic oil s. (TOS)
   Treacher Collins s.
   trisomy D s.
   Trousseau s.
   Turner s.
   twiddler's s.
   Uhl s.
   Ullmann s.
   VACTERL s.
   vasculocardiac s. of
    hyperserotonemia
   vasovagal s.
   VATER association s.
   velocardiofacial s.
   vena cava s.
   venolobar s.
   Vernet s.
   Villaret s.
   Vogt-Koyanagi-Harada s.
   Waardenburg s.

Ward-Romano s.
wasting s.
Watson s.
Weber-Osler-Rendu s.
Werner s.
West s.
white clot s.
Williams s.
Williams-Campbell s.
Wilson-Mikity s.
Wiskott-Aldrich s.
Wolff-Parkinson-White s.
s. X
XO s.
XXXX s.
XXXY s.
yellow nail s.
Yentl s.
Young s.
synechia, pl. **synechiae**
s. pericardii
synergism
synergistic
Synergyst
S. DDD pacemaker
S. II pacemaker
syngenesioplastic transplant
synpneumonic empyema
synthase
glycogen s.
synthesis
thromboxane s.
synthetase
pantothenate s.
synvinolin
syphilis
bejel s.
cardiovascular s.
tertiary s.
syphilitic
s. aortic aneurysm
s. aortic valvulitis
s. aortitis
s. arteritis
s. endarteritis
s. endocarditis

s. laryngitis
s. myocarditis
Syracol-CF
syringe
anaerobic Pulsator s.
Concord line draw s.
Namic angiographic s.
Osciflator balloon inflation s.
Pulsator s.
Raulerson s.
Ultraject prefilled s.
syrup
albuterol sulfate s.
Carbodec S.
Cardec-S S.
Co-Xan s.
Decofed S.
Extra Action Cough S.
Hydramyn S.
Kenacort S.
Rondec S.
system
Abiomed biventricular
support s.
ABL 625 s.
ABL 520 blood gas
measurement s.
ACS Concorde over-the-wire
catheter s.
Acuson cardiovascular s.
adrenergic nervous s.
Advanced Cardiovascular S.'s
(ACS)
Advanced Catheter S.'s (ACS)
Aladdin infant flow s.
Alcon Closure S.
ANCOR imaging s.
Angio-Jet rapid
thrombectomy s.
annular phased array s.
(APAS)
Arcomax FMA cardiac
angiography s.
Argyle-Turkel safety
thoracentesis s.
Aria CPAP s.
Atakr s.

NOTES

S

481

system *(continued)*
atrioventricular conduction s.
Atrium Blood Recovery s.
automated cervical cell
screening s.
automatic exposure s.
autonomic nervous s.
Autotrans s.
autotransfusion s.
BACTEC s.
Bard cardiopulmonary
support s.
Bard percutaneous
cardiopulmonary support s.
Baylor autologous
transfusion s.
Beta-Cath s.
BiliBlanket phototherapy s.
Biodex S.
Biosound Phase 2
ultrasound s.
Bonchek-Shiley vein
distention s.
BosPac cardiopulmonary
bypass s.
brachiocephalic s.
BRAT s.
Burette multiple patient
delivery s.
Cadence tiered therapy
defibrillator s.
Capintec VEST s.
cardiac conduction s.
CardiData Prodigy s.
Cardiofreezer cryosurgical s.
cardioscope U s.
cardiovascular s.
Cardiovascular Angiography
Analysis S. (CAAS)
Cardiovit AT-10
ECG/spirometry
combination s.
CASE computerized exercise
EKG s.
catheter-snare s.
catheter-tip micromanometer s.
Cath-Finder catheter tracking s.
Cell Saver autologous blood
recovery s.
Cell Saver Haemonetics
Autotransfusion s.
Cenflex central monitoring s.
cine-pulse s.

CineView Plus Freeland s.
Circulaire aerosol drug
delivery s.
circulatory support s.
CMS AccuProbe 450 s.
Cobe Spectra apheresis s.
codominant s.
COER-24 delivery s.
CO_2ject s.
complement s.
complete pacemaker patient
testing s. (CPPTS)
conduction s.
coordinate s.
COROSCOP C cardiac
imaging s.
CPS s.
Cragg Endopro s.
C-VEST radiation detector s.
CVIS/InterTherapy intravascular
ultrasound s.
cytochrome P450 s.
Dallas Classification S.
DAR breathing s.
DCI-S automated coronary
analysis s.
Desilets introducer s.
Diasonics/Sonotron Vingmed
CFM 800 imaging s.
dilator-sheath s.
Dinamap s.
DPAP interactive airway
management s.
2-D TEE s. Ultra-Neb 99
DUPEL drug delivery s.
Dymer excimer delivery s.
echocardiographic automated
boundary detection s.
echocardiographic scoring s.
Echovar Doppler s.
electrode s.
Elscint tomography s.
endocrine s.
Endotak lead s.
EnGuard double-lead ICD s.
EnGuard pacing and
defibrillation lead s.
EPT-1000 cardiac ablation s.
Erie S.
Estes point s.
Estes-Romhilt EKG point-
score s.
Fiberlase s.

fiberoptic catheter delivery s.
fibrinolytic s.
Finger Phantom pulse oximeter
testing s.
fixed-wire balloon dilatation s.
Flowtron DVT pump s.
FMA cardiovascular imaging s.
Frank EKG lead placement s.
Frank XYZ orthogonal lead s.
gastrointestinal therapeutic s.
(GITS)
gated s.
General Electric Advantx s.
GenESA closed-loop
delivery s.
Guidant TRIAD three-electrode
energy defibrillation s.
Gyroscan HP Philips 15S
whole-body s.
Haemolite autologous blood
recovery s.
Haemonetics Cell Saver s.
HeartMate implantable
pneumatic left ventricular
assist s.
HEARTrac I Cardiac
Monitoring s.
hematopoietic s.
Hewlett-Packard 5 MHz
phased-array TEE s.
Hewlett-Packard Sonos 1000,
1500 ultrasound s.
hexaxial reference s.
His-Purkinje s.
Hombach lead placement s.
Horizon AutoAdjust CPAP s.
Horizon nasal CPAP s.
IDIS s.
Image-View s.
Imatron C-100 s.
implantable left ventricular
assist s. (IPLVAS)
INCA s.
Infiniti catheter introducer s.
infra-Hisian conduction s.
Innovator Holter s.
integrated lead s.

INTEGRIS cardiac imaging s.
Intra-Op autotransfusion s.
Irri-Cath suction s.
Irvine viable organ-tissue
transport s. (IVOTTS)
isocenter s.
Jinotti closed suctioning s.
kallikrein-bradykinin s.
Kiethly-DAS series 500 data-
acquisition s.
King double umbrella
closure s.
KK s.
lead s.
left ventricular assist s.
(LVAS)
Leocor hemoperfusion s.
Leukotrap red cell storage s.
Liposorber LA-15 s.
Luxtec fiberoptic s.
Magnum-Meier s.
Marquette Case-12
electrocardiographic s.
Marquette Case-12 exercise s.
Mason-Likar 12-lead EKG s.
M/D 4 defibrillator s.
MedGraphics Cardio O2 s.
Medi-Facts s.
Medi-Tech catheter s.
Medtronic Interactive
Tachycardia Terminating s.
Medtronic Transvene
endocardial lead s.
Meier-Magnum s.
Metrix atrial defibrillation s.
MicroHartzler ACS balloon
catheter s.
micromanometer catheter s.
MIDA 1000 monitoring s.
Mobin-Uddin filter s.
Monaldi drainage s.
Mullins sheath s.
Myocardial Infarction Data
Acquisition S. (MIDAS)
nervous s.
nonthoracotomy defibrillation
lead s.

S

NOTES

system *(continued)*
Novacor left ventricular
assist s.
Nu-Trake Weiss emergency
airway s.
Omni tract retractor s.
OptiHaler drug delivery s.
orthogonal lead s.
over-the-wire balloon
dilatation s.
Oximetrix 3 S.
Oxycure topical oxygen s.
Oxyfill oxygen refilling s.
Oxy-Ultra-Lite ambulatory
oxygen s.
Paceart complete pacemaker
patient testing s.
pacemaker code s.
parasympathetic nervous s.
Patil stereotactic s.
PCA s.
PCD Transvene implantable
cardioverter-defibrillator s.
PDB preperitoneal distention
balloon s.
Pelorus stereotactic s.
peripheral access s. (PAS)
Peripheral AngioJet s.
peripheral atherectomy s.
phased array s.
plasma coagulation s.
Pleur-evac autotransfusion s.
Port-A-Cath implantable
catheter s.
Portex Soft-Seal cuff s.
Presto-Flash spirometry s.
Presto spirometry s.
Prevue s.
programmable implantable
medication s. (PIMS)
PulseDose portable compressed
oxygen s.'s
PulseSpray infusion s.
Purkinje s.
Q-cath catheterization
recording s.
Rasor Blood Pumping s.
Remac s.
Renaissance spirometry s.
renin-angiotensin-aldosterone s.
(RAAS)
renin-angiotensin-aldosterone s.
(RAAS)

reticuloendothelial s.
RFb s.
Romhilt-Estes point scoring s.
Rotacs s.
rotational atherectomy s. (RAS)
R-Port implantable vascular
access s.
Rx5000 cardiac pacing s.
RX stent delivery s.
SAM s.
Sandman s.
saphenofemoral s.
sarcotubular s.
Schneider-Meier-Magnum s.
Sequel compression s.
Sequestra 1000 s.
sheath and dilator s.
SICOR cardiac catheterization
recording s.
Simpson Coronary
AtheroCath s.
Simpson-Robert vascular
dilation s.
SinuScope s.
SKY epidural pain control s.
Snuggle Warm convective
warming s.
Sonos 500 imaging s.
SpiroSense s.
sympathetic nervous s.
sympathoadrenal s.
Symphony patient
monitoring s.
T s.
TAM s.
transtelephonic ambulatory
monitoring system
ThAIRapy vest airway
clearance s.
TheraPEP positive expiratory
pressure therapy s.
Thora-Klex chest drainage s.
Thoratec VAD S.
Thrombolytic Assessment s.
(TAS)
Thumper CPR s.
Total Synchrony S.
TRAKE-fit s.
transluminal lysing s.
transtelephonic ambulatory
monitoring s. (TAM system)
Traveler portable oxygen s.
triaxial reference s.

TRON 3 VACI cardiac
imaging s.
two-bottle thoracic drainage s.
Ultraflex esophageal stent s.
Unilink s.
USCI Probe balloon-on-a-wire
dilatation s.
Vapor-Phase heated
humidification s.
Vario s.
VDD pacing s.
Ventak PRx defibrillation s.
Ventak PRx III/Endotak s.
Ventritex TVL s.
vessel occlusion s.
Veterans Affairs Medical
Center scoring s.
Viagraph EKG s.
video s.
Vingmed CFM 800
echocardiographic s.
White s.
Xillix ACCESS s.
Xillix LIFE-Lung s.
XYZ lead s.
Yellow IRIS s.

systemic
s. blood flow (SBF)
s. circulation
s. collateral
s. heart
s. hemodynamic parameters
s. hemodynamics
s. infection
s. inflammatory response
syndrome (SIRS)
s. lupus erythematosus (SLE)
s. mean arterial pressure
(SMAP)
s. necrotizing vasculitis
s. to pulmonary artery
anastomosis
s. to pulmonary connection
s. to pulmonary shunt
s. vascular hypertension
s. vascular resistance (SVR)

s. vascular resistance index
(SVRI)
s. venous hypertension
s. venous return

systole
aborted s.
s. alternans
anticipated s.
atrial s.
auricular s.
cardiac s.
electrical s.
electromechanical s.
frustrate s.
hemic s.
isovolumic s.
late s.
premature s.
ventricular s.
ventricular ectopic s.

systolic
s. anterior motion (SAM)
s. apical impulse
s. apical murmur
s. blood pressure (SBP)
s. bruit
s. click
s. click-murmur syndrome
s. current
s. current of injury
s. doming
s. ejection murmur (SEM)
s. ejection period (SEP)
s. ejection rate (SER)
s. function
s. gallop
s. gallop rhythm
s. gradient
s. heart failure
s. honk
s. hypertension
S. Hypertension in the Elderly
S. Hypertension in the Elderly
Program (SHEP)
s. left ventricular pressure
s. pressure time index (SPTI)
s. regurgitant murmur

NOTES

S

485

systolic *(continued)*
s. reserve
s. shock
s. thrill
s. time interval (STI)
s. trough
s. velocity ratio
s. whipping
s. whoop
systolometer

T

T artifact
T cell defect
T cells
T loop
T sign
T system
T tube
T vector
T wave
T wave alternans
T wave flattening

T2

T2 relaxation time
T2 weighted image

T₄

thyroxine

T₁

duration of inspiration

T_E

duration of expiration

t

t test

T1 weighted image
TA

tantalum

¹⁷⁸TA

tantalum-178

tabacosis
tabby

t. cat heart
t. cat striation

tabetic cuirass
table

anterior t.
Diamond-Forrester t.
Kaplan-Meier life t.
Siemens open heart t.

tablet

Actifed Allergy T.
Afrin T.
Aristocort T.
Brontex T.
Carbiset-TR T.
Carbodec TR T.
Cardizem T.
Kenacort T.
Nitrong Oral T.
Phyllocontin T.
Summagraphics digitizing t.

tabourka

bruit de t.

Tac-3
TAC atherectomy catheter
tache

t. blanche
t. laiteuse

tachyarrhythmia

supraventricular t.
ventricular t.

tachyarrhythmic substrate
tachybrady arrhythmia
tachybradycardia syndrome
tachycardia

accelerated idioventricular t.
alternating bidirectional t.
antidromic circus-movement t.
atrial t. (AT)
atrial chaotic t.
atrial ectopic t. (AET)
atrial paroxysmal t.
atrial reentry t.
atrial ventricular nodal
  reentry t.
atrial ventricular
  reciprocating t. (AVRT)
atrioventricular junctional
  reciprocating t.
atrioventricular nodal t.
  (AVNT)
atrioventricular nodal
  reentrant t. (AVNRT)
atrioventricular reciprocating t.
atypical atrioventricular nodal
  reentrant t. (AAVNRT)
auricular t.
automatic atrial t. (AAT)
automatic ectopic t.
A-V junctional t.
A-V nodal reentry t.
A-V node reentrant t.
A-V reciprocating t.
bidirectional ventricular t.
bundle-branch reentrant t.
chaotic atrial t.
circus-movement t.
Coumel t.
t. cycle length
double t.
drug-refractory t.

tachycardia *(continued)*
  ectopic atrial t. (EAT)
  endless-loop t.
  t. en salves
  entrainment of t.
  essential t.
  exercise-induced ventricular t.
  fetal t.
  idiopathic ventricular t. (IVT)
  idioventricular t.
  incessant t.
  inducible polymorphic
    ventricular t.
  intra-atrial reentrant t.
  junctional t. (JT)
  junctional ectopic t. (JET)
  junctional reciprocating t.
  macroreentrant atrial t.
  Mahaim-type t.
  malignant ventricular t.
  monoform t.
  monomorphic ventricular t.
  multifocal atrial t. (MAT)
  multiform t.
  narrow-complex t.
  nodal paroxysmal t.
  nodal reentrant t.
  nonparoxysmal atrioventricular
    junctional t.
  nonsustained ventricular t.
    (NSVT)
  orthodromic A-V reentrant t.
  orthodromic circus
    movement t.
  orthodromic reciprocating t.
    (ORT)
  orthostatic t.
  pacemaker-mediated t. (PMT)
  parasystolic ventricular t.
  paroxysmal atrial t. (PAT)
  paroxysmal junctional t.
  paroxysmal nodal t.
  paroxysmal reentrant
    supraventricular t.
  paroxysmal sinus t.
  paroxysmal supraventricular t.
    (PSVT)
  paroxysmal ventricular t.
  t. pathway mapping
  permanent junctional
    reciprocating t. (PJRT)
  pleomorphic t.
  polymorphous ventricular t.

  primary ventricular t. (PVT)
  rapid nonsustained
    ventricular t.
  reciprocating macroreentry
    orthodromic t.
  reentrant atrial t.
  reentrant supraventricular t.
  reflex t.
  refractory t.
  repetitive monomorphic
    ventricular t.
  repetitive paroxysmal
    ventricular t.
  resting t.
  right ventricular outflow
    tract t.
  salvo of ventricular t.
  S-A nodal reentrant t.
  self-terminating t.
  sinus nodal reentrant t.
  sleeping t.
  slow-fast t.
  spontaneous reentrant sustained
    ventricular t.
  supraventricular t. (SVT)
  sustained monomorphic
    ventricular t. (SMVT)
  t. traumosa exophthalmica
  ventricular t. (VT)
  wide QRS t.
  t. window
  Wolff-Parkinson-White
    reentrant t.
tachycardia-bradycardia syndrome
tachycardiac
tachycardia-dependent aberrancy
tachycardia-induced cardiomyopathy
tachycardia-polyuria syndrome
tachycardic
tachycrotic
tachydysrhythmia
Tachylog pacemaker
tachypacing
tachyphylactic
tachyphylaxis
tachypnea
  nervous t.
tachyrhythmia
tachysystole
tack
  Effler t.
tacrolimus
Tactiflex

Tactilaze angioplasty
tactile fremitus
TAD
    T. guidewire
tag
    epicardial fat t.
    pleural t.
Tagarno 3SD cineangiography
    projector
TAH
    total artificial heart
        Berlin TAH
        CardioWest TAH
        Penn State TAH
        Vienna TAH
tail sign
TAIM
    Trial of Antihypertensive
    Interventions and Management
Taiwan acute respiratory (TWAR)
Takayasu
    T. aortitis
    T. arteritis
    T. disease
    idiopathic arteritis of T.
    T. syndrome
Takayasu-Onishi disease
talc
    t. operation
    t. pleurodesis
    t. pneumoconiosis
    t. poudrage
    t. slurry
talcosis
Tambocor
tambour
    bruit de t.
    t. sound
TAMI
    Thrombolysis and Angioplasty in
    Myocardial Infarction
    TAMI protocol
Tamm-Horsfall protein
tamponade, tamponage
    acute t.
    atypical t.
    balloon t.

    cardiac t.
    chronic t.
    esophageal t.
    esophagogastric t.
    heart t.
    low-pressure t.
    pericardial t.
    Rose t.
    subacute t.
    traumatic t.
TAM system
TAN
    total adenine nucleotides
tandem
    T. cardiac device
    t. lesion
tangential percussion
Tangier disease
TANI
    total axial node irradiation
tannates
    methyclothiazide and
        cryptenamine t.
Tanner operation
tantalum (TA)
    t. balloon-expandable stent
        with helical coil
    t. bronchogram
    powdered t.
    t. stent
tantalum-178 (^{178}TA)
    t. generator
TAP
    transesophageal atrial pacing
tap
    bloody t.
    mitral t.
    pericardial t.
    pleural t.
Tapcath esophageal electrode
tape
    ColorZone t.
    umbilical t.
tapered
    t. movable core curved wire
    guide
    T. Torque guidewire

NOTES

Taper guidewire
Taperseal hemostatic device
tapotage
Tapsul pill electrode
TAPVC
    total anomalous pulmonary venous
        connection
TAPVD
    total anomalous pulmonary venous
        drainage
TAPVR
    total anomalous pulmonary venous
        return
Taq
    T. DNA polymerase
    T. extender
TAR
    thrombocytopenia-absent radius
        TAR syndrome
tar
    coal t.
Tarabine PFS
tardive
    t. cyanosis
tardus
    pulsus t.
    pulsus parvus et t.
target
    dyspnea t.
    t. heart rate (THR)
    t. lesion
    t. site
    T. Tip lead
Tarone-Ware nonparametric linear
rank test
tartrate
    metoprolol t.
    phenindamine t.
    vinorelbine t.
    zolpidem t.
TAS
    Thrombolytic Assessment system
Tascon prosthetic valve
Ta segment
task
    metabolic equivalents of t.
        (MET, METs)
TAT
    thrombin-antithrombin
Tatlockia micdadei
taurinum
    cor t.

TAUSA
    Thrombolysis and Angioplasty in
        Unstable Angina
Taussig-Bing
    T.-B. anomaly
    T.-B. disease
    T.-B. heart
    T.-B. syndrome
TAV
    transvenous aortovelography
Tavist
taxonomic
taxonomy
Taybi syndrome
Tay-Sachs disease
Tazicef
Tazidime
TB
    tuberculosis
TBARS
    thiobarbituric acid reactive substance
TBV
    total blood volume
Tc
    technetium
Tc-99
    Tc-99 sestamibi
    Tc-99 sestamibi scintigraphy
^{99m}Tc, Tc-99m
    technetium-99m
TCAD
    transplant coronary artery disease
TCG
    time compensation gain
Tc-99m (*var. of* ^{99m}Tc)
TCOM
    transcutaneous oxygen monitor
TCPC
    total cavopulmonary connection
TCT
    transcatheter therapy
tcu-PA
    2-chain urokinase plasminogen
        activator
TDI
    toluene diisocyanate
TE
    echo delay time
TEA
    thromboendarterectomy
    transluminal extraction atherectomy

tea
    pectoral t.
    t. taster's cough
teacher's node
TEAM
    Thrombolytic Trial of Eminase in
    Acute Myocardial Infarction
TEAP
    transesophageal atrial pacing
tear
    Boerhaave t.
    intimal t.
    Mallory-Weiss t.
    medial t.
    neointimal t.
teardrop heart
teboroxime
    t. imaging
    t. scan
    technetium-99m t.
tebo scan
TEC
    transluminal endarterectomy catheter
    transluminal extraction catheter
    TEC atherectomy device
technetium (Tc)
    t. hexakis 2-methoxyisobutyl
    isonitrile (Tc-99 sestamibi)
technetium-99m (^{99m}Tc, Tc-99m)
    t. furofosmin
    t. hexamibi scan
    t. imaging
    t. methoxyisobutyl isonitrile
    t. methylene diphosphonate
    t. MIBI
    t. MIBI imaging
    t. pyrophosphate
    t. sestamibi stress test
    t. stannous pyrophosphate
    scintiscan
    t. teboroxime
    t. tetrafosmin
    t. tetrofosmin
technetium-sestamibi
technetium-teboroxime
technique
    ablative t.

airway occlusion t.
Amplatz t.
antegrade double balloon/double
  wire t.
antegrade/retrograde
  cardioplegia t.
anterior sandwich patch t.
anterograde transseptal t.
anti-aliasing t.
Araki-Sako t.
atrial-well t.
background subtraction t.
Bentall inclusion t.
bootstrap two-vessel t.
Brecher and Cronkite t.
button t.
catheterization t.
chloramine-T t.
clearance t.
clonogenic t.
Copeland t.
coronary flow reserve t.
cough CPR t.
crash t.
Crawford graft inclusion t.
Creech t.
cryosurgical t.
cutdown t.
digital subtraction t.
dilator and sheath t.
direct insertion t.
DOC exchange t.
Doppler auto-correlation t.
Dotter t.
Dotter-Judkins t.
double-dummy t.
double-wire t.
Douglas bag t.
dye dilution t.
ECG signal-averaging t.
en bloc, no-touch t.
entangling t.
exchange t.
Exorcist t.
Fick t.
first-pass t.
flow mapping t.

T

NOTES

technique *(continued)*
flush and bathe t.
forced oscillation t. (FOT)
forward triangle t.
gated t.
George Lewis t.
gloved fist t.
Goris background subtraction t.
grabbing t.
Grüntzig t.
guidewire t.
hydrogen inhalation t.
immunostaining t.
indicator dilution t.
indocyanine green indicator
  dilution t.
J loop t.
Judkins t.
Judkins-Sones t.
Kern t.
kissing balloon t.
Lown t.
Marbach-Weil t.
McGoon t.
Merendino t.
minimal leak t.
modified brachial t.
modified Seldinger t.
Mullins blade t.
Nikaidoh-Bex t.
no-leak t.
Oxford t.
percutaneous t.
Porstmann t.
pressure half-time t.
radiographic t.
radionuclide t.
Rashkind balloon t.
relaxation t.
Ricketts-Abrams t.
Rosalki t.
scatterplot smoothing t.
Schonander t.
Schoonmaker-King single
  catheter t.
Sealy-Laragh t.
Seldinger percutaneous t.
Sewall t.
Sheehan and Dodge t.
skewer t.
snare t.
Sones t.
sonication t.

Sparks mandrel t.
static dilation t.
Stewart-Hamilton cardiac
  output t.
thermal dilution t.
thermodilution t.
Trusler aortic valve t.
two-patch t.
upgated t.
velocity catheter t.
Waldhausen subclavian flap t.
wax-matrix t.
xenon washout t.
Zavala t.
technology
phased array t.
PulseDose oxygen delivery t.
TED
thromboembolic disease
TED antiembolism stockings
TEDD
total end-diastolic diameter
tedding device
Tedral
TEE
transesophageal echocardiography
OmniPlane TEE
TEEP
transesophageal echocardiography
  with pacing
Tefcor movable core straight wire
guide
Teflon
T. catheter
T. coating
T. graft
T. intracardiac patch
T. pledget
T. pledget suture buttress
T. TFE SubLite Wall tubing
Teflon-coated
T.-c. guidewire
Tega-Vert Oral
Tegopen
TEGwire
T. balloon dilatation catheter
T. guide
T.E.H.
theophylline, ephedrine, and
  hydroxyzine
Teichholz
T. ejection fraction
T. formula

teichoic acid antibody
teicoplanin
glycopeptide t.
Telachlor Oral
Teladar
telangiectasia, pl. **telangiectases**
hemorrhagic t.
hereditary hemorrhagic t.
Teldrin oral
telecardiogram
telecardiophone
Telectronics
T. ATP implantable cardioverter-defibrillator
T. Guardian ATP 4210 device
T. Guardian ATP II ICD
T. leads
telecurietherapy
telediastolic
telelectrocardiogram
telemetry
cardiac t.
multiple-parameter t. (MPT)
telescope
Storz bronchoscopic t.
telesystolic
Teletrast gauze
Teline Oral
telopeptide
type I collagen t. (ICTP)
TEM
transtelephonic exercise monitor
temafloxacin
Temco hoist
temperature
core t.
t., pulse, and respiration (TPR)
temperature-sensing pacemaker
temporal
t. arteritis
t. dispersion
t. resolution
temporary
t. pacemaker placement
t. pacing
t. pervenous lead

t. unilateral pulmonary artery occlusion
Ten
T. balloon
T. system balloon catheter
tenacious sputum
Tenathan
tendinea
macula t.
tendineae
chordae t.
tendinosum
xanthoma t.
tendinous
t. spot
t. xanthoma
t. zones of heart
tendon
false t.
t. of Todaro, Todaro t.
tendophony, tenophony
Tenex
Tenif
teniposide
Tennant distress scale
Tennis Racquet angiographic catheter
tenonometer
tenophony (*var. of* tendophony)
Tenoretic
Tenormin
Tenox
tense
t. edema
t. pulse
tensile stress
Tensilon
T. injection
tension
alveolar carbon dioxide t.
alveolar oxygen t.
arterial carbon dioxide t.
carbon dioxide t.
left ventricular t.
myocardial t.
oxygen t.
t. pneumopericardium

T

NOTES

tension *(continued)*
  t. pneumothorax
  wall t.
tension-length relation
tension-time index
tent
  CAM t.
  croup t.
  Croupette child t.
  mist t.
  oxygen t.
  pleural t.'s
  Silon t.
  steam t.
tenting
  t. of hemidiaphragm
  t. sign
  t. of skin
Tenzel calipers
teratoma
  pericardial t.
  t. tumor
terazosin
  t. hydrochloride
terbutaline
  t. sulfate
tercile value
terconazole
terephthalate
  polyethylene t. (PET)
terfenadine
terikalant
terminal
  t. aorta
  t. cisterna
  t. edema
  t. endocarditis
  t. groove
  t. pneumonia
  t. Purkinje fibers
  Wilson central t.
terminalis
  crista t.
  sulcus t.
termination
  underdrive t.
terodiline
Terramycin
  T. I.M. injection
  T. Oral
terreus
  Aspergillus t.

terror
  night t.'s
tertiary
  t. contractions
  t. syphilis
Terumo
  T. dialyzer
  T. guidewire
  T. m wire
  T. Radiofocus sheath
  T. SP coaxial catheter
  T. SP hydrophilic-polymer-
    coated microcatheter
TES
  transcutaneous electrical stimulation
TESD
  total end-systolic diameter
tesla
Tessalon Perles
test, testing
  abdominal jugular t.
  acetylcholine t.
  acid infusion t.
  adenosine thallium t.
  Adson t.
  Advanced Care cholesterol t.
  aerobic exercise stress t.
  ajmaline t.
  AlaSTAT latex allergy t.
  Allen t.
  Amplicor *Mycobacterium*
    tuberculosis t.
  Amplified *Mycobacterium*
    tuberculosis Direct t.
  Anderson t.
  anoxemia t.
  Apo E t.
  Apt t.
  Arloing-Courmont t.
  arm exercise stress t.
  arm-tongue time t.
  Astrand bicycle exercise
    stress t.
  ASTZ t.
  atrial pacing stress t.
  atropine t.
  Balke exercise stress t.
  Balke-Ware t.
  Bernstein t.
  bicycle ergometer exercise
    stress t.
  Blake exercise stress t.
  blanch t.

blot t.
Blumenau t.
Bonferroni t.
Bordet-Gengou t.
breath excretion t.
breath-holding t.
breath pentane t.
Brodie Trendelenburg
  tourniquet t.
bronchial challenge t.
bronchoprovocation t.
broth t.
Bruce exercise stress t.
CAMP t.
Cardiolite stress t.
cardiopulmonary exercise t.
  (CPET, CPX test)
carotid sinus t.
Casoni t.
chi-square t.
Cochran t.
coin t.
cold pressor t.
complement-fixation t.
Coombs t.
CPX t.
    cardiopulmonary exercise test
Craig t.
Crampton t.
cuff t.
Davidson protocol exercise t.
Dehio t.
dexamethasone suppression t.
dipyridamole handgrip t.
dobutamine stress t.
double triangular t.
DPPC t.
DR-70 tumor marker t.
Duncan multiple range t.
Dunnett t.
duodenal string t.
electrophysiologic t.
ELISPOT t.
Ellestad exercise stress t.
ergonovine provocation t.
Escherich t.
ether t.

exercise stress t. (EST)
exercise tolerance t. (ETT)
exercise treadmill t. (ETT)
external rotation, abduction,
  stress t. (EAST)
extrastimulus t.
Farr t.
Fisher exact t.
foam stability t.
Fowler single-breath t.
Friedman t.
FTA-ABS t.
Gibbon-Landis t.
Goethlin t.
Gradational Step exercise
  stress t.
Graded Exercise exercise
  stress t.
Hallion t.
Ham t.
Hamburger t.
head-down tilt t.
head-up tilt t.
head-up tilt-table t. (HUTTT)
Heaf t.
Henle-Coenen t.
hepatojugular reflux t.
Hess capillary t.
high-altitude simulation t.
  (HAST)
Hines-Brown t.
Hitzenberg t.
HIVAGEN t.
Hotelling T2 t.
Howell t.
hypoxemia t.
IgG avidity t.
isometric handgrip t.
isoproterenol stress t.
isoproterenol tilt-table t.
J point treadmill t.
Kattus exercise stress t.
Kleihauer t.
Kleihauer-Betke t.
Kruskal-Wallis t.
Kveim antigen skin t.
Kveim-Stilzbach t.

NOTES

test *(continued)*
Lautier t.
LDL Direct blood t.
Lee-Desu log rank t.
lepromin t.
Levy Chimeric Faces T.
Lewis-Pickering t.
Liebermann-Burchard t.
Lignieres t.
liver function t. (LFT)
Livierato t.
log-rank t.
Machado-Guerreiro t.
Mann-Whitney t.
Mantel-Haenszel t.
Mantoux t.
Master exercise stress t.
Master two-step exercise t.
Matas t.
McNemar t.
Mester t.
methacholine t.
MHA-TP t.
MIBI stress t.
10-minute supine/30-minute
tilt t.
6-Minute Walk T.
Monotest CK-MB NAC-act t.
Moschcowitz t.
MUGA exercise stress t.
Muller t.
Multiple Sleep Latency T.
(MSLT)
Multistage Maximal Effort
exercise stress t.
MycoAKT latex bead
agglutination t.
Nagle exercise stress t.
Nathan t.
Naughton graded exercise
stress t.
Newman-Keuls t.
Nickerson-Kveim t.
noninvasive t.
Norris t.
Ochsner-Mahorner t.
Optichin disk t.
Pachon t.
paired *t* t.
p24 antigen t.
paracoccidioidin skin t.
peppermint t.
Persantine-isonitrile stress t.

Perthes t.
Peto-Prentice log-rank t.
Phalen stress t.
Physical Work Capacity
exercise stress t.
pilocarpine iontophoresis t.
planar thallium t.
plantar ischemia t.
Plesch t.
Portmanteau t.
PPD skin t.
PPL skin t.
primed lymphocyte t.
provocation t.
pulmonary function t. (PFT)
Q-Stress treadmill stress t.
Quick t.
radioallergosorbent t. (RAST)
Reflotron bedside
theophylline t.
reverse transcriptase polymerase
chain reaction t.
Roos t.
Rumpel-Leede t.
Sabin-Feldman dye t.
Salkowski t.
Sandrock t.
Schapiro-Wilks t.
Scheffé t.
Schellong t.
Schiff t.
Schlichter t.
Schultze t.
Schwartz t.
serological t.
sestamibi stress t.
shake t.
Sheffield exercise stress t.
single-breath nitrogen
washout t.
single-stage exercise stress t.
Snider match t.
sniff t.
Spearman rho t.
Spectral Cardiac STATus T.
SpectRx t.
split-function lung t.
Stamey t.
Sterneedle tuberculin t.
stress t.
Stroop color word conflict t.
Student *t* t.
Student-Newman-Keuls t.

surf t.
sweat chloride t.
symptom-limited treadmill exercise t.
t t.
Tarone-Ware nonparametric linear rank t.
technetium-99m sestamibi stress t.
thallium-201 exercise stress t.
TheoFAST t.
thermodilution t.
thyroid function t.
tilt t.
tilt-table t. (TTT)
tine t.
tolazoline t.
treadmill exercise stress t.
Trendelenburg t.
treponemal t.
Tris-buffer infusion t.
tuberculin t.
Tuffier t.
Tukey t.
two-step exercise t.
unpaired *t* t.
Valsalva t.
VDRL t.
Visov t.
Vitalometer t.
Vitalor screening pulmonary function t.
Vollmer t.
volume-challenge t.
von Recklinghausen t.
walking ventilation t.
water-gurgle t.
Weinberg t.
Weyl t.
whiff t.
Widal t.
Wideroe t.
Wilcoxon rank sum t.
Wilks-Schapiro t.
William t.
Winslow t.
X-Scribe stress t.

Youman-Parlett t.
Zwenger t.
tester
    Quik-Chek external pacer t.
testosterone
tetanus
tethering
tetracaine hydrochloride
Tetracap Oral
tetracrotic
tetracycline
tetrad
    Fallot t.
    t. spell
tetrahedon chest
tetrahydrobiopterin
tetrahydrochloride
    diaminobenzidine t.
Tetralan Oral
tetralogy
    Eisenmenger t.
    t. of Fallot
    Fallot pink t.
Tetram Oral
Tetramune
tetranitrate
    erythrityl t.
    pentaerythritol t.
tetrapolar esophageal catheter
tetrazolium
    nitroblue t.
tetrodotoxin
tetrofosmin
    technetium-99m t.
tet spell
Texas influenza
TGA
    transposition of great arteries
TGC
    time-gain compensation
    time-gain control
T-Gesic
TGF
    transforming growth factor
TGV
    thoracic gas volume
    transposition of great vessels

T

NOTES

ThAIRapy
  T. vest
  T. vest airway clearance
    system
thalassemia
  sickle cell-t.
thalidomide
Thalitone
thallium (Tl)
  t. electrocardiogram
  t. perfusion imaging
  t. washout
thallium-201 (^{201}Tl)
  t. exercise stress test
  t. perfusion scintigraphy
  t. planar scintigraphy
  t. SPECT scintigraphy
thallous chloride Tl-201
Thal procedure
THC:YAG laser
thebesian
  t. circulation
  t. foramina
  t. valve
  t. vein
Theden method
Theis rib retractor
Theo-24
Theobid
theobromine
Theochron
Theoclear L.A.
Theo-Dur
TheoFAST test
Theo-G
Theolair
Theolate
theophylline
  t., ephedrine, and hydroxyzine
    (T.E.H.)
  t., ephedrine, and phenobarbital
  t. and guaifenesin
theorem
  Bayes t.
  Bernoulli t.
theory
  Bayliss t.
  Cannon t.
  cross-linkage t.
  dipole t.
  immunological t.
  Melzack-Wall gate t.
  myogenic t.

  neuroendocrine t.
  neurogenic t.
  Ornish t.
  reentry t.
  response-to-injury t.
  sliding filament t.
  Spitzer t.
Theospan-SR
Theovent
Theo-X
TheraCys
Theramin Expectorant
TheraPEP
  T. positive expiratory pressure
    therapy system
  T. pre-respiratory therapy
    treatment
therapeutic
  t. dissection
  t. endpoint
  t. pneumothorax
therapy
  angina-guided t.
  antialdosterone t.
  antiarrhythmic t.
  anticoagulant t.
  antiendotoxin t.
  antimicrobial t.
  antiplatelet t.
  augmentation t.
  behavioral t.
  beta-blocker t.
  cerebral protective t.
  Clinitron air-fluidized t.
  collapse t.
  deep chest t.
  device t.
  electroconvulsive t.
  embolization t.
  empiric t.
  fibrinolytic t.
  fluid t.
  Healing and Early Afterload
    Reducing T. (HEART)
  immunosuppression t.
  ischemia-guided medical t.
  long-term oxygen t. (LTOT)
  Lymphapress compression t.
  oral anticoagulant t.
  oxygen t.
  photodynamic t.
  prophylactic t.
  radiation t.

rheologic t.
shock t.
step-down t.
thrombolytic t.
transcatheter t. (TCT)
warfarin t.
TheraSnore oral appliance
thermal
    t. angiography
    t. dilution technique
    t. memory stent
thermal/perfusion balloon
  angioplasty (TPBA)
Thermedics
    T. cardiac device
    T. HeartMate 10001P left
      anterior assist device
thermic fever
thermistor
    t. plethysmography
    t. thermodilution catheter
Thermocardiosystems left ventricular
  assist device
thermodilution
    t. balloon catheter
    t. cardiac output
    t. catheter introducer kit
    coronary sinus t.
    Kim-Ray t.
    t. measurement
    t. method
    t. technique
    t. test
thermography
    infrared t.
thermometer
    IVAC electronic t.
    Thermoscan Pro-1-Instant t.
thermoplastic
thermoresistable
    Mycobacterium t.
Thermoscan Pro-1-Instant
  thermometer
thermosetting resin
Thermos pacemaker
ThermoVent heat and moisture
  exchanger

The Sickness Impact Profile
thiabendazole
thiacetazone
thiamine deficiency
thiamylal sodium
thiazide diuretic
thickened pericardium
thickening
    cardiac wall t.
    diffuse intimal t.
    endocardial t.
    intimal t.
    leaflet t.
    pleural t.
    wall t.
thickness
    intimal-medial t. (IMT)
    relative wall t. (RWT)
    wall t.
thick and sticky mucus
thigh balloon
thigh-high antiembolic stockings
thimble valvotomy
thinning
    infarct t.
    shear t.
    ventricular wall t.
thin-section CT
thin-slice CT scan
thin-walled
    t.-w. catheter
    t.-w. needle
thioamide
thiobarbituric
    t. acid-reactive
    t. acid reactive substance
    (TBARS)
thiocyanate
Thiomerin
thionamide
thiopental
    t. sodium
thiopentone sodium
thioridazine
    t. hydrochloride
thiotepa

T

NOTES

499

third-degree heart block
third heart sound (S₃)
Thoma ampulla
Thomas shunt
Thom flap laryngeal reconstruction
  method
Thompson-Hatina method
Thomsen disease
thoracalgia
thoracalis
  aorta t.
thoracentesis
  Argyle-Turkel t.
  blind t.
  t. needle
thoraces (*pl. of* thorax)
thoracic
  t. aorta
  t. aortic aneurysm
  t. aortic dissection
  t. arch aortography
  t. asphyxiant dystrophy
  t. axis
  t. cage
  t. crisis
  t. duct
  t. electrical bioimpedance
  t. empyema
  t. endometriosis syndrome
  t. esophagus
  t. gas volume (TGV)
  t. impedance
  t. incisure
  t. inlet
  t. limb
  t. nerve
  t. outlet syndrome
  t. respiration
  t. squeeze
  t. vertebral body
  t. vessel
thoracica
  aorta t.
thoracic-pelvic-phalangeal dystrophy
thoracicus
  ductus t.
thoracis
  compages t.
  paracentesis t.
thoracoabdominal
  t. aortic aneurysm
  t. dyssynchrony
  t. paradox

thoracocardiography
thoracocentesis
thoracodorsal
  t. artery
thoracodynia
thoracolumbar
thoracophrenolaparotomy
thoracoplasty
  costoversion t.
  Delorme t.
  Fowler t.
  Schede t.
  Wilms t.
Thoracoport placement
thoracoschisis
thoracoscope
  Coryllos t.
  Jacobaeus t.
  Jacobaeus-Unverricht t.
  rigid t.
thoracoscopic talc insufflation
thoracoscopy
Thoracoseal drainage
thoracosternotomy
thoracostomy
  closed chest t.
  tube t.
  t. tube
thoracotome
  Bettman-Fovash t.
thoracotomy
  t. incision
  Lewis t.
Thora-Drain III chest drainage
Thora-Klex
  T.-K. chest drainage system
  T.-K. chest tube
Thora-Port
thoracoscope
  Boutin t.
thoracoscopic
  t. apical pleurectomy
  t. talc pleurodesis
Thoratec
  T. cardiac device
  T. pump
  T. VAD System
  T. ventricular assist device
thorax, pl. thoraces
  amazon t.
  t. asthenicus
  barrel-shaped t.
  cholesterol t.

frozen t.
t. paralyticus
Peyrot t.
pyriform t.
Thorazine
Thorel
T. bundle
T. pathway
Thornell microlaryngoscopy
Thorotrast
thorough-fare channel
THR
target heart rate
threads
mucous t.
thready pulse
three-block claudication
three-chambered heart
three-channel electrocardiogram
three-dimensional
t.-d. echocardiography (3DE)
t.-d. Fourier transform (3DFT)
three-pillow orthopnea
three-turn epicardial lead
three-way stopcock
thresher's lung
threshing fever
threshold
aerobic t.
anaerobic t.
anginal perceptual t.
atrial capture t.
atrial defibrillation t.
cough t.
defibrillation t.
fibrillation t.
flicker fusion t.
ischemic t.
lactate t.
lead t.
nociceptive t.
pacemaker t.
t. pacing
pacing t.
t. percussion
stimulation t.

ventilation t.
ventilatory t.
ventricular capture t.
work t.
threw an embolus
thrill
aneurysmal t.
aortic t.
arterial t.
coarse t.
dense t.
diastolic t.
parasternal systolic t.
precordial t.
presystolic t.
purring t.
systolic t.
throb
thrombasthenia
Thrombate III
thrombectomize
thrombectomy
percutaneous rotational t.
(PRT)
thrombi (*pl. of* thrombus)
intramural t.
LAA t.
thrombin
clot-bound t.
t. generation
thrombin-antithrombin (TAT)
t.-a. III complex
Thrombinar
Thrombinex
thrombin-soaked Gelfoam
thrombin, topical
thromboangiitis
t. obliterans
thromboaortopathy
occlusive t.
thromboarteritis
thromboclasis
thromboclastic
thrombocytapheresis
thrombocythemia
thrombocytopenia

T

NOTES

501

thrombocytopenia-absent
  t.-a. radius (TAR)
  t.-a. radius syndrome
thrombocytosis
thromboelastogram
thromboelastograph
thromboembolectomy
thromboembolic
  t. disease (TED)
  t. pulmonary hypertension
thromboembolism
  pulmonary t.
  venous t.
thromboendarterectomy (TEA)
thromboendarteritis
thromboendocarditis
Thrombogen
thrombogenic
thrombogenicity
thromboglobulin
  beta t.
thromboid
thrombolic
thrombolizer
  Angiocor rotational t.
thrombolus
thrombolysis
  T. and Angioplasty in
    Myocardial Infarction (TAMI)
  T. and Angioplasty in
    Unstable Angina (TAUSA)
  Antithrombotics in the
    Prevention of Reocclusion in
    Coronary T. (APRICOT)
  coronary t.
  Hirudin in T. (HIT)
  T. in Myocardial Infarction
    (TIMI)
  Prourokinase and t-PA
    Enhancement of T.
    (PATENT)
  selective intracoronary t.
    (SICT)
  Should We Intervene
    Following T. (SWIFT)
thrombolytic
  t. agent
  T. Assessment system (TAS)
  t. therapy
  T. Trial of Eminase in Acute
    Myocardial Infarction (TEAM)
thrombomodulin

thrombophlebitis
  t. migrans
  t. saltans
thromboplastin
  partial t. time (PTT)
  t. time (TT)
thrombopoietin (TPO)
ThromboScan MRI
thrombosed
thrombosis, pl. thromboses
  agonal t.
  Anticoagulants in the
    Secondary Prevention of
    Events in Coronary T.
    (ASPECT)
  aortic t.
  aortoiliac t.
  arterial t.
  atrophic t.
  brachial artery t.
  cardiac t.
  catheter-induced t.
  cavernous sinus t.
  central splanchnic venous t.
    (CSVT)
  cerebral t.
  cerebrovascular t.
  coagulation t.
  compression t.
  coronary artery t.
  creeping t.
  deep venous t. (DVT)
  dilation t.
  effort-induced t.
  embolic t.
  femoral artery t.
  femoral venous t.
  iliac vein t.
  infective t.
  Integrelin to Manage Platelet
    Aggregation to Prevent
    Coronary T. (IMPACT)
  intramural t.
  jumping t.
  laser-induced t.
  marantic t., marasmic t.
  mural t.
  Paget-Schroetter venous t.
  plate t.
  platelet t.
  portal vein t.
  propagating t.
  prosthetic valve t.

puerperal t.
Ribbert t.
sinus t.
traumatic t.
venous t.
thrombostasis
Thrombostat
Thrombotest
thrombotic
    t. endocarditis
    t. microangiopathy
    t. thrombocytopenic purpura
    (TTP)
Thrombo-Wellcotest method
thromboxane
    t. A_2
    t. receptor antagonist
    t. synthesis
    t. synthetase inhibitor
thrombus, pl. thrombi
    agglutinative t.
    agonal t.
    annular t.
    antemortem t.
    atrial t.
    ball t.
    ball valve t.
    blood plate t., blood platelet t.
    calcified t.
    coral t.
    currant jelly t.
    fibrin t.
    globular t.
    t. grade
    hyaline t.
    infective t.
    intracardiac t.
    intravascular t.
    laminated t.
    lateral t.
    marantic t., marasmic t.
    migratory t.
    mixed t.
    mural t.
    obstructive t.
    occluding t.
    occlusive t.

organized t.
pale t.
parietal t.
pedunculated t.
plate t.
platelct t.
postmortem t.
t. precursor protein (TpT)
T. Precursor Protein
    immunoassay
primary t.
progressive t.
propagated t.
red t.
right atrial t.
saddle t.
secondary t.
straddling t.
stratified t.
t. stripper
traumatic t.
valvular t.
ventricular t.
white t.
**through-and-through myocardial
    infarction**
through-the-wall mattress suture
Thruflex balloon
ThruLumen lumen
thrush
    t. breast
    t. breast heart
thrust
    cardiac t.
thulium:YAG laser angioplasty
thumbprint bronchus sign
thump
    chest t.
    precordial t.
Thumper CPR system
thumpversion
thymectomy
    video-assisted thoracoscopic t.
thymic
    t. asthma
    t. cyst
thymoma

T

NOTES

thymopentin
thymostimuline
thymusectomy
Thyro-Block
thyrocardiac
    t. disease
thyroid
    aberrant t.
    accessory t.
    t. antibody
    t. bruit
    t. cachexia
    t. disease
    t. extract
    t. function test
    intrathoracic t.
    t. isthmus
    lingual t.
    t. notch
    t. panel
    retrosternal t.
    t. storm
    substernal t.
    t. tumor
thyroidectomy
thyroiditis
    chronic lymphocytic t.
    de Quervain t.
    Hashimoto t.
    Riedel t.
    woody t.
thyroid-stimulating hormone (TSH)
thyrointoxication
thyromegaly
thyroprival
thyrotoxic heart disease
thyrotoxicosis
thyrotoxin
    t. radioisotope assay
thyrotropin
thyrotropin-releasing hormone
response
thyroxine, thyroxin (T₄)
ᴅ-thyroxine
ʟ-thyroxine
TI-201
    thallous chloride TI-201
TIA
    transient ischemic attack
tiamenidine
tiapamil
Tiazac
    T. extended-release capsules

TIBBS
    Total Ischemic Burden Bisoprolol
    Study
Tibbs arterial cannula
TIBET
    Total Ischaemic Burden European
    Trial
tibial
    t. artery
    t. pulse
tibioperoneal vessel angioplasty
Ticar
ticarcillin
    t. and clavulanic acid
    t. disodium
ticarcillin/clavulanate
TICE BCG
tick
    t. anticoagulant peptide
    t. paralysis
Ticlid
ticlopidine hydrochloride
Ti-Cron suture
tic-tac
    t.-t. rhythm
    t.-t. sounds
tidal
    t. air
    t. volume (TV, Vᴛ)
    t. wave
    t. wave pulse
tiered-therapy antiarrhythmic device
Tietze syndrome
tiger
    t. heart
    t. lily heart
tight
    t. asthmatic
    t. junction
    t. stenosis
tightness
    chest t.
tight-to-shaft Aire-Cuf tracheostomy
tube
Tilade
    T. Inhalation Aerosol
    T. inhaler
Tildiem
tilt
    t. test
    t. vitals
tilting-disk
    t.-d. aortic valve prosthesis

t.-d. occluder
t.-d. prosthetic valve
tilt-table test (TTT)
time
acceleration t.
acquisition t.
activated clotting t. (ACT)
activated partial
thromboplastin t. (aPTT)
A-H conduction t.
arm-tongue t.
atrioventricular t.
bypass t.
capacitor forming t.
carotid ejection t.
charge t.
circulation t.
clot retraction t.
coagulation t.
t. compensation gain (TCG)
conduction t.
corrected sinus node
recovery t.
cross-clamp t.
dead t.
deceleration t.
detect t.
t. domain
t. domain signal-averaged
electrocardiogram
donor organ ischemic t.
doubling t.
Duke bleeding t.
echo delay t. (TE)
ejection t.
esophageal transit t.
euglobulin clot lysis t.
flushing t.
forced expiratory t. (FET)
H-R conduction t.
H-V conduction t.
intra-atrial conduction t.
isovolumic relaxation t. (IVRT)
Ivy bleeding t.
left ventricular ejection t.
(LVET)

lysis t.
magnetic relaxation t.
maximum walking t.
median survival t. (MST)
P-A conduction t.
pain-free walking t. (PFWT)
partial thromboplastin t. (PTT)
P-H conduction t.
prothrombin t. (PT)
prothrombin time/partial
thromboplastin t. (PT/PTT)
quick prothrombin t.
relaxation t.
repetition t. (TR)
rise t.
saturation t.
sinoatrial conduction t. (SACT)
sinoatrial recovery t. (SART)
sinus node recovery t. (SNRT)
spin-lattice t.
spin-spin t.
thromboplastin t. (TT)
transmitral E-wave
deceleration t.
T2 relaxation t.
ventilator t.
ventricular activation t. (VAT)
time-activity curve
time-averaged peak velocity
Timecelles
Sinufed T.
time-cycled ventilation
timed
t. forced expiratory volume
t. vital capacity
time-domain analysis
time-gain
t.-g. compensation (TGC)
t.-g. control (TGC)
Timentin
time-resolved imaging by automatic
data segmentation (TRIADS)
time-to-peak contrast
time-varied
t.-v. gain (TVG)
t.-v. gain control (TVGC)

NOTES

T

TIMI
　　Thrombolysis in Myocardial
　　Infarction
　　TIMI classification
Timolide
timolol
　　t. maleate
Timoptic Ophthalmic
timori
　　Brugia t.
TINA monitor
tine test
tinkle
　　Bouillaud t.
　　metallic t.
TintElize PAI-1 ELISA kit
tip
　　Andrews suction t.
　　Luer-Lok needle t.
　　Medtronic t.
　　t. occluder
　　papillary muscle t.
　　Polaris Mansfield/Webster
　　　deflectable t.
tip-deflecting wire
TIPS
　　transjugular intrahepatic
　　portosystemic shunt
tirofiban
Tissot spirometer
tissue
　　t. ablation
　　adipose t.
　　atrioventricular conduction t.
　　autodigestion of connective t.
　　t. bank
　　caseated t.
　　connective t.
　　t. Doppler imaging
　　t. factor
　　His-Purkinje t.
　　interfascicular fibrous t.
　　myocardial t.
　　t. necrosis
　　nodal t.
　　perinodal t.
　　t. plasminogen activator (t-PA)
　　t. preservation
　　t. valve
tissue-specific antibodies
tissue-type plasminogen activator

titanium
　　t. cage
　　T. VasPort
titer
　　antiheart antibody t.
　　anti-Rho-D t.
　　bactericidal t.
　　Lyme t.
　　serum bactericidal t. (SBT)
titration
Titrator
Tl
　　thallium
²⁰¹Tl
　　thallium-201
TLC
　　total lung capacity
TLI
　　total lymphoid irradiation
TMP-SMX
　　trimethoprim-sulfamethoxazole
TMR
　　transmyocardial revascularization
　　Heart Laser for TMR
TNF
　　tumor necrosis factor
TNM
　　tumor, nodes, metastasis
　　TNM classification
　　TNM staging
to-and-fro
　　t.-a.-f. murmur
　　t.-a.-f. sound
tobacco heart
tobramycin
　　nebulized t.
tocainide
　　t. hydrochloride
Todaro
　　tendon of T., T. tendon
　　T. triangle
Todd-Hewitt broth
Todd units
Tofranil
Togaviridae virus
TOHP
　　Trials of Hypertension Prevention
toilet, toilette
　　bronchial t.
　　pulmonary t.
　　respiratory t.
　　tracheobronchial t.

toilet-seat
t.-s. angina
t.-s. syncope
tolazamide
tolazoline
t. hydrochloride
t. test
tolbutamide
tolerance
hemodynamic t.
Tolinase
toluene
t. diisocyanate (TDI)
Tolu-Sed DM
tomograph
ECAT III positron t.
tomographic
high resolution thin section
computed t.
t. radionuclide ventriculography
tomography
atrial bolus dynamic
computer t.
axial computed t. (ACT)
biplanar t.
cine computed t.
computed t. (CT)
computerized axial t. (CAT)
electron beam computed t.
(EBCT)
gated computed t.
high resolution computed t.
(HRCT)
optical coherence t. (OCT)
positron emission t. (PET)
quantitative computed t. (QCT)
rapid acquisition computed
axial t. (RACAT)
seven-pinhole t.
single-photon emission t.
(SPET)
single-photon emission
computed t. (SPECT)
slant-hole t.
ultrafast computed t. (UFCT)

xenon-enhanced computed t.
(XECT)
x-ray cine computed t.
TomTec echo platform
tone
bronchial smooth muscle t.
heart t.'s
Traube double t.
Williams tracheal t.
tongs
Trippi-Wells t.
tongue
smoker's t.
t. traction
Tonocard
tonometer
air-puff t.
Gärtner t.
Tono-Pen t.
tonometered whole blood
tonometry
applanation t.
Tono-Pen tonometer
tonoscillograph
tonsillaris
angina t.
tonsillar pillar
tonsillitis
caseous t.
chronic catarrhal t.
diphtherial t.
tonsilloadenoidectomy
tool
Avenue insertion t.
QuantX color quantification t.
top-hat supra-annular aortic valve
topical
Bactroban T.
Benadryl T.
t. cooling
Efudex T.
Fluoroplex T.
Gelfoam T.
t. hypothermia
Mycostatin T.
Nilstat T.
Nystex T.

T

NOTES

507

topical *(continued)*
    Oxsoralen T.
    thrombin, t.
Toposar
    T. injection
Toprol XL
Torcon NB selective angiographic catheter
Torek resection of thoracic esophagus
Torktherm torque control catheter
Tornalate
Tornwaldt cyst
toroidal valve
Toronto
    T. Alexithymia Scale
    T. Lung Transplant Group
    T. SPV aortic valve
    T. SPV bioprosthesis
torpedo-shaped pattern
torque
    clockwise t.
    t. control
    t. control balloon catheter
    t. vise
torquer
    Clip On t.
torquing ability
torr
    t. pressure
    t. unit
Torricelli
    T. law
    T. model
    T. orifice equation
torsade de pointes
torsemide
tortuosity
tortuous
    t. veins
    t. vessel
Torula histolytica
Torulopsis glabrata
torulosis
torus aorticus
TOS
    toxic oil syndrome
Toshiba
    T. biplane transesophageal transducer
    T. electrocardiography machine
tosylate
    bretylium t.

Totacillin
total
    t. acidity
    t. adenine nucleotides (TAN)
    t. alternans
    t. anomalous pulmonary venous connection (TAPVC)
    t. anomalous pulmonary venous drainage (TAPVD)
    t. anomalous pulmonary venous return (TAPVR)
    t. artificial heart (TAH)
    t. axial node irradiation (TANI)
    t. blood volume (TBV)
    t. cavopulmonary connection (TCPC)
    t. circulatory arrest
    T. Cross balloon catheter
    t. end-diastolic diameter (TEDD)
    t. end-systolic diameter (TESD)
    T. Ischaemic Burden European Trial (TIBET)
    T. Ischemic Burden Bisoprolol Study (TIBBS)
    t. lung capacity (TLC)
    t. lymphoid irradiation (TLI)
    t. patient shock count
    t. peripheral resistance (TPR)
    t. peripheral resistance index (TPRI)
    t. pulmonary resistance
    t. Synchrony System
Tote-A-Neb nebulizer
touch shock count
Toupet hemifundoplication
Tourguide guiding catheter
tourniquet
    Bethune lobectomy t.
    Carr lobectomy t.
    Esmarch t.
    Medi-Quet t.
    pneumatic t.
    Rumel t.
    Shenstone t.
Touro LA
Tower stent
toxemia
toxemic pneumonia
toxic
    t. agent
    t. delirium

t. myocarditis
t. oil syndrome (TOS)
t. shock

toxicity
amphetamine t.
anthracycline t.
antimony t.
dextroamphetamine t.
digitalis t.
digoxin t.
emetine t.
fluoride t.
hydrocarbon t.
phenylpropanolamine t.
plant t.

toxin
adenylate cyclase t.
t. exposure
pertussis t.
RNA glycosidase t.

toxin-insensitive current
Toxocara
T. canis
toxoid
diphtheria and tetanus t.
Toxoplasma gondii
toxoplasmosis
ToxR protein
TP
TP interval
TP segment
t-PA
tissue plasminogen activator
TPBA
thermal/perfusion balloon
angioplasty
T-piece
Ayers T-p.
T-p. oxygen
TPO
thrombopoietin
T-P-Q segment
TPR
temperature, pulse, and respiration
total peripheral resistance
TPRI
total peripheral resistance index

TpT
thrombus precursor protein
TQ segment
TR
repetition time
tricuspid regurgitation
trabeculae carneae
trabecular hypertrophy
trabecula septomarginalis
trabeculation
TRACE
Trandolapril Cardiac Evaluation
trace
t. metal
T. vein stripper
tracer
carbon-11 palmitic acid
radioactive t.
frequency t.
iodine-123 heptadecanoic acid
radioactive t.
TrachCare
T. multi-access catheter
Neonatal Y T.
trachea
bifurcation of t.
carina of t.
scabbard t.
steepling of t.
tracheae
bifurcatio t.
tracheal
t. aspirate
t. bronchus
t. button
t. deviation
t. intubation
t. mucus velocity
t. rales
t. rings
t. sound
t. steepling
t. tug
trachealis
angina t.
tracheitis

T

NOTES

tracheobronchial
  t. amyloidosis
  t. lavage
  t. toilet
  t. tree
  t. tuberculosis
tracheobronchitis
tracheobronchoscopy
tracheoesophageal
  t. junction
  t. puncture
Tracheolife HME
tracheomalacia
tracheopathia osteoplastica
tracheopharyngeal
tracheophonesis
tracheophony
tracheoscope
  Storz t.
  Storz-Shapshay t.
tracheostenosis
tracheostomy
  t. button
  t. cuff
  flap t.
  Great Ormond Street t.
  Montgomery t.
  percutaneous dilational t.
  (PDT)
  t. stoma
tracheotome
  Salvatore-Maloney t.
tracheotomy
Trach-Mist
trachomatis
  Chlamydia t.
Trach-Talk
trachyphonia
tracing
  carotid pulse t.
  diamond-shaped t.
  jugular venous pulse t.
  pressure t.
  pulse t.
trackability
Tracker-18 Soft Stream side-hole microinfusion catheter
tracking
  spatial t.
tracks
  tram t.
Trac Plus catheter
Tracrium

tract
  atriodextrofascicular t.
  atriofascicular t.
  atrio-Hisian bypass t.
  atrionodal bypass t.
  bypass t.
  concealed bypass t.
  gastrointestinal t.
  inflow t.
  James accessory t.'s
  left ventricular outflow t.
  (LVOT)
  nodo-Hisian bypass t.
  nodoventricular t.
  outflow t.
  respiratory t.
  right ventricular outflow t.
  (RVOT)
  Wolff-Parkinson-White bypass t.
traction
  t. aneurysm
  t. bronchiectasis
  Crego t.
  tongue t.
trailing edge
training effect
trains
  drive t.
  t. of ventricular pacing
trainwheel rhythm
trait
  sickle cell t.
TRAKE-fit system
Trakstar balloon catheter
tram
  t. lines
  t. tracks
Trandate
  T. injection
  T. Oral
trandolapril
  T. Cardiac Evaluation
  (TRACE)
tranexamic acid
Tranquility Quest
tranquilizer
trans
  t. fat
  t. fatty acids
transaminase
  glutamic-oxaloacetic t. (GOT)

serum glutamic-oxaloacetic t.
(SGOT)
serum glutamic-pyruvic t.
(SGPT)
transaortic valve gradient
transatrial pacing
transaxial
  t. plane
  t. slice
transaxillary apical bullectomy
transbrachial aortography
transbronchial
  t. lung biopsy
  t. needle aspiration
transcapillary refill
transcatheter
  t. ablation
  t. closure
  t. embolization
  t. therapy (TCT)
  t. umbrella
Transcop
transcranial
  t. contrast Doppler sonography
  t. Doppler probe
transcription
  gene t.
transcutaneous
  t. echo
  t. electrical stimulation (TES)
  t. extraction catheter
  t. oxygen monitor (TCOM)
Transdermal
  Catapres-TTS T.
Transdermal-NTG Patch
Transderm-Nitro
  T.-N. Patch
transducer
  Acuson V5M multiplane
  TEE t.
  annular array t.
  t. aperture
  Bentley t.
  charge-coupled device t.
  Cordis Sentron t.
  Deltran disposable t.
  diaphragm t.

Diasonics t.
Doppler t.
echocardiographic t.
Gould Statham pressure t.
Mikro-Tip t.
Millar Mikro-Tip catheter
  pressure t.
M-mode t.
Pedoff continuous wave t.
phased array sector t.
phonocardiographic t.
pressure t.
quartz t.
Spectranetic P23 Statham t.
Toshiba biplane
  transesophageal t.
ultrasound t.
variomatrix t.
V510B Biplane TEE t.
Vingmed CFM 750 t.
V5M Multiplane t.
transendothelial
transesophageal
  t. atrial pacing (TAP, TEAP)
  t. atrial stimulation (TRAS)
  t. contrast echocardiography
  t. dobutamine stress
  echocardiography
  t. echo
  t. echocardiography (TEE)
  t. echocardiography with
  pacing (TEEP)
  t. echo probe
  t. probe
transfer
  adenovirus-mediated gene t.
  chordal t.
  ex vivo gene t.
  vascular gene t.
  in vivo gene t.
transferase
transform
  fast-Fourier t.
  Fourier t.
  three-dimensional Fourier t.
  (3DFT)
transforming growth factor (TGF)

NOTES

511

transfusion
    autologous t.
    Baylor rapid autologous t.
    (BRAT)
    donor-specific t.
    exchange t.
transfusional hemosiderosis
transient
    calcium t.
    t. depolarization
    t. heart block
    t. inward current
    t. ischemia
    t. ischemic attack (TIA)
    t. leukocytosis
    t. mesenteric ischemia
    t. pericarditis
    t. response imaging (TRI)
    t. syncope
    t. tachypnea of newborn
    (TTNB)
transition
    forced ischemia-reperfusion t.
    sympathovagal t.
transitional
    t. cell
    t. cell carcinoma
    t. cell zone
    t. respiration
transjugular intrahepatic
  portosystemic shunt (TIPS)
translesional spectral flow velocity
translocation
    Nikaidoh t.
translocator
    adenine nucleotide t.
    adenosine nucleotide t. (ANT)
translumbar aortography
transluminal
    t. angioplasty catheter
    t. coronary angioplasty
    t. endarterectomy catheter
    (TEC)
    t. extraction atherectomy
    (TEA)
    t. extraction catheter (TEC)
    t. lysing system
transmembrane
    t. calcium flux
    t. potential
    t. signaling
    t. voltage

transmission
    air-borne t.
    genetic t.
transmitral
    t. Doppler E:A ratio
    t. E:A ratio
    t. E-wave deceleration time
transmitted murmur
transmural
    t. myocardial infarction
    t. pressure
    t. steal
transmyocardial
    t. laser revascularization
    t. pacing stylet
    t. perfusion pressure
    t. revascularization (TMR)
Transonic flowmeter
transplant, transplantation
    allogeneic t.
    bilateral lung t. (BLT)
    bilateral sequential lung t.
    bone marrow t.
    cardiac t.
    t. coronary artery disease
    (TCAD)
    double lung t.
    en bloc bilateral lung t.
    heart t.
    heart-lung t. (HLT)
    heterologous cardiac t.
    heterotopic cardiac t.
    heterotopic heart t. (HHT)
    homologous cardiac t.
    International Society for Heart
    and Lung T. (ISHLT)
    Lower-Shumway cardiac t.
    lung t. (LTx)
    orthotopic cardiac t.
    orthotopic heart t. (OHT)
    t. pneumonia
    rejection cardiomyopathy t.
    renal t.
    single-lung t. (SLT)
    syngenesioplastic t.
transport
    oxygen t.
transposition
    t. of arterial stems
    t. assessment
    t. complex
    t. of great arteries (TGA)
    t. of great vessels (TGV)

transradial approach
transsarcolemmal calcium current
Trans-Scan
    T.-S. 2100 noninvasive
      physiological monitor
transseptal
    t. angiocardiography
    t. catheter
    t. left heart catheterization
    t. puncture
transstenotic pressure gradient
  measurement
transtelephonic
    t. ambulatory monitoring
      system (TAM system)
    t. arrhythmia monitoring
      (TTM)
    t. exercise monitor (TEM)
transthoracic
    t. echocardiography (TTE)
    t. needle aspiration (TTNA)
    t. needle aspiration biopsy
    t. pacemaker
    t. pacing stylet
transtracheal
    t. aspiration
    t. oxygen catheter
transudate
transudative pleural effusion
transvalensis
    Nocardia t.
transvalvular
    t. aortic gradient
    t. flow
Transvene
    Medtronic T.
    T. nonthoracotomy implantable
      cardioverter-defibrillator
    T. tripolar electrode
Transvene-RV lead
transvenous
    t. aortovelography (TAV)
    t. defibrillator lead
    t. device
    t. electrode
transventricular mitral valve
  commissurotomy

transverse
    t. incision
    t. section of heart
    t. tubule
transversus
    situs t.
transxiphoid approach
tranylcypromine
trap-door approach
trapezius
    t. ridge sign
trapped gas volume
Trapper catheter exchange device
trapping
    air t.
TRAS
    transesophageal atrial stimulation
trash foot
Trasicor
Trasylol
Trates
Traube
    T. bruit
    T. double tone
    T. dyspnea
    T. heart
    T. murmur
    T. semilunar space
    T. sign
trauma
    blunt t.
traumatic
    t. aortic aneurysm
    t. aortic disruption
    t. aortography
    t. apnea
    t. asphyxia
    t. emphysema
    t. fistula
    t. heart disease
    t. pericarditis
    t. pneumonia
    t. rupture
    t. tamponade
    t. thrombosis
    t. thrombus

T

NOTES

Traveler
  T. portable oxygen system
  Pulmo-Aide T.
Travenol infusion pump
trazodone
  t. hydrochloride
Treacher Collins syndrome
treadmill
  arm ergometry t.
  t. echocardiography
  t. electrocardiogram
  exercise t.
  t. exercise stress test
  Marquette t.
  Q-Stress t.
  self-powered t.
  Tunturi Jogger-2 self-
    powered t.
treadmill-induced angina
treatment
  Albertini t.
  antianginal t.
  Brehmer t.
  DeBove t.
  Forlanini t.
  Frankel t.
  hypertension optimal t. (HOT)
  Koga t.
  McPheeters t.
  Nauheim t.
  nonpharmacologic measure
    of t.
  Nordach t.
  Oertel t.
  Schott t.
  stand-alone laser t.
  TheraPEP pre-respiratory
    therapy t.
  Tuffnell t.
Trecator-SC
Tredex bicycle
tree
  bronchial t.
  endobronchial t.
  tracheobronchial t.
tree-in-winter appearance
trefoil
  t. balloon
  t. balloon catheter
  t. Schneider balloon
tremor
  flapping t.

tremulus
  pulsus t.
trench lung
Trendar
Trendelenburg
  T. operation
  T. position
  T. test
trendscriber
Trental
trepidatio cordis
treponemal
  t. antibody
  t. test
Treponema pallidum
trepopnea
treppe
  negative t.
  t. phenomenon
  positive t.
TRI
  transient response imaging
triad
  acute compression t.
  adrenomedullary t.
  Andersen t.
  t. asthma
  Beck t.
  Cushing t.
  Fallot t.
  Grancher t.
  Hull t.
  Kartagener t.
  Osler t.
  Virchow t.
triadic junction
TRIADS
  time-resolved imaging by automatic
    data segmentation
trial
  T. of Antihypertensive
    Interventions and Management
    (TAIM)
  Antihypertensive Lipid
    Lowering Heart Attack T.
    (ALLHAT)
  Atenolol Silent Ischemia T.
    (ASIST)
  Australian Therapeutic T.
  Balloon versus Optimal
    Atherectomy T. (BOAT)
  BENESTENT t.

Canadian Amiodarone
  Myocardial Infarction
  Arrhythmia T. (CAMIAT)
Canadian Coronary
  Atherectomy T. (CCAT)
Canadian Coronary
  Atherosclerosis Intervention T.
  (CCAIT)
Cardiac Arrhythmia
  Suppression T. (CAST)
Coronary Angioplasty versus
  Excisional Atherectomy T.
  (CAVEAT)
Coronary Primary
  Prevention T. (CPPT)
Dutch Ibopamine
  Multicenter T. (DIMT)
Emory Angioplasty versus
  Surgery T. (EAST)
European Carotid Surgery T.
  (ECST)
Fluvastatin Long-Term
  Extension T. (FLUENT)
Grampian Region Early
  Anistreplase T. (GREAT)
Heparin Aspirin Reperfusion T.
  (HART)
T.'s of Hypertension
  Prevention (TOHP)
Leicester Intravenous
  Magnesium Intervention T.
  (LIMIT)
Multicenter Diltiazem Post-
  Infarction T. (MDPIT)
Multi-Hospital Eastern Atlantic
  Restenosis T. (M-HEART)
Multiple Risk Factor
  Intervention T. (MRFIT)
Nordic Enalapril Exercise T.
  (NEET)
North American Symptomatic
  Carotid Endarterectomy T.
  (NASCET)
randomized t.'s
Regionally Organized Cardiac
  Key European T. (ROCKET)
SAVE t.

Secondary Prevention
  Reinfarction Israeli
  Nifedipine T. (SPRINT)
Simvastatin/Enalapril Coronary
  Atherosclerosis Regression T.
  (SCAT)
Total Ischaemic Burden
  European T. (TIBET)
VA Symptomatic T.
triamcinolone
Triaminic
  T. AM Decongestant Formula
  T. Expectorant
triamterene
  hydrochlorothiazide and t.
triangle
  aortic t.
  axillary t.
  Burger scalene t.
  Calot t.
  cardiohepatic t.
  carotid t.
  clavipectoral t.
  Einthoven t.
  Gerhardt t.
  infraclavicular t.
  Jackson safety t.
  Koch t.
  t. of Koch
  Rauchfuss t.
  sternocostal t.
  subclavian t.
  Todaro t.
Triatoma infestans
triatrial heart
triatriatum
  cor t.
triaxial reference system
triazolam
trichinosis
trichlormethiazide
Trichosporon
Tri-Clear Expectorant
Tricodur
  T. Epi compression support
  bandage

T

NOTES

Tricodur *(continued)*
 T. Omos compression support
  bandage
 T. Talus compression support
  bandage
tricrotic
tricrotism
tricrotous
tricuspid
 t. atelectasis
 t. atresia
 t. incompetence
 t. insufficiency
 t. murmur
 t. opening snap
 t. position
 t. regurgitation (TR)
 t. restenosis
 t. stenosis
 t. valve
 t. valve annuloplasty
 t. valve annulus
 t. valve area
 t. valve closure sound
 t. valve disease
 t. valve doming
 t. valve flow
 t. valve prolapse
 t. valve vegetation
 t. valvular leaflet
 t. valvuloplasty
tricyclic antidepressant
Tridil
 T. injection
triethiodide
 gallamine t.
trifascicular block
Tri-flow incentive spirometry
trigeminal
 t. cough
 t. pulse
 t. rhythm
trigeminus
 pulsus t.
trigeminy
Trigger
 Smart T.
triggered
 t. activity
 atrial demand-t. (AAT)
 t. pacing
triglyceride level
triglyceride-rich lipoproteins (TRL)

triglycerides
 medium chain t.
 serum t.
trigone
Triguide catheter
Tri-Hydroserpine
Tri-Immunol
triiodothyronine
trilazad mesylate
trileaflet
triloculare
 cor t.
trilocular heart
trilogy
 T. DC, DR, SR pulse
  generator
 t. of Fallot
 Fallot t.
Trimadeau sign
trimazosin
Tri-Met apnea monitor
trimethaphan
 t. camsylate
trimethoprim
 t. sulfate
trimethoprim-sulfamethoxazole
 (TMP-SMX)
trimetrexate
 t. glucuronate
trimipramine maleate
Trimox
Trimpex
trinucleotide
 cytosine-thymine-guanine t.
triolet
 bruit de t.
Trios M pacemaker
Tripedia
tripelennamine
tripe palm
trip-hammer pulse
triphenyl
 T. Expectorant
triphenyl tetrazolium chloride
 (TTC)
triphenyltetrazolium staining method
triphosphatase
 adenosine t. (ATPase)
triphosphate
 adenosine t. (ATP)
 guanosine t. (GTP)
 inositol t.

purine nucleotides adenosine t.
uridine t.

triple
t. rhythm
t. stimulus
triple-balloon valvuloplasty
triple-bandpass filter
triple-humped pressure pulse
**triple-lumen balloon flotation
thermistor catheter**
triplets
tripolar
t. defibrillation coil electrode
t. lead
t. w/Damato curve catheter
**TriPort hemostasis introducer
sheath kit**
Trippi-Wells tongs
triprolidine
Tris-buffer infusion test
trisection
pulse t.
tris(hydroxymethyl)aminomethane
trisomy
t. 13, 18, 21
t. D syndrome
Triumph VR pacemaker
TRL
triglyceride-rich lipoproteins
Trocal
trocar
Axiom thoracic t.
B-D Potain thoracic t.
Bueleau empyema t.
Hurwitz thoracic t.
trochocardia
trochorizocardia
Troisier sign
troleandomycin
**TRON 3 VACI cardiac imaging
system**
trophic changes
trophoblastic tumor
tropical
t. endomyocardial fibrosis
t. pulmonary eosinophilia
tropomyosin

troponin C, I, T
trospectomycin sulfate
trough
t. dosing
t. level
peak and t.
systolic t.
X-descent t.
Y-descent t.
trough-and-peak levels
troughing
venous t.
trousers
air t.
MAST t.
military anti-shock t. (MAST)
pneumatic t.
Trousseau syndrome
**TR-R9 antithrombin receptor
polyclonal antibody**
Tru-Cut biopsy needle
true
t. aortic aneurysm
t. asthma
t. cyst
T. Form support stockings
t. vs. false aneurysm
aortography
true-negative test result
true-positive test result
TrueTorque wire guide
Truflex
trumpet
angel's t.
trunci (*pl. of* truncus)
truncoaortic sac
truncoconal area
truncus, pl. **trunci**
t. arteriosus
Trunecek
T. sign
T. symptom
trunk
bifurcation of pulmonary t.
t. forward flexion
Truphylline Suppository

T

NOTES

517

Trusler
T. aortic valve technique
T. rule for pulmonary artery banding
T. technique of aortic valvuloplasty
TruZone peak flow meter
Trypanosoma
T. *brucei*
T. *cruzi*
T. *gambiense*
T. *rhodesiense*
trypanosomiasis
American t.
trypsin
t., balsam peru, and castor oil
TSH
thyroid-stimulating hormone
TT
thromboplastin time
TTC
triphenyl tetrazolium chloride
TTC stain
TTE
transthoracic echocardiography
TTM
transtelephonic arrhythmia monitoring
TTNA
transthoracic needle aspiration
TTNB
transient tachypnea of newborn
TTP
thrombotic thrombocytopenic purpura
TTS catheter
TTT
tilt-table test
TU
TU complex
TU wave
Tubbs dilator
tube
AccuMark calibrated infant feeding t.
Aire-Cuf tracheostomy t.
American tracheotomy t.
Andrews-Pynchon t.
angled pleural t.
Argyle Sentinel Seal chest t.
Arm-a-Med endotracheal t.
Atkins-Cannard tracheal t.
Baylor cardiovascular sump t.

Bivona Fome-Cuff t.
Bivona TTS tracheostomy t.
Blue Line cuffed endotracheal t.
bronchial t.
Broncho-Cath double-lumen endotracheal t.
bulboventricular t.
Caluso PEG t.
Carabelli t.
Carden bronchoscopy t.
Carlens double-lumen endotracheal t.
Celestin esophageal t.
Charnley drain t.
Chaussier t.
chest t.
Chevalier Jackson tracheal t.
Cole pediatric t.
Cole uncuffed endotracheal t.
Cooley sump t.
cuffed endotracheal t.
cuffed tracheostomy t.
Deane t.
DIC tracheostomy t.
Doesel-Huzly bronchoscopic t.
double-lumen endobronchial t.
Dow Corning t.
Durham t.
endocardial t.
endotracheal t.
Endotrol endotracheal t.
Endotrol tracheal t.
Ewald t.
fenestrated tracheostomy t.
fluffy-cuffed t.
Fome-Cuf tracheostomy t.
Fuller bivalve trach t.
Gabriel Tucker t.
glutaraldehyde-tanned bovine collagen t.
Gore-Tex t.
Guisez t.
Haldane-Priestley t.
Hi-Lo Jet tracheal t.
Holter t.
Hyperflex tracheostomy t.
Jackson cane-shaped tracheal t.
J-shaped t.
Keofeed feeding t.
Kuhn t.
Lanz low-pressure cuff endotracheal t.

Laryngoflex reinforced endotracheal t.
Lennarson t.
Lepley-Ernst tracheal t.
Lindholm tracheal t.
Lo-Pro tracheal t.
Lore-Lawrence trachea t.
Luer tracheal t.
Mackler t.
Magill Safety Clear Plus endotracheal t.
Montgomery Safe-T-t.
Mosher life-saving tracheal t.
Mousseau-Barbin esophageal t.
Nachlas t.
nasogastric t.
nasotracheal t.
Olympus One-Step Button t.
oroendotracheal t.
Pitt talking tracheostomy t.
pleural t.
Polisar-Lyons tracheal t.
polyvinyl chloride t.
Portex Per-Fit tracheostomy t.
primordial catheter t.
Quinton t.
RAE endotracheal t.
right-angle chest t.
Ruschelit polyvinyl chloride endotracheal t.
Sandoz suction/feeding t.
Sarns intracardiac suction t.
scavenging t.
Sensiv endotracheal t.
Shiley tracheostomy t.
Softech endotracheal t.
Souttar t.
T t.
t. thoracostomy
thoracostomy t.
Thora-Klex chest t.
tight-to-shaft Aire-Cuf tracheostomy t.
UTTS endotracheal t.
Vacutainer t.
Vinyon-N cloth t.
Vivonex Moss t.

water-seal chest t.
wire-wound endotracheal t.
x-ray t.
Z-wave t.
TubeChek esophageal intubation detector
tuberculin
Koch t.
t. test
tuberculoid myocarditis
tuberculoma
tuberculosilicosis
tuberculosis (TB)
active t.
acute miliary t.
adult t.
aerogenic t.
anthracotic t.
atypical t.
avian t.
basal t.
t. of bones and joints
cerebral t.
cestodic t.
childhood t.
t. colliquativa
t. cutis
disseminated t.
extrapulmonary t.
exudative t.
hematogenous t.
hilus t.
t. indurativa
inhalation t.
t. of larynx
t. lichenoides
t. of lungs
t. miliaris disseminata
miliary t.
multidrug-resistant t. (MDR-TB)
Mycobacterium t.
open t.
oral t.
orificial t.
papulonecrotic t.
postprimary t.
primary t.

T

NOTES

tuberculosis *(continued)*
   productive t.
   pulmonary t.
   reactivation t.
   reinfection t.
   renal t.
   surgical t.
   tracheobronchial t.
tuberculostatic
tuberculous
   t. arteritis
   t. caseation
   t. chemotherapy
   t. empyema
   t. empyesis
   t. endocarditis
   t. laryngitis
   t. pericarditis
   t. pleurisy
   t. pneumonia
tuberoeruptive xanthoma
tuberous
   t. sclerosis
   t. xanthoma
Tubersol
tubing
   Teflon TFE SubLite Wall t.
tubocurarine
   t. chloride
tubular
   t. breath sounds
   t. necrosis
   t. respiration
tubule
   distal convoluted t.
   proximal convoluted t.
   transverse t.
tucker
   Cooley cardiac t.
   Crafoord-Cooley t.
Tucker bronchoscope
Tuffier test
Tuffnell treatment
tug, tugging
   tracheal t.
Tukey-Kramer posttest
Tukey test
tularemia
   oropharyngeal t.
tularemic pneumonia
tularensis
   Francisella t.

tumor
   t. blush
   carcinoid t.
   cardiac t.
   chromaffin cell t.
   clear cell t.
   craniopharyngeal duct t.
   t. embolism
   extrathoracic t.
   germ cell t.
   granular cell t.
   Hürthle cell t.
   t. marker
   mesenchymal-derived t.
   mesodermal t.
   migrated t.
   myxoma t.
   t. necrosis factor (TNF)
   neuroendocrine t.
   neurogenic t.
   papillary t.
   paraganglioma t.
   pericardiac t.
   phantom t.
   t. plop
   t. plop sound
   polycystic t.
   Purkinje t.
   Rathke pouch t.
   sarcomatous t.
   sugar t.
   teratoma t.
   thyroid t.
   trophoblastic t.
tumor, nodes, metastasis (TNM)
tumorogenic
tumultus cordis
tunic
   Bichat t.
   vascular t.
tunnel
   Kawashima intraventricular t.
   percutaneous t.
   subsartorial t.
tunneler
   CPI t.
   Crafoord t.
   Eidemiller t.
   Kelly-Wick vascular t.
   Oregon t.
Tunturi
   T. EL400 bicycle ergometer

T. Jogger-2 self-powered treadmill
Tuohy-Borst
 T.-B. adapter
 T.-B. introducer
tuple-1 gene
turbinate
turbulence
turbulent
 t. diastolic mitral inflow
 t. jet
turgor
 coronary vascular t.
 skin t.
Turner syndrome
Tusibron-DM
Tuss
 HycoClear T.
Tussigon
Tussionex
Tussi-Organidin DM NR
tussive
 t. fremitus
 t. squeeze
 t. syncope
Tuttle thoracic forceps
TV
 tidal volume
TVG
 time-varied gain
TVGC
 time-varied gain control
TWAR
 Taiwan acute respiratory
 TWAR agent
 TWAR disease
 TWAR pneumonia
Twee alternating cut-off compressor stockings
twiddler's syndrome
Twin
 Bennett T.
 T. Jet nebulizer
two-block claudication
two-bottle thoracic drainage system
two-chamber view
two-dimensional (2-D)

t.-d. echocardiography (2DE)
 t.-d. integrated backscatter
two-flight exertional dyspnea
two-flights-of-stairs claudication
two-patch technique
two-pillow orthopnea
two-stage
 ultrathin-walled t.-s. (UTTS)
two-step exercise test
two-turn epicardial lead
Tylenol
tympanitic sound
tympany
 bell t.
type
 t. A, B behavior
 Ambrose plaque t.
 cardioinhibitory t.
 cell t.
 t. 1, 2, 3, 4 dextrocardia
 t. I collagen telopeptide (ICTP)
 t. I glycogen storage disease
 t. I, II dip
 t. III procollagen
 t. II pneumocytes
typhoid
 t. fever
 t. pleurisy
 t. pneumonia
typhus
 African tick t.
 Queensland tick t.
 scrub t.
typical small cell
typing
 human lymphocyte antigen t.
Typ Vasocope III Doppler probe
tyramine
Tyrode solution
tyrosine
Tyshak
 T. balloon
 T. catheter
T-Y stent

T

NOTES

U

U loop
U sutures
U virus
U wave
U wave alternans
U wave inversion

ubiquinone
ubiquitin
UD-CG 212
UFCT
ultrafast computed tomography
UHFV
ultrahigh-frequency ventilation
Uhl

U. anomaly
U. disease
U. malformation
U. syndrome

ulcer

decubitus u.
diabetic u.
foot u.
peptic u.
stasis u.
venous u.

ulcerans

Mycobacterium u.

ulcerative endocarditis
ulcerogangrenous
ulceromembranous
ulcerosa

angina u.
pharyngitis u.

Uldall subclavian hemodialysis catheter
Ullmann syndrome
ULP

ultra-low profile
ULP catheter

ULR

guaifenesin, phenylpropanolamine, and phenylephrine

ultimum moriens
Ultracef
ultracentrifugation
UltraCision ultrasonic knife
Ultracor prosthetic valve

ultrafast

u. computed tomographic scanner
u. computed tomography (UFCT)
U. CT scanner

Ultraflex

U. esophageal stent system
U. self-expanding stent

ultrahigh-frequency ventilation (UHFV)
Ultraject prefilled syringe
ultra-low

u.-l. profile (ULP)
u.-l. profile fixed-wire balloon dilatation catheter

Ultra Low resistance voice prosthesis
ultrarapid subthreshold stimulation
Ultra-Select nitinol PTCA guidewire
ultrasonic

u. cardiography
u. nebulizer

ultrasonography

B-mode u.
compression u.
Doppler u.
duplex pulsed-Doppler u.
high-resolution B-mode u.
intracaval endovascular u. (ICEUS)

ultrasonoscope

Acuson XP-5 u.

ultrasound

ADR Ultramark 4 u.
Aloka u.
u. angiography
B-mode u.
cardiac u.
u. cardiography
colorvascular Doppler u.
continuous-wave Doppler u.
U. Contrast Microsphere
Doppler u.
duplex u.
echo-guided u.
gray-scale u.
u. holography
Interspec XL u.
Intertherapy intravascular u.

U

ultrasound *(continued)*
>   intracoronary u. (ICUS)
>   intraluminal u. (ILUS)
>   intravascular u. (IVUS)
>   Irex Exemplar u.
>   power Doppler u.
>   Shimadzu cardiac u.
>   u. transducer
>   VingMed u.

ultrasound-guided bronchoscopy
ultrastructure
Ultra-Thin balloon catheter
ultrathin-walled two-stage (UTTS)
ultraviolet laser
Ultravist
>   U. contrast
>   U. injection

umbilical
>   u. artery
>   u. tape
>   u. vein

umbilicalis
>   arteritis u.

umbrella
>   atrial septal defect u.
>   Bard Clamshell septal u.
>   Bard PDA u.
>   Clamshell septal u.
>   u. closure
>   double u.
>   u. filter
>   patent ductus arteriosus u.
>   PDA u.
>   Rashkind double u.
>   transcatheter u.

UMI
>   U. catheter
>   U. needle
>   U. transseptal Cath-Seal
>   catheter introducer

U-Mid-O₂ Jet Set
Unasyn
underdrive
>   u. pacing
>   u. termination

underperfused myocardium
undersensing
>   pacemaker u.

underwater seal drainage
undifferentiated
>   u. carcinoma
>   u. small cell carcinoma

undulating pulse

unequal pulse
Unicard
unicommissural
unidirectional block
Uni-Dur
**unifocal ventricular ectopic beat
  (UVEB)**
unilateral
>   u. emphysema
>   u. hyperlucency of the lung
>   u. nonfunctioning lung

Unilink
>   U. anastomotic device
>   U. system

Unilith pacemaker
unilocular cyst
Unipass endocardial pacing lead
Unipen
>   U. injection
>   U. Oral

Uniphyl
unipolar
>   u. connector
>   u. defibrillation coil electrode
>   u. electrocardiogram
>   u. Itrel 1 pulse generator
>   u. limb leads
>   u. Pisces Sigma
>   u. precordial lead

**UniPort hemostasis introducer
  sheath kit**
Unipres
Uni-Pro
Unisperse blue dye
Unistasis valve
unit
>   BCD Plus cardioplegic u.
>   BICAP u.
>   Biosound 2000 II
>   ultrasound u.
>   BiPAP u.
>   Bipolar Circumactive Probe
>   B u. (BICAP)
>   Collins Eagle I spirometry u.
>   coronary care u. (CCU)
>   digital fluoroscopic u.
>   ECG triggering u.
>   enhanced external
>   counterpulsation u.
>   FreeDop portable Doppler u.
>   Hounsfield u.
>   hybrid u.
>   intrapleural sealed drainage u.

kallidinogenase inactivator u.
kallikrein inactivating u.'s
  (KIU)
Karmen u.'s
Kreiselman u.
life change u.
LIZ-88 ablation u.
million international u.'s (MIU)
mobile coronary care u.
peripheral resistance u. (PRU)
R u.
Solcotrans autotransfusion u.
Sullivan nasal variable positive
  airway pressure u.
Surgitron u.
Todd u.'s
torr u.
Wood u.'s
United
  U. Network for Organ Sharing
    (UNOS)
  U. States Catheter &
    Instrument Company
  U. States Pharmacopeia (USP)
Uni-Tussin DM
Unity-C cardiac pacemaker
Unity VDDR pacemaker
univariate predictor
Univasc
Uni-Vent
univentricular
  u. atrioventricular connection
  u. heart
universalis
  adiposis u.
universal pacemaker
University
  U. of Akron artificial heart
  U. of Wisconsin solution
Uniweave catheter
Unna paste boot
UNOS
  United Network for Organ Sharing
unpaired *t* **test**
unroofed
Unschuld sign

unstable
  u. angina
  u. plaque
up
  pinked u.
uPA
  urokinase-type plasminogen
    activator
upgated technique
upgoing Babinski
upper
  u. airway obstruction
  u. lobe bronchus
  u. nodal extrasystole
  u. respiratory infection (URI)
UPPP
  uvulopalatopharyngoplasty
up-regulation
upright exercise
upstairs-downstairs heart
upstream airways
upstroke
  carotid u.
  diastolic u.
  u. pattern on apexcardiogram
    (dP/dt)
  u. velocity
uptake
  glucose u.
  I-123 MIBG u.
    iodine-123
      metaiodobenzylguanidine
      uptake
  iodine-123
    metaiodobenzylguanidine u.
    (I-123 MIBG uptake)
  lung u.
  maximum oxygen u.
  myocardial oxygen u.
  N-13 ammonia u.
  oxygen u.
uptake-1
  norepinephrine u.
uptake-mismatch pattern
urate
urea

U

NOTES

ureae
　　Actinobacillus u.
Urecholine
ureidopenicillin
uremia
uremic
　　u. pericarditis
　　u. pneumonitis
Uresil
　　U. embolectomy thrombectomy
　　　catheter
　　U. radiopaque silicone band
　　　vessel loops
urgency
　　hypertensive u.
URI
　　upper respiratory infection
uric acid
uridine triphosphate
urinary catheter
urine volume
Uri-Tet Oral
Urobak
urocanic acid
Urografin-76
urokinase
urokinase-type plasminogen activator
　　(uPA)
Uro-Mag
Uroplus DS
urticaria
　　aquagenic u.
　　pressure u.

USAFSAM treadmill protocol
USCI
　　USCI catheter
　　USCI Goetz bipolar electrode
　　USCI Hyperflex guidewire
　　USCI introducer
　　USCI NBIH bipolar electrode
　　USCI Probe balloon-on-a-wire
　　　dilatation system
　　USCI Sauvage EXS side-limb
　　　prosthesis
　　USCI shunt
use dependence
U-shaped catheter loop
USP
　　United States Pharmacopeia
ustus
　　Aspergillus u.
usurpation
Utah total artificial heart
UTTS
　　ultrathin-walled two-stage
　　　UTTS endotracheal tube
UVEB
　　unifocal ventricular ectopic beat
uvulopalatopharyngoplasty (UPPP)
uvulopalatoplasty
　　laser-assisted u. (LAUP)

V

    V lead
    V wave

V$_A$

    alveolar ventilation per minute

V$_D$

    physiological dead space ventilation
      per minute

V$_E$

    minute ventilation

V$_{MAX}$

    maximal velocity

V$_T$

    tidal volume

V510B Biplane TEE transducer
V5M Multiplane transducer
V-A

    ventriculoatrial
      V-A conduction
      V-A interval

VA

    variant angina
      VA Symptomatic Trial

VAC

    ventriculoatrial conduction

vaccae

    Mycobacterium v.

vaccine

    ActHIB v.
    diphtheria, tetanus toxoids, and
      acellular pertussis v.
    diphtheria, tetanus toxoids, and
      whole-cell pertussis v.
    diphtheria, tetanus toxoids, and
      whole-cell pertussis vaccine
      and haemophilus b
      conjugate v.
    haemophilus b conjugate v.
    HbOC v.
    Imovax v.
    inactivated poliovirus v.
    influenza virus v.
    lipopolysaccharide v.
    meningococcal v.
    pneumococcal v.
    PRP-D v.
    PRP-OMPC v.
    14-valent v.

vaccinia

Vac-Pak-II ultra-lite portable
** aspirator**
VACTERL

    vertebral, vascular, anal, cardiac,
      tracheoesophageal, renal, and limb
      anomalies
    VACTERL syndrome

Vacu-Aide
Vacutainer tube
vacuus

    pulsus v.

VAD

    ventricular assist device

vagal

    v. attack
    v. block
    v. body
    v. bradycardia
    v. escape
    v. neural crest
    v. reaction
    v. reflex
    v. response
    v. stimulation

vagolytic

    v. property

vagomimetic

    v. intervention

vagus

    v. arrhythmia
    v. nerve
    v. pneumonia
    v. pulse

Vairox high compression vascular
** stockings**
14-valent vaccine
vallecular dysphagia
Valley fever
Valleylab Force 2
Valsalva

    V. maneuver
    ruptured sinus of V.
    V. sinus, sinus of V.
    V. test

valsalviana

    dysphagia v.

value

    Astrup blood gas v.
    index v.
    JTc v.

V

value *(continued)*
  negative predictive v. (NPV)
  Pearson-Clopper v.
  predictive v.
  QRS-T v.
  reference v.
  resting v.
  tercile v.
Valugraph
  Mijnhard V.
valve
  abnormal cleavage of
    cardiac v.
  Abrams-Lucas flap heart v.
  Angell-Shiley bioprosthetic v.
  Angell-Shiley xenograft
    prosthetic v.
  Angiocor prosthetic v.
  aortic v.
  artificial cardiac v.
  atrial v.
  atrioventricular v.
  ball v.
  ball-cage v.
  ball-in-cage prosthetic v.
  ball-occluder v.
  Baxter mechanical v.
  Beall mitral v.
  Beall-Surgitool ball-cage
    prosthetic v.
  Beall-Surgitool disk
    prosthetic v.
  Bianchi v.
  Bicarbon Sorin v.
  Bicer-val prosthetic v.
  bicommissural aortic v. (BAV)
  bicuspid aortic v.
  bileaflet tilting-disk
    prosthetic v.
  Biocor prosthetic v.
  bioprosthetic heart v.
  bioprosthetic prosthetic v.
  Bio-Vascular prosthetic v.
  Björk-Shiley mitral v.
  Björk-Shiley monostrut v.
  Björk-Shiley prosthetic v.
  Blom-Singer v.
  bovine heart v.
  bovine pericardial v.
  Braunwald-Cutter ball
    prosthetic v.
  caged ball v.
  calcified aortic v.

  Capetown aortic prosthetic v.
  CarboMedics bileaflet prosthetic
    heart v.
  CarboMedics top-hat supra-
    annular v.
  cardiac v.
  Carpentier-Edwards mitral
    annuloplasty v.
  Carpentier-Edwards
    pericardial v.
  Carpentier-Edwards porcine
    prosthetic v.
  Carpentier-Edwards porcine
    supra-annular v.
  Carpentier pericardial v.
  C-C heart v.
  CirKuit-Guard pressure
    relief v.
  cleft mitral v.
  congenital anomaly of
    mitral v.
  Cooley-Bloodwell-Cutter v.
  Cooley-Cutter disk
    prosthetic v.
  Coratomic prosthetic v.
  crisscross atrioventricular v.
  Cross-Jones disk prosthetic v.
  Cross-Jones mitral v.
  cryopreserved homograft v.
  Cutter-Smeloff disk v.
  Cutter-Smeloff mitral v.
  DeBakey-Surgitool prosthetic v.
  v. debris
  Delrin heart v.
  diastolic fluttering aortic v.
  disk-cage v.
  Duostat rotating hemostatic v.
  Duraflow heart v.
  Duromedics mitral v.
  eccentric monocuspid tilting-
    disk prosthetic v.
  Edmark mitral v.
  Edwards-Duromedics bileaflet
    heart v.
  Edwards heart v.
  eustachian v.
  flail mitral v.
  flair v.
  floppy mitral v. (FMV)
  four-legged cage v.
  GateWay Y-adapter rotating
    hemostatic v.

glutaraldehyde-tanned bovine
heart v.
glutaraldehyde-tanned porcine
heart v.
Gott butterfly heart v.
Guangzhou GD-1 prosthetic v.
Hall-Kaster prosthetic v.
Hall prosthetic heart v.
Hancock modified orifice v.
Hancock porcine v.
Hans Rudolph nonbreathing v.
Hans Rudolph three-way v.
Harken ball v.
heart v.
Heimlich chest drainage v.
Heimlich heart v.
Hemex prosthetic v.
hemostasis v.
hockey-stick tricuspid v.
Hufnagel prosthetic v.
Ionescu-Shiley pericardial v.
Ionescu trileaflet v.
Jatene-Macchi prosthetic v.
Kay-Shiley caged-disk v.
Lillehei-Kaster pivoting-disk
prosthetic v.
Liotta-BioImplant LPB
prosthetic v.
Magovern-Cromie ball-cage
prosthetic v.
mechanical v.
Medtronic-Hall monocuspid
tilting-disk v.
Medtronic-Hall prosthetic
heart v.
Medtronic Intact v.
Medtronic prosthetic v.
MH v.
mitral v. (MV)
Mitroflow pericardial heart v.
Mitroflow pericardial
prosthetic v.
Monostrut Björk-Shiley v.
Montgomery speaking v.
native v.
noncalcified v.
Omnicarbon prosthetic heart v.

Omniscience tilting-disk v.
v. orifice area
parachute mitral v.
Passy-Muir tracheostomy
speaking v.
PEEP v.
Pemco prosthetic v.
porcine prosthetic v.
prosthetic aortic v.
prosthetic cardiac v.
Provox speaking v.
Puig Massana-Shiley
annuloplasty v.
pulmonary autograft v.
pulmonic v.
v. replacement
v. rupture
semilunar v.
Shiley convexoconcave heart v.
Shiley Phonate speaking v.
Singer-Blom v.
Smeloff-Cutter ball-cage
prosthetic v.
Smeloff heart v.
Sorin prosthetic v.
Starr-Edwards ball-and-cage v.
Starr-Edwards mitral v.
Starr-Edwards prosthetic v.
Starr-Edwards Silastic v.
Stellite ring material of
prosthetic v.
stentless porcine aortic v.
stent-mounted allograft v.
stent-mounted heterograft v.
St. Jude bileaflet prosthetic v.
St. Jude Medical bileaflet
tilting-disk aortic v.
St. Jude mitral v.
St. Jude prosthetic aortic v.
straddling atrioventricular v.
straddling tricuspid v.
Surgitool prosthetic v.
v. of Sylvius
Tascon prosthetic v.
thebesian v.
tilting-disk prosthetic v.
tissue v.

NOTES

valve *(continued)*
    top-hat supra-annular aortic v.
    toroidal v.
    Toronto SPV aortic v.
    tricuspid v.
    Ultracor prosthetic v.
    Unistasis v.
    Vascor porcine prosthetic v.
    v. vegetation
    v. of Vieussens, Vieussens v.
    Wessex prosthetic v.
    Xenomedica prosthetic v.
    Xenotech prosthetic v.
valvectomy
valvoplasty
valvotomy, valvulotomy
    aortic v.
    aortic v.
    balloon aortic v. (BAV)
    balloon mitral v. (BMV)
    balloon pulmonary v.
    balloon tricuspid v.
    double-balloon v.
    Inoue balloon mitral v.
    v. knife
    Longmire v.
    mitral balloon v. (MBV)
    mitral valve v.
    percutaneous mitral balloon v.
      (PMBV)
    repeat balloon mitral v.
    single-balloon v.
    thimble v.
valvular
    v. aortic stenosis
    v. calcification
    v. dysfunction
    v. endocarditis
    v. heart disease
    v. incompetence
    v. insufficiency
    v. orifice
    v. pneumothorax
    v. prolapse
    v. pulmonic stenosis
    v. regurgitation
    v. sclerosis
    v. thrombus
valvulitis
    aortic v.
    chronic v.
    mitral v.

rheumatic v.
    syphilitic aortic v.
valvuloplasty
    aortic v.
    bailout v.
    balloon v. (BV)
    balloon aortic v. (BAV)
    balloon mitral v. (BMV)
    balloon pulmonary v. (BPV)
    Carpentier tricuspid v.
    double-balloon v.
    intracoronary thrombolysis
      balloon v.
    mitral v.
    multiple-balloon v.
    percutaneous balloon aortic v.
    percutaneous balloon mitral v.
    percutaneous balloon
      pulmonic v.
    percutaneous mitral v. (PMV)
    percutaneous mitral balloon v.
      (PMBV)
    percutaneous transluminal
      balloon v.
    pulmonary v.
    single-balloon v.
    tricuspid v.
    triple-balloon v.
    Trusler technique of aortic v.
valvulotome
    Bakst v.
    bread knife v.
    Carmody v.
    Hall v.
valvulotomy *(var. of* valvotomy)
VAMC prognostic score
vampire bat plasminogen activator
van
    V. Andel catheter
    v. den Bergh disease
    v. Gieson stain
    V. Hoorne canal
    V. Slyke analysis
    V. Tassel angled pigtail
      catheter
vanadium
vanadiumism
Vancenase
    V. AQ Inhaler
    V. Pockethaler
Vanceril
    V. Oral Inhaler

Vancocin
    V. injection
    V. Oral
Vancoled injection
vancomycin
    v. hydrochloride
Vanex-LA
vanishing lung
Vansil
Vantin
Vaponefrin
vaporizer
    Cool-vapor v.
    Fluotec v.
    Israel Benzedrine v.
    Maxi-Myst v.
vapor massage
Vapor-Phase heated humidification system
vapotherapy
VAPS
    volume-assured pressure support
Vaquez disease
Varco thoracic forceps
variability
    baseline v.
    beat-to-beat v.
    cardiac v.
    heart rate v. (HRV)
variable
    v. coupling
    v. deceleration
    v. positive airway pressure (VPAP)
    v. threshold angina
variables
    impedance v.
    Newton law of motion and v.
variance
    analysis of v. (ANOVA)
    ball v.
    multivariate analysis of v. (MANOVA)
variant
    v. angina (VA)
    v. angina pectoris
    Miller Fisher v.

variation
    circadian v.
variceal
    v. ligation
    v. sclerosing
    v. sclerotherapy
varicella
    v. pneumonia
    v. zoster (VZ)
varicella-zoster
    v.-z. immunoglobulin (VZIG)
    v.-z. virus
varices (*pl. of* varix)
varicose
    v. vein
    v. vein stripping and ligation
varicosity
    saphenous vein v.
Variflex catheter catheter
variomatrix transducer
Vario system
variotii
    Paecilomyces v.
Varivas R denatured homologous vein graft
varix, pl. varices
    cirsoid v.
    downhill esophageal varices
    esophageal varices
VAS
    visual analogue scale
vasa vasorum
Vas-Cath catheter
Vascor
    V. porcine prosthetic valve
Vascoray
VascuClamp
    V. minibulldog vessel clamp
    V. vascular clamp
VascuCoil peripheral vascular stent
Vascu-Flo carotid shunt
vascular
    v. access catheter
    v. bed
    v. bundle
    v. cell adhesion molecule-1 (VCAM-1)

V

NOTES

vascular *(continued)*
  v. choir
  v. clamp
  v. clip
  v. compromise
  v. ectasia
  v. endothelial growth factor
    (VEGF)
  v. funnel
  v. gene transfer
  v. graft prosthesis
  v. groove
  v. hemostatic device (VHD)
  v. impedance
  v. incident
  v. injury
  v. insult
  v. markings
  v. murmur
  v. pattern
  v. peripheral resistance
  v. redistribution
  v. reflex
  v. resistance index
  v. ring
  v. ring division
  v. sclerosis
  v. sheath
  v. sling
  v. smooth muscle cells
    (VSMC)
  v. spasm
  v. spider
  v. stenosis
  v. stiffness
  v. tunic
  v. zone
vascularity
vascularization
vasculature
  pulmonary v.
vasculitis
  allergic v.
  Henoch-Schönlein v.
  hypersensitivity v.
  leukocytoblastic v.
  livedo v.
  necrotizing v.
  nodular v.
  pulmonary v.
  segmented hyalinizing v.
  systemic necrotizing v.

vasculocardiac
  v. syndrome of
    hyperserotonemia
vasculogenesis
vasculogenic impotence
vasculopathy
  allograft v.
  cardiac allograft v. (CAV)
  cerebral v.
  graft v.
  hypertensive v.
Vascushunt
Vascutek
  V. gelseal vascular graft
  V. knitted vascular graft
  V. woven vascular graft
Vaseretic
vasoactive
  v. drug
  v. intestinal peptides (VIP)
  v. mediator
vasoconstriction
  hypoxic pulmonary v. (HPV)
  pulmonary v.
vasoconstrictor
  v. center
  v. peptide
vasodepression
vasodepressor-cardioinhibitory
  syncope
vasodepressor substance
Vasodilan
vasodilation, vasodilatation
  coronary v.
  reflex v.
vasodilator
  v. agent
  v. center
  v. reserve
vasogenic
  v. edema
  v. shock
Vasoglyn
vasoinhibitor
vasomotion
  coronary v.
vasomotor
  v. angina
  v. paralysis
vasomotoria
  angina pectoris v.
vasopressin
  arginine v. (AVP)

vasopressin
  arginine v. (AVP)
vasopressor
  v. deficiency
  v. reflex
vasoregulatory asthenia
vasorelaxation
vasoresponse
vasorum
  aortic vasa v.
  vasa v.
VasoSeal vascular hemostasis device
vasospasm
  coronary v.
  ergonovine-induced v.
vasospastic angina
Vasotec
  V. I.V.
  V. Oral
vasotonic angina
vasovagal
  v. attack
  v. hypotension
  v. reaction
  v. syncope
  v. syndrome
Vasoxyl
VasPort
  Titanium V.
Vas recorder
VAT
  ventricular activation time
  VAT pacemaker
  VAT pacing
VATER
  vertebral defects, imperforate anus,
  transesophageal fistula, and radial
  and renal dysplasia
  VATER association syndrome
  VATER complex ·
VATS
  video-assisted thoracic surgery
Vaughan
  Singh-V. Williams
  antiarrhythmic drug
  classification
  Singh-V. Williams
  class effect
  Singh-V. Williams
  classification of arrhythmias

VC
  vital capacity
V/C
  ventilation-to-circulation
  V/C ratio
VCAM-1
  vascular cell adhesion molecule-1
VCDF
  volume-cycled decelerating-flow
  ventilation
VCF
  velocity of circumferential fiber
  shortening
VCG
  vectorcardiography
V-Cillin K Oral
VCO$_2$
  venous carbon dioxide production
VCV
  ventricular conduction velocity
VDD
  VDD pacing
  VDD pacing system
V-Dec-M
VDRL
  Venereal Disease Research
  Laboratories
  VDRL test
VEB
  ventricular ectopic beat
VE-cMRI
  velocity-encoded cine-magnetic
  resonance imaging
vector
  v. cardiography
  v. electrocardiogram
  instantaneous v.
  v. loop
  manifest v.
  mean manifest v.
  P v.
  QRS v.
  spatial v.
  ST v.
  T v.

V

NOTES

Veetids Oral
vegetal bronchitis
vegetation
  aortic valve v.
  bacterial v.
  endocardial v.
  leaflet v.
  prosthetic valve v.
  pulmonary valve v.
  tricuspid valve v.
  valve v.
  ventricular septal defect v.
vegetative
  v. endocarditis
  v. lesion
VEGF
  vascular endothelial growth factor
VeHF
  Veterans Heart Failure
  VeHF study
veiled puff
veiling glare
vein
  allantoic v.
  anomalous pulmonary v.
  autogenous v.
  axillary v.
  azygos v.
  basilic v.
  Boyd perforating v.
  brachial v.
  brachiocephalic v.
  cardiac v.
  cardinal v.
  cephalic v.
  common femoral v.
  coronary v.
  cryopreserved v.
  Dodd perforating v.
  external jugular v.
  facial v.
  femoral v.
  v. graft
  v. graft cannula
  v. graft ring marker
  hemiazygos v.
  hepatic v.
  human umbilical v. (HUV)
  iliac v.
  innominate v.
  internal jugular v.
  interventricular v.'s
  jugular v.

  left internal jugular v.
  levoatriocardinal v.
  Marshall oblique v.
  nest of v.'s
  omphalomesenteric v.
  portal v.
  profunda femoris v.
  pulmonary v.
  renal v.
  Retzius v.'s
  reverse saphenous v.
  saphenous v.
  sausaging of v.
  subclavian v.
  thebesian v.
  tortuous v.'s
  umbilical v.
  varicose v.
  ventricular v.
  vitelline v.
Veingard
  V. dressing
Velban
Velcro rales
Velex woven Dacron vascular graft
velocardiofacial syndrome
velocimeter
  FloMap v.
velocimetry
  Doppler v.
velocity
  aortic jet v.
  v. catheter technique
  v. of circumferential fiber
    shortening (VCF)
  conduction v.
  coronary blood flow v.
    (CBFV)
  ejection v.
  end-diastolic v.
  flow v.
  instantaneous spectral peak v.
  left ventricular outflow tract v.
  maximal v. (V_{MAX})
  peak A v.
  peak E v.
  peak systolic v.
  pulse wave v. (PWV)
  shortening v.
  time-averaged peak v.
  tracheal mucus v.
  translesional spectral flow v.
  upstroke v.

ventricular conduction v. (VCV)
velocity-encoded cine-magnetic resonance imaging (VE-cMRI)
velolaryngeal endoscope
velopharyngeal insufficiency
Velosef
Velosulin Human
velour collar graft
Velpeau hernia
vena
    v. contracta
vena cava, pl. **venae cavae**
    v.c. cannula
    v.c. clip
    foramen venae cavae
    inferior v.c. (IVC)
    v.c. obstruction
    Spencer plication of v.c.
    superior v.c. (SVC)
    v.c. syndrome
venacavogram
Vena Tech LGM filter
venectasia
Venereal Disease Research Laboratories (VDRL)
venereum
    lymphogranuloma v. (LGV)
VenES II Medical stockings
Venflon needle
venipuncture
venoarterial shunting
venoconstriction
venodilation
Venodyne external pneumatic compression System EPS-410
Venofit medical compression stockings
Venoflex medical compression stockings
Venoglobulin-I, -S
venogram
venography
    contrast v.
venolobar syndrome
venom
    arthropod v.

    bee v.
    black widow spider v.
    scorpion v.
    snake v.
    spider v.
veno-occlusive disease
venopressor
venorespiratory reflex
Venoscope
    Landry Vein Light V.
venosity
venostasis
venosum
    cor v.
venosus
    ductus v.
    pulsus v.
    sinus v.
venous
    v. access
    v. admixture
    v. cannula
    v. capacitance bed
    v. carbon dioxide production (VCO_2)
    v. collateral
    v. congestion
    v. Corrigan wave
    v. cutdown
    v. digital angiogram
    v. embolism
    v. engorgement
    v. flow measurement
    v. grooves
    v. heart
    v. hum
    v. hyperemia
    v. hypertension
    v. intravasation
    v. lakes
    v. mesenteric vascular occlusion
    v. murmur
    v. phase
    v. pressure
    v. pressure gradient support stockings

NOTES

V

venous *(continued)*
    v. pulse
    v. puncture
    v. return
    v. return curve
    v. runoff
    v. saturation
    v. sheath
    v. smooth muscle
    v. spasm
    v. spread
    v. stasis
    v. thromboembolism
    v. thrombosis
    v. troughing
    v. ulcer
    v. valvular insufficiency
    v. web
venous intravasation
venovenostomy
venovenous dye dilution curve
Ventaire
Ventak
    V. AICD pacemaker
    V. defibrillator
    V. ECD
    V. P3 AICD
    V. PRx defibrillation system
    V. PRx III/Endotak system
vented-electric HeartMate LVAD
ventilated alveoli
ventilation
    airway pressure release v. (APRV)
    alveolar v.
    artificial v.
    assist/control mode v.
    assisted v.
    v. bronchoscope
    v. collateralization
    continuous-flow v.
    continuous mandatory v.
    control-mode v.
    v. equivalent
    forced mandatory intermittent v. (FMIV)
    high-frequency v. (HFV)
    high-frequency jet v. (HFJV)
    high-frequency oscillatory v.
    high-frequency positive pressure v. (HFPPV)
    intermittent demand v. (IDV)

intermittent mandatory v. (IMV)
intermittent positive pressure v. (IPPV)
inverse-ratio v. (IRV)
v. mask
maximal v. (MV)
maximum voluntary v. (MVV)
mechanical v. (MV)
minute v. (V_E)
mouth-to-mouth v.
partial liquid v.
pressure-controlled inverse ratio v. (PCIRV)
pressure-regulated volume control v. (PRVC)
pressure support v.
proportional assist v. (PAV)
v. scintigraphy
split-lung v.
synchronized intermittent mandatory v. (SIMV)
v. threshold
time-cycled v.
ultrahigh-frequency v. (UHFV)
volume-cycled decelerating-flow v. (VCDF)
ventilation/perfusion (V/Q)
    v. defect
    v. imaging
    v. lung scan (V/Q lung scan)
    v. mismatch
    v. ratio
    v. relation
    v. scan
ventilation-to-circulation (V/C)
ventilator
    Adult Star 1010 v.
    Bear 1, 2 adult volume v.
    Bear Cub infant v.
    Bennett MA-1, PR-2 v.
    Bennett pressure-cycled v.
    Bio-Med MVP-10 pediatric v.
    Bird 8400STi v.
    Bird VDR v.
    blow-by v.
    Bourns-Bear I v.
    Bourns infant v.
    Critical Care V.
    cuirass v.
    v. dependency
    E-150 Breeze v.
    Hamilton v.

high-frequency jet v.
high-frequency oscillation v.
ICV-10 v.
Infrasonics v.
IVAC v.
v. management
MicroVent v.
Monaghan 300 v.
MVV v.
Ohio critical care v.
Pneumotron v.
pneuPAC v.
pressure v.
pressure-cycled v.
Puritan-Bennett v.
Searle volume v.
Sechrist IV-100 infant v.
Servo v. 300
Siemens v.
Smart Trigger Bear 1000 v.
v. time
Vix infant v.
volume v.
volume-cycled v.
Wave VM200 v.
v. weaning
ventilator-associated pneumonia
ventilator-induced
v.-i. pneumopericardium
v.-i. pneumothorax
ventilatory
v. capacity
v. equivalent
v. support
v. threshold
Venti mask
Ventolin
V. Nebules
V. Rotacaps
VenTrak respiratory mechanics monitor
ventricle
double-inlet v.
double-outlet left v.
double-outlet right v. (DORV)
hypoplasia of right v.

ischemic contracture of the
left v.
left v. (LV)
L-looping of the v.
Mary Allen Engle v.
right v. (RV)
single v.
suicide v.
volume-overloaded left v.
ventricular
v. aberration
v. activation time (VAT)
v. afterload
v. aneurysm
v. angiography
v. arrhythmia
v. assist device (VAD)
v. asynchronous pacemaker
v. bigeminy
v. biopsy
v. bradycardia
v. canal
v. capture
v. capture threshold
v. conduction
v. conduction velocity (VCV)
v. contour
v. contractility
v. couplet
v. demand-inhibited pacemaker
v. demand-triggered pacemaker
v. depolarization abnormality
v. diastole
v. diastolic pressure
v. dilation
v. distensibility
v. drive
v. ectopic beat (VEB)
v. ectopic systole
v. ectopy
v. effective refractory period
(VERP)
v. end-diastolic volume
v. endoaneurysmorrhaphy
v. end-systolic pressure-volume
relation
v. escape

V

NOTES

ventricular *(continued)*
  v. escape beat
  v. extrasystole
  v. fibrillation (VF)
  v. filling
  v. filling pressure
  v. flutter
  v. function
  v. function curve
  v. fusion beat
  v. geometry
  v. gradient
  v. hypertrophy
  v. inflow anomaly
  v. inflow tract obstruction
  v. inhibited pulse generator
  v. interdependence
  v. inversion
  v. mapping
  v. milk spots
  v. myxoma
  v. outflow tract obstruction
  v. pacing
  v. perforation
  v. performance
  v. plateau
  v. ponderance
  v. power
  v. preexcitation
  v. preload
  v. premature beat (VPB)
  v. premature complex (VPC)
  v. premature contraction (VPC)
  v. premature depolarization (VPD)
  v. pressure-volume loop
  v. pulse amplitude
  v. pulse width
  v. reentry
  v. relaxation
  v. remodeling
  v. response
  v. rhythm
  v. sensing configuration
  v. sensitivity
  v. septal defect (VSD)
  v. septal defect murmur
  v. septal defect vegetation
  v. septal rupture
  v. septum
  v. situs solitus
  v. standstill
  v. synchronous pulse generator
  v. systole
  v. tachyarrhythmia
  v. tachycardia (VT)
  v. tachycardia cycle length (VTCL)
  v. tachycardia/ventricular fibrillation (VT/VF)
  v. thrombus
  v. triggered pulse generator
  v. vein
  v. wall motion
  v. wall shortening
  v. wall stress
  v. wall thinning
  v. wave
ventricularization
ventricular-programmed stimulation
ventriculoarterial
  v. concordance
  v. coupling
  v. discordance
ventriculoatrial (V-A)
  v. conduction (VAC)
ventriculocyte
ventriculographic catheter
ventriculography
  biplane v.
  contrast v.
  equilibrium multigated radionuclide v.
  left v.
  quantitative left v.
  radionuclide v. (RNV)
  rest-exercise equilibrium radionuclide v.
  tomographic radionuclide v.
ventriculophasic
ventriculopuncture
ventriculoradial dysplasia
ventriculoscopy
ventriculoseptal defect (VSD)
ventriculotomy
  encircling endocardial v.
  partial encircling endocardial v.
Ventritex
  V. Cadence device
  V. Cadence ICD
  V. Cadence implantable cardioverter-defibrillator
  V. TVL system
Venture demand oxygen delivery device
Ventureyra ventricular catheter

Venturi
V. effect
V. forces
V. insufflator
V. jet adapter
V. mask
V. spirometer
V. Venti-mask Mark 2
V. wave
venule
VePesid
V. injection
V. Oral
vera
polycythemia v.
verapamil
v. hydrochloride
PPR v.
veratridine
Verbatim balloon catheter
Vercyte
Verelan
VeriFlex
V. cardiac device
V. guidewire
vermicular pulse
verminous
v. aneurysm
v. bronchitis
Vermizine
Vermox
vernal edema of lung
Vernet syndrome
Verneuil canal
veronii
Aeromonas v.
VERP
ventricular effective refractory
period
verruca, pl. **verrucae**
verrucosa
arteritis v.
Phialophora v.
verrucous
v. carcinoma
v. carditis
v. endocarditis

verruga peruana
Versacaps
Versatrax II 7000A pacemaker
Versed
versicolor
Aspergillus v.
Verstraeten bruit
vertebral
v. artery bypass graft
v. defects, imperforate anus,
transesophageal fistula, and
radial and renal dysplasia
(VATER)
v., vascular, anal, cardiac,
tracheoesophageal, renal, and
limb anomalies (VACTERL)
vertebrobasilar occlusive disease
vertical
v. heart
v. long-axis view
vertigo
laryngeal v.
very-low-density lipoprotein (VLDL)
vesicle
intermediary v.
vesicular
v. breath sounds
v. bronchiolitis
v. bronchitis
v. emphysema
v. murmur
v. rales
vesiculobronchial
vesiculobullous
vesiculocavernous respiration
vesnarinone
vessel
bouquet of v.'s
capacitance v.
v. clamp
collateral v.
conductance v.
coronary resistance v.
corrected transposition of the
great v.'s
v. dilator
feeder v.

V

NOTES

vessel *(continued)*
    femoral v.
    ghost v.
    great v.
    infarct-related v.
    intramyocardial prearteriolar v.
    v. lumen
    native v.
    v. occlusion system
    recruitable collateral v.
    renal blood v.
    resistance v.
    retinal v.
    splanchnic v.
    thoracic v.
    tortuous v.
    transposition of great v.'s
    (TGV)
Vessel-Clude
Vesseloops
    V. rubber band
Vesselpaw
VEST
    V. ambulatory nuclear detector
    V. ambulatory ventricular
    function monitor
    V. left ventricular function
    detector
vest
    Bremer AirFlo V.
    Mark VII cooling v.
    ThAIRapy v.
vestibular laryngitis
vestibule
    Sibson v.
vestigial fold
Veterans
    V. Administration Cooperative
    study
    V. Affairs Medical Center
    scoring system
    V. Heart Failure (VeHF)
VF
    ventricular fibrillation
V-Gan injection
VHD
    vascular hemostatic device
V-H interval
viability
    myocardial v.
Viagraph EKG system
Viamonte-Hobbs dye injector

Vibramycin
    V. injection
    V. Oral
Vibra-Tabs
vibration
    chest percussion and v.
    v. disease
vibrational angioplasty
Vibrio
    V. cholerae
    V. parahaemolyticus
vibrocardiogram
vicarious respiration
Vickers Ventimask Mark 2 mask
Vicks
    V. DayQuil Sinus Pressure &
    Congestion Relief
    V. 44D Cough & Head
    Congestion Relief
    V. Formula 44
    V. 44 Non-Drowsy Cold &
    Cough Liqui-Caps
Vicks 44E
Vicodin
Vicor pacemaker
video
    v. camera
    v. densitometry
    v. imaging
    v. loop
    v. monitor
    v. system
videoangiography
    digital v.
video-assisted
    v.-a. thoracic surgery (VATS)
    v.-a. thoracoscopic thymectomy
videodensitometry
videohydrothoracoscope
    Circon v.
videointensity
videotape recorder
Videx Oral
Vienna TAH
Vieussens
    circle of V.
    valve of V., V. valve
view
    apical four-chamber v.
    apical two-chamber v.
    Baltaxe v.
    caudocranial hemiaxial v.
    coned-down v.

craniocaudal v.
field of v. (FOV)
five-chamber v.
five-view chest x-ray with AP, PA, lateral, and both oblique v.'s
four-chamber v.
four-view chest x-ray with PA and lateral, and both oblique v.'s
hemiaxial v.
horizontal long-axis v.
ice-pick v.
laid-back v.
long axial oblique v.
long-axis v.
orthogonal v.
parasternal v.
parasternal long-axis v.
parasternal short-axis v.
RAO v.
sagittal v.
scout v.
short-axis parasternal v.
sitting-up v.
subcostal v.
suprasternal v.
swimmer's v.
two-chamber v.
vertical long-axis v.
weeping willow v.
view-aliasing artifact
Viggo-Spectramed catheter
vigilance response
Villaret syndrome
villosa
pericarditis v.
villosum
cor v.
Vim-Silverman needle
vinblastine sulfate
Vincasar PFS injection
Vincent angina
vincristine
v. sulfate
vindesine
Vineberg procedure

Vingmed
V. CFM-700
V. CFM 800 echocardiographic system
V. CFM 750 transducer
V. ultrasound
vinorelbine tartrate
vinyl chloride
Vinyon-N cloth tube
VIP
vasoactive intestinal peptides
Viper PTA catheter
viral
v. bronchiolitis
v. cardiomyopathy
v. hepatitis
v. myocarditis
v. pericarditis
v. pneumonia
v. respiratory infection
Virazole Aerosol
Virchow triad
viridans
Aerococcus v.
v. endocarditis
Streptococcus v.
Viringe vascular access flush device
virology
Virtis blender
virulence
virus
Amapari v.
Arenaviridae v.
Astroviridae v.
v. bronchopneumonia
CA v.
Calciviridae v.
Coe v.
Columbia S.K. v.
Coronaviridae v.
Coxsackie A, B, B3, B4 v.
Ebola v.
ECHO v.
enteric cytopathogenic human orphan virus
EMC v.
encephalomyocarditis v.

NOTES

V

virus *(continued)*
    enteric cytopathogenic human
        orphan v. (ECHO virus)
    Epstein-Barr v. (EBV)
    Filoviridae v.
    Hantaan v.
    herpes simplex v. (HSV)
    human immunodeficiency v.
        (HIV)
    human T-cell
        leukemia/lymphoma v.
        (HTLV)
    human T-cell lymphotropic v.
        (HTLV)
    Kotonkan v.
    Lassa v.
    Lipovnik v.
    Marburg v.
    Mayaro v.
    Muerto Canyon v.
    Orthomyxoviridae v.
    parainfluenza v.
    Paramyxoviridae v.
    Picornaviridae v.
    REO v.
    respiratory syncytial v. (RSV)
    Rift Valley fever v.
    Ross River v.
    Semliki Forest v.
    Sendai v.
    Sindbis v.
    syncytial v.
    Togaviridae v.
    U v.
    varicella-zoster v.
viscera (*pl. of* viscus)
visceral
    v. heterotaxy
    v. larva migrans
    v. peel
    v. pericardiectomy
    v. pericardium
    v. pleura
    v. pleurisy
visceroatrial
    v. situs
    v. situs solitus
**viscerobronchial cardiovascular
    anomaly**
viscerocardiac reflex
viscid mucus

viscometer
    Brookfield v.
    Ostwald v.
viscosity
    blood v.
viscous
viscus, pl. **viscera**
vise
    hemodynamic v.
    torque v.
Visicath endoscope
Visken
Visov test
Vista 4, T, TRS pacemaker
visual analogue scale (VAS)
visualization
    fluoroscopic v.
Vitacuff
Vitagraft
    V. arteriovenous shunt
    V. vascular graft
vital
    v. capacity (VC)
**Vital-Cooley microvascular needle
    holder**
Vitalograph
    V. pulmonary monitor
    V. spirometer
vitalography
Vitalometer test
Vitalor
    V. incentive spirometer
    V. screening pulmonary
        function test
**Vital-Ryder microvascular needle
    holder**
vitals
    tilt v.
**vitamin B, B_1, B_6, B_{12}, C, D, E,
    K**
vitamin K antagonist
Vita-Stat automatic device
Vitatron
    V. catheter electrode
    V. Diamond ICD
    V. Diamond pacemaker
    V. leads
vitelline vein
vitiligo
    symmetric v.
vitreous opacity
vitro
    in v.

vitronectin
Viva
    Air V.
Vivactil
Vivalan
Vivalith II pulse generator
vivo
    ex v.
    in v.
Vivonex
    V. Moss tube
    V. Plus nutritional supplement
Vix infant ventilator
VLDL
    very-low-density lipoprotein
Vmax
V. Mueller catheter
VO_2
    oxygen consumption
    oxygen consumption per minute
    peak exercise oxygen consumption
    volume oxygen consumption
    VO_2 max
vocal fremitus
vocational rehabilitation
Voda catheter
Vogt-Koyanagi-Harada syndrome
voice
    amphoric v.
    cavernous v.
    double v.
    eunuchoid v.
    hot potato v.
voix de polichinelle
Volkmann ischemic paralysis
Vollmer test
Volmax
volt
    electron v. (eV)
    kiloelectron v. (keV)
    megaelectron v. (MeV)
voltage
    Cornell v.
    v. criteria
    v. equilibrium
    Gubner-Ungerleider v.
    root-mean-square v.

    Sokolow-Lyon v.
    transmembrane v.
voltage-dependent
    v.-d. block
    v.-d. calcium channel
volume
    blood v.
    cardiac v.
    circulation v.
    compressible v.
    conductance stroke v.
    v. depletion
    v. of distribution
    dP/dt_{MAX}-end-diastolic v.
    effective circulating blood v.
    end-diastolic v. (EDV)
    end-systolic v. (ESV)
    expiratory reserve v. (ERV)
    forced expiratory v. (FEV)
    high lung v.
    inspiratory reserve v. (IRV)
    intravascular v.
    left ventricular end-diastolic v.
    left ventricular stroke v.
    v. load hypertrophy
    v. loading
    lung v.
    mandatory minute v. (MMV)
    maximal expiratory flow v. (MEFV)
    mean corpuscular v. (MCV)
    v. overload
    v. oxygen consumption (VO_2)
    plasma v.
    presystolic pressure and v.
    pulmonary blood v. (PBV)
    relative cardiac v.
    residual v. (RV)
    v. stiffness
    stroke v. (SV)
    v. thickness index (VTI)
    thoracic gas v. (TGV)
    tidal v. (TV, V_T)
    timed forced expiratory v.
    total blood v. (TBV)
    trapped gas v.
    urine v.

V

NOTES

volume *(continued)*
   v. ventilator
   ventricular end-diastolic v.
volume-assured pressure support (VAPS)
volume-challenge test
volume-cycled
   v.-c. decelerating-flow ventilation (VCDF)
   v.-c. ventilator
volume-overloaded left ventricle
Volumeter
   Drager V.
volume-time curve
volumetric infusion pump
volutrauma
von
   v. Claus chronometric method
   V. Lackum surcingle
   v. Recklinghausen disease
   v. Recklinghausen test
   v. Willebrand disease
   v. Willebrand factor
VOO
   V. pacemaker
   V. pacing
voodoo death
Voorhees bag
voxel gray scale
V-Pace transluminal pacing lead
VPAP
   variable positive airway pressure
VPB
   ventricular premature beat
VPC
   ventricular premature complex
   ventricular premature contraction
VPD
   ventricular premature depolarization
V/Q
   ventilation/perfusion
   V/Q defect
   V/Q lung scan

   V/Q mismatch
   V/Q quotient
VSD
   ventricular septal defect
   ventriculoseptal defect
   Eisenmenger VSD
   pinhole VSD
V-slope method
VSMC
   vascular smooth muscle cells
VT
   ventricular tachycardia
VTCL
   ventricular tachycardia cycle length
VTI
   volume thickness index
VT/VF
   ventricular tachycardia/ventricular fibrillation
vulgaris
   Proteus v.
vulnerable
   v. period
   v. phase
Vumon injection
V-Vac suction apparatus
VVD mode pacemaker
VVI
   V. pacemaker
   V. pacing
VVIR
   V. pacemaker
   V. pacing
VVI-RR pacing
VVI/VVIR pacing
V_1 to V_6 leads
VVT pacing
VZ
   varicella zoster
VZIG
   varicella-zoster immunoglobulin
VZV

Waardenburg syndrome
wafer
    Coloplast w.
waist
    cardiac w.
    w. of catheter
    w. of heart
waisting
    w. of balloon
Waldenström macroglobulinemia
Waldeyer tonsillar ring
Waldhausen subclavian flap
    technique
WALK
    Walking with Angina-Learning is
    Key
    WALK program
Walker-Murdoch wrist sign
walking
    w. pneumonia
    w. ventilation test
    W. with Angina-Learning is
    Key (WALK)
walk-through angina
wall
    w. amplitude
    anterior w. (AW)
    chest w.
    inferobasal w.
    lateral w. (LW)
    left ventricular w.
    w. motion
    w. motion abnormality
    w. motion analysis
    w. motion score
    w. motion score index
    (WMSI)
    w. motion study
    posteroseptal w.
    w. stress
    w. structure
    w. tension
    w. thickening
    w. thickness
Wallace Flexihub central venous
    pressure cannula
Wallstent
    W. flexible, self-expanding
    wire-mesh stent

Schneider W.
    W. spring-loaded stent
Walter Reed classification
wandering
    w. baseline
    w. goiter
    w. heart
    w. pacemaker
    w. pneumonia
Wangiella
Wang transbronchial needle
Ward-Romano syndrome
Wardrop method
warfarin
    w. sodium
    w. therapy
warmer
    blood w.
warm nodule
warm-up phenomenon
Warthin-Starry-staining bacilli
wash bath
washings
    bronchial w.
    bronchoalveolar w.
    bronchopulmonary w.
    w. and brushings
    lung w.
washout
    helium w.
    w. phase
    w. phenomenon
    thallium w.
Wasserman needle
Wasserman-positive pulmonary
    infiltrate
wasting
    potassium w.
    salt w.
    w. syndrome
watch-crystal fingernail
water
    w. brash
    extravascular lung w.
    w. retention
    w. wheel murmur
water-bottle heart
water-gurgle test
water-hammer pulse
Waterman bronchoscope

545

water-seal
    w.-s. chest tube
    w.-s. drainage
watershed
    w. infarct
    w. infarction
    w. region
Waterston
    W. extrapericardial anastomosis
    W. groove
    W. operation
    W. shunt
Waterston-Cooley procedure
watertight seal
waterwheel sound
Watson
    W. heart valve holder
    W. syndrome
watt-seconds
wave
    A w.
    a w.
    w. amplitude
    arterial w.
    atrial repolarization w.
    bifid P w.'s
    brain w.
    C w.
    c w.
    cannon a w.
    catacrotic w.
    catadicrotic w.
    c-v systolic w.
    D w.
    delta w.
    dicrotic w.
    diphasic P w.
    diphasic T w.
    E w.
    electrocardiographic w.
    E wave to A w. (E/A)
    f w.
    fibrillary w.'s
    fibrillatory w.
    flipped T w.
    flutter-fibrillation w.'s
    giant a w.
    giant v w.
    H w.
    inverted T w.
    J w.
    Osborne w.
    overflow w.

    P w.
    peaked P w.
    percussion w.
    peristaltic w.
    polymorphic slow w.
    postextrasystolic T w.
    precordial A w.
    pressure w.
    propagation of R w.
    pseudonormalization of T w.
    pulse w.
    Q w.
    QS w.
    R w.
    rapid filling w.
    recoil w.
    regurgitant w.
    retrograde P w.
    RF w.
    S w.
    sawtooth w.
    seismic w.
    sine w.
    ST w.
    ST-T w.
    T w.
    tidal w.
    TU w.
    U w.
    V w.
    venous Corrigan w.
    ventricular w.
    Venturi w.
    W. VM200 ventilator
    x w.
    y w.
    y descent w.
waveform
    Edmark monophasic w.
    Gurvich biphasic w.
    Lown-Edmark w.
    pressure w.
    quasi-sinusoidal biphasic w.
    spectral w.
wavelength
waveshape
wave-speed mechanism
wavy
    w. fiber
    w. respiration
wax-matrix technique
weakness
wean

weaning
> ventilator w.

Weavenit
> W. patch graft
> W. prosthesis

web
> esophageal w.
> laryngeal w.
> pulmonary arterial w.
> venous w.

Weber-Christian disease
Weber experiment
Weber-Janicki cardiopulmonary exercise protocol
Weber-Osler-Rendu syndrome
web-spacer
> C-bar w.-s.

Webster
> W. halo catheter
> W. orthogonal electrode catheter

Wedensky effect
wedge
> W. angiogram
> arterial w.
> ball w.
> w. biopsy
> w. excision
> mediastinal w.
> w. pressure
> w. pressure balloon catheter
> w. pulmonary angiography
> pulmonary artery w. (PAW)

weeping
> w. dermatitis
> w. willow view

Wegener granulomatosis
Weibel-Palade bodies
Wei-Lachin statistic
Weil disease
Weil-Felix reaction
Weill sign
Weinberg test
Weiss logarithmic method
Welcker method
well
> pericardial w.

well-differentiated carcinoma
Wenckebach
> W. atrioventricular block
> W. A-V block
> W. cycle
> W. period
> W. periodicity block
> W. phenomenon
> W. sign

Werlhof disease
Werner syndrome
Wernicke aphasia
Wesolowski vascular prosthesis
Wessex prosthetic valve
West
> W. of Scotland Coronary Prevention Study (WOSCOPS)
> W. syndrome

Westberg space
Westergren
> W. erythrocyte sedimentation rate
> W. method

westermani
> *Paragonimus w.*

Westermark sign
Western
> W. blot
> W. red cedar

Westminster drug-free protocol
Westrim LA
wet
> w. beriberi
> w. cough
> w. lung
> w. pleurisy
> w. rales
> w. swallow

Wexler catheter
Weyl test
wheal and flare
Wheatstone bridge
wheat weevil disease
wheeze
> asthmoid w.
> monophonic w.

NOTES

W

wheezing
bronchial w.
expiratory w.
wheezy
whiff test
whip
catheter w.
whipping
systolic w.
Whipple disease
whispered bronchophony
whispering
w. pectoriloquy
w. resonance
Whisper Mist humidifier
whistling rales
white
w. asphyxia
w. blood cell count
w. clot syndrome
w. lung
w. pneumonia
w. spot
w. sputum
W. system
w. thrombus
white-coat
w.-c. angina
w.-c. hypertension
Whitfield ointment
WHO
World Health Organization
whole
w. blood buffer base
w. blood cardioplegia
w. body hyperthermia
Wholey
W. Hi-Torque Floppy
guidewire
W. Hi-Torque modified J
guidewire
W. Hi-Torque standard
guidewire
whoop
systolic w.
whooping
w. cough
w. murmur
whorl motion
Wichmann asthma
Wickwitz esophageal stricture
Widal test

wide
w. complex rhythm
w. QRS tachycardia
Wideroe test
width
atrial pulse w.
pulse w.
ventricular pulse w.
Wiener filter
Wigle scale
Wigraine
Wiktor coronary stent
Wilcoxon rank sum test
Wilkie disease
Wilks lambda criterion
Wilks-Schapiro test
Willett-Stampfer method
William
W. Harvey arterial blood filter
W. Harvey cardiotomy
reservoir
W. test
Williams
W. cardiac device
W. phenomenon
W. sign
W. syndrome
W. tracheal tone
Williams-Campbell syndrome
Williamson sign
Willis
circle of W.
Willock respiratory jacket
Wilms thoracoplasty
Wilson
W. block
W. central terminal
W. disease
W. lead
Wilson-Cook papillotome
Wilson-Kimmelsteil disease
Wilson-Mikity syndrome
Wilson-White method
Wilton-Webster coronary sinus thermodilution catheter
Windkessel effect
window
acoustic w.
aortic w.
aorticopulmonary w.
aortic pulmonary w.
aortopulmonary w.
cycle-length w.

Hanning w.
imaging w.
Parzen w.
pericardial w.
pleuropericardial w.
pulmonary parenchymal w.
tachycardia w.
windowed balloon
windpipe
windsock
w. aneurysm
w. sign
winged baseplate
Winiwarter-Buerger disease
Winslow test
winter
w. bronchitis
w. cough
w. vomiting disease
Wintrich sign
Wintrobe sedimentation rate
wire (*See also* guidewire)
ACS microglide w.
Amplatz torque w.
atrial pacing w.
auger w.
central core w.
control w.
Cragg Convertible w.
Cragg FX w.
Cragg infusion w.
crenulated tantalum w.
curved J-exchange w.
delivery w.
Eder-Puestow w.
flow w.
w. guide
Hancock temporary cardiac
pacing w.
high-torque w.
Hi-Per Flex exchange w.
w. holder
w. insertion
J w.
J exchange w.
Katzen infusion w.
Killip w.

Linx extension w.
magnet w.
w. mesh self-expandable stent
RadiMedical fiberoptic pressure-
monitoring w.
rotablator w.
Sadowsky hook w.
Stertzer-Myler extension w.
Terumo m w.
tip-deflecting w.
wire-guided oval intracostal dilator
wire-loop lesion
wire-wound endotracheal tube
wiring
sternal w.
w. of sternum
Wirsung dilation
wiry pulse
Wiskott-Aldrich syndrome
Wizard
W. cardiac device
W. disposable inflation device
WMSI
wall motion score index
WOB
work of breathing
Wolff-Parkinson-White (WPW)
W.-P.-W. bypass tract
W.-P.-W. reentrant tachycardia
W.-P.-W. syndrome
Wolvek
W. sternal approximation
fixation instrument
W. sternal approximator
Womack procedure
wood
W. lamp
w. pulp worker's lung
W. units
W. units index
wooden resonance
wooden-shoe heart
Woodworth phenomenon
woody
w. edema
w. thyroiditis
Wooler-type annuloplasty

NOTES

W

woolsorter's pneumonia
work
    w. of breathing (WOB)
    w. capacity
    w. rehabilitation
    w. status
    stroke w.
    w. threshold
World Health Organization (WHO)
WOSCOPS
    West of Scotland Coronary
    Prevention Study
wound
    blowing w.
    bullet w.
    entrance w.
    exit w.
    gunshot w.
    knife w.
    stab w.
    sucking w.
woven
    w. coronary artery disease
    w. Dacron tube graft
    w. Teflon prosthesis

W pattern
WPW
    Wolff-Parkinson-White
wrap
    cardiac muscle w.
    no-phase w.
wrap-around ghosting artifact
wrapping
    aneurysm w.
Wright
    W. peak flow
    W. peak flow meter
    W. respirometer
    W. spirometer
    W. stain
Wrisberg ganglion
Wuchereria bancrofti
Wu-Hoak hypothesis
Wycillin injection
Wydora
Wymox
Wytensin

X

X axis
X wave of Ohnell

x

x depression
x descent
x wave

xamoterol
xanthelasma
xanthine

x. oxidase
x. oxidase reaction

xanthogranuloma
xanthoma

eruptive x.
palmar x.
planar x.
x. striatum palmare
x. tendinosum
tendinous x.
tuberoeruptive x.
tuberous x.

xanthomatosis
xanthomatous
Xanthomonas maltophilia
X-descent trough
Xe

xenon
133Xe

xenon-133
127Xe

xenon-127
XeCl

xenon chloride
XeCl excimer laser

XECT

xenon-enhanced computed
tomography

xenobiotic
xenodiagnosis
xenograft

bovine pericardial heart
valve x.
stentless porcine x.

Xenomedica prosthetic valve
xenon (Xe)

x. chloride (XeCl)
x. chloride excimer laser

x. lung ventilation imaging
x. washout technique

xenon-127 (127Xe)
xenon-133 (133Xe)
xenon-enhanced computed
tomography (XECT)
xenopi

Mycoplasma x.

Xenopus oocytes
Xenotech prosthetic valve
xenotransplant
Xeroform gauze
xerosis
xerotrachea
Xillix

X. ACCESS system
X. LIFE-Lung system

xinafoate

salmeterol x.

xipamide
xiphisternal

x. crunching sound
x. process

xiphisternum
xiphocostal
xiphodynia
xiphoid

x. angle
x. cartilage
x. process

xiphoiditis
X-linked

X.-l. dilated cardiomyopathy

XO syndrome
x-ray

babygram x.-r.
x.-r. beam filtration
chest x.-r.
x.-r. cine computed
tomography
x.-r. generator
Scanning-Beam Digital x.-r.
sinus x.-r.
x.-r. tube

X-Scribe stress test
XT cardiac device
X-Trode electrode catheter
XXXX syndrome
XXXY syndrome
Xylocaine

X

xylol pulse indicator
xylosoxidans
　Achromobacter x.
　Alcaligenes x.

XYZ lead system
X, Y, Z recordings

Y

Y axis
Y connector
Y stent

y

y depression of jugular venous pulse
y descent
y descent of jugular venous pulse
y descent wave
y wave
Y2B8 antibody
Yacoub and Radley-Smith classification
YAG
   yttrium-aluminum-garnet
   YAG laser
Yamasa assay kit
Yankauer
   Y. bronchoscope
   Y. pharyngeal speculum
Yates correction

yaws
Y-descent trough
Yeager formula
yellow
   y. cross
   y. fever
   Y. IRIS system
   y. nail syndrome
   y. sputum
Yentl syndrome
Yersinia
   Y. enterocolitica
   Y. pseudotuberculosis
YM 151
YM934
Yodoxin
yohimbine hydrochloride
Youden index
Youlten nasal inspiratory peak flow meter
Youman-Parlett test
Young syndrome
yuppie influenza

Z

Z band
Z line
Z point
Z stent

z

z point pressure
zabicipril
Zaditen
Zagam
Zahn

Z. lines
pockets of Z.
Zaire subtype
zalcitabine (ddC)
Zalkind lung retractor
Zang space
Zaroxolyn
Zartan
zatebradine
Zavala

Z. lung biopsy needle
Z. technique
Zavod bronchospirometry catheter
Zebeta
zebra artifact
ZEEP

zero end-expiratory pressure
Zefazone
Zener diode
Zenker diverticulum
Zenotech graft material
Zephrex
Zerit
zero

z. end-expiratory pressure
(ZEEP)
z. end-inspiratory pressure
zero-order kinetics
Zestoretic
Zestril
Ziac
zidovudine
Ziehl-Neelsen stain
zig-zag stent
Zilactin-L
zileuton
Zimberg esophageal hiatal retractor
Zimmer antiembolism support
stockings

Zimmermann arch
Zinacef

Z. injection
zinc

z. finger gene
z. fume fever
z. gelatin
Zinecard
ZIP

zoster immune plasma
zipper

Z. anti-disconnect device
z. scar
Zithromax

Z. Z-Pak
Z-Med catheter
ZOC

Seloken ZOC
Zocor
zofenopril
zofenoprilic acid
Zolicef
Zoll

Z. NTP noninvasive pacemaker
Z. PD1200 external
defibrillator
Zollinger-Gilmore intraluminal vein
stripper
zolpidem tartrate
zone

echo z.
Fraunhofer z.
Fresnel z.
H z.
protective z.
slow z.
subcostal z.
subendocardial z.
tendinous z.'s of heart
transitional cell z.
vascular z.
ZORprin
zoster

herpes z.
z. immune plasma (ZIP)
varicella z. (VZ)
Zosyn
Z-Pak

Zithromax Z-P.

Zucker
 Z. multipurpose bipolar
  catheter
 Z.-Myler cardiac device
Zuckerkandl bodies
Zutphen study

Z-wave tube
Zwenger test
Zydone
Zygomycetes
zygomycosis
Zyrtec

Anatomical Illustrations

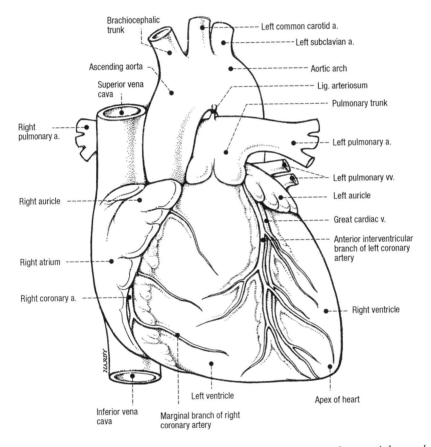

Figure 1. *Anterior view of the heart showing coronary arteries, auricles and great vessels.*

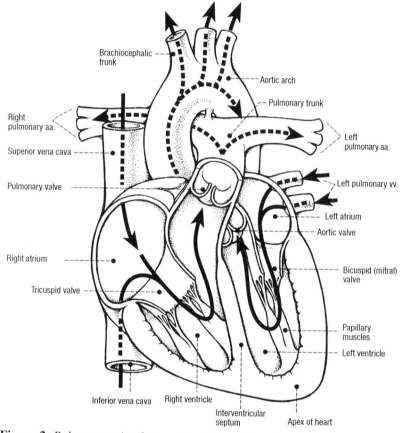

Figure 2. *Pulmonary circulation.* Blood circulation through the heart chambers and major vessels is shown.

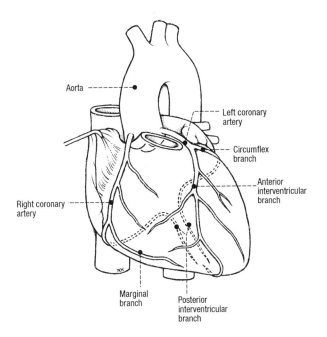

Aorta

Left coronary
artery

Circumflex
branch

Anterior
interventricular
branch

Right coronary
artery

Marginal
branch

Posterior
interventricular
branch

Figure 3. *Anterior view of the heart with coronary arteries.*

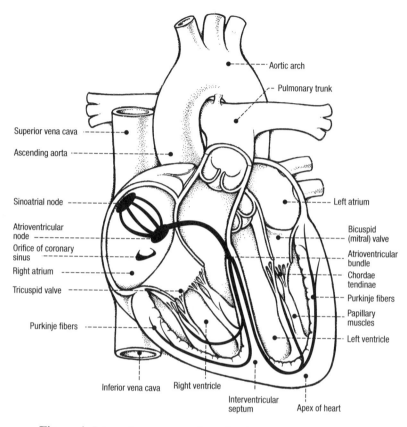

Figure 4. *Internal anatomy and conducting system of the heart.*

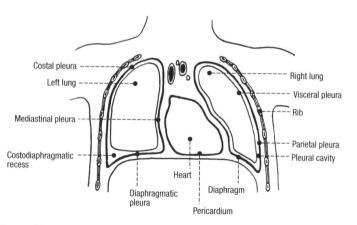

Figure 5. *Frontal section of thorax showing pleural relationships.* From Chung KW. Gross anatomy, 2nd ed. Baltimore: Williams & Wilkins, 1991.

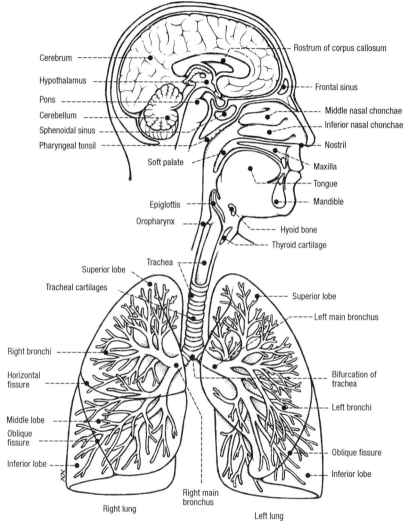

Figure 6. *Anterior (thorax) and mid-sagittal view (head) showing respiratory anatomy.*

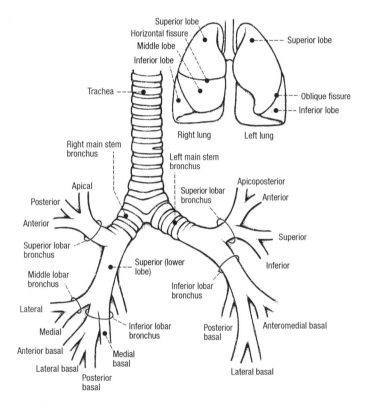

Figure 7. *Anterior view of trachea and bronchi with lobes of liver.*

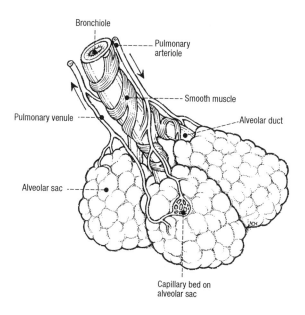

Figure 8. *Alveoli.* The flow of deoxygenated blood towards the alveolar sacs is shown. At the capillary beds they exchange carbon dioxide for oxygen before returning via the pulmonary venule to the heart.

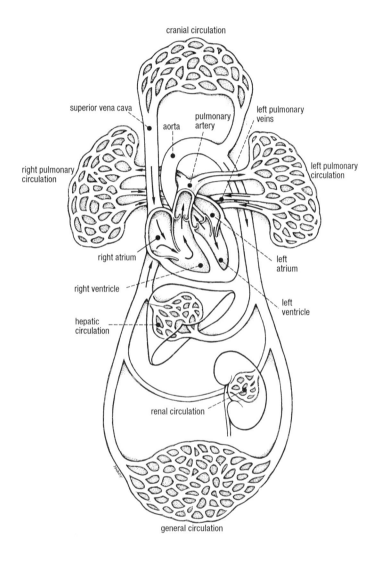

Figure 9. *Blood circulation.* During pulmonary circulation deoxygenated blood is pumped from the heart to the lungs where it exchanges carbon dioxide for oxygen before returning to the heart. Oxygenated blood leaves the heart via the great vessels and travels to the various parts of the body.

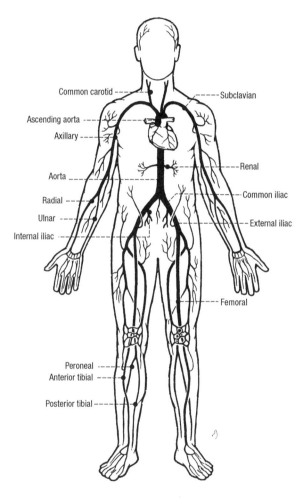

Figure 10. *Major arteries of the body.*

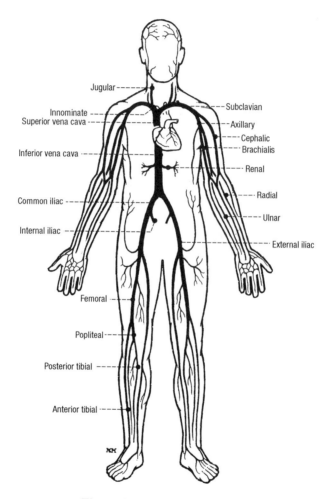

Figure 11. *Major veins of the body.*

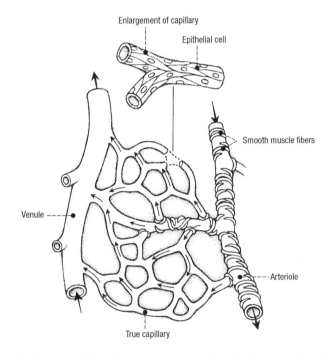

Figure 12. *Capillary bed.* The flow of oxygenated blood via the arteriole towards the capillaries is shown. Deoxygenated blood then returns to the heart via the venule.

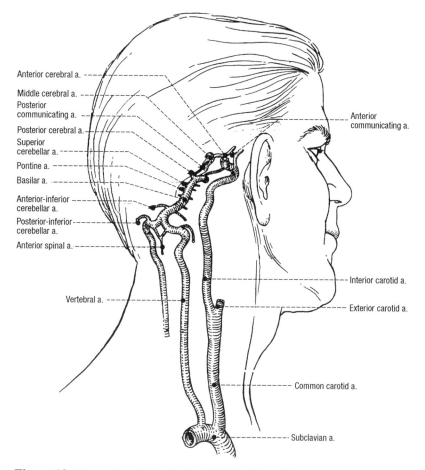

Figure 13. *Formation of the circle of Willis.* From Chung KW. Gross anatomy, 2nd ed. Baltimore: Williams & Wilkins, 1991.

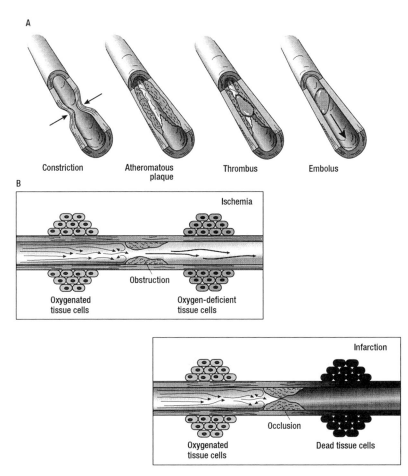

Figure 14. *Blood flow reduction.* A. Examples of conditions causing reduction of blood flow. B. Effects of reductions of blood flow. From Willis MC. Medical Terminology, Baltimore: Williams & Wilkins, 1996.

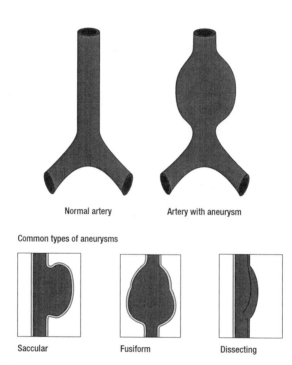

Normal artery   Artery with aneurysm

Common types of aneurysms

Saccular   Fusiform   Dissecting

Figure 15. *Common types of aneurysms.* From Willis MC. Medical Terminology, Baltimore: Williams & Wilkins, 1996.

Cardiology Drugs by Indication

Adams-Stokes Syndrome
Adrenalin
epinephrine
isoproterenol
Isuprel

Angina
acebutolol hydrochloride
Adalat
Adalat CC
amlodipine
atenolol
bepridil hydrochloride
Betachron E-R
Calan
Cardene
Cardene SR
Cardilate
Cardizem CD
Cardizem Injectable
Cardizem SR
Cardizem Tablet
Corgard
Dilacor XR
diltiazem
Duotrate
erythrityl tetranitrate
felodipine
Inderal
Inderal LA
Isoptin
Lopressor
metoprolol tartrate
nadolol
nicardipine hydrochloride
nifedipine
Norvasc
pentaerythritol tetranitrate
Peritrate
Peritrate SA

Plendil
Procardia
Procardia XL
propranolol hydrochloride
Sectral
Tenormin
Toprol XL
Vascor
verapamil hydrochloride
Verelan

Arrhythmias
amiodarone hydrochloride
Betachron E-R
Betapace Oral
bretylium tosylate
Bretylol
Calan
Cardioquin Oral
Cordarone
Crystodigin
digitoxin
digoxin
disopyramide phosphate
encainide hydrochloride
Enkaid
Ethmozine
flecainide
Inderal
Inderal LA
Isoptin
Lanoxicaps
Lanoxin
lidocaine hydrochloride
moricizine hydrochloride
Norpace
phenytoin
propafenone hydrochloride
propranolol hydrochloride
Quinaglute Dura-Tabs

Quinalan Oral
Quinidex Extentabs
quinidine
Quinora Oral
Rythmol
sotalol hydrochloride
Tambocor
tocainide hydrochloride
Tonocard
verapamil hydrochloride
Verelan
Xylocaine

Bradycardia
aminophylline
atropine sulfate
isoproterenol
Isuprel

Calcium Channel Blocker Toxicity
calcium gluceptate
calcium gluconate
Kalcinate

Cardiac Decompensation
dobutamine hydrochloride
Dobutrex Injection

Cardiac Ischemia
abciximab
ReoPro

Cardiogenic Shock
Crystodigin
digitoxin
digoxin
dobutamine hydrochloride
Dobutrex Injection
dopamine hydrochloride
Intropin Injection
Lanoxicaps
Lanoxin

Cardiomyopathy
Betachron E-R
Inderal

Inderal LA
propranolol hydrochloride

Cardiomyopathy (Drug-induced)
dexrazoxane
Zinecard

Cerebrovascular Accident (CVA)
Ticlid
ticlopidine hydrochloride

Claudication
pentoxifylline
Trental

Congestive Heart Failure
Alazine Oral
Altace Oral
amiloride hydrochloride
amrinone lactate
Apresazide
Apresoline Injection
Apresoline Oral
bepridil hydrochloride
bumetanide
Bumex
Capoten
Capozide
captopril
captopril and hydrochlorothiazide
Crystodigin
Demadex Injection
Demadex Oral
Deponit Patch
digitoxin
digoxin
dopamine hydrochloride
Dyrenium
enalapril
flosequinan
furosemide
hydralazine and hydrochlorothiazide
hydralazine hydrochloride

Hydrazide
Hy-Zide
Inocor
Intropin Injection
Lanoxicaps
Lanoxin
Lasix Injection
Lasix Oral
Manoplax
Midamor
milrinone lactate
Minipress
Minitran Patch
Nitro-Bid I.V. Injection
Nitro-Bid Ointment
Nitro-Bid Oral
Nitrocine Oral
Nitrodisc Patch
Nitro-Dur Patch
Nitrogard Buccal
nitroglycerin
Nitroglyn Oral
Nitrolingual Translingual Spray
Nitrol Ointment
Nitrong Oral Tablet
Nitropress
nitroprusside sodium
Nitrostat Sublingual
prazosin hydrochloride
Primacor
ramipril
torsemide
Transdermal-NTG Patch
Transderm-Nitro Patch
triamterene
Tridil Injection
Vascor
Vasotec I.V.
Vasotec Oral

Deep Vein Thrombosis (DVT)
dalteparin
enoxaparin sodium
Fragmin

heparin
Hep-Lock Injection
Liquaemin Injection
Lovenox Injection

Disseminated Intravascular Coagulation (DIC)
enoxaparin sodium
heparin
Hep-Lock Injection
Liquaemin Injection
Lovenox Injection

Ductus Arteriosus
Indocin I.V. Injection
indomethacin

Ductus Arteriosus (Temporary Maintenance of Patency)
alprostadil
Caverject Injection
Prostin VR Pediatric Injection

Embolism (Arterial)
enoxaparin sodium
heparin
Hep-Lock Injection
Liquaemin Injection
Lovenox Injection

Embolism (Myocardial)
Abbokinase Injection
Activase Injection
alteplase, recombinant
Anacin
anistreplase
Arthritis Foundation Pain Reliever
A.S.A.
Ascriptin
aspirin
Asprimox
Bayer Aspirin
Bayer Buffered Aspirin
Bayer Low Adult Strength

Bufferin
Coumadin
dicumarol
dipyridamole
Easprin
Ecotrin
Eminase
Empirin
enoxaparin sodium
Extra Strength Bayer Enteric 500
   Aspirin
Gensan
Halfprin 81
heparin
Hep-Lock Injection
Kabikinase
Liquaemin Injection
Lovenox Injection
Measurin
Persantine
Sofarin
St. Joseph Adult Chewable Aspirin
Streptase
streptokinase
urokinase
warfarin sodium
ZORprin

Endocarditis, Acute, I.V. Drug Abuse

Garamycin Injection
gentamicin sulfate
Jenamicin Injection
Lyphocin Injection
Vancocin Injection
Vancocin Oral
Vancoled Injection
vancomycin hydrochloride

Endocarditis, Acute Native Valve

Lyphocin Injection
Vancocin Injection
Vancocin Oral
Vancoled Injection
vancomycin hydrochloride

Endocarditis, Prosthetic Valve

Garamycin Injection
gentamicin sulfate
Jenamicin Injection
Lyphocin Injection
Vancocin Injection
Vancocin Oral
Vancoled Injection
vancomycin hydrochloride

Endocarditis, Subacute Native Valve

ampicillin
Garamycin Injection
gentamicin sulfate
Jenamicin Injection
Lyphocin Injection
Marcillin
Omnipen
Omnipen-N
penicillin g, parenteral, aqueous
Pfizerpen Injection
Polycillin
Polycillin-N
Principen
Totacillin
Totacillin-N
Vancocin Injection
Vancocin Oral
Vancoled Injection
vancomycin hydrochloride

Fibrillation (Atrial)

Betachron E-R
Cardioquin Oral
Cardizem CD
Cardizem Injectable
Cardizem SR
Cardizem Tablet
Crystodigin
digitoxin
digoxin

Dilacor XR
diltiazem
Inderal
Inderal LA
Lanoxicaps
Lanoxin
procainamide hydrochloride
Procan SR
Pronestyl
Pronestyl-SR
propranolol hydrochloride
Quinaglute Dura-Tabs
Quinalan Oral
Quinidex Extentabs
quinidine
Quinora Oral

Fibrillation (Atrial, Paroxysmal)
Calan
Cardioquin Oral
Isoptin
Quinaglute Dura-Tabs
Quinalan Oral
Quinidex Extentabs
quinidine
Quinora Oral
verapamil hydrochloride
Verelan

Fibrillation (Ventricular)
amiodarone hydrochloride
Anestacon
bretylium tosylate
Bretylol
Cordarone
Dermaflex Gel
Dilocaine
Duo-Trach
lidocaine hydrochloride
LidoPen
Nervocaine
Octocaine
procainamide hydrochloride
Procan SR

Pronestyl
Pronestyl-SR
propafenone hydrochloride
Rythmol
Xylocaine
Zilactin-L

Flutter (Atrial)
Betachron E-R
Calan
Cardizem CD
Cardizem Injectable
Cardizem SR
Cardizem Tablet
Crystodigin
digitoxin
digoxin
Dilacor XR
diltiazem
Inderal
Inderal LA
Isoptin
Lanoxicaps
Lanoxin
propranolol hydrochloride
verapamil hydrochloride
Verelan

Heart Block
Adrenalin
epinephrine
isoproterenol
Isuprel

Hemorrhage
Adrenalin
AlphaNine
Amen Oral
Amicar
aminocaproic acid
aprotinin
AquaMEPHYTON Injection
Avitene
Aygestin
cellulose, oxidized

Curretab Oral
Cycrin Oral
Depo-Provera Injection
Duralutin Injection
epinephrine
Estrovis
factor ix complex (human)
gelatin, absorbable
Gelfilm Ophthalmic
Gelfoam Topical
Gesterol Injection
Helistat
Hemotene
hydroxyprogesterone caproate
Hy-Gestrone Injection
Hylutin Injection
Hyprogest Injection
Konakion Injection
Konyne 80
medroxyprogesterone acetate
Mephyton Oral
microfibrillar collagen hemostat
Micronor
Mononine
norethindrone
Norlutate
Norlutin
NOR-Q.D.
Oxycel
phytonadione
Pro-Depo Injection
Prodrox Injection
Profilnine Heat-Treated
progesterone
Proplex T
Provera Oral
quinestrol
sodium tetradecyl sulfate
Sotradecol Injection
Surgicel
Thrombinar
thrombin, topical
Thrombogen

Thrombostat
Trasylol

Hemorrhage (Prevention)
Cyklokapron Injection
Cyklokapron Oral
tranexamic acid

Hypercholesterolemia
cholestyramine resin
Choloxin
Colestid
colestipol hydrochloride
dextrothyroxine sodium
fluvastatin
Lescol
Lorelco
lovastatin
Mevacor
Pravachol
pravastatin sodium
probucol
Questran
Questran Light
simvastatin
Zocor

Hyperlipidemia
Atromid-S
cholestyramine resin
Choloxin
clofibrate
Colestid
colestipol hydrochloride
dextrothyroxine sodium
Gemcor
gemfibrozil
Lopid
Lorelco
lovastatin
Mevacor
Niacels
niacin
Nicobid

Nicolar
Nicotinex
probucol
Questran
Questran Light
simvastatin
Slo-Niacin
Zocor

Hypertension

Accupril
acebutolol hydrochloride
Adalat
Adalat CC
Alazide
Alazine Oral
Aldactazide
Aldoclor
Aldomet
Aldoril
Altace Oral
amlodipine
amlodipine and benazepril
amrinone lactate
Apresazide
Apresoline Injection
Apresoline Oral
Arfonad Injection
atenolol
atenolol and chlorthalidone
benazepril hydrochloride
bepridil hydrochloride
Betachron E-R
betaxolol hydrochloride
Betimol Ophthalmic
Betoptic Ophthalmic
Betoptic S Ophthalmic
bisoprolol and hydrochlorothiazide
bisoprolol fumarate
Blocadren Oral
Brevibloc Injection
Calan
Cam-ap-es

Capoten
Capozide
captopril
captopril and hydrochlorothiazide
Cardene
Cardene SR
Cardizem CD
Cardizem Injectable
Cardizem SR
Cardizem Tablet
Cardura
carteolol hydrochloride
Cartrol Oral
carvedilol
Catapres Oral
Catapres-TTS Transdermal
chlorothiazide and methyldopa
chlorothiazide and reserpine
clonidine
clonidine and chlorthalidone
Combipres
Coreg
Corgard
Cozaar
diazoxide
Dilacor XR
diltiazem
Diupres-250
Diupres-500
Diutensin
doxazosin
DynaCirc
enalapril
enalapril and hydrochlorothiazide
Enduronyl
Enduronyl Forte
esmolol hydrochloride
Eutron
felodipine
fosinopril
guanabenz acetate
guanadrel sulfate
guanethidine monosulfate

guanfacine hydrochloride
H.H.R.
hydralazine and hydrochlorothiazide
hydralazine hydrochloride
hydralazine, hydrochlorothiazide, and
reserpine
Hydrap-ES
Hydrazide
hydrochlorothiazide and reserpine
hydrochlorothiazide and
spironolactone
hydroflumethiazide and reserpine
Hydro-Fluserpine
Hydropres
Hydro-Serp
Hydroserpine
Hylorel
Hyperstat I.V.
Hytrin
Hyzaar
Hy-Zide
Inderal
Inderal LA
Inderide
Inocor
Inversine
Ismelin
Isoptin
isradipine
Kerlone Oral
labetalol hydrochloride
lisinopril
Loniten
Lopressor
losartan and hydrochlorothiazide
losartan potassium
Lotensin
Lotrel
Marpres
mecamylamine hydrochloride
methyclothiazide and cryptenamine
tannates
methyclothiazide and deserpidine

methyclothiazide and pargyline
methyldopa
methyldopa and hydrochlorothiazide
metoprolol tartrate
Minipress
Minizide
Minodyl
minoxidil
moexipril hydrochloride
Monopril
nadolol
nicardipine hydrochloride
nifedipine
Nitropress
nitroprusside sodium
Normodyne Injection
Normodyne Oral
Norvasc
Ocupress Ophthalmic
pindolol
Plendil
prazosin and polythiazide
prazosin hydrochloride
Prinivil
Priscoline Injection
Procardia
Procardia XL
Proglycem Oral
propranolol and hydrochlorothiazide
propranolol hydrochloride
quinapril hydrochloride
ramipril
Renormax
reserpine
Rogaine
Salutensin
Salutensin-Demi
Sectral
Ser-A-Gen
Ser-Ap-Es
Serathide
Serpalan
spirapril

Spironazide
Spirozide
Tenex
Tenoretic
Tenormin
terazosin
timolol
Timoptic Ophthalmic
Timoptic-XE Ophthalmic
tolazoline hydrochloride
Toprol XL
Trandate Injection
Trandate Oral
Tri-Hydroserpine
trimethaphan camsylate
Unipres
Univasc
Vascor
Vaseretic 5–12.5
Vaseretic 10–25
Vasotec I.V.
Vasotec Oral
verapamil hydrochloride
Verelan
Visken
Wytensin
Zebeta
Zestril
Ziac

Hypertension (Arterial)
Levatol
penbutolol sulfate

Hypertension (Coronary)
Deponit Patch
Minitran Patch
Nitro-Bid I.V. Injection
Nitro-Bid Ointment
Nitro-Bid Oral
Nitrocine Oral
Nitrodisc Patch
Nitro-Dur Patch
Nitrogard Buccal

nitroglycerin
Nitroglyn Oral
Nitrolingual Translingual Spray
Nitrol Ointment
Nitrong Oral Tablet
Nitrostat Sublingual
Transdermal-NTG Patch
Transderm-Nitro Patch
Tridil Injection

Hypertension (Paroxysmal)
phentolamine mesylate
Regitine

Hypertriglyceridemia
Gemcor
gemfibrozil
Lopid
Niacels
niacin
Nicobid
Nicolar
Nicotinex
Slo-Niacin

Hypertrophic Cardiomyopathy
Adalat
Adalat CC
nifedipine
Procardia
Procardia XL

Hypoprothrombinemia
AquaMEPHYTON Injection
Konakion Injection
Mephyton Oral
phytonadione

Hypotension
Adrenalin
Aramine
dopamine hydrochloride
ephedrine sulfate
epinephrine

Intropin Injection
isoproterenol
Isuprel
Levophed Injection
metaraminol bitartrate
methoxamine hydrochloride
norepinephrine bitartrate
Vasoxyl

Ischemia

Cerespan Oral
Ethaquin
Ethatab
ethaverine hydrochloride
Ethavex-100
Genabid Oral
Isovex
papaverine hydrochloride
Pavabid Oral
Pavased Oral
Pavatine Oral
Paverolan Oral
pentoxifylline
Trental

Mitral Valve Prolapse

Betachron E-R
Inderal
Inderal LA
propranolol hydrochloride

Myocardial Infarction

Activase Injection
alteplase, recombinant
Anacin
anistreplase
Arthritis Foundation Pain Reliever
A.S.A.
Ascriptin
aspirin
Asprimox
atenolol
Bayer Aspirin
Bayer Buffered Aspirin
Bayer Low Adult Strength

Betachron E-R
Betimol Ophthalmic
Blocadren Oral
Bufferin
Corgard
Coumadin
dipyridamole
Easprin
Ecotrin
Eminase
Empirin
enoxaparin sodium
Extra Strength Bayer Enteric 500
    Aspirin
Gensan
Halfprin 81
heparin
Hep-Lock Injection
Inderal
Inderal LA
Kabikinase
Liquaemin Injection
Lopressor
Lovenox Injection
Measurin
metoprolol tartrate
nadolol
Persantine
propranolol hydrochloride
Sofarin
St. Joseph Adult Chewable Aspirin
Streptase
streptokinase
Tenormin
timolol
Timoptic Ophthalmic
Timoptic-XE Ophthalmic
Toprol XL
warfarin sodium
ZORprin

Myocardial Reinfarction

Anacin
Arthritis Foundation Pain Reliever

A.S.A.
Ascriptin
aspirin
Asprimox
Bayer Aspirin
Bayer Buffered Aspirin
Bayer Low Adult Strength
Betachron E-R
Betimol Ophthalmic
Blocadren Oral
Bufferin
dipyridamole
Easprin
Ecotrin
Empirin
Extra Strength Bayer Enteric 500
    Aspirin
Gensan
Halfprin 81
Inderal
Inderal LA
Lopressor
Measurin
metoprolol tartrate
Persantine
propranolol hydrochloride
St. Joseph Adult Chewable Aspirin
timolol
Timoptic Ophthalmic
Timoptic-XE Ophthalmic
Toprol XL
ZORprin

Organ Transplant
muromonab-CD3
Orthoclone OKT3
Prograf
tacrolimus

Pericarditis
Acthar
Adlone Injection
Amcort
A-methaPred Injection

Aristocort Forte
Aristocort Intralesional Suspension
Aristocort Tablet
Aristospan
Articulose-50 Injection
betamethasone
Celestone
Celestone Soluspan
Cortef
corticotropin
cortisone acetate
Cortone Acetate Injection
Cortone Acetate Oral
Decadron
Decadron Phosphate
Decaject
Decaject-LA
Delta-Cortef Oral
Deltasone Oral
depMedalone Injection
Depoject Injection
Depo-Medrol Injection
Depopred Injection
dexamethasone
Dexasone
Dexasone L.A.
Dexone
Dexone LA
D-Med Injection
Duralone Injection
Haldrone
Hexadrol
Hexadrol Phosphate
H.P. Acthar Gel
Hydeltrasol Injection
Hydeltra-T.B.A. Injection
hydrocortisone
Hydrocortone Acetate
Hydrocortone Phosphate
I-Methasone
Kenacort Syrup
Kenacort Tablet
Kenalog Injection

Key-Pred Injection
Key-Pred-SP Injection
LactiCare-HC
Liquid Pred Oral
Medralone Injection
Medrol Oral
methylprednisolone
Meticorten Oral
M-Prednisol Injection
paramethasone acetate
Pediapred Oral
penicillin g, parenteral, aqueous
Pfizerpen Injection
Predaject Injection
Predalone Injection
Predcor Injection
Predicort-50 Injection
Prednicen-M Oral
prednisolone
Prednisol TBA Injection
prednisone
Prelone Oral
Procort
Selestoject
Solu-Cortef
Solu-Medrol Injection
Solurex
Solurex L.A.
Sterapred Oral
Tac-3

Peripheral Vascular Disease (PVD)
Cyclan
cyclandelate
Cyclospasmol

Peripheral Vasospastic Disorders
Priscoline Injection
tolazoline hydrochloride

Persistent Fetal Circulation (PFC)
Priscoline Injection
tolazoline hydrochloride

Persistent Pulmonary Hypertention of the Newborn (PPHN)
Priscoline Injection
tolazoline hydrochloride

Persistent Pulmonary Vasoconstriction
Priscoline Injection
tolazoline hydrochloride

Pheochromocytoma
Betachron E-R
Demser
Dibenzyline
Inderal
Inderal LA
metyrosine
Minipress
phenoxybenzamine hydrochloride
phentolamine mesylate
prazosin hydrochloride
propranolol hydrochloride
Regitine

Pheochromocytoma (Diagnosis)
Catapres Oral
clonidine

Platelet Aggregation (Prophylaxis)
Anacin
Arthritis Foundation Pain Reliever
A.S.A.
Ascriptin
aspirin
Asprimox
Bayer Aspirin
Bayer Buffered Aspirin
Bayer Low Adult Strength
Bufferin
dipyridamole
Easprin
Ecotrin

Empirin
Extra Strength Bayer Enteric 500
   Aspirin
Gensan
Halfprin 81
Measurin
Persantine
St. Joseph Adult Chewable Aspirin
ZORprin

Polycythemia Vera
busulfan
mechlorethamine hydrochloride
Mustargen Hydrochloride
Myleran
pipobroman
Vercyte

Primary Pulmonary Hypertension (PPH)
epoprostenol sodium
Flolan Injection

Purpura (Thrombocytopenic)
Gamimune N
Gammagard S/D
immune globulin, intravenous
Oncovin Injection
Polygam S/D
Sandoglobulin
Venoglobulin-I
Venoglobulin-S
Vincasar PFS Injection
vincristine sulfate

Rheumatic Fever
Acthar
Adlone Injection
Amcort
A-methaPred Injection
Anacin
Argesic-SA
Aristocort Forte
Aristocort Intralesional Suspension
Aristocort Tablet

Aristospan
Artha-G
Arthritis Foundation Pain Reliever
Articulose-50 Injection
A.S.A.
Ascriptin
aspirin
Asprimox
Bayer Aspirin
Bayer Buffered Aspirin
Bayer Low Adult Strength
Beepen-VK Oral
betamethasone
Betapen-VK Oral
Bicillin C-R 900/300 Injection
Bicillin C-R Injection
Bicillin L-A Injection
Bufferin
Celestone
Celestone Soluspan
Cortef
corticotropin
cortisone acetate
Cortone Acetate Injection
Cortone Acetate Oral
Decadron
Decadron Phosphate
Decaject
Decaject-LA
Delta-Cortef Oral
Deltasone Oral
depMedalone Injection
Depoject Injection
Depo-Medrol Injection
Depopred Injection
dexamethasone
Dexasone
Dexasone L.A.
Dexone
Dexone LA
Disalcid
D-Med Injection
Duralone Injection

Easprin
Ecotrin
E.E.S. Oral
Empirin
E-Mycin Oral
Eryc Oral
EryPed Oral
Ery-Tab Oral
Erythrocin Oral
erythromycin
Extra Strength Bayer Enteric 500
   Aspirin
Gensan
Haldrone
Halfprin 81
Hexadrol
Hexadrol Phosphate
H.P. Acthar Gel
Hydeltrasol Injection
Hydeltra-T.B.A. Injection
hydrocortisone
Hydrocortone Acetate
Hydrocortone Phosphate
Ilosone Oral
I-Methasone
Kenacort Syrup
Kenacort Tablet
Kenalog Injection
Key-Pred Injection
Key-Pred-SP Injection
LactiCare-HC
Ledercillin VK Oral
Liquid Pred Oral
Marthritic
Measurin
Medralone Injection
Medrol Oral
methylprednisolone
Meticorten Oral
Mono-Gesic
M-Prednisol Injection
paramethasone acetate
PCE Oral

Pediapred Oral
penicillin g benzathine
penicillin g benzathine and procaine
   combined
penicillin v potassium
Pen.Vee K Oral
Permapen Injection
Predaject Injection
Predalone Injection
Predcor Injection
Predicort-50 Injection
Prednicen-M Oral
prednisolone
Prednisol TBA Injection
prednisone
Prelone Oral
Procort
Robicillin VK Oral
Salflex
Salgesic
salsalate
Salsitab
Selestoject
Solu-Cortef
Solu-Medrol Injection
Solurex
Solurex L.A.
Sterapred Oral
St. Joseph Adult Chewable Aspirin
Tac-3
V-Cillin K Oral
Veetids Oral
ZORprin

Stevens-Johnson Syndrome

Acthar
Adlone Injection
Amcort
A-methaPred Injection
Aristocort Forte
Aristocort Intralesional Suspension
Aristocort Tablet
Aristospan

Articulose-50 Injection
betamethasone
Celestone
Celestone Soluspan
Cortef
corticotropin
cortisone acetate
Cortone Acetate Injection
Cortone Acetate Oral
Decadron
Decadron Phosphate
Decaject
Decaject-LA
Delta-Cortef Oral
Deltasone Oral
depMedalone Injection
Depoject Injection
Depo-Medrol Injection
Depopred Injection
dexamethasone
Dexasone
Dexasone L.A.
Dexone
Dexone LA
D-Med Injection
Duralone Injection
Haldrone
Hexadrol
Hexadrol Phosphate
H.P. Acthar Gel
Hydeltrasol Injection
Hydeltra-T.B.A. Injection
hydrocortisone
Hydrocortone Acetate
Hydrocortone Phosphate
I-Methasone
Kenacort Syrup
Kenacort Tablet
Kenalog Injection
Key-Pred Injection
Key-Pred-SP Injection
LactiCare-HC
Liquid Pred Oral

Medralone Injection
Medrol Oral
methylprednisolone
Meticorten Oral
M-Prednisol Injection
paramethasone acetate
Pediapred Oral
Predaject Injection
Predalone Injection
Predcor Injection
Predicort-50 Injection
Prednicen-M Oral
prednisolone
Prednisol TBA Injection
prednisone
Prelone Oral
Procort
Selestoject
Solu-Cortef
Solu-Medrol Injection
Solurex
Solurex L.A.
Sterapred Oral
Tac-3

Syncope
Adrenalin
ammonia spirit, aromatic
Aromatic Ammonia Aspirols
epinephrine
isoproterenol
Isuprel

Tachycardia (Atrial, Paroxysmal)
Calan
Cardioquin Oral
Crystodigin
digitoxin
digoxin
edrophonium chloride
Enlon Injection
Isoptin
Lanoxicaps

Lanoxin
Quinaglute Dura-Tabs
Quinalan Oral
Quinidex Extentabs
quinidine
Quinora Oral
Reversol Injection
Tensilon Injection
verapamil hydrochloride
Verelan

Tachycardia (Supraventricular)

Brevibloc Injection
Calan
Cardioquin Oral
esmolol hydrochloride
Isoptin
procainamide hydrochloride
Procan SR
Pronestyl
Pronestyl-SR
Quinaglute Dura-Tabs
Quinalan Oral
Quinidex Extentabs
quinidine
Quinora Oral
verapamil hydrochloride
Verelan

Tachycardia (Supraventricular, Paroxysmal)

Adenocard
Adenoscan
adenosine
Calan
Cardioquin Oral
Cardizem CD
Cardizem Injectable
Cardizem SR
Cardizem Tablet
Dilacor XR
diltiazem

Isoptin
methoxamine hydrochloride
procainamide hydrochloride
Procan SR
Pronestyl
Pronestyl-SR
Quinaglute Dura-Tabs
Quinalan Oral
Quinidex Extentabs
quinidine
Quinora Oral
Vasoxyl
verapamil hydrochloride
Verelan

Tachycardia (Ventricular)

amiodarone hydrochloride
Betachron E-R
bretylium tosylate
Bretylol
Cordarone
encainide hydrochloride
Enkaid
Ethmozine
flecainide
Inderal
Inderal LA
isoproterenol
Isuprel
lidocaine hydrochloride
methoxamine hydrochloride
mexiletine
Mexitil
moricizine hydrochloride
procainamide hydrochloride
Procan SR
Pronestyl
Pronestyl-SR
propafenone hydrochloride
propranolol hydrochloride
Rythmol
Tambocor
Vasoxyl
Xylocaine

Tachycardia (Ventricular, Paroxysmal)
Cardioquin Oral
disopyramide phosphate
Norpace
Quinaglute Dura-Tabs
Quinalan Oral
Quinidex Extentabs
quinidine
Quinora Oral

Tetrology of Fallot
Betachron E-R
Inderal
Inderal LA
propranolol hydrochloride

Thrombolytic Therapy
Abbokinase Injection
Activase Injection
alteplase, recombinant
anistreplase
Eminase
Kabikinase
Streptase
streptokinase
urokinase

Thrombophlebitis, Suppurative
Lyphocin Injection
Vancocin Injection
Vancocin Oral
Vancoled Injection
vancomycin hydrochloride

Thrombosis (Arterial)
Kabikinase
Streptase
streptokinase

Thrombosis (Venous)
Coumadin
dalteparin
dextran

dicumarol
enoxaparin sodium
Fragmin
Gentran
heparin
Hep-Lock Injection
Liquaemin Injection
LMD
Lovenox Injection
Macrodex
Rheomacrodex
Sofarin
warfarin sodium

Tissue Graft
muromonab-CD3
Orthoclone OKT3

Transient Ischemic Attack (TIA)
Anacin
Arthritis Foundation Pain Reliever
A.S.A.
Ascriptin
aspirin
Asprimox
Bayer Aspirin
Bayer Buffered Aspirin
Bayer Low Adult Strength
Bufferin
Easprin
Ecotrin
Empirin
enoxaparin sodium
Extra Strength Bayer Enteric 500
   Aspirin
Gensan
Halfprin 81
heparin
Hep-Lock Injection
Liquaemin Injection
Lovenox Injection
Measurin
St. Joseph Adult Chewable Aspirin
ZORprin

Varicose Ulcers

Granulex
trypsin, balsam peru, and castor
   oil

Varicose Veins

Gelucast
morrhuate sodium
Scleromate
sodium tetradecyl sulfate
Sotradecol Injection
zinc gelatin

Vasoactive Intestinal Peptide-Secreting Tumor (VIP)

octreotide acetate
Sandostatin

Vascular Disorders

isoxsuprine hydrochloride
Vasodilan

Ventricular Contractions, Premature

acebutolol hydrochloride
Cardioquin Oral
disopyramide phosphate
encainide hydrochloride
Enkaid
lidocaine hydrochloride
mexiletine
Mexitil
Norpace
procainamide hydrochloride
Procan SR
Pronestyl
Pronestyl-SR
Quinaglute Dura-Tabs
Quinalan Oral
Quinidex Extentabs
quinidine
Quinora Oral
Sectral
Xylocaine

Common Terms by Procedure

Cardiac Catheterization Terms

angled pigtail catheter
angulation
aortic pullback pressure
aspirated and flushed
atherosclerotic aortic disease
atherosclerotic narrowing
atrioventricular node (AVN)
AVN — atrioventricular node
CABG — coronary artery bypass
  graft
CHD — coronary heart disease
cineangiogram
circumflex (CX)
CK — creatine kinase
coronary artery bypass graft (CABG)
coronary heart disease (CHD)
creatine kinase (CK)
CX — circumflex
diaphragm
digital compression
first obtuse marginal artery (OM-1)
flash-lamp excited pulsed dye
floppy guidewire
fluoroscopic visualization
fusiform aneurysm
global left ventricular ejection
  fraction
gradient
guidewire
GUSTO protocol
Hartzler dilatation catheter
Hemashield
hematoma
heparin
heparinized saline
iatrogenic atrial septal defect
Inoue balloon catheter
intraluminal

Judkins-Sones technique of cardiac
  catheterization
LAO — left anterior oblique
LAO position
late reperfusion
left anterior oblique (LAO)
left dominant coronary circulation
left internal mammary artery (LIMA)
left ventricle (LV)
left ventricular end-diastolic pressure
  (LVEDP)
LIMA — left internal mammary
  artery
LV — left ventricle
LVEDP — left ventricular end-
  diastolic pressure
millijoule (mJ)
mitral valve area (MVA)
mitral valve gradient (MVG)
mJ — millijoule
modified Bruce protocol
MVA — mitral valve area
MVG — mitral valve gradient
New York Heart Association
  (NYHA)
New York Heart Association
  classification
no-reflow phenomenon
NYHA — New York Heart
  Association
occlusion
OM-1 — first obtuse marginal artery
OM-2 — second obtuse marginal
  artery
opacify
ostial lesion
ostium
oxygen saturation

peak systolic aortic pressure (PSAP)
peak systolic gradient (PSG)
percutaneous mitral balloon
   valvotomy
percutaneous mitral valvuloplasty
   (PMV)
peripheral atherosclerotic disease
PMV — percutaneous mitral balloon
   valvuloplasty
port
projection
PSAP — peak systolic aortic pressure
PSG — peak systolic gradient
PSG pressure
pullback pressure
ramus intermedius artery
RAO — right anterior oblique
RAO angulation

RAO position
right anterior oblique (RAO)
scattergram
second obtuse marginal artery (OM-2)
sheath
side port
single-photon emission
sinus node (SN)
SN — sinus node
stenosis
technetium-99m imaging
thallium-201 stress test
thin-walled needle
thrombolytic agent
USCI catheter
venous sheath
visualization

Percutaneous Transluminal Coronary Angioplasty Terms

angioplasty
arterial sheath
ASC Alpha balloon
ASC RX perfusion balloon catheter
atheroblation laser
atrioventricular node (AVN)
AVN — atrioventricular node
balloon-centered argon laser
balloon pump
Baxter Intrepid balloon
CABG — coronary artery bypass
    graft
cardiac chamber
cardiac output
CHD — coronary heart disease
cinediagnostic
circumflex (CX)
CK —creatine kinase
coronary artery bypass graft (CABG)
coronary heart disease (CHD)
creatine kinase (CK)
CX — circumflex
excimer laser coronary angioplasty
    (ELCA)
first obtuse marginal artery (OM-1)
flash-lamp excited pulsed dye
floppy
fluorescence-guided "smart" laser
fraction
French JR4 Schneider catheter
French SAL catheter
French sheath
fusiform aneurysm
global left ventricular ejection
    fraction
Goodale-Lubin catheter
guider
guide wire
guiding catheter
Hadow balloon
Hartzler dilatation catheter

helium-cadmium diagnostic laser
Hemashield
hemiaxial view
high-flow catheter
Hi-Per Flex wire
Hi-Torque floppy with Propel
holmium laser
hot-tip laser probe
iatrogenic atrial septal defect
Inoue balloon catheter
intra-aortic balloon
intraluminal
intravascular ultrasound (IVUS)
introducer
IVUS — intravascular ultrasound
J-guide wire
JR4 catheter
JR5 catheter
Judkins-Sones technique
Kay balloon
laser
late reperfusion
left internal mammary artery (LIMA)
left ventricle (LV)
left ventricular end-diastolic pressure
    (LVEDP)
lens
LIMA — left internal mammary
    artery
Linx extension wire
LV — left ventricle
LVEDP — left ventricular end-
    diastolic pressure
manifold
MB fraction
Medi-Tech balloon catheter
millijoule (mJ)
mitral valve area (MVA)
mitral valve gradient (MVG)
mJ — millijoule
MVA — mitral valve area

MVG — mitral valve gradient
Mylar catheter
Nd:YAG laser —
  neodymium:yttrium-aluminum-
  garnet laser
Nestor-3 guiding catheter
New York Heart Association
  (NYHA)
New York Heart Association
  classification
NL3 guider
NoProfile balloon
no-reflow phenomenon
NYHA — New York Heart
  Association
occlusion
Olbert balloon
OM-1 — first obtuse marginal artery
OM-2 — second obtuse marginal
  artery
opacify
ostium
peak systolic aortic pressure (PSAP)
peak systolic gradient (PSG)
percutaneous mitral balloon
  valvotomy
percutaneous mitral balloon
  valvuloplasty (PMV)
Phantom guide wire
PMV — percutaneous mitral balloon
  valvuloplasty
probe
probe-patent graft
Propel
PSAP — peak systolic aortic pressure

PSG — peak systolic gradient
PSG pressure
pullback pressure
pump
radiocontrast dye
ramus intermedius artery
Rotablator
rotational ablation laser
sapphire lens
scattergram
second obtuse marginal artery (OM-2)
Seldinger technique
silk guide wire
single-photon emission
sinus node (SN)
Skinny balloon catheter
Slinky balloon
SN — sinus node
spectroscopy-directed laser
spirometer
stenosis
stenotic lesion
TEC — transluminal endarterectomy
  catheter
technetium-99m imaging
thallium-201 stress test
thrombolytic agent
tip-deflecting wire
Tissot spirometer
transluminal endarterectomy catheter
  (TEC)
ultrasound
USCI introducer
Zucker catheter

Carotid Endarterectomy Terms

anastomosis
angiography
ansa cervicalis
artcriotomy
backbleeding
backbled
bifurcation
blunt eversion carotid endarterectomy
carotid artery
carotid Doppler
carotid sheath
cerebral perfusion
common carotid artery
debris
ductus clamp
external jugular vein
facial vein
heparinization
hypoglossal nerve
internal carotid artery
internal jugular vein
intima
intimal flap

Javid clamp
Javid shunt
jugular vein
lingual artery
lumen
luminal narrowing
Model 40–400 Pruitt-Inahara shunt
plaque
platysma
protamine sulfate
reversible ischemic neurologic defect
  (RIND)
RIND — reversible ischemic
  neurologic defect
Rumel tourniquet
stenosis
stenotic lesion
sternocleidomastoid
superior carotid artery
superior thyroid artery
umbilical tape
vascular tape

Coronary Artery Bypass Graft Terms

anastomosed
anastomosis
Argyle chest tube
arterial inflow line
blood cardioplegia
body cooling
buttonhole openings
cardiopulmonary bypass
circumflex coronary artery
cross-clamp time
cross-clamped
Dexon suture
distal anastomoses
end-to-side
fibrillating
harvested
heparin
heparinized
hypothermia
iced slush
internal jugular vein
internal mammary artery
left ventricle
mediastinum

myocardial protection
obtuse marginal branch
partial occluding clamp
pericardial well
pericardium
posterior descending artery
protamine sulfate
radial artery line
reverse portion saphenous vein
right atrium
saphenous vein
Sewall technique
side-to-side
skin staples
stab wound incision
sternal wire sutures
sternotomy incision
sternum
Swan-Ganz catheter
temporary AV sequential pacer wires
venous outflow line
vent line
venting of air
weaned off bypass

Pulmonary Function Test Terms

ABG — arterial blood gas
arterial blood gas (ABG)
bronchospasm
bronchospastic component
carboxyhemoglobin
configuration
coving
diffusing capacity of lungs for carbon
  monoxide (DLCO)
DLCO — diffusing capacity of lungs
  for carbon monoxide
expiratory limb
FEF — forced expiratory flow
FEV_1 — forced expiratory volume in
  one second
FEV_1:FVC ratio - forced expiratory
  volume in one second to forced
  vital capacity ratio
flow volume loop
forced expiratory flow (FEF)
forced expiratory volume in one
  second (FEV_1)
forced expiratory volume in one
  second to forced vital capacity ratio
  (FEV_1:FVC ratio)
forced vital capacity (FVC)

FVC — forced vital capacity
hypoxemia
increment
large airway
lung mechanics
lung volume
maximum voluntary ventilation
  (MVV)
MVV — maximum voluntary
  ventilation
obstructive component
respiratory volume to total lung
  capacity ratio (RV:TLC)
respiratory volume (RV)
restrictive airways disease
restrictive lung disorder
RV — respiratory volume
RV:TLC ratio — respiratory volume
  to total lung capacity ratio
small airway
spirometry
supernormal
timed vital capacity (TVC)
TLC — total lung capacity
total lung capacity (TLC)
TVC — timed vital capacity

Flexible Fiberoptic Bronchoscopy Terms

acid-fast bacillus (AFB)
AFB — acid-fast bacillus
aspirate
aspiration
biopsy forceps
Bird ventilator
bronchial brushing
bronchial washing
brushings
cell button
culture and sensitivity
Cytobrush
cytology
endotracheal tube
flexible fiberoptic bronchoscope

fungus
Gram stain
high-flow oxygen
left apical posterior subsegment
left main stem bronchus
left side B6
lung biopsy
mucous plugging
right main stem bronchus
secretions
subsegment
suctioning
ventilation
washings

Appendix 4
Sample Reports

Sample Cardiac Catheterization with Left Ventriculography and Selective Right and Left Coronary Arteriography

TITLE OF OPERATION: 1) Left heart catheterization
2) Left ventriculography
3) Selective right and left coronary arteriography

PROCEDURE IN DETAIL: The patient was premedicated and taken to the cardiac catheterization laboratory where the right groin was prepped and draped in the usual sterile fashion. Local anesthesia was achieved using 1% lidocaine. The right femoral artery was cannulated with an 18-gauge thin-walled needle. A flexible guide wire was introduced into the right femoral artery and advanced to the level of the diaphragm under fluoroscopic guidance. A #7 French pigtail catheter was advanced over the guide wire to the level of the diaphragm under fluoroscopy. Heparin was then administered. Aortic pressure was recorded and a sample obtained for oxygen saturation study. The catheter was then carefully advanced across the aortic valve and into the left ventricular cavity where pressure was again documented. Left ventriculography was performed in both RAO and LAO projections. After left ventriculography, left ventricular end-diastolic pressure was recorded as well as aortic pressure after careful pullback demonstrated there was no aortic valvular gradient. The catheter was withdrawn and exchanged for a #7 French JL4 left coronary catheter which was advanced over the guide wire, aspirated, and flushed. The catheter was then carefully advanced through the left coronary ostium and selective left coronary arteriography was performed and documented in multiple projections. After adequate visualization of the left coronary system, the catheter was withdrawn and exchanged for a #7 French JR4 coronary catheter. The catheter was exchanged, advanced, aspirated, and flushed in similar fashion. The catheter was then used for right coronary visualization, and carefully advanced to the right coronary ostium where right coronary arteriography was performed in several projections. The catheter was then withdrawn as was the vascular sheath and protamine sulfate was administered IV. Hemostasis was achieved by digital compression. There was no hematoma and the distal pulses were all intact at the conclusion of the study. The patient left the cardiac catheterization laboratory in satisfactory condition.

Sample Percutaneous Coronary Artery Angioplasty

TITLE OF OPERATION: Percutaneous Coronary Artery Angioplasty

PROCEDURE IN DETAIL: Using local Xylocaine anesthesia and the percutaneous technique, a #8 French USCI dilator with sheath was placed into the right femoral vein. Subsequently a #7 French Zucker catheter was inserted into the venous sheath and advanced into the main pulmonary artery. The Zucker catheter was checked for pacemaker purposes in the right ventricle. Next, using local Xylocaine anesthesia and the Seldinger technique, a #8 French USCI dilator with sheath was placed into the right femoral artery. A #8 French USCI size 4 left coronary artery catheter was inserted into the femoral arterial sheath and advanced to the ostium of the left coronary artery. Multiple cinediagnostic angiograms of the left coronary artery were performed. A #2.5 French USCI balloon angioplasty catheter was inserted into the femoral guide catheter and advanced across the obstruction in the circumflex coronary artery. After multiple low-pressure inflations the obstruction was reduced to less than 15%, and the patient was doing well. The catheters and sheaths were removed and hemostasis achieved by means of digital pressure. Both right and left distal pulses were intact at the conclusion of the procedure. The patient was sent to the recovery room in satisfactory condition.

Sample Carotid Endarterectomy

TITLE OF OPERATION: Right carotid endarterectomy

PROCEDURE IN DETAIL: The patient was taken to the operating room where satisfactory general orotracheal anesthesia was obtained and the patient was prepped and draped in the usual fashion. A right longitudinal neck incision was made and carried down through the platysma muscles. The anterior border of the sternocleidomastoid muscle and internal jugular vein were dissected free. The transverse facial vein was taken down between clamps and ligated. The common carotid, internal carotid, and external carotid arteries were then dissected free and encircled with vascular tapes. Systemic heparinization was accomplished by administering 5000 units of intravenous heparin. Approximately five minutes later, ductus clamps were placed, first on the external carotid, and then on the common carotid. Occlusion of the lingual artery as well as the superior artery of the thyroid was performed. An arteriotomy was performed in the lateral aspect of the common carotid artery all the way up to the internal carotid artery, passing beyond the point where arteriosclerotic plaque was present. Beyond this point, nice smooth artery was visualized. The occluded area revealed about 90% stenosis of the bifurcation by an ulcerated plaque with a great deal of associated debris. Passing beyond the plaque, a Javid clamp was inserted in the usual manner, and upon release of the clamp, flow was reestablished into the internal carotid through the Javid shunt. An arteriotomy was then carried out, completely cleaning out the bifurcation as well as the internal and external carotid arteries. The arteriotomy was closed using a continuous running 6–0 Prolene suture. Initial suturing was performed by using the Javid shunt as a stent. Upon finishing half the suture line, the shunt was removed and the remainder of the arteriotomy was closed with the same suture material. Blood-tight anastomosis was achieved at the end of the procedure. The heparin was reversed by the administration of protamine and the wound closed in the usual fashion using a continuous running stitch of 3–0 Dexon to approximate the fascia and continuous running stitch of 4–0 nylon for the skin. The patient was transferred to the recovery room in good condition.

Sample Coronary Artery Bypass Graft

TITLE OF OPERATION: Coronary Artery Bypass Graft x Four, Using Reverse Saphenous Vein and Left Internal Mammary Artery

PROCEDURE IN DETAIL: The patient was anesthetized, adequately prepped and draped. The anesthesiologist placed a right radial artery monitor line and a Swan-Ganz catheter to the right internal jugular vein. The chest was opened through a midline sternotomy incision. The left internal mammary artery was dissected by means of the Sewall technique. The saphenous vein for bypass purposes was harvested from the right leg. The pericardium was opened and a pericardial well created. The patient was heparinized. An arterial inflow line was introduced through the ascending aorta, a venous outflow line through the right atrium, and the left ventricle was entered through the right superior pulmonary vein. The patient was then placed on cardiopulmonary bypass and with the heart fibrillating, the ascending aorta was cross-clamped. Blood cardioplegia myocardial protection with iced slush was instituted. Using the reverse portion of the saphenous vein, three distal anastomoses were accomplished between this vein and the diagonal coronary, the obtuse marginal #2 of the circumflex coronary artery, and the posterior descending right coronary artery. The left internal mammary artery was then anastomosed end-to-side to the left anterior descending coronary artery. Following completion of all distal anastomoses, the cross-clamp was released and a partial occluding clamp was placed on the ascending aorta. Three buttonhole openings were made in the ascending aorta and the three proximal anastomoses were accomplished between the vein grafts and the ascending aorta. Air was next vented from the vein grafts and flow was reestablished through the newly created saphenous vein bypass grafts. The patient was then weaned successfully off cardiopulmonary bypass. The left ventricular vent line was removed as were the venous outflow lines and the arterial inflow lines. Heparin was reversed by the administration of protamine sulfate. The mediastinum and left chest were then drained with Argyle chest tubes which were brought out through separate stab wound incisions. The wound was closed in layers. The sternum was approximated with buried sternal wire sutures, subcutaneous tissues with Dexon sutures, and the skin with skin staples. The leg incision was likewise closed in layers, subcutaneous tissues with 2–0 Dexon sutures and the skin with skin staples. Temporary AV sequential pacer wires had been placed in the right atrium and were brought out through separate stab wound incisions. The patient tolerated the procedure well and was taken to the intensive care unit in stable condition.

Sample Pulmonary Function Test

TITLE OF PROCEDURE: Pulmonary Function Test

PROCEDURE IN DETAIL: Lung mechanics by spirometry reveals diminished forced vital capacity. There is a moderate reduction in the FVC and a severe reduction in the FEV_1. The FEV_1:FVC ratio is markedly diminished. Timed vital capacity is supernormal. MVV is reduced. The forced expiratory flow rates are markedly to severely reduced. Lung volumes reveal diminished total lung capacity. RV:TLC ratio is high. DLCO is normal. Flow volume loop configuration appears somewhat erratic but there is minimal coving at the terminal end of the expiratory limb. Arterial blood gases reveal hypoxemia and an increased content of carboxyhemoglobin, indicating that the patient is a smoker. The combination of reduced total lung capacity with increment in timed vital capacity speaks probably for a restrictive lung disorder with some obstructive component in both large and small airways with reversible bronchospasm.

Sample Flexible Fiberoptic Bronchoscopy with Brushings, Washings, and Endobronchial Lung Biopsy

TITLE OF PROCEDURE: 1) Flexible fiberoptic bronchoscopy
2) Left upper lobe brushings and washings
3) Endobronchial lung biopsy

PROCEDURE IN DETAIL: The flexible fiberoptic bronchoscope was passed through the endotracheal tube which had been placed by the anesthesiologist. High-flow oxygen was instituted and the scope was passed uneventfully. Excessive secretions were seen in both the left and right main stem bronchus. Mucous plugging in the right lower lobe bronchus was suctioned and erythema in the subsegment raised the suspicion of possible aspiration. The carina was sharp and not splayed. The left lower lobe and left side B6 were essentially normal but a huge mucous plug was seen almost obscuring the left apical posterior subsegment. Attempts to dislodge this obstruction could not be achieved by suctioning and brushing, but this was achieved to a certain extent by mechanical removal of the clot with biopsy forceps. Forceps were introduced and reintroduced at least three times until peripheral subsegmental anatomy of the left upper lobe posterior segment could be visualized. After the huge mucous plug was removed, brushing was again done of the site. Bronchial brushings were sent for cytology, and washings sent for Gram stain, culture and sensitivity, fungus, AFB, and cytology. The patient tolerated the procedure well and left the endoscopy suite in satisfactory condition.